Sepsis: Clinical Diagnosis and Treatment

Sepsis: Clinical Diagnosis and Treatment

Edited by Scarlett Beckinsale

hayle
medical

New York

Hayle Medical,
750 Third Avenue, 9th Floor,
New York, NY 10017, USA

Visit us on the World Wide Web at:
www.haylemedical.com

ISBN: 978-1-63241-517-2

Trademark Notice: Registered trademark of products or corporate names are used only for explanation and identification without intent to infringe.

Cataloging-in-Publication Data

Sepsis : clinical diagnosis and treatment / edited by Scarlett Beckinsale.
    p. cm.
Includes bibliographical references and index.
ISBN 978-1-63241-517-2
1. Septicemia. 2. Septicemia--Diagnosis. 3. Septicemia--Treatment. I. Beckinsale, Scarlett.
RC182.S4 S47 2018
616.944--dc23

Table of Contents

Preface

Sometimes our body's reaction to infection can result in damage to internal tissues and organs. Such a condition is referred to as sepsis. Some of the symptoms of sepsis are high fever, increased heart and breathing rate, etc. This book is compiled in such a manner, that it will provide in-depth knowledge about the diagnosis and treatment of sepsis. Those in search of information to further their knowledge will be greatly assisted by this book.

The researches compiled throughout the book are authentic and of high quality, combining several disciplines and from very diverse regions from around the world. Drawing on the contributions of many researchers from diverse countries, the book's objective is to provide the readers with the latest achievements in the area of research. This book will surely be a source of knowledge to all interested and researching the field.

In the end, I would like to express my deep sense of gratitude to all the authors for meeting the set deadlines in completing and submitting their research chapters. I would also like to thank the publisher for the support offered to us throughout the course of the book. Finally, I extend my sincere thanks to my family for being a constant source of inspiration and encouragement.

Editor

Neurological Complications after Neonatal Bacteremia: The Clinical Characteristics, Risk Factors, and Outcomes

Shih-Ming Chu[1,3], Jen-Fu Hsu[1,3], Chiang-Wen Lee[4,5], Reyin Lien[1,3], Hsuan-Rong Huang[1,3], Ming-Chou Chiang[1,3], Ren-Huei Fu[1,3], Ming-Horng Tsai[2,3,4]*

1 Division of Pediatric Neonatology, Department of Pediatrics, Chang Gung Memorial Hospital, Taoyuan, Taiwan, 2 Division of Neonatology and Pediatric Hematology/Oncology, Department of Pediatrics, Chang Gung Memorial Hospital, Yunlin, Taiwan, 3 College of Medicine, Chang Gung University, Taoyuan, Taiwan, 4 Department of Nursing, Division of Basic Medical Sciences, and Chronic Diseases and Health Promotion Research Center, Chang Gung University of Science and Technology, Chia-Yi, Taiwan, 5 Research Center for Industry of Human Ecology, Chang Gung University of Science and Technology, Taoyuan, Taiwan

Abstract

Background: Neonates with bacteremia are at risk of neurologic complications. Relevant information warrants further elucidation.

Study Design: This was a retrospective cohort study of neonates with bacteremia-related neurologic complications (BNCs) in a tertiary-level neonatal intensive care unit (NICU). A systemic chart review was performed conducted to identify clinical characteristics and outcomes. A cohort of related conditions was constructed as the control group. Logistic regression analysis was used to identify independent risk factors for BNC.

Results: Of 1037 bacteremia episodes, 36 (3.5%) had BNCs. Twenty-four cases of BNCs were related to meningitis, five were presumed meningitis, and seven occurred after septic shock. The most common causative pathogens were Group B streptococcus (41.7%) and *E. coli* (16.7%). The major BNCs consisted of seizures (28), hydrocephalus (20), encephalomalacia (11), cerebral infarction (7), subdural empyema (6), ventriculitis (8), and abscess (4). Eight (22.8%) neonates died and six (16.7%) were discharged in critical condition when the family withdrew life-sustaining treatment. Among the 22 survivors, eight had neurologic sequelae upon discharge. After multivariate logistic regression analysis, neonates with meningitis caused by Group B streptococcus (adjusted odds ratio [OR]: 8.90, 95% confidence interval [CI]: 2.20–36.08; $p = 0.002$) and combined meningitis and septic shock (OR, 5.94; 95% CI: 1.53–23.15; $p = 0.010$) were independently associated with BNCs.

Conclusions: Neonates with bacteremia-related neurologic complications are associated with adverse outcomes or sequelae. Better strategies aimed at early detection and reducing the emergence of neurologic complications and aggressive treatment of Group B streptococcus sepsis are needed in neonates with meningitis and septic shock.

Editor: Patrick M. Schlievert, University of Iowa Carver College of Medicine, United States of America

Funding: The authors have no support or funding to report.

Competing Interests: The authors have declared that no competing interests exist.

* Email: mingmin.tw@yahoo.com.tw

Introduction

Neonatal bacteremia remains one of the major infectious problems in the neonatal intensive care unit (NICU) [1,2], with mortality rates of 10%–30% [3–5]. It is also associated with increased medical costs, prolonged hospital stay and potentially poor long-term neurodevelopmental outcomes [6–8]. Neonatal bacterial meningitis is a severe infectious disease that often occurs concomitantly with the onset of bacteremia, especially those caused by Group B streptococcus (GBS), *E. coli* or other Gram-negative pathogens [9–11]. Neonatal meningitis has been associated with a variety of neurologic complications including seizure, hydrocephalus, arachnoiditis, subdural empyema, and encephalopathy [12–15].

Neurological complications after neonatal bacteremia with or without meningitis are important, because they can be life-threatening and may require neurosurgical treatment. There are a large number of studies on the incidence, risk factors, microbiology, and mortality of neonatal bacteremia or meningitis [1–8], but there is paucity of literature regarding acute and subacute neurological morbidities caused by neonatal bacteremia. Moreover, an episode of bacteremia presenting with severe sepsis or septic shock may be associated with neurological sequelae, probably due to brain hypoperfusion, transient hypoxia, or metabolic acidosis [16]. Prompt identification and aggressive intervention for these neurological complications will result in a more favorable outcome. In this study, we examined the occurrence, characteristics, risk factors and treatment for acute neurological complications after bacteremia in neonates.

Materials and Methods

Study design, setting, and patients

A database search of all positive blood culture-proven neonatal bloodstream infections at the NICU of Chang Gung Memorial Hospital (CGMH) between January 2004 and December 2011 was performed. The NICU is an academic, tertiary-level medical center with a total of 49 beds equipped with mechanical ventilator and 28 beds with special care nurseries. Bacteremia-associated neurological complication (BNC) was defined as any newly neurological symptoms or signs and abnormalities on neuroimaging study (Transcranial ultrasound, computed tomography [CT] scan or magnetic resonance imaging [MRI]) that occurred soon after an episode of bacteremia, or judged by a clinical neonatologist to be directly resulted from an episode of bacteremia. Fulminant episodes of neonatal bacteremia with early mortality within 48 hours from onset were not enrolled. This study was approved by the institutional review board of CGMH, with a waiver of informed consent. However, all patient records/information was anonymized and de-identified prior to analysis.

Case finding

The hospital records of all neonates with bloodstream infection were reviewed for evidence of neurological complications. Patients were selected to undergo detailed chart review when: 1) a lumbar puncture or neuroimaging study was performed; 2) a neurologic consultation was arranged; 3) a seizure was documented in the discharge or progression note; 4) a neurologic surgery, such as ventriculoperitoneal shunting or extraventricular drainage, was performed; or 5) experience of severe sepsis or septic shock during hospital course.

Study definitions

Neonatal bacteremia (or bloodstream infection). Neonatal bacteremia was defined as according to the criteria from the Centers for Disease Control (CDC) and Prevention [17]. Early-onset sepsis and late-onset sepsis were defined as the presence of clinical sepsis and at least one positive blood culture obtained before and after the first 72 hours of life, respectively [6–8]. Blood cultures positive for organisms generally considered as contaminants, including corynebacterium, propionibacterium, penicillium, and diphtheroids, were excluded from analysis. Records of patients with blood culture positive for CoNS were reviewed, and the CDC criteria for CoNS bacteremia were strictly applied [17].

Chronic medical conditions. All comorbidities of prematurity, including respiratory distress syndrome (RDS), intraventricular hemorrhage (IVH), bronchopulmonary dysplasia (BPD), and periventricular leukomalacia (PVL) were based on the latest updated diagnostic criteria in the standard textbook of neonatology [18]. Congenital anomalies in this study included all neonates with either documented or undocumented syndrome, chromosome abnormalities, and genetic or metabolic disorders, but not simple cleft palate or polydactyly.

Bacteremia-related neurological complications included:

1) Seizure: neonates without an underlying seizure disorder, brain pathology, or significant metabolic disturbance who had a repeated seizure attack or an abnormal epileptiform discharges on the electroencephalography after bacteremia that required regular anticonvulsants medications.

2) Post-infectious encephalopathy: Neonates who had consciousness change after stabilization of vital signs that lasted >24 hours after the onset of bacteremia.

3) Hydrocephalus and/or ventriculomegaly: documented by transcranial ultrasound after the onset of bacteremia, and in neonates without previous brain pathology.

4) The presence of any newly focal infections, including subdural empyema, arachnoiditis, ventriculitis, and spinal abscess or brain abscess.

5) Other neurologic complications: included neonates with encephalomalacia or cerebral infarction due to hypotension.

Data collection

This neonatal database was fed by the neonatologist specialist every weekday since 2003 and contained information on basic demographic characteristics, records of all complications of prematurity and all nosocomial infections, summary of hospital courses, and final diagnosis of all patients. For all enrolled cases and controls, detailed data were retrieved by a systemic review of the medical record by using a structured data collection form. Two independent investigators (Dr. H.-R.H. and Dr. J.-F.H.) searched for the following variables: 1) presence and duration of altered mental status; 2) seizure activity along the entire hospital courses, or during or within 48 hours after onset of bacteremia; 3) results of cerebrospinal fluid analysis and findings of neuroimaging studies; and 4) antimicrobial regimens, treatment and hospital course, and clinical outcomes. In patients with a BNC, it was confirmed by a pediatric infectious disease specialist and a pediatric neurologist.

Enrollment of the control group

All neonatal bacteremia, including early-onset sepsis and late-onset sepsis, were retrospectively reviewed to identify the characteristics that predisposed neonates at risk of developing BNCs. After identifying the subgroups vulnerable to have BNCs, those without BNCs after bacteremia were enrolled as the controls. All demographic data, clinical presentations, treatment and outcomes were compared between cases (neonates with BNC) and the controls.

Statistical analysis

Tests of significance between means and proportions were carried out using either χ^2 or Student t test, respectively. All p values were two tailed, and were considered to be statistically significant if the value was <0.05. Categorical data was tested for odds ratios (ORs). Unadjusted and adjusted OR and corresponding 95% confidence intervals (CIs) were derived to examine the risk factors for the development of BNC. We performed a multivariate analysis using a logistic regression model to examine the interaction among gestational age, which was defined as a categorical variable, and meningitis and septic shock. Only variables with a p value<0.1 will be enrolled into the final multivariate logistic regression model. All statistical calculations were performed using SPSS software version 15.0 (SPSS, Chicago, IL).

Results

During the study period, 1037 episodes of neonatal bacteremia and 57 episodes of meningitis were identified in 769 patients in our NICU. After onset of bacteremia, neurological complications were identified in 36 (3.5%) patients (episodes) by brain sonography (n = 36) and/or CT scan (n = 36) and/or brain MRI (n = 33) and/or lumbar puncture (n = 31). When compared with neonatal bacteremia without neurological complications (Table 1), BNCs had a high percentage (23/36, 63.9%) of occurring in the late-preterm (gestational age 33–36 weeks) or term-born infants, and had an earlier onset of bacteremia, although the rate of early-onset sepsis was comparable. The causative pathogens in the neonatal bacteremia with BNCs were also significantly different from those without BNCs (Table 1). Furthermore, patients with bacteremia and BNCs were usually associated with more severe clinical manifestations and significantly higher severity of illness (judged by NTISS scores) [19] (Table 1).

The basic demographics of neonates with BNCs are summarized in Table 2. In these patients with BNCs, 24 patients (66.7%) had meningitis, five (13.9%) had negative CSF cultures but at least one individual CSF marker of meningitis, and seven (19.4%) had neurological sequelae after septic shock or severe sepsis. The BNCs included seizure (n = 28, 77.8%), ventriculomegaly (n = 26, 72.2%), hydrocephalus (n = 20, 55.6%), encephalomalacia (n = 11, 30.6%), cerebral infarction (n = 7, 19.4%), subdural empyema (n = 6, 16.7%), abscess (n = 4, 11.1%), ventriculitis (n = 8, 22.2%) and subdural effusion (n = 11, 30.6%).

The most common causative pathogens were GBS (15/36, 41.7%) and *E. coli* (6/36, 16.7%). Among neonates with meningitis, the most common pathogen was GBS (14, 58.3%). Other pathogens included *E. coli* (3), *K. pneumoniae* (1), *Chryseobacterium meningosepticum* (1), *L. monocytogenes* (1),

Salmonella group D (1), *P. aeruginosa* (1), *E. cloacae* (1), and coagulase negative Staphylococcus (1). All of the meningitis events were concomitant with the onset of bacteremia, except for one case of Salmonella group D meningitis that occurred at one week after onset of bacteremia. In these patients, pre-existing neurological comorbidities were noted in only five patients, including IVH Gr II (2), IVH Gr III (2), and one patient had IVH Gr IV and hypoxic ischemic encephalopathy due to perianal asphyxia.

The time to diagnosis of all BNCs from onset of bacteremia with and without meningitis until BNCs is summarized in Figure 1. The median time from the onset of sepsis to neurologic symptoms was 10 days (range, 0–82 days, interquartile range [IQR], 3–24 days), with different symptoms highly correlated with their onsets. Seizure accounted for the earliest onset of neurological symptoms (median time from sepsis, 1 days, range: 0–14 days), and encephalomalacia and cerebral infarction were often the last to be detected (median time from onset of sepsis, 27 days, IQR, 20–56 days). The clinical features during this period included seizure (77.8%), feeding intolerance (86.1%), fever (11.1%), respiratory failure (19.4%), increased intracranial pressure (72.2%), bulging anterior fontanel (27.8%), and lethargy (22.2%). Among the 28 neonates with seizure, six patients had seizure as the initial

Table 1. Clinical and laboratory features in neonates with bacteremia-associated neurological complications among 1037 episodes of bacteremia in the neonatal intensive care unit.

Characteristics	Bacteremia episodes with neurological complications (n = 36)	Bacteremia episodes without neurological complications (n = 1001)	P value
Birth body weight (g), median (IQR)	2520.0 (1535.0–3017.5)	1340.0 (941.5–2032.5)*	<0.001
Gestational age (weeks), median (IQR)	36.0 (29.3–38.8)	30.0 (27.0–35.0)*	<0.001
Age at onset of bacteremia (days), median (IQR)	20.5 (6.0–30.3)	25.0 (14.0–50.0)	0.008
Early-onset sepsis,& n (%)	5 (13.9)	80 (8.0)	0.209
Late-onset sepsis,& n (%)	31 (86.1)	921 (92.0)	
Causative Pathogens, n (%)			<0.001
Group B Streptococcus	15 (41.7)	33 (3.3)	
Escherichia coli	6 (16.7)	79 (7.9)	
Other Gram-positive pathogens	5 (13.9)	544 (54.3)	
Other Gram-negative pathogens	10 (27.8)	248 (24.8)	
Fungus	0 (0)	52 (5.2)	
Polymicrobial pathogens	0 (0)	45 (4.5)	
Clinical manifestations, n (%)			
Septic shock	18 (50.0)	166 (16.6)	<0.001
Coagulopathy or gastrointestinal bleeding	20 (58.3)	242 (24.2)	<0.001
Disseminated intravascular coagulopathy	12 (33.3)	89 (8.9)	<0.001
Respiratory distress¶	27 (75.0)	605 (60.5)	0.084
Requirement of blood transfusion#	24 (66.7)	374 (37.4)	0.001
Concurrent meningitis	24 (66.7)	33 (3.3)	<0.001
NTISS score at most severe day of bacteremia, mean±standard deviation	18.9±6.13	16.7±4.92	0.006
Outcomes, n (%)			
Sepsis attributable mortality	14/36 (38.9)	68/1001 (6.8)	<0.001
Overall mortality	14/36 (38.9)	90/769 (11.7)*	<0.001

*Data are 713 unique patients with late onset sepsis and 56 unique patients with early-onset sepsis.
¶Indicating those required mechanical ventilators, including intubation or continuous positive airway pressure, during the treatment courses of bacteremia.
&Early-onset sepsis and late-onset sepsis are defined as clinical sepsis with positive blood culture obtained before and after first 72 hours of life, respectively.
#Indicating requirement of blood transfusions of red blood cell, platelet, or fresh frozen plasma.
IQR: interquartile range, NTISS: Neonatal Therapeutic Intervention Scoring System[19].

Table 2. Pathogens, clinical manifestations, and demographics of neonates with bacteremia-associated neurological complications.

Characteristics	Total cases (n = 36)	Meningitis (n = 24)	Presumed Meningitis (n = 5)	Septic shock (n = 7)
Birth weight (g), median (IQR)	2520.0 (1535.0–3017.5)	2700.0 (2236.0–3127.5)	2100.0 (1360.0–2679.5)	1125.0 (800–2330.0)
Gestational age (weeks), median (IQR)	36.0 (29.3–38.8)	37.5 (33.5–39.8)	34.0 (29.0–37.5)	29.0 (25.0–36.0)
Gender (male/female), n (%)	19 (52.8)/17 (47.2)	15 (62.5)/9 (37.5)	2 (40.0)/3 (60.0)	2 (28.6)/5 (71.4)
Age of bacteremia onset (days), median (IQR)	20.5 (6.0–30.3)	21.5 (6.0–33.3)	10.0 (5.5–21.5)	21.0 (4.0–31.0)
Pathogens, n (%)				
Group B Streptococcus	15 (41.7)	14 (58.3)	1 (20.0)	0 (0)
Escherichia coli	6 (16.7)	3 (12.5)	3 (60.0)	0 (0)
Other Gram-positive pathogens	5 (13.9)	2 (8.3)	0 (0)	3 (42.9)
Other Gram-negative pathogens	10 (27.8)	5 (20.8)	1 (20.0)	4 (57.1)
Neurological complications after bacteremia				
Seizure	28 (77.8)	19 (79.2)	4 (80.0)	5 (71.4)
Ventriculomegaly/Hydrocephalus	26 (72.2)/20 (55.6)	17 (70.8)/12 (50.0)	4 (80.0)/4 (80.0)	5 (71.4)/4 (57.1)
Increased intracranial pressure (IICP)	26 (72.2)	17 (70.8)	4 (80.0)	5 (71.4)
Subdural effusion	11 (30.6)	8 (33.3)	1 (20.0)	2 (28.6)
Encephalomalacia	11 (30.6)	7 (29.1)	2 (40.0)	2 (28.6)
Ventriculitis	8 (22.2)	5 (20.8)	2 (40.0)	1 (14.3)
Subdural empyema	6 (16.7)	6 (25.0)	0 (0)	0 (0)
Abscess[#]	4 (11.1)	4 (16.7)	0 (0)	0 (0)
Cerebral infarction	7 (19.4)	4 (16.7)	1 (20.0)	2 (28.6)
Intracranial hemorrhage[¶]	7 (19.4)	4 (16.7)	1 (20.0)	2 (28.6)
Periventricular leukomalacia	4 (11.1)	2 (8.3)	0 (0)	2 (28.6)
Condition at discharge, n (%)				
Survival	22 (61.1)	17 (70.8)	2 (40.0)	3 (42.9)
Discharge without neurological sequelae	14 (38.9)	10 (41.7)	2 (40.0)	2 (28.6)
Discharge with neurological sequelae	8 (22.2)	7 (29.2)	0 (0)	1 (14.3)
Mortality	8 (22.2)	4 (16.7)	2 (40.0)	2 (28.6)
Withdraw life-sustaining treatment	6 (16.7)	3 (12.5)	1 (20.0)	2 (28.6)

[#]Including subdural abscess (2), and spinal cord abscess (2), and brain abscess (1).
[¶]Including intraventricular hemorrhage (3), subependymal hemorrhage (3), subarachnoid hemorrhage (1), and hemorrhage on bilateral globus pallidus (1).
IQR: interquartile range.

symptom of bacteremia and seven (25%) were poorly controlled despite the administration of antiepileptic drugs for more than 48 hours. Nine patients had electrolyte imbalance, three patients developed central diabetes insipidus, and one had syndrome of inappropriate antidiuretic hormone secretion (SIADH).

Initial antibiotics that covered both Gram-positive and Gram-negative organisms were used for all thirty-six patients. Only two cases (pathogens: *C. meningosepticum* and *P. aeruginosa*) did not receive appropriate antibiotics within 24 hours after bacteremia onset. They were treated with penicillin, one of third generation cephalosporin (cefotaxime or ceftazidime), or carbapenem, based on the results and antimicrobial susceptibility patterns of blood and CSF cultures. The mean duration of antimicrobial therapy was 23.2 ± 11.8 days (range, 7 to 38 days). Eighteen (50%) patients received neurosurgical treatment, including extraventricular drainage tube placement (n = 9), ventriculoperitoneal shunt (n = 9), subdural drainage (n = 3) and subdural-peritoneal shunt (n = 2). Four patients required multiple neurosurgical interventions.

Focal infectious complications occurred in fifteen patients, including seven had ventriculitis, four had subdural empyema, two had subdural abscess, one had subdural empyema plus brain abscess, and the last one had subdural empyema plus spinal cord abscess and arachnoiditis. All of these BNCs occurred after meningitis (12 patients with the following causative pathogens: GBS [6], *E. coli* [3], Salmonella group D [1], *P. aeruginosa* [1], and *C. meningosepticum* [1]) or presumed meningitis (3 cases). These BNCs were found at 4–22 days (median: 7 days) after the onset of bacteremia. Cranial MRI was performed in all of these patients and included diffusion-weighted imaging (DWI) hyperintense and apparent diffusion coefficient (ADC) hypointense signal in 6 cases with subdural empyema. Four patients with ventriculitis and six patients with subdural empyema or abscess received surgical drainage, while aggressive treatment was withdrawn in two critically-ill patients upon their parents' request. Of the eight patients who survived after surgical treatment, three had neurological sequelae at discharge. Subdural effusion was noted

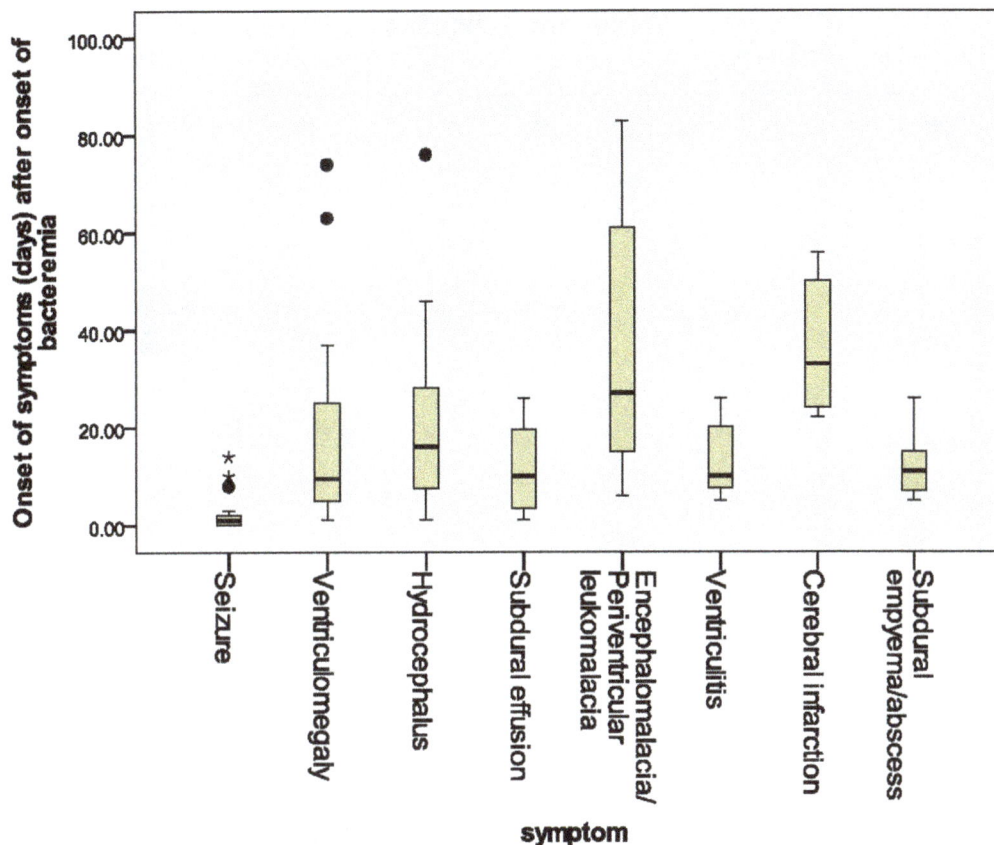

Figure 1. Time to diagnosis of various bacteremia-related neurological complications in the neonatal intensive care unit. Bacteremia onset was defined as when the blood culture sampling was obtained, whereas onset of neurological complication was defined at the symptom presentation or diagnosis by neuroimaging studies.

in another six patients in whom the brain MRI showed hypointensity on DWI.

The BNCs of seven patients resulted from septic shock and brain hypoperfusion. They had no evidence of bacterial meningitis, but lumbar puncture was performed in only three patients. Their neurologic symptoms included seizure (5), subdural effusion (2), increased intracranial pressure (5), ventriculomegaly (5), and hydrocephalus (4). Only one patient received surgical intervention. An unfavorable outcome was observed in five patients, including death (2), withdraw of life-sustaining treatment (2), and neurological sequelae (1). Only two patients finally survived without neurological sequelae upon discharge.

Overall, there was a significantly worse outcome in our cohort of neonates with BNCs (both $p<0.001$ by log rank test when compared with neonates without BNCs after bacteremia and meningitis, respectively) (Figure 2). Fourteen (63.6%) of twenty-two survivors who received complete treatment had a favorable outcome without neurological sequelae upon discharge. Eight neonates had motor disabilities at discharge, including opisthotonus posture, drop foot, ankle clonus, and poor feeding and swallowing discoordination. A total of eight patients died, and six patients were discharged after families gave up aggressive treatment and withdrew their life-support. A higher rate of an unfavorable outcome was observed in neonates with acute neurological complications compared to those with meningitis but without acute neurological complications (72% vs. 17%; $p<0.001$).

Because BNCs tended to occur in neonatal bacteremia with concomitant meningitis or septic shock, the relevant subgroup without BNCs constituted the controls. The possible risk factors for BNC are shown in Table 3. By univariate analysis, the risk for BNC varied by gestational age, with full term neonates at greatest risk (OR, 7.08; 95% CI, 2.10–23.90). Pre-existing neurological sequelae were not risk factors for BNC. GBS infection and neonatal meningitis with septic shock increased the likelihood of developing BNCs. After multivariate logistic regression analysis, these two factors remained independently associated with the development of BNCs (adjusted OR: 8.90, 95% CI: 2.20–36.08; $p = 0.002$, and adjusted OR, 5.94; 95% CI: 1.53–23.15, $p = 0.010$, respectively) (Table 3).

Discussion

This study demonstrates that although neurological complications occur only in 3.5% of neonatal bacteremia, they are highly associated with unfavorable outcomes (61.1% had mortality or neurological sequelae). These neurological complications may result from either direct bacterial invasion, sepsis-associated encephalopathy [20], or both. In neonatal bacteremia with concomitant meningitis, 24 (42.1%) cases developed at least one neurological complication in the acute or subacute phase, leading to a complicated clinical course. In neonatal bacteremia with meningitis, GBS and combined septic shock are independently associated with an 8.9- and a 5.9-fold increased risk of developing

Survival Functions

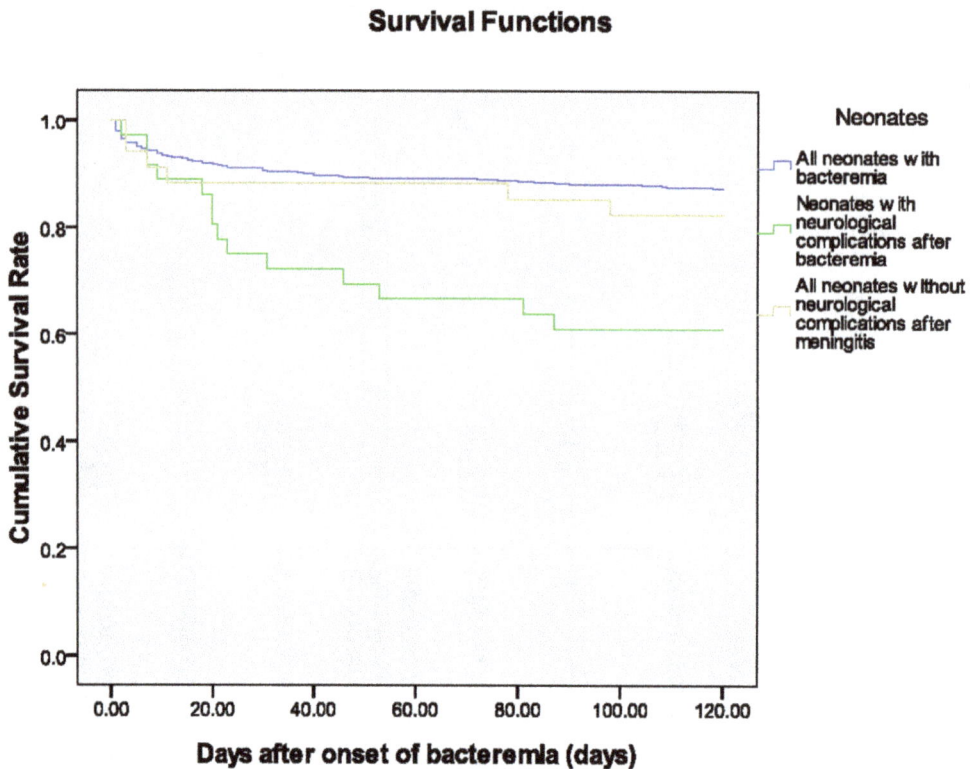

Figure 2. The Kaplan-Meier survival curve of neonates with bacteremia-related neurological complications (BNCs), and those discharged in a critical condition after withdrawing life-sustaining treatments were considered dead at the day of discharge.

BNCs. Thus, cranial imaging to detect focal infectious complications or brain pathology is indicated [21].

In contrast to previous studies that have focused on sequelae after childhood meningitis [22,23], this is the first study investigating neurological complications after bacteremia in the NICU. Meningitis in neonates is associated with a significantly higher rate of acute and subacute neurological complications than in children, which is reported to be around 6.8%–24.0% [22,23]. Among the BNCs, ventriculitis, subdural empyema and subdural fluid collection were more common in the younger age group based on the current study findings and previous literature [22–26]. Mild, transient hydrocephalus and ventriculitis are present in

Table 3. Risk factors for neurological complications in neonatal bacteremia with meningitis or septic shock.

Variable	N (%) (total n = 144)	Unadjusted OR (95% CI)	Multivariate logistic regression analysis	
			Adjusted OR (95% CI)	P value
Gestational age				
≤27 weeks	39 (27.1)	1 (ref.)	-	-
28–32 weeks	41 (28.4)	2.12 (0.58–7.71)	-	-
33–36 weeks	26 (18.1)	3.22 (0.84–12.43)	-	-
≥37 weeks	38 (26.4)	7.08 (2.10–23.90)	3.23 (0.81–12.97)	0.098
Male gender	86 (59.7)	0.68 (0.32–1.46)	-	-
Pathogens				
Overall	144 (100)	1 (ref.)		
Group B streptococcus	23 (15.8)	16.13 (4.56–56.99)	8.90 (2.20–36.08)	0.002
Gram-negative bacilli	73 (50.7)	2.41 (0.82–7.10)	2.31 (0.75–7.13)	0.145
Multi-drug resistant bacteria*	10 (6.9)	1.89 (0.71–5.44)	-	-
Pre-existing neurological sequelae	27 (18.8)	0.63 (0.22–1.81)	-	-
Combined meningitis and septic shock	14 (9.7)	10.00 (2.90–34.44)	5.94 (1.53–23.15)	0.010

*Indicating Gram-negative bacilli was resistant to at least three or more of the following antimicrobial categories: carbapenems, penicillins, broad-spectrum cephalosporins, monobactams, aminoglycosides and fluorquinolones.

most patients with meningitis [25,26], but they tend to be more persistent or progressive in young infants with immature neurological development.

Nearly two-thirds of BNCs occur in the late-preterm or full-term infants. Although GBS is well known as the most important pathogen of neonatal early-onset sepsis, 80% (12/15) of our GBS-related BNCs are late-onset sepsis and the majority (13/15, 86.7%) occurred in neonates with a gestational age of ≥33 weeks. A recent prospective report has found that term-born infants have more GBS late-onset sepsis and meningitis compared to preterm infants had [27], even though the incidence is relatively lower in term-born infants (0.24 and 1.4 per 1000 live births for term and preterm newborns, respectively). Given the substantial burden of late-onset GBS disease, an effective prevention strategy should be enforced to reduce maternal colonization and transmission [27,28].

Based on the time frame of BNC occurrences, nearly half of ventriculomegaly, hydrocephalus, cerebral infarction and encephalomalacia were detected at more than one month after bacteremia or meningitis onset. However, focal infectious complications tended to be detected within half a month after meningitis onset. It can be surmised that these focal infectious complications are the direct extension or persistence of bacterial invasion, and pathological brain would result from subacute neurological damages. The association of these focal infectious complications with an even higher rate of adverse outcome warrants greater awareness. Moreover, some may be delayed diagnosed, because the clinical symptoms are subtle or similar to other BNCs like hydrocephalus or ventriculomegaly. Better strategies aimed at reducing the occurrence of BNCs, such as correct treatment of bacteremia, and more frequent follow-up with neuroimaging studies for early detection of these intracranial lesions are therefore needed.

Risk factors associated with the development of BNCs have not been previously described. Full-term neonates are at an increased risk for BNCs compared to premature infants. However, gestational age-related risks of BNCs are attributable to the high frequency of Group B streptococcus infection in full-term infants. In addition, the presence of pre-existing neurologic sequelae is not independently associated with the development of BNCs, which undoubtedly reduces the possibility of selection bias among the controls. It is reasonable that Group B streptococcus contributes independently to BNCs since Group B streptococcus is the leading cause of meningitis in neonates. Recent studies have found that its special mechanism involves the penetration of the blood-brain barrier [29,30].

Our study has several important limitations. The clinical features of the patients were retrospectively collected and the sample size was not large enough for a good statistical analysis. It is sometimes difficult to judge whether neonates with pre-existing neurologic sequelae from extreme prematurity had BNCs or progression of neurological deficit after an episode of bacteremia. Furthermore, lack of long-term follow-up for the survivors results in the unavailability of information regarding their neurodevelopmental outcomes.

In conclusion, approximately one-fourth of neonates with meningitis or septic shock experience neurologic complications despite prompt instigation of effective antibiotic therapy. Due to the high risk of adverse outcomes after the development of neurologic complications, it is important that physicians can highly alert the possibility of BNCs after bacteremia, especially those caused by Group B streptococcus, and aim to detect neurological complications early at onset of bacteremia to address already present complications and diminish damage and/or progression. Better strategies aimed at reducing the occurrence, aggressive treatment of Group B streptococcus bacteremia, and more frequent cranial ultrasound follow-up are strongly recommended for the screening of infants with bacterial meningitis.

Acknowledgments

The abstract has been previously published as a conference abstract (http://www.jns-journal.com/article/S0022-510X%2813%2902380-0/fulltext) and accepted as the poster presentation in XXIst World congress of neurology (WCN 2013). Vienna, Austria in September 21–26, 2013.

All authors thank Mrs. Chiao-Ching Chiang for keeping the database of our NICU, and all nursing staff working in our NICUs for keeping extremely detailed patient records, which contributed greatly to the completion of this research.

Author Contributions

Conceived and designed the experiments: SMC MHT. Performed the experiments: CWL. Wrote the paper: SMC. Contributed the patients and collected the data: RL JFH SMC MCC RHF HRH. Final approval of this paper: MHT.

References

1. Ho JJ (2001) Late onset infection in very low birth weight infants in Malaysian level 3 neonatal nurseries. Malaysian Very Low Birth Weight Study Group. Pediatr Infect Dis J 20: 557–560.
2. Weston EJ, Pondo T, Lewis MM, Martell-Cleary P, Morin C, et al. (2011) The burden of invasive early-onset neonatal sepsis in the United States, 2005–2008. Pediatr Infect Dis J 30: 937–941.
3. Stoll BJ, Hansen N, Fanaroff AA, Wright LL, Carlo WA, et al. (2002) Late-onset sepsis in very low birth weight neonates: the experience of the NICHD Neonatal Research Network. Pediatrics 110: 285–291.
4. Stoll BJ, Hansen NI, Sánchez PJ, Faix RG, Poindexter BB, et al. (2011) Early onset neonatal sepsis: the burden of group B Streptococcal and E. coli disease continue. Pediatrics 127: 817–826.
5. Makhoul IR, Sujov P, Smolkin T, Lusky A, Reichman B (2002) Epidemiological, clinical, and microbiological characteristics of late-onset sepsis among very low birth weight infants in Israel: a national survey. Pediatrics 109: 34–39.
6. Atif ML, Sadaoui F, Bezzaoucha A, Kaddache CA, Boukari R, et al. (2008) Prolongation of hospital stay and additional costs due to nosocomial bloodstream infection in an Algerian neonatal care unit. Infect Control Hosp Epidemiol 29: 1066–1170.
7. Stoll BJ, Hansen NI, Adams-Chapman I, Fanaroff AA, Hintz SR, et al. (2004) Neurodevelopmental and growth impairment among extremely low-birth-weight infants with neonatal infection. JAMA 292: 2357–2365.
8. Schlapbach LJ, Aebischer M, Adams M, Natalucci G, Bonhoeffer J, et al. (2011) Impact of sepsis on neurodevelopmental outcome in a Swiss National Cohort of extremely premature infants. Pediatrics 128: e348–e357.
9. Gaschignard J, Lew C, Romain O, Cohen R, Bingen E, et al. (2011) Neonatal bacterial meningitis: 444 cases in 7 years. Pediatr Infect Dis J 30: 212–217.
10. Trijbels-Smeulders MA, Kimpen JL, Kollée LA, Bakkers J, Melchers W, et al. (2006) Serotypes, genotypes, and antibiotic susceptibility profiles of group B streptococci causing neonatal sepsis and meningitis before and after introduction of antibiotic prophylaxis. Pediatr Infect Dis J 25: 945–948.
11. May M, Daley AJ, Donath S, Isaacs D, Australasian Study Group for Neonatal Infections (2005) Early onset neonatal meningitis in Australia and New Zealand, 1992–2002. Arch Dis Child Fetal Neonatal Ed. 90: F324–327.
12. Carter JE, Laurini JA, Evans TN, Estrada B (2008) Neonatal candida parasilosis meningitis and empyema related to epidural migration of a central venous catheter. Clin Neurol Neurosurg 110: 614–618.
13. de Goede CG, Jardine PE, Eunson P, Renowden S, Sharples P, et al. (2006) Severe progressive late onset myelopathy and arachnoiditis following neonatal meningitis. Eur J Paediatr Neurol 10: 31–36.
14. Chang YC, Huang CC, Wang ST, Chio CC (1997) Risk factor of complications requiring neurosurgical intervention in infants with bacterial meningitis. Pediatr Neurol 17: 144–149.
15. Liu ZH, Chen NY, Tu PH, Lee ST, Wu CT (2010) The treatment and outcome of postmeningitic subdural empyema in infants. J Neurosurg Pediatr 6: 38–42.
16. Nakanishi H, Yamanaka S, Koriyama T, Shishida N, Miyagi N, et al. (2010) Clinical characterization and long-term prognosis of neurological development in preterm infants with late-onset circulatory collapse. J Perinatol 30: 751–756.

17. Horan TC, Andrus M, Dudeck MA (2008) CDC/NHSN surveillance definition of health care-associated infection and criteria for specific types of infections in the acute care setting. Am J Infect Control 36: 309–332.

18. Taeusch HW, Ballard RA, Gleason CA (2006) Avery's Diseases of the Newborn. 8th Edition.

19. Gray JE, Richardson DK, McCormick MC, Workman-Daniels K, Goldmann DA (1992) Neonatal therapeutic intervention scoring system: a therapy-based severity-of-illness index. Pediatrics 90: 561–567.

20. Gofton TE, Young GB (2012) Sepsis-associated encephalopathy. Nat Rev Neurol 8: 557–566.

21. Hughes DC, Raghavan A, Mordekar SR, Griffiths PD, Connolly DJ (2010) Role of imaging in the diagnosis of acute bacterial meningitis and its complications. Postgrad Med J 86: 478–485.

22. Vasilopoulou VA, Karanika M, Theodoridou K, Katsioulis AT, Theodoridou MN, et al. (2011) Prognostic factors related to sequelae in childhood bacterial meningitis: data from a Greek meningitis registry. BMC Infect Dis 11: 214.

23. Ramakrishnan M, Ulland AJ, Steinhardt LC, Moïsi JC, Were F, et al. (2009) Sequelae due to bacterial meningitis among African children: a systematic literature review. BMC Med 14: 47.

24. Jim KK, Brouwer MC, van der Ende A, van de Beek D (2012) Subdural empyema in bacterial meningitis. Neurology 79: 2133–2139.

25. van de Beek D, de Gans J, Tunkel AR, Wijdicks EF (2006) Community-acquired bacterial meningitis in adults. N Engl J Med 354: 44–53.

26. Mohan S, Jain KK, Arabi M, Shah GV (2012) Imaging of meningitis and ventriculitis. Neuroimaging Clin N Am 22: 557–583.

27. Berardi A, Rossi C, Lugli L, Creti R, Bacchi Reggiani ML, et al. (2013) Group B streptococcus late-onset disease: 2003–2010. Pediatrics 131: e361–368.

28. Jordan HT, Farley MM, Craig A, Mohle-Boetani J, Harrison LH, et al. (2008) Revisiting the need for vaccine prevention of late-onset neonatal group B streptococcal disease: a multistate, population-based analysis. Pediatr Infect Dis J 27: 1057–1064.

29. Magalhães V, Andrade EB, Alves J, Ribeiro A, Kim KS, et al. (2013) Group B streoptococcus hijacks the host plasminogen system to promote brain endothelial cell invasion. PLoS One 8: e63244.

30. van Sorge NM, Quach D, Gurney MA, Sullam PM, Nizet V, et al. (2009) The group B streptococcal serine-rich repeat 1 glycoprotein mediates penetration of the blood-brain barrier. J Infect Dis 199: 1479–1487.

2

Sustained Elevation of Resistin, NGAL and IL-8 Are Associated with Severe Sepsis/Septic Shock in the Emergency Department

Stephen P. J. Macdonald[1,2,3], **Shelley F. Stone**[1,2]*, **Claire L. Neil**[1,2], **Pauline E. van Eeden**[1,2], **Daniel M. Fatovich**[1,2,4], **Glenn Arendts**[1,2,4], **Simon G. A. Brown**[1,2,4]

1 Centre for Clinical Research in Emergency Medicine, Harry Perkins Institute of Medical Research, Perth, Australia, **2** Discipline of Emergency Medicine, School of Primary, Aboriginal and Rural Health Care, University of Western Australia, Perth, Australia, **3** Emergency Department, Armadale Health Service, Perth, Australia, **4** Emergency Department, Royal Perth Hospital, Perth, Australia

Abstract

Objective: To identify biomarkers which distinguish severe sepsis/septic shock from uncomplicated sepsis in the Emergency Department (ED).

Methods: Patients with sepsis underwent serial blood sampling, including arrival in the ED and up to three subsequent time points over the first 24 hours. Messenger RNA (mRNA) levels of 13 genes representing arms of the innate immune response, organ dysfunction or shock were measured in peripheral blood leucocytes using quantitative PCR, and compared with healthy controls. Serum protein concentrations of targets differentially expressed between uncomplicated sepsis and severe sepsis/septic shock were then measured at each time point and compared between the two patient groups.

Results: Of 27 participants (median age 66 years, (IQR 35, 78)), 10 had uncomplicated sepsis and 17 had sepsis with organ failure (14 septic shock; 3 had other sepsis-related organ failures). At the time of first sample collection in the ED, gene expression of Interleukin (IL)-10 and Neutrophil Gelatinase Associated Lipocalin (NGAL) were significantly higher in severe sepsis than uncomplicated sepsis. Expression did not significantly change over time for any target gene. Serum concentrations of IL-6, IL-8, IL-10, NGAL and Resistin were significantly higher in severe sepsis than uncomplicated sepsis at the time of first sample collection in the ED, but only IL-8, NGAL and Resistin were consistently higher in severe sepsis compared to uncomplicated sepsis at all time points up to 24 h after presentation.

Conclusions: These mediators, produced by both damaged tissues and circulating leukocytes, may have important roles in the development of severe sepsis. Further work will determine whether they have any value, in addition to clinical risk parameters, for the early identification of patients that will subsequently deteriorate and/or have a higher risk of death.

Editor: Cordula M. Stover, University of Leicester, United Kingdom

Funding: SB is supported by a NHMRC Career Development Fellowship Award ID1023265. Additional funding was received from the Royal Perth Hospital Medical Research Foundation and the University of Western Australia. The funders had no role in study design, data collection and analysis, decision to publish or preparation of the manuscript.

Competing Interests: The authors have declared that no competing interests exist.

* Email: Shelley.Stone@uwa.edu.au

Introduction

Sepsis is a significant global health problem with high rates of morbidity and mortality [1], and accounts for a significant proportion of Intensive Care Unit (ICU) admissions [2,3]. The incidence of sepsis increases with age, and elderly patients are more likely to suffer death or permanent disability as a result of sepsis [4,5]. Sepsis-associated organ dysfunction and shock are major contributors to poor outcome. The pathophysiology of sepsis is complex, with both pro-inflammatory and anti-inflammatory pathways activated [6]. The immune response is thought to depend upon both pathogen factors (load and virulence) and host factors (genetics, age and co-morbid disease burden).

The Emergency Department (ED) is the initial point of contact for most patients with community-acquired sepsis. An accurate assessment to identify actual or impending organ dysfunction or shock at this early stage may influence outcome since this is the major driver of mortality in sepsis. The distinction between uncomplicated sepsis (infection + SIRS) and severe sepsis/septic shock is clinically important in the ED in terms of early treatment and correct patient disposition. Measuring one inflammatory/immunological marker at a single time point has been shown to have little value [3,7,8,9,10,11,12], however a "panel" of biomarkers may provide better prediction of illness severity and clinical outcome [13,14,15,16,17]. A recent study validating a risk stratification tool found that measurement of five candidate biomarkers, admission lactate concentration, age and chronic disease burden was required to reliably estimate the probability of mortality in adults with sepsis. [18] Other studies of biomarker panels are limited by a number of factors including single time point sample collection and/or collection of samples at time points many hours after initial presentation. [16,19,20,21]

The aim of this study was therefore to identify, in patients with uncomplicated sepsis and severe sepsis, differences in biomarkers representing key elements of the innate immune response and organ dysfunction very early in the course of disease. For candidate biomarkers, we assessed both differential gene expression in circulating peripheral blood leukocytes (PBL) and serum concentrations of expressed protein. For biomarkers differentially expressed between the two patient groups, we also aimed to explore changes over time.

Methods

Setting

Study participants were enrolled in our prospective, observational Critical Illness and Shock Study (CISS) between April 2011 and July 2012 in the Emergency Departments of one tertiary referral hospital and one community general hospital in Perth, Western Australia. The CISS methodology has been previously described [22]. Briefly, CISS is based on a convenience sample of ED patients recruited during rostered research nurse hours, 0700 to 2100 most days of the week. CISS enrolment criteria include physiological evidence of shock or respiratory failure.

Ethics approval and consent

Ethics approval was obtained from the Human Research Ethics Committees at each hospital. Because the need for emergency care took priority, waiver of initial consent was approved under the provision of paragraph 2.3.6 of the National Health and Medical Research Council Ethical Conduct guidelines (2007). Once treatment was started, fully informed written consent was obtained as soon as possible and patients were given the option of declining further involvement and having all research samples collected up to that point destroyed.

Case selection

CISS entry criteria required 'shock' (SBP<90, OR MAP<65 OR HR>SBP i.e. shock index>1, or lactate>4 mmol/l) or hypoxaemic respiratory failure (requirement of>6 L/min O_2 to maintain saturations>90% or PaO_2(mmHg)/FiO_2 <200 if ventilated/venture mask). These physiological criteria were intentionally over-inclusive to maximize the recruitment of suitable patients in the dynamic ED environment and resulted in the inclusion of some patients with transient abnormal observations and a subsequently benign clinical course. We selected cases from the CISS database that; (i) satisfied a clinical definition of sepsis; likely or confirmed infection (identified by the clinical decision to administer intravenous antibiotics in the ED) along with two or more systemic inflammatory response syndrome (SIRS) criteria – temperature>38 or <36°C, HR>90 beats/min, RR>20 breaths/min or white cell count>12 or <4×10⁹/L, and (ii) had blood samples available from when enrolment criteria were met in ED (T0), and at least 2 subsequent time points within 24 hours of admission.

We excluded cases transferred from other hospitals, as these patients had often been unwell for an extended period of time, cases where sepsis was judged not to be the primary cause of illness and cases in which extracted mRNA failed our quality or quantity

requirements (see below). A summary flowchart of the participant screening and enrolment process is shown in Figure S1.

Case classification

To test our hypothesis of differential biomarker profiles associated with organ dysfunction, cases were reviewed by two physician investigators (SPJM, GA) and classified into two severity groups, uncomplicated sepsis and severe sepsis including septic shock. This was based on clinical and laboratory features, according to standard consensus criteria. [23] *Uncomplicated sepsis* was defined as a SOFA score of <2 and no requirement for organ support. *Severe sepsis* was defined as the presence of sepsis related organ dysfunction with a SOFA score on admission of ≥2. *Septic shock* was defined as persistence of a systolic BP < 90 mmHg after a minimum 20 ml/kg isotonic crystalloid bolus, OR a serum lactate of ≥4 mmol/L. This clinical classification was undertaken separately and blinded to the laboratory analyses.

Clinical data collection, follow up and outcome

Baseline clinical data included haemodynamic and respiratory parameters, electrolytes, renal function, full blood count, blood gas (venous or arterial) analysis and serum lactate. Charlson Comorbidity Index (CCI) [24], mortality in ED sepsis (MEDS) and sequential organ failure assessment (SOFA) scores were calculated. Participants were followed to 30 days from admission. Hospital length of stay, admission to intensive care and all cause mortality were recorded.

Blood sampling and sample storage

Blood samples were collected as soon as practicable after enrolment criteria were met in the ED, (T0) and between 1–2, 3–6 and 12–30 hours post-T0. At each time, 2×4 ml EDTA plasma tube, 1×3.5 ml serum tube and 2×2.5 ml Blood RNA PAXgene tubes (PreAnalytiX GmbH, Switzerland) were collected. The RNA PAXgene tubes were placed immediately at 4°C then transferred to −20°C within 72 hours, before final storage at −80°C. Serum and EDTA plasma were collected and stored immediately at −80°C.

Biomarker selection

Targets representing key arms of the innate immune response, organ dysfunction and shock were selected. These included pathogen-associated molecular pattern (PAMP) receptors that activate the innate immune system (Toll-Like Receptors TLR2 and TLR4), a general marker of immune cell activation (Urokinase Plasminogen Activator Receptor (UPAR)), pro- and anti-inflammatory cytokines and chemokines (Interleukin (IL)-6, IL-8, IL-10, Monocyte Chemotactic Protein-1 (MCP-1) and Macrophage Inhibitory Protein-1β (MIP-1β)), a marker of apoptosis (Fas ligand (FasL)), the vasodilatory peptide Adrenomedullin (ADM) which may play a protective role after hypoxic tissue injury, the inflammatory biomarker Resistin that upregulates Vascular Cell Adhesion Molecule-1 (VCAM-1) expression on endothelial cells, and a marker of acute kidney injury (Neutrophil Gelatinase-Associated Lipocalin (NGAL)).

Changes in gene expression and protein levels over time were compared between patients with uncomplicated sepsis and severe sepsis/septic shock, and with a cohort of age and sex-matched healthy controls.

Extraction and quality control of RNA

RNA was extracted using PAXgene Blood RNA Extraction Kits (PreAnalytiX GmbH, Switzerland) by automation with the

Qiacube instrument (Qiagen, Australia). The purity and integrity of the RNA was assessed on a NanoDrop (Thermo Scientific, Australia) and Bioanalyzer (Agilent). Samples with RIN<7 and total RNA <1 µg were excluded. As a result, the quality of included samples was very high (median OD 260/280 ratio of 2.1 (IQR 2.0–2.1); median RIN 8.2 (IQR 7.9–8.6).

Synthesis of cDNA

Complimentary DNA (cDNA) was synthesized using 1 µg RNA, 200 ng random primers and 10 mM dNTPs (Invitrogen Life Technologies, Australia), incubated at 65°C for 5 min. A mastermix of superscript III reverse transcriptase (200 units), first-strand buffer, 40 units of RNase inhibitor and 100 mM dithiothreitol (Invitrogen Life Technologies, Australia) were added and incubated at 25°C for 5 min then at 50°C for 50 min. Followed by heat inactivation at 70°C for 15 min. RNase H (1 unit; New England BioLabs, USA) was added and incubated for 20 min at 37°C. Storage of cDNA was at −20°C.

Quantitative PCR (qPCR)

The measurement of mRNA levels of target genes was performed following MIQE guidelines [25]. PCR reactions were performed in a total volume of 10 µl, comprising 37.5 ng of each primer (Table S1), 0.5 µl of ResoLight Dye (Roche Diagnostics, Australia), 1 µl of 10x PCR buffer, 5 mM MgCl$_2$, 0.2 mM dNTPs, 0.33 Units Platinum Taq DNA Polymerase (Invitrogen Life Technologies) and 2 µl of 1/10 cDNA. Cycling conditions were: 50°C for 2 min, 95°C for 10 min, followed by 40 cycles of 95°C for 15 sec, annealing temp (Table S1) for 15 sec and 72°C for 15 sec. A dissociation curve was established as follows: Samples were ramped from 60°C to 95°C stepwise at 0.05°C per second. Reactions were performed in triplicate and were optimized for temperature and magnesium concentration (Rotorgene 6000; Applied Biosystems, Viia 7). Dissociation profiles were used to check for single product amplification.

Template cloning for standard curve preparation. RNA extracted from PBLs stimulated overnight with phorbol myristate acetate (PMA) was used to prepare cDNA. Amplification of targets of interest was carried out using the same primers used for qPCR and products were ligated into pGEM-T Easy (Promega, Australia). JM109 Competent cells (Promega, Australia) were transformed with the construct, ampicillin resistant colonies were grown in liquid culture and plasmid DNA was prepared using the QIAprep Spin Miniprep Kit (Qiagen, Australia). Sequences not amplified in this manner were synthetically produced by Integrated DNA Technologies. Cloned sequences were verified on both strands by Sanger sequencing. Plasmids were linearised with AatII (New England Biolabs, USA) and standard curves were prepared immediately prior to each run.

Analysis using qBase plus. Viia7 software determined Cq values using the Baseline Threshold algorithm. Three reference genes, GAPDH, HPRT and YWHAZ, were determined as appropriate to normalize Cq data using qBase plus software, v. 2.6 (Biogazelle, Belgium). Replicates that varied by greater than 0.8 Cq were excluded.

Measuring serum protein levels (CBA/ELISA)

Serum concentrations of IL-6, IL-10, IL-8 and MCP-1 were measured by Cytometric Bead Array (CBA) Flex Sets as described previously. [26] Briefly, CBA Flex Sets employ a bead population with distinct fluorescence intensity for both APC and APC-Cy7 for each individual biomarker measured. Serum concentrations of NGAL and Resistin were measured using ELISAs from R&D Systems according to the manufacturer's instructions. Intra and interassay CVs were 6.55% and 8.77% for the Resistin ELISA and 6.74% and 8.22% for the NGAL ELISA.

Statistical Analysis

Data are presented as median (interquartile range). Because of the skewed distribution of biomarker levels in both healthy controls and patients non-parametric tests were applied. When results were available from three groups the Kruskal-Wallis test was used, followed by application of a Bonferroni correction to post hoc multiple pairwise comparisons performed using the Wilcoxon rank-sum (Mann-Whitney) test. When results were available from two groups only, the Wilcoxon rank-sum (Mann-Whitney) test was performed. P-values presented in bold in the tables are those that remain significant after Bonferroni correction. Correlations were assessed with Spearman rank correlation with Bonferroni adjustments applied for multiple simultaneous testing. The Skillings-Mack test was used to test for differences over time within each patient group Statistical analysis was performed with Stata version 10.1 (StataCorp, College Station, Texas).

Results

Patients

The clinical characteristics for each group are presented in summary form in Table 1. Additional clinical data for individual participants is presented in Table S2. Of 27 patients, 10 had uncomplicated sepsis and 17 had sepsis with organ failure (14 with shock and 3 with other organ failures). As expected, patients with severe sepsis/septic shock were older, had greater comorbid burden and higher rates of ICU admission and mortality. The median time from arrival in the ED to initial blood sample collection (T0) was 58 minutes (IQR 29–95 minutes).

Differential expression of genes in sepsis compared to healthy controls

Results are presented as a Calculated Normalised Relative Quantity (CNRQ), the relative gene expression compared to the three reference genes (GAPDH, YWHAZ, HPRT) for each sample (qBasePlus, Biogazelle). At T0, there was a significant difference in gene expression across all three study groups for all target genes except MIP-1β and UPAR (p<0.035 for all comparisons, Kruskal-Wallis) (Table 2). Compared to healthy controls, IL-10, Resistin and ADM expression was higher in both uncomplicated sepsis and those with severe sepsis/septic shock (p = 1.0×10^{-4}, p = 1.9×10^{-6}; p = 0.001, p = 2.4×10^{-5} and p = 0.005, p = 0.013, respectively, Mann Whitney), whereas FasL and IL-6 expression were lower (p = 0.005, p = 0.004 and p = 4.0×10^{-4}, p = 5.3×10^{-6}, respectively, Mann Whitney) (Table 2). Two genes were differentially expressed in severe sepsis/septic shock but not in uncomplicated sepsis; MCP-1 expression was lower than healthy controls (p = 0.002, Mann Whitney), whereas NGAL expression was higher (p = 7.0×10^{-4}, Mann Whitney). Three genes were differentially expressed in uncomplicated sepsis patients but not in severe sepsis; IL-8 expression was lower than healthy controls (p = 5.0×10^{-4}, Mann Whitney), whereas TLR2 and TLR4 expression was higher (p = 0.013 and p = 0004, respectively, Mann Whitney).

Differential expression of genes in severe sepsis/septic shock compared to uncomplicated sepsis

Only NGAL had significantly higher expression at T0 in patients with severe sepsis/septic shock compared to patients with uncomplicated sepsis (p = 0.007, Mann-Whitney) (Table 2). IL-10

Table 1. Participant baseline clinical characteristics.

	Uncomplicated sepsis	Severe sepsis/shock	P value	All
N	10	17	-	**27**
Age (years)	43 (25, 75)	67 (59, 80)	0.04	**66 (35, 78)**
M/F	6/4	11/6	0.56	**17/10**
Temp (°C)	38.8 (38.3, 40)	37.9 (36.6, 38.8)	0.13	**38.5 (37.2, 39.9)**
Pulse Rate/min	111 (85, 123)	110 (87, 130)	0.65	**110 (85, 125)**
Resp Rate/min	22 (18, 32)	24 (18, 30)	0.98	**24 (18, 30)**
MAP (mmHg)	75 (69, 88)	63 (60, 77)	0.04	**69 (63, 86)**
WCC (x10⁹/L)	11.9 (9.4, 14.3)	12.8 (8.2, 15.3)	0.98	**12.5 (9.1, 14.7)**
Lactate (mmol/L)	1.5 (0.9, 2.1)	3.7 (2.5, 5.9)	<0.001	**2.5 (1.7, 4.3)**
SOFA score	0 (0, 1)	7 (5, 9)	<0.001	**3 (1, 8)**
MEDS score	3 (0, 7)	11 (8, 11)	0.002	**8 (3, 11)**
CCI	0 (0, 1)	1 (1, 2)	0.04	**1 (0, 2)**
ICU admit (%)	1 (10)	12 (71)	0.004	**13 (48)**
Length of stay (days)	5 (3, 6)	10 (6, 17)	0.037	**7 (4, 15)**
Death within 30 days N (%)	0 (0)	3 (18)	0.27	**3 (11)**

Unless otherwise stated values are median (IQR). MAP, mean arterial pressure; WCC, total White blood Cell Count; SOFA, sequential organ failure assessment; MEDS, Mortality in Emergency Department Sepsis: CCI, Charlson Comorbidity Index; ICU, Intensive Care Unit.

and Resistin mRNA levels were also elevated at T0 in severe sepsis/septic shock patients compared to those with uncomplicated sepsis but these differences were not statistically significant after Bonferroni correction (p = 0.035 and p = 0.056, respectively, Mann Whitney) (Table 2).

Changes in gene expression over time

To determine if target gene expression changed significantly over time in patients presenting to the ED with sepsis, results were divided into four sample timing groups: T0 (time of first blood sample), T1-2 (samples collected between 51–125 minutes post-T0), T3-6 (samples collected between 165–365 minutes post-T0) and T12-30 (samples collected between 790–1605 minutes post-T0). If two samples were collected from an individual patient within these time frames, the result from the earliest time point was included for analysis. Target gene expression was stable over time in both patient groups, with the exception of IL-6 mRNA expression changing significantly over time in patients with uncomplicated sepsis (p = 0.019, Skillings-Mack) and UPAR in severe sepsis/septic shock (p = 0.024, Skillings-Mack) (Table S3).

Serum concentrations of Resistin, NGAL, IL-6, IL-10, IL-8 and MCP-1

Based on qPCR results, we analysed serum concentrations of six potential biomarkers in both patient groups (n = 27) and age/sex matched healthy controls (n = 13). At T0, serum concentrations of Resistin, NGAL, IL-6, IL-10, IL-8 and MCP-1 were significantly different across all three study groups (p < 0.02 for all comparisons, Kruskal-Wallis) (Table 3). Serum concentrations of Resistin, NGAL, IL-6 and IL-10 were higher in all sepsis cases compared to healthy controls (p ≤ 0.003 for all comparisons, Mann Whitney) (Table 3). Patients with severe sepsis/septic shock, but not uncomplicated sepsis, had significantly higher serum concentrations of IL-8 and MCP-1 compared to healthy controls (p = 5.6×10⁻⁶ and p = 0.004, respectively, Mann Whitney).

At T0, serum concentrations of Resistin, NGAL, IL-6, IL-10 and IL-8 were significantly higher in patients with severe sepsis/

septic shock compared to patients with uncomplicated sepsis (p = 4.5×10⁻⁵,   p = 2.5×10⁻⁴,   p = 0.002,   p = 0.018   and p = 9.0×10⁻⁴ respectively, Mann Whitney) (Table 3). Serum concentrations of MCP-1 did not differ between the two patient groups. Serum concentrations of Resistin and NGAL at T0 correlated significantly with patient SOFA scores (R = 0.71, p = 0.011 and R = 0.67, p = 0.039, respectively, Spearman test with Bonferroni adjustment).

Serum concentrations of Resistin, NGAL and IL-8 were significantly different between the two patient groups at all time points (p < 0.05 for all comparisons, Mann-Whitney) (Table 4). In patients with uncomplicated sepsis, the only statistically significant change was a decrease in IL-10 over time (p = 0.016, Skillings-Mack) (Table 4). However, in patients with severe sepsis/septic shock, there were statistically significant changes over time in serum concentrations of Resistin, IL-6, IL-10, IL-8 and MCP-1 (p = 0.024, p = 3.5×10⁻⁶, p = 5.0×10⁻⁴, p = 0.002, p = 0.049, Skillings-Mack). Serum concentrations of NGAL remained stable in patients with both uncomplicated sepsis and severe sepsis/septic shock over the first ~24 hours after ED arrival (p = 0.119 and p = 0.237, respectively, Skillings-Mack) (Table 4).

Correlation of mRNA expression and serum protein concentrations

When comparing all samples from all patients at all timepoints, only Resistin and NGAL mRNA levels correlated with serum protein   concentrations   (R = 0.52,   p < 0.001   and   R = 0.36, p = 0.022, respectively, Spearmans with Bonferroni adjustment). Serum levels of all biomarkers measured correlated positively with each other with p < 0.003 for all comparisons except MCP-1 versus IL-10 where the p-value was 0.03.

Discussion

In this study we used quantitative PCR to identify potential candidate genes differentially expressed in circulating leucocytes early in the ED in severe sepsis compared to uncomplicated sepsis

Table 2. Target gene expression at T0 in healthy controls, uncomplicated sepsis and severe sepsis/shock.

Target gene expression [#]	Healthy Controls (n = 19) Median (IQR)	Uncomplicated Sepsis (n = 10) Median (IQR)	Severe Sepsis/Septic Shock (n = 17) Median (IQR)	p[1]	p[2]	p[3]	p[4]
IL-10	−0.75 (−0.92, −0.67)	−0.19 (−0.26, 0.005)	0.22 (−0.14, 0.48)	1.0×10^{-4}	$\mathbf{1.0 \times 10^{-4*}}$	$\mathbf{1.9 \times 10^{-6}}$	0.035
Resistin	−0.70 (−0.93, −0.44)	−0.21 (−0.42, 0.14)	0.22 (−0.21, 0.75)	1.0×10^{-4}	**0.001**	$\mathbf{2.4 \times 10^{-5}}$	0.056
Adrenomedullin	−0.40 (−0.59, −0.006)	0.23 (−0.05, 0.44)	0.02 (−0.29, 0.30)	0.005	**0.005**	**0.013**	0.219
FasL	0.53 (0.37, 0.70)	0.08 (−0.33, 0.34)	−0.11 (−0.44, 0.44)	0.003	**0.005**	**0.004**	0.651
IL-6	0.49 (0.28, 0.54)	−0.09 (−0.33, 0.14)	−0.04 (−0.37, 0.16)	1.0×10^{-4}	$\mathbf{4.0 \times 10^{-4}}$	$\mathbf{5.3 \times 10^{-6}}$	0.920
MCP-1	0.60 (0.43, 0.69)	0.47 (−0.33, 0.94)	−0.12 (−0.57, 0.50)	0.011	0.363	**0.002**	0.205
NGAL	−0.43 (−0.57, −0.14)	−0.56 (−0.61, −0.05)	0.38 (−0.23, 0.73)	0.001	0.819	$\mathbf{7.0 \times 10^{-4}}$	**0.007**
IL-8	0.30 (0.21, 0.48)	−0.63 (−0.79, −0.002)	−0.26 (−0.41, 0.58)	0.003	$\mathbf{5.0 \times 10^{-4}}$	0.064	0.108
TLR2	−0.18 (−0.35, −0.07)	0.14 (−0.13, 0.29)	−0.07 (−0.25, 0.21)	0.033	**0.013**	0.070	0.451
TLR4	−0.34 (−0.44, −0.04)	0.06 (−0.15, 0.39)	0.05 (−0.35, 0.17)	0.019	**0.004**	0.103	0.292
MIP-1β	0.25 (−0.03, 0.33)	−0.15 (−0.36, 0.26)	−0.18 (−0.54, 0.89)	0.389			
UPAR	−0.05 (−0.08, 0.20)	0.11 (−0.12, 0.43)	−0.07 (−0.42, 0.46)	0.586			

[1] p value for difference across all three groups (Kruskal-Wallis)
[2] p-value for the difference between uncomplicated sepsis and healthy controls (Mann Whitney)
[3] p-value for the difference between severe sepsis/septic shock and healthy controls (Mann Whitney)
[4] p value for the difference between uncomplicated and severe sepsis/septic shock (Mann Whitney)
* P-values in **bold** remain significant after Bonferonni correction (p<0.017)
# results are presented as Calculated Normalised Relative Quantity (CNRQ)

Table 3. Serum biomarker concentrations in healthy controls, uncomplicated sepsis and severe sepsis/septic shock at T0.

Biomarker	Healthy Controls (n=13) Median (IQR)	Uncomplicated sepsis (n=10) Median (IQR)	Severe sepsis/septic shock (n=17) Median (IQR)	p^1	p^2	p^3	p^4
Resistin (ng/ml)	12.6 (8.6, 14.3)	36.5 (31.8, 51.1)	118 (88.2, 182)	1.0×10^{-4}	2.0×10^{-4}	3.8×10^{-6}	4.5×10^{-5}
NGAL (ng/ml)	114 (96, 135)	249 (222, 318)	476 (383, 843)	1.0×10^{-4}	**0.001**	5.6×10^{-6}	2.5×10^{-4}
IL-6 (pg/ml)	0.0 (0.0, 7.1)	235 (99.3, 634)	5224 (592, 19,790)	1.0×10^{-4}	4.4×10^{-5}	3.3×10^{-6}	**0.002**
IL-10 (pg/ml)	0.0 (0.0, 5.9)	19.1 (7.5, 40.2)	117 (26.3, 560)	1.0×10^{-4}	**0.003**	2.0×10^{-4}	0.018
IL-8 (pg/ml)	21.1 (18.3, 26.4)	44.3 (17.8, 205)	757 (221, 1898)	1.0×10^{-4}	0.107	5.6×10^{-6}	9.0×10^{-4}
MCP-1 (pg/ml)	231 (163, 267)	497 (152, 1899)	2947 (259, 9722)	0.017	0.385	**0.004**	0.132

[1] p value for difference across all three groups (Kruskal-Wallis)
[2] p-value for the difference between uncomplicated sepsis and healthy controls (Mann Whitney)
[3] p-value for the difference between severe sepsis/septic shock and healthy controls (Mann Whitney)
[4] p-value for the difference between uncomplicated and severe sepsis/septic shock (Mann Whitney)
* P-values in **bold** remain significant after Bonferonni correction (p<0.017)

and healthy controls. We then measured serum protein levels at multiple time points over the first 24 h of hospital stay, and identified consistently significant differences in levels of Resistin, NGAL and IL-8 between the groups at all time points.

Sepsis is a dynamic condition and patients present to the ED at various stages in their illness evolution. An essential task is to risk stratify patients to direct timely care and correct disposition. Biomarkers of organ dysfunction may more accurately detect patients with severe sepsis or shock before this manifests either clinically or with conventional markers such as creatinine or lactate. Our study obtained serial blood samples commencing early in the ED and over the subsequent 24 hours. We found that while expression of our chosen target genes in PBL did not significantly change over time, almost all of the measured proteins in serum did, specifically in the severe sepsis/septic shock group. This has clinical and research implications since timing of sampling may be critical. For example, if patients are recruited into studies in the ICU, measured levels of cytokines may be markedly different to those on arrival prior to resuscitation. A reliable serum marker for severe sepsis should differentiate patients with organ dysfunction/shock regardless of the timing of sampling and resuscitation status of the patient. Of the six serum proteins we measured based upon the results of our qPCR analysis, only three – Resistin, NGAL and IL-8 differentiated severe sepsis from uncomplicated sepsis at all time points and only NGAL remained stable over time in both patient groups. It is unlikely that any single marker will be sufficiently accurate for clinical purposes. For this reason it is suggested that a multi-marker "panel" may be more useful. [14]

Resistin, first described in 2001 as an adipocyte-secreted hormone causing insulin resistance in type-2 diabetes, has since been found to be an important pro-inflammatory cytokine in humans, secreted principally by monocytes and epithelial cells. [27,28] In a study of patients with severe sepsis and septic shock, resistin was found to correlate strongly with disease severity, as well as with levels of inflammatory cytokines, lactate D-dimer and creatinine. [29] Another study found that resistin levels were higher among ICU patients with sepsis compared to non-infected controls, and this was unrelated to preexisting diabetes or obesity. [30]

NGAL, a member of the lipocalin family of proteins, is expressed by neutrophils and a number of epithelial cells. It has emerged as an early marker of acute kidney injury in a range of critical illness settings, including in sepsis. [31,32] Among ED patients with sepsis elevated NGAL on admission was predictive of subsequent renal injury. [33] In a multi-centre study a biomarker panel of NGAL along with IL-1ra and protein C was predictive of severe sepsis, septic shock and death among ED patients with suspected sepsis. [14] Analysis of gene expression patterns from blood samples from septic and non-septic patients in a meta-analysis has also suggested that NGAL is a strong candidate gene for predicting SIRS patients that may progress to sepsis. [34]

A defining characteristic of severe sepsis may be recruitment of circulating immune cells to produce inflammatory mediators, in addition to local tissue production. It is notable that, for both NGAL and resistin, as well as serum concentrations being higher, gene expression was also greater in circulating leukocytes of patients with severe sepsis compared to uncomplicated sepsis.

The serum levels of individual cytokines are expected to vary enormously between individuals due to differential timing of release, metabolism and the complex interplay between the vast array of biomarkers released during sepsis. [35] In a recent study, Lvovschi et al determined that cytokine levels either individually or in combination do not appear useful for differentiating severe

Table 4. Serum biomarker levels in uncomplicated sepsis and severe sepsis/septic shock over time.

	Uncomplicated sepsis (n = 10*)	Severe sepsis/septic shock (n = 17*)			
	Median (IQR)	Median (IQR)	p¹	p²	p³
Resistin (ng/ml)					
T0	36.5 (31.8, 51.1)	118 (88.2, 182)	**4.5×10⁻⁵**	0.064	0.024
1–2 hours post-T0	36.8 (27.2, 41.4)	99 (69.2, 149)	**1.0×10⁻⁴**		
3–6 hours post-T0	49.0 (37.6, 54.0)	135 (90.2, 161)	**7.0×10⁻⁴**		
12–30 hours post-T0	50.8 (29.3, 81.3)	122 (83.0, 163)	**0.011**		
NGAL (ng/ml)					
T0	249 (222, 318)	476 (383, 843)	**2.5×10⁻⁴**	0.119	0.237
1–2 hours post-T0	243 (187, 307)	506 (388, 791)	**2.0×10⁻⁴**		
3–6 hours post-T0	259 (232, 324)	534 (402, 798)	**0.003**		
12–30 hours post-T0	415 (232, 537)	607 (461, 737)	0.044		
IL-6 (pg/ml)					
T0	235 (99.3, 634)	5224 (592, 19,790)	**0.002**	0.803	3.5×10−6
1–2 hours post-T0	176 (51, 977)	4088 (430, 13,270)	**0.005**		
3–6 hours post-T0	321 (76.6, 669)	2253 (370, 6652)	0.023		
12–30 hours post-T0	82.2 (41.3, 320)	262 (106, 1635)	0.096		
IL-10 (pg/ml)					
T0	19.1 (7.5, 40.2)	117 (26.3, 560)	0.018	0.016	5×10⁻⁴
1–2 hours post-T0	31.6 (9.3, 78.4)	138 (28.2, 424)	0.071		
3–6 hours post-T0	12.7 (1.6, 16.2)	165 (20.5, 532)	0.031		
12–30 hours post-T0	9.8 (2.3, 18.6)	24.4 (6.5, 131)	0.095		
IL-8 (pg/ml)					
T0	44.3 (17.8, 205)	757 (221, 1898)	**9.0×10⁻⁴**	0.540	0.002
1–2 hours post-T0	91.7 (24.0, 167)	677 (231, 1196)	**0.002**		
3–6 hours post-T0	114 (32.2, 175)	736 (243, 974)	**0.002**		
12–30 hours post-T0	56.8 (15.1, 187)	287 (140, 451)	**0.011**		
MCP-1 (pg/ml)					
T0	497 (152, 1899)	2947 (259, 9722)	0.132	0.591	0.049
1–2 hours post-T0	588 (107, 1471)	2115 (513, 6367)	0.071		
3–6 hours post-T0	579 (156, 783)	1654 (647, 2722)	0.036		
12–30 hours post-T0	426 (90.0, 1239)	517 (268, 1646)	0.335		

¹p value for the difference between uncomplicated and severe sepsis/septic shock (Mann Whitney). P values in **bold** remain significant after Bonferroni correction (p< 0.013).
²p value for change over time for uncomplicated sepsis (Skillings Mack)
³p value for change over time for severe sepsis/septic shock (Skillings Mack)
*At T0 and 1–2 hours post-T0, data was available from n = 10 uncomplicated sepsis and n = 17 severe sepsis/septic shock patients, at 3–6 hours post-T0, data was available from n = 8 uncomplicated sepsis and n = 17 severe sepsis/septic shock and at 12–30 hours post-T0 data was available from n = 6 uncomplicated sepsis and n = 13 severe sepsis/septic shock.

sepsis from uncomplicated sepsis in the ED. [36] We found that, although serum levels of IL-6, IL-10 and IL-8 were significantly elevated in severe sepsis/septic shock compared to uncomplicated sepsis up to 6–8 hours post-ED arrival, significant changes in serum levels over time, especially in patients with severe sepsis, means clinical use of these markers as a routine test to predict sepsis severity or progression may be limited.

Notable strengths of this study are the recruitment of patients very early in the course of their hospital management, with serial sampling over time. As well as addressing the issue of 'lead time' when patients are recruited into biomarker studies in ICU, often many hours after presentation, we also included patients not admitted to the ICU, reflecting real-world experience of sepsis in

the ED. We approached the selection of biomarkers by two methods, using qPCR to identify differential gene activation in leucocytes between two clinically relevant phenotypic groups, then confirming these results by measuring the serum protein products of those genes. There are also several limitations to the study. Patients were selected by convenience sampling and the availability of sufficient quality mRNA for qPCR analysis. In addition, the study sample was a subgroup of a larger ED critical illness study and may not necessarily be representative of the ED sepsis population. Our selection of serum markers was informed by the results of the qPCR analysis of leucocyte mRNA, meaning we may have excluded important markers produced predominantly by tissues. The small number of patients and multiple statistical tests increases the risk of chance 'positive' findings of association between groups. The small numbers also precluded undertaking any regression analyses; given the high degree of correlation between the markers this is necessary to determine the independent predictive value of any given marker. Finally, when interpreting the analyses over time it is important to note that not all patients had complete samples at all time points which may have led to bias in the later time-point comparisons.

Our findings indicate a potential role for IL-8, Resistin and NGAL to differentiate patients with severe sepsis from those with a more benign course, however whether this might be of any use in addition to clinical parameters is unknown. The next step is to attempt to replicate these findings in a larger prospective cohort and so refine and validate a panel of biomarkers which will complement clinical assessment to identify high risk patients in the ED.

Supporting Information

Figure S1 A summary flowchart of the participant screening and enrolment process.

Table S1 Primer sequences for qPCR expression analysis.

Table S2 Clinical characteristics.

Table S3 Target gene expression in uncomplicated and severe sepsis over time by qPCR.

Acknowledgments

We acknowledge the research nursing staff at Royal Perth and Armadale Hospitals for identifying patients for the study and collecting and processing blood samples, including Ellen MacDonald (Clinical Nurse Manager), Helen Hammersley, Clare Nash, Jen Wurmel, Naomi Sweeting, Lilian Offer, Alysse Pownall and Shiree Walker. The authors acknowledge the facilities, scientific and technical assistance of the Australian Microscopy & Microanalysis Research Facility at the Centre for Microscopy, Characterisation & Analysis, The University of Western Australia, a facility funded by The University, State and Commonwealth Governments. The authors would also like to thank Mrs Sally Burrows for providing expert statistical advice.

Author Contributions

Conceived and designed the experiments: SM SS CN PvE SB. Performed the experiments: CN. Analyzed the data: SM SS SB. Wrote the paper: SM SS DF GA SB. Recruited patients and reviewed clinical data: SM DF GA SB.

References

1. Dellinger RP, Levy MM, Carlet JM, Bion J, Parker MM, et al. (2008) Surviving Sepsis Campaign: international guidelines for management of severe sepsis and septic shock: 2008. [Erratum appears in Intensive Care Med. 2008 Apr;34(4):783-5]. Intensive Care Medicine 34: 17–60.

2. Bagshaw SM, Webb SA, Delaney A, George C, Pilcher D, et al. (2009) Very old patients admitted to intensive care in Australia and New Zealand: a multi-centre cohort analysis. Crit Care 13: R45.

3. Carson SS (2003) The epidemiology of critical illness in the elderly. Crit Care Clin 19: 605–617, v.

4. Martin GS, Mannino DM, Moss M (2006) The effect of age on the development and outcome of adult sepsis. [see comment]. Critical Care Medicine 34: 15–21.

5. Strehlow MC, Emond SD, Shapiro NI, Pelletier AJ, Camargo CA Jr (2006) National study of emergency department visits for sepsis, 1992 to 2001. Annals of Emergency Medicine 48: 326–331.

6. Angus DC, van der Poll T (2013) Severe sepsis and septic shock. N Engl J Med 369: 840–851.

7. Brenner T, Hofer S, Rosenhagen C, Steppan J, Lichtenstern C, et al. (2010) Macrophage migration inhibitory factor (MIF) and manganese superoxide dismutase (MnSOD) as early predictors for survival in patients with severe sepsis or septic shock. J Surg Res 164: e163–171.

8. Christ-Crain M, Morgenthaler NG, Struck J, Harbarth S, Bergmann A, et al. (2005) Mid-regional pro-adrenomedullin as a prognostic marker in sepsis: an observational study. Crit Care 9: R816–824.

9. Gustafsson A, Ljunggren L, Bodelsson M, Berkestedt I (2012) The Prognostic Value of suPAR Compared to Other Inflammatory Markers in Patients with Severe Sepsis. Biomark Insights 7: 39–44.

10. Pierrakos C, Vincent JL (2010) Sepsis biomarkers: a review. Crit Care 14: R15.

11. Nakamura T, Sato E, Fujiwara N, Kawagoe Y, Suzuki T, et al. (2009) Circulating levels of advanced glycation end products (AGE) and interleukin-6 (IL-6) are independent determinants of serum asymmetric dimethylarginine (ADMA) levels in patients with septic shock. Pharmacol Res 60: 515–518.

12. Gille-Johnson P, Hansson KE, Gardlund B (2012) Clinical and laboratory variables identifying bacterial infection and bacteraemia in the emergency department. Scand J Infect Dis 44: 745–752.

13. Bozza FA, Salluh JI, Japiassu AM, Soares M, Assis EF, et al. (2007) Cytokine profiles as markers of disease severity in sepsis: a multiplex analysis. Crit Care 11: R49.

14. Shapiro NI, Trzeciak S, Hollander JE, Birkhahn R, Otero R, et al. (2009) A prospective, multicenter derivation of a biomarker panel to assess risk of organ dysfunction, shock, and death in emergency department patients with suspected sepsis. Crit Care Med 37: 96–104.

15. Ip M, Rainer TH, Lee N, Chan C, Chau SS, et al. (2007) Value of serum procalcitonin, neopterin, and C-reactive protein in differentiating bacterial from viral etiologies in patients presenting with lower respiratory tract infections. Diagn Microbiol Infect Dis 59: 131–136.

16. Punyadeera C, Schneider EM, Schaffer D, Hsu HY, Joos TO, et al. (2010) A biomarker panel to discriminate between systemic inflammatory response syndrome and sepsis and sepsis severity. J Emerg Trauma Shock 3: 26–35.

17. Kofoed K, Andersen O, Kronborg G, Tvede M, Petersen J, et al. (2007) Use of plasma C-reactive protein, procalcitonin, neutrophils, macrophage migration inhibitory factor, soluble urokinase-type plasminogen activator receptor, and soluble triggering receptor expressed on myeloid cells-1 in combination to diagnose infections: a prospective study. Crit Care 11: R38.

18. Wong HR, Lindsell CJ, Pettila V, Meyer NJ, Thair SA, et al. (2014) A multibiomarker-based outcome risk stratification model for adult septic shock*. Crit Care Med 42: 781–789.

19. Lichtenstern C, Brenner T, Bardenheuer HJ, Weigand MA (2012) Predictors of survival in sepsis: what is the best inflammatory marker to measure? Curr Opin Infect Dis 25: 328–336.

20. Travaglino F, De Berardinis B, Magrini L, Bongiovanni C, Candelli M, et al. (2012) Utility of Procalcitonin (PCT) and Mid regional pro-Adrenomedullin (MR-proADM) in risk stratification of critically ill febrile patients in Emergency Department (ED). A comparison with APACHE II score. BMC Infect Dis 12: 184.

21. Freund Y, Delerme S, Goulet H, Bernard M, Riou B, et al. (2012) Serum lactate and procalcitonin measurements in emergency room for the diagnosis and risk-stratification of patients with suspected infection. Biomarkers.

22. Arendts G, Stone SF, Fatovich DM, van Eeden P, MacDonald E, et al. (2012) Critical illness in the emergency department: lessons learnt from the first 12 months of enrolments in the Critical Illness and Shock Study. Emerg Med Australas 24: 31–36.

23. Levy MM, Fink MP, Marshall JC, Abraham E, Angus D, et al. (2003) 2001 SCCM/ESICM/ACCP/ATS/SIS International Sepsis Definitions Conference. Intensive Care Med 29: 530–538.

24. Charlson ME, Pompei P, Ales KL, MacKenzie CR (1987) A new method of classifying prognostic comorbidity in longitudinal studies: development and validation. J Chronic Dis 40: 373–383.

25. Bustin SA, Benes V, Garson JA, Hellemans J, Huggett J, et al. (2009) The MIQE guidelines: minimum information for publication of quantitative real-time PCR experiments. Clin Chem 55: 611–622.

26. Stone SF, Cotterell C, Isbister GK, Holdgate A, Brown SG (2009) Elevated serum cytokines during human anaphylaxis: Identification of potential mediators of acute allergic reactions. J Allergy Clin Immunol 124: 786–792 e784.

27. Pang SS, Le YY (2006) Role of resistin in inflammation and inflammation-related diseases. Cell Mol Immunol 3: 29–34.

28. Aziz M, Jacob A, Yang WL, Matsuda A, Wang P (2013) Current trends in inflammatory and immunomodulatory mediators in sepsis. J Leukoc Biol 93: 329–342.

29. Sunden-Cullberg J, Nystrom T, Lee ML, Mullins GE, Tokics L, et al. (2007) Pronounced elevation of resistin correlates with severity of disease in severe sepsis and septic shock. Crit Care Med 35: 1536–1542.

30. Koch A, Gressner OA, Sanson E, Tacke F, Trautwein C (2009) Serum resistin levels in critically ill patients are associated with inflammation, organ dysfunction and metabolism and may predict survival of non-septic patients. Crit Care 13: R95.

31. Constantin JM, Futier E, Perbet S, Roszyk L, Lautrette A, et al. (2010) Plasma neutrophil gelatinase-associated lipocalin is an early marker of acute kidney injury in adult critically ill patients: a prospective study. Journal of Critical Care 25: 176 e171–176.

32. Lentini P, de Cal M, Clementi A, D'Angelo A, Ronco C (2012) Sepsis and AKI in ICU Patients: The Role of Plasma Biomarkers. Crit Care Res Pract 2012: 856401.

33. Shapiro NI, Trzeciak S, Hollander JE, Birkhahn R, Otero R, et al. (2010) The diagnostic accuracy of plasma neutrophil gelatinase-associated lipocalin in the prediction of acute kidney injury in emergency department patients with suspected sepsis. Ann Emerg Med 56: 52–59 e51.

34. Lindig S, Quickert S, Vodovotz Y, Wanner GA, Bauer M (2013) Age-independent co-expression of antimicrobial gene clusters in the blood of septic patients. Int J Antimicrob Agents 42 Suppl: S2–7.

35. Herzum I, Renz H (2008) Inflammatory markers in SIRS, sepsis and septic shock. Curr Med Chem 15: 581–587.

36. Lvovschi V, Arnaud L, Parizot C, Freund Y, Juillien G, et al. (2011) Cytokine profiles in sepsis have limited relevance for stratifying patients in the emergency department: a prospective observational study. PLoS One 6: e28870.

3

Formal Modelling of Toll like Receptor 4 and JAK/STAT Signalling Pathways: Insight into the Roles of SOCS-1, Interferon-β and Proinflammatory Cytokines in Sepsis

Rehan Zafar Paracha[1], Jamil Ahmad[2]*, Amjad Ali[1]*, Riaz Hussain[3], Umar Niazi[4], Samar Hayat Khan Tareen[2], Babar Aslam[1]

1 Atta-Ur-Rahman School of Applied Biosciences (ASAB), National University of Sciences and Technology (NUST), Islamabad, Pakistan, 2 Research Center for Modeling and Simulation (RCMS), National University of Sciences and Technology (NUST), Islamabad, Pakistan, 3 Shifa College of Pharmaceutical Sciences, Shifa Tameer-e-Millat University, Islamabad, Pakistan, 4 IBERS, Aberystwyth University, Edward Llwyd Building, Penglais Campus, Aberystwyth, Ceredigion, Wales, United Kingdom

Abstract

Sepsis is one of the major causes of human morbidity and results in a considerable number of deaths each year. Lipopolysaccharide-induced sepsis has been associated with TLR4 signalling pathway which in collaboration with the JAK/STAT signalling regulate endotoxemia and inflammation. However, during sepsis our immune system cannot maintain a balance of cytokine levels and results in multiple organ damage and eventual death. Different opinions have been made in previous studies about the expression patterns and the role of proinflammatory cytokines in sepsis that attracted our attention towards qualitative properties of TLR4 and JAK/STAT signalling pathways using computer-aided studies. René Thomas' formalism was used to model septic and non-septic dynamics of TLR4 and JAK/STAT signalling. Comparisons among dynamics were made by intervening or removing the specific interactions among entities. Among our predictions, recurrent induction of proinflammatory cytokines with subsequent downregulation was found as the basic characteristic of septic model. This characteristic was found in agreement with previous experimental studies, which implicate that inflammation is followed by immunomodulation in septic patients. Moreover, intervention in downregulation of proinflammatory cytokines by SOCS-1 was found desirable to boost the immune responses. On the other hand, interventions either in TLR4 or transcriptional elements such as NFκB and STAT were found effective in the downregulation of immune responses. Whereas, IFN-β and SOCS-1 mediated downregulation at different levels of signalling were found to be associated with variations in the levels of proinflammatory cytokines. However, these predictions need to be further validated using wet laboratory experimental studies to further explore the roles of inhibitors such as SOCS-1 and IFN-β, which may alter the levels of proinflammatory cytokines at different stages of sepsis.

Editor: Francesco Pappalardo, University of Catania, Italy

Funding: This work was supported by research grants from Higher Education Commission of Pakistan (Grant No. 20-1464/R&D/09/5252) and COMSTECH-TWAS (Grant No. 09-047RG/ITC/AS_C) (Standing Committee on Scientific and Technological Cooperation (COMSTECH) and The Academy of Sciences for the Developing World (TWAS)). The funders had no role in study design, data collection and analysis, decision to publish, or preparation of the manuscript.

Competing Interests: The authors have declared that no competing interests exist.

* Email: dr.ahmad.jamil@gmail.com (JA); amjad_uni@yahoo.com (AA)

Introduction

Sepsis is a serious medical condition associated with complications of an exacerbated human immune response against endotoxin/lipopolysaccharides (LPS) mediated severe infections [1]. It can lead to endotoxin shock, organ damage, morbidity and eventual death [2,3]. The incidence of sepsis is growing regardless of advances in the therapeutic and supportive treatments [4,5]. In 1992, nearly 500,000 cases of sepsis were found in the United States among which 35% of the patients led to mortality [6]. In 2001, around 750,000 cases of sepsis with 28.6% mortality rate per annum was recorded [7]. In a trend analysis from 1993 to 2003, a significant increase in the cases of severe sepsis and hospitalization was reported [8], which is still rising [9].

Pro- and anti-inflammatory cytokines are groups of proteins, which mediate endogenous inflammation and immunomodulation, respectively. Proinflammatory cytokines (PICyts) including tumour necrosis factor (TNF)-α, interferon (IFN)-γ, interleukin (IL)-la, IL-1β and IL-6 induce a series of immune responses to overcome the pathogen load [10]. In contrast, anti-inflammatory cytokines such as transforming growth factor (TGF)-β, IL-4, IL-10, IL-13 and other cytokine inhibitors including soluble tumour necrosis factor receptor (sTNFR)-I and II, IL-lra, or soluble IL-1 receptors (sIL-1r) modulate the immune responses and can induce temporary immunosuppression in septic patients [11].

Our understandings about the contributory role of pro- and anti-inflammatory immune responses in sepsis evolved with the passage of time and highlighted disparities among the scientific findings. Earlier animal studies suggested that proinflammatory responses were the major cause of the systemic inflammatory response syndrome (SIRS) and mortality, whereas anti-inflammatory responses were associated with comparatively less severe complications [12]. In contrast, recently submitted suggestions disprove previous studies and indicated that the anti-inflammatory responses and immunosuppression might in fact be responsible for compensatory anti-inflammatory response syndrome (CARS), severe sepsis, organ damage and subsequent mortality [13–17]. Moreover, other studies implicated that pro- and anti-inflammatory responses are correlated with each other and provide opportunities for septic patients for the management of pathogens and hyperinflammation at different levels of sepsis [18,19].

Toll like receptors (TLRs) are pattern recognition receptors and play their important role in the induction of innate immunity against endotoxins [20]. Previous studies have demonstrated that the expression levels of TLR4 were elevated on human monocytes in healthy volunteers challenged with LPS [21] as well as in septic patients [22,23]. Activation of TLR4 leads to the production of pro- and anti-inflammatory cytokines by inducing two different signalling pathways [24]. TLR4 is unique among other TLRs due to its ability to induce myeloid differentiation primary response gene (MyD)88 and TIR-domain-containing-adapter-inducing interferon-β (TRIF) dependent pathways [25]. These two pathways culminate in the generation of PICyts and Interferon-β (IFN-β), respectively. Along with the production of IFN-β, TRIF dependent signalling has also been implicated to induce the NFκB activation through TRAF6 [26]. On the other hand, IFN-β has been implicated in the modulation of late hyperinflammation in sepsis [27]. Figure 1 is the simple representation of the TLR4 and Janus kinase (JAK)/signal transducer and activator of transcription (STAT) (JAK/STAT) signalling pathways adapted from previous experimental studies and databases associated with biological signalling [28–34].

MyD88 dependent pathway activates due to the formation of a complex between MyD88, TLR4 and toll-interleukin 1 receptor (TIR) domain containing adaptor protein (TIRAP also known as MAL). This pathway culminates in the activation of NFκB with subsequent production of PICyts [35]. In contrast, the TRIF dependent pathway is activated by the formation of a complex between TRIF, TRIF related adaptor molecule (TRAM or TICAM2) and TLR4 [36]. This complex results in the activation of transcriptional regulator interferon regulatory factor 3 (IRF3) with subsequent transcription of IFN-β [37]. Moreover, the TRIF dependent pathway has also been implicated for the delayed activation of NFκB, through TRIF mediated TRAF6 activation, however, MyD88 dependent pathway is reported for its explicit contribution in the production of PICyts [38]. PICyts and IFN-β mediated JAK/STAT signalling is essential for the induction of pro- or anti-inflammatory immune responses, respectively [31,39]. PICyts and IFN-β stimulate JAKs with subsequent translocation of STATs into the nucleus where it transcribes necessary genes responsible to react appropriately against the pathogen or inflammation [30,31].

TLR4 mediated immune responses are downregulated by several negative feedback mechanisms [40]. Regulation of TLR4 mediated signalling maintain homeostasis between infectious challenge and hyperinflammatory responses [41]. Negative regulatory proteins such as suppressor of cytokine signalling-1 (SOCS-1), A20 zinc finger protein and sterile alpha-and armadillo-motif-containing protein (SARM) are well reported for their inhibitory roles in TLR4 signalling [42–44]. Recently, IFN-β is found associated with the induction of TH1 to TH2 response shift to reduce the levels of circulating PICyts [27,45–47]. Various experiments on SOCS-1 knockout cells highlighted that SOCS-1 is necessary to protect against endotoxemia and hyperinflammation by inhibiting PICyts and IFN-β mediated JAK/STAT signalling, respectively [48–50].

In this study, we devised qualitative (discrete) model of TLR4 and JAK/STAT signalling, which was constructed by using the well-known mathematical formalism of René Thomas [51–53].

Construction of the models according to this formalism do not require quantitative data (the expression of entities and kinetic rate parameters of reactions), which is often difficult to obtain for the biological regulatory networks (BRNs) [54]. Construction of the qualitative model requires only the qualitative thresholds and logical parameters, which can be easily adjusted (see Definitions in Material and Methods section). The qualitative model encompasses all the possible qualitative states or levels of entities present in a BRN. The dynamics of the BRN are captured by the state graph (representing the states and trajectories) where important behaviours can be seen as cyclic paths and paths diverging towards stable states. These cycles and stable states represent the activation profiles of the entities, respectively. The advantage of the state graph is that it can represent a state space in any dimension as a discrete abstraction, while in other approaches, like ordinary differential equations, this may be very challenging. Comparison of the qualitative model with its differential equation counterpart is given by René Thomas et al. in [55] to prove that both approaches are equivalent, however, the qualitative modelling is more suitable for model checking based reasoning to infer unknown parameters [56].

In our previous study, TLR4 mediated MyD88 dependent pathway was studied, with a particular focus on the role of Bruton's tyrosine kinase and MAL in the production of hyperinflammatory responses especially in the case of cerebral malaria [57]. The current study presents the dynamics of the TLR4 and JAK/STAT signalling pathway by updating our previous study with new interactions and entities to gain an insight into a different pathological condition of sepsis. Additionally, the current study also provides an understanding about the importance of signalling downregulated by SOCS-1, IFN-β, A20 and SARM. Moreover, modelling of interventions in signalling were used to understand the roles of NFκB, PICyts, IFN-β, JAK/STAT and SOCS-1 in immune responses [55].

The BRN of TLR4-JAK/STAT (Figure 2) in this study implicates that TLR4, IFN-β, JAK/STAT and SOCS-1 mediated signalling perform their roles in a recursive manner. Intervention in the SOCS-1 mediated downregulation of PICyts is associated with the production of overactive immune response, whereas, interventions either in TLR4 or NFκB-JAK/STAT signalling is connected with downregulation of overactive immune responses. Additionally, IFN-β downregulates PICyts in the earlier phase of signalling, whereas SOCS-1 regulates the levels of cytokines in late phase. On this account, levels of PICyts fluctuate within different qualitative levels during sepsis and may provide the basis for the differences in scientific findings [18,19]. However, these predictions were generated by the use of computer-aided models and need to be further validated in wet laboratory experiments.

Materials and Methods

The formalism of René Thomas

Traditionally, biological systems are modelled using ordinary differential equations, which require time derivatives of expression levels, temperature, physical state and kinetic rates of entities, etc. [58]. Due to the complexity of the biological systems, each variable with all of its parameters are either system specific or rarely known. For this reason, computer-aided qualitative modelling of biological systems is generally preferred to understand the dynamics of the BRN at a preliminary level, which can then be validated using *in vitro* experiments.

In 1970, René Thomas introduced Boolean logic for the qualitative modelling of BRNs, which was later generalised to kinetic logic [59–66]. Using kinetic logic, possible dynamics of a

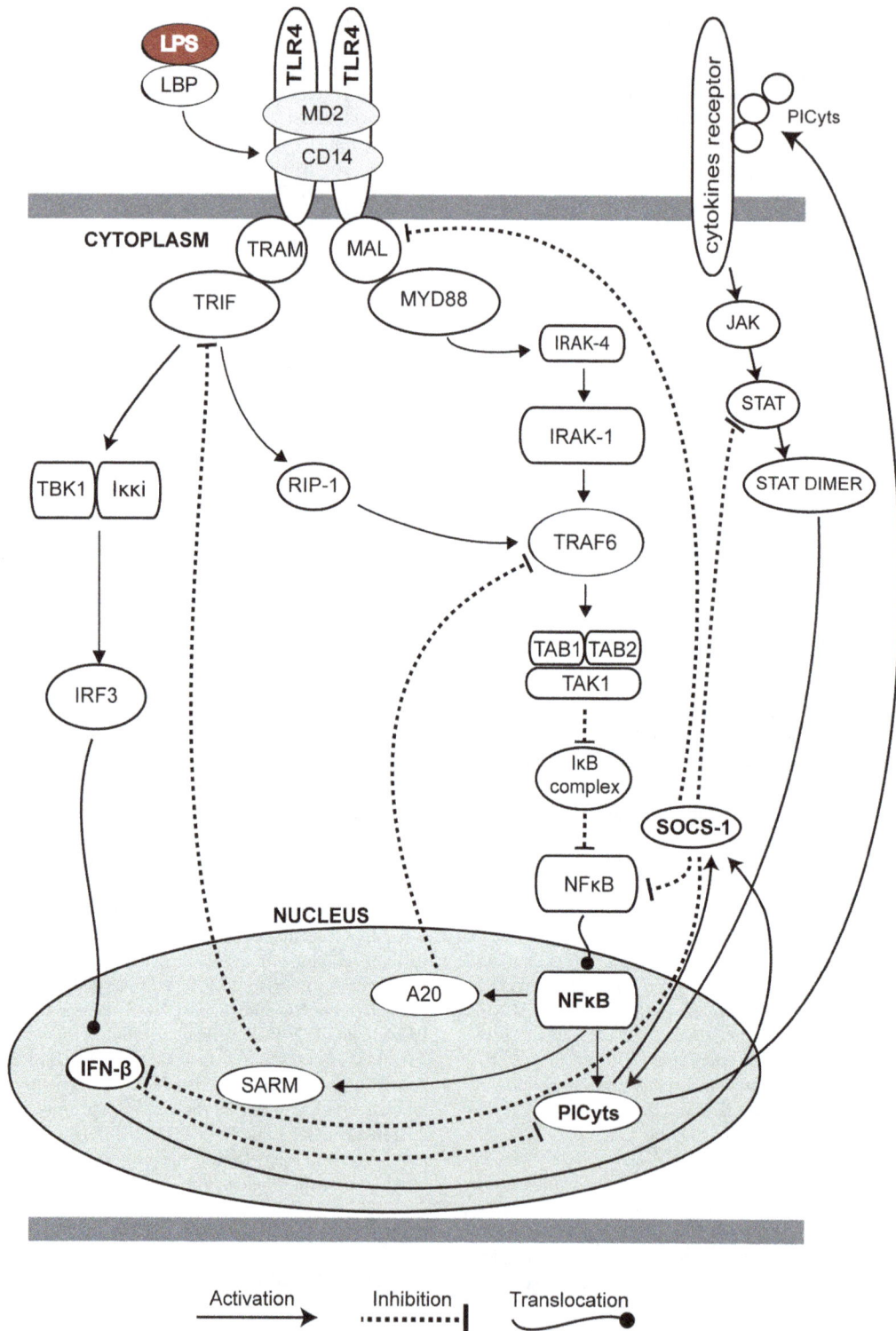

Figure 1. TLR4 and JAK/STAT signalling pathway. Overview of TLR4 and JAK/STAT signalling pathway adopted from previous experimental studies and databases associated with signalling pathways [20,28–33]. TLR4 activates two separate signalling pathways, including MyD88 and TRIF dependent pathways [103]. TIRAP/Mal and TRAM are recruited by TLR4 as adaptor proteins to activate MyD88 and TRIF dependent pathways, respectively [35,103]. Following MYD88 activation, IRAK4 is phosphorylated by MyD88-MAL complex, which ultimately results in the phosphorylation of IRAK1 protein. Phosphorylated IRAK1 activates TRAF6 [104] which after forming a complex with TAK1-TAB1/2 activates Iκκ complex [105]. Iκκα and Iκκβ catalyse the phosphorylation of IκB, resulting in its dissociation from NFκB. Afterwards NFκB translocate into nucleus [106] and transcribes PICyts which results in the subsequent induction of SOCS-1 [48,107]. Along with PICyts, SARM and A20 are also transcribed by NFκB which inhibit TRIF and TRAF6, respectively [44,108]. Interaction of SOCS-1 with MAL results in its polyubiquitylation and degradation of MAL [42]. SOCS-1 also result in the degradation of NFκB after binding with its p65 subunit [109]. Moreover, it is also responsible for inhibiting PICyts mediated JAK/STAT signalling [110]. The alternate pathway for the MyD88 independent induction of NFκB is TRIF which associates with RIP-1 and induce TRAF6 [111]. Cytoplasmic

domain of TLR4 associates with TRAM and TRIF, and interacts with a complex of TBK1 and Iκκi to induce phosphorylation of IRF3 [103]. After dimerization, phosphorylated IRF3 translocate into nucleus which results in the production of type I IFNs. IFN-β is responsible for the downregulation of PICyts through a shift of TH1 to TH2 responses and induce immune regulation. Recently SOCS-1 mediated downregulation of IFN-β has been observed [50].

BRN can be determined in a scalable but rigorous manner. Kinetic logic provided its effectiveness in preference to the Boolean logic by the successful modelling of different BRNs [67]. Effectiveness of the kinetic logic has been proved by analysing lambda phage genetic switch, differentiation process in helper T cells, control of organ differentiation in Arabidopsis thaliana flowers and segmentation during embryogenesis in *Drosophila melanogaster* [51–53]. The kinetic logic formalism is an influential method for examining BRNs in which interactions among entities are well reported. Use of logical parameters consistent with threshold values eliminate the necessity of various parameters of expression, temperature, physical state and kinetic rates etc. Moreover, this approach has the ability to model the system close to the approximations obtained by differential equations [55].

Semantics of the Kinetic Logic Formalism

The semantics of the kinetic logic formalism [55] have been discussed in our previous work [57], where we have explained the following formal definitions by considering an example of a toy BRN composed of three entities (shown as Figure 6 in the previous study). The definitions and the terms necessary to understand the semantics used in this study have been mentioned below, adapted from our previous study [57].

Definition 1 (Directed Graph). "A directed graph is an ordered pair $D(V,E)$, where:

- V is the set of all nodes and
- $E \subseteq V \times V$ is the set of ordered pairs called edges or arcs"

An edge e.g. (a,b) is directed from an entity or node "a" to "b", where "a" is the tail and "b" is the head of that respective edge. In a directed graph, $D^-(x)$ and $D^+(x)$ denote the set of predecessors and successors of a specific node $x \in V$, respectively".

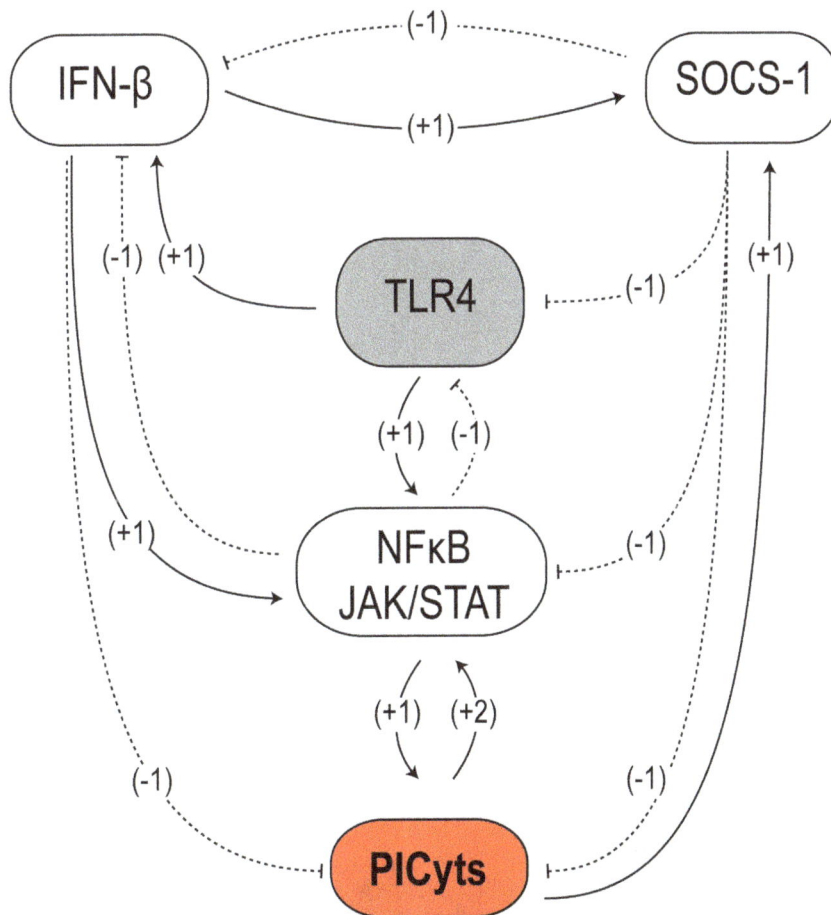

Figure 2. The BRN of TLR4 and JAK/STAT signalling pathway. The reduced BRN of TLR4 and JAK/STAT signalling pathway is derived from Figure 1. Nodes represent entities, whereas interactions between them are shown as edges. Sign on the edges represent the type of interaction between nodes i.e. positive for activation (solid arrows) and negative for inhibition (dotted arrows). Integers "1" and "2" on the edges represent the threshold levels of entities (see Material and Methods section).

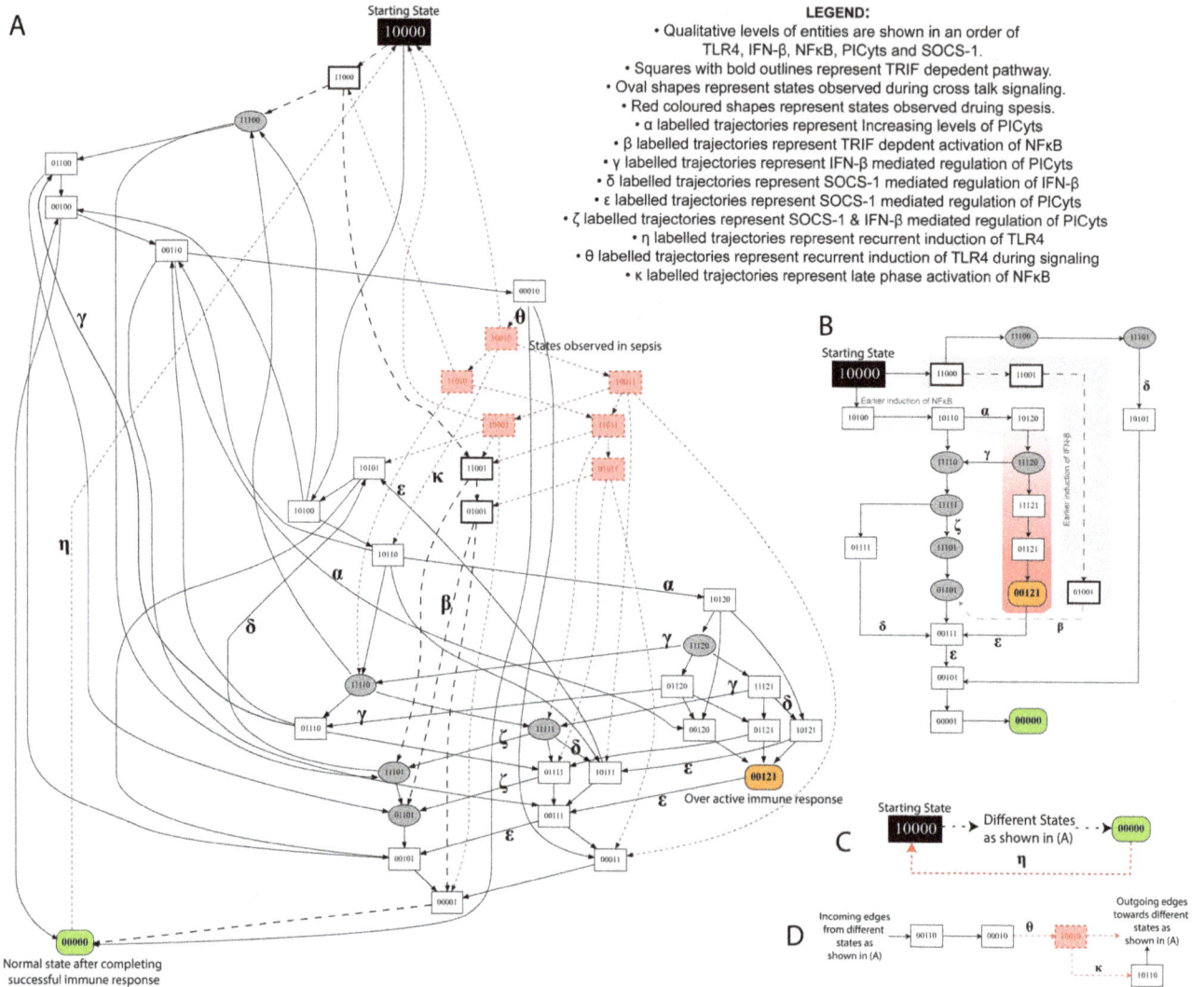

Figure 3. State graph of TLR4 and JAK/STAT signalling during non-septic and septic conditions. (A) Each node represents a particular state observed during signalling associated with non-septic and septic conditions. Integers "0", "1" and "2" within the nodes represent qualitative levels of proteins in the order of TLR4, IFN-β, NFκB, PICyts and SOCS-1. Inactive entities are represented by integer "0" whereas active and overactive entities are represented by integers "1" and "2", respectively. Nodes and trajectories, which were specifically observed during signalling dynamics associated with sepsis, are shown in red, whereas common nodes and trajectories found in both conditions are shown in black. Trajectories start from state "10000", representing the activation of TLR4, and ultimately lead towards "00000", which is a stable state in non-septic condition. On the other hand, a trajectory labelled with "η" from state "00000" to starting state "10000" results in a cyclic path during signalling dynamics associated with sepsis. MyD88 and TRIF dependent signalling are shown as black lines and dashed arrows, respectively. Nodes, which represent crosstalk of both signalling pathways i.e. IFN-β and NFκB with qualitative level "1" are presented in oval shapes. Arrows labelled with Greek small letters are used to represent trajectories associated with different signalling events (see legend in the figure). The conditions necessary to produce a state graph shown in the figure are given in Table 1. (B–D) specific states and trajectories which can possibly represent the complete state graph given in (A).

Definition 2 (Biological Regulatory Network). "A BRN is a labelled directed graph $D(V,E)$, where V is a set of nodes which represents biological entities and $E \subseteq V \times V$ is a set of all possible edges, which represent the interaction between entities".

- Each edge can be labelled with a pair of variables (σ, ψ), where σ represents the qualitative threshold levels and is a positive integer and ψ is "+" or "−" representing the type of interaction, which can either be "activation" or "inhibition", respectively.

- Each node e.g. "a" has a limit (l_a), in its threshold level, which is equal to its out-degree (the total number of outgoing edges from "a"). This relation can be presented by $\forall b \in D^+(a)$ and

$\sigma_{ab} \in \{1,2,3,....,r_a\}$ where $r_a \leq l_a$ which means that the threshold levels of entity "a" can be set within a range "1" to "total number of outgoing edges" and because it has only one outgoing edge towards predecessor "b" so the threshold level which can be set for it can be only be "1".

- Each entity, e.g. "a", has its abstract expression in the set $Z_a = \{0,1,2,...,r_a\}$.

Definition 3 (States). "The state of a BRN is a tuple $s \in M$, where M in terms of entity "a" is:

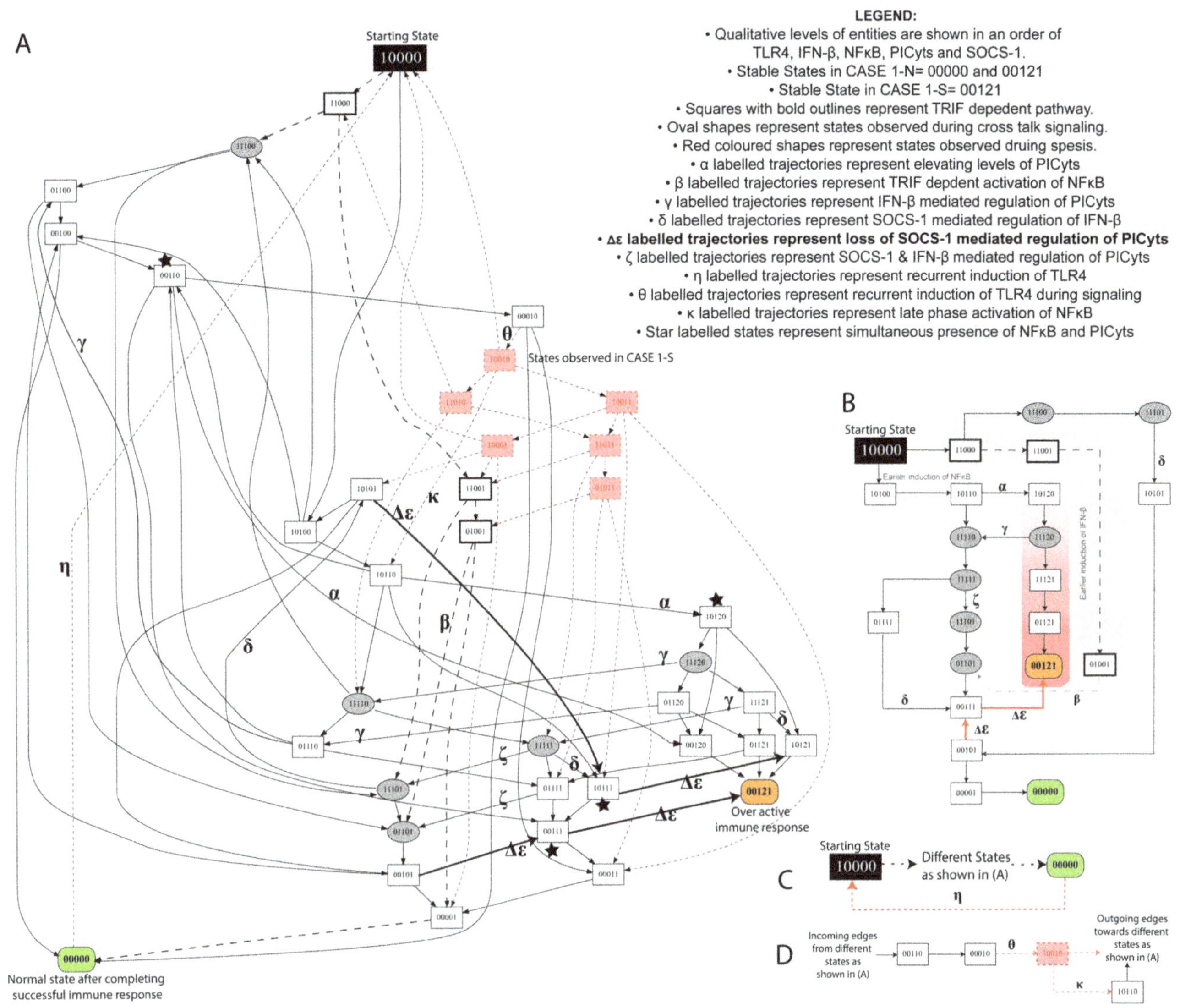

Figure 4. State graph of CASE 1-N and 1-S. (A) Each node represents a particular state observed during signalling associated with CASE 1-N and CASE 1-S. Integers "0", "1" and "2" within the nodes represent qualitative levels of proteins in the order of TLR4, IFN-β, NFκB, PICyts and SOCS-1. Inactive entities are represented by integer "0" whereas active and overactive entities are represented by integers "1" and "2", respectively. States and trajectories, which were specifically observed during signalling dynamics associated with CASE 1-S, are shown in red, whereas common states and trajectories found in both CASES are shown in black. Trajectories start from state "10000", representing the activation of TLR4 and ultimately lead towards "00000" and "00121", which are stable states in CASE 1-N. On the other hand, only one stable state "00121" was observed during signalling dynamics associated with CASE 1-S and a trajectory labelled with "η" from state "00000" to starting state "10000" results in cyclic path. Trajectories associated with loss of SOCS-1 mediated downregulation of PICyts in CASE 1-N and CASE 1-S are presented as bold arrows labelled with symbol "Δε". Nodes are labelled with stars in which NFκB and PICyts were active simultaneously and have the probability to lead towards overactive immune response. MyD88 and TRIF dependent signalling are shown as black lines and dashed arrows, respectively. Nodes, which represent crosstalk of both signalling pathways i.e. IFN-β and NFκB with qualitative level "1" are presented in oval shapes. Arrows labelled with Greek small letters are used to represent trajectories associated with different signalling events (see legend in the figure). The conditions necessary to produce a state graph are shown in the figure are given in Table 3. (B–D) specific states and trajectories which can possibly represent the complete state graph given in (A).

$$M = \Pi_{a \in V} Z_a$$

The qualitative states are represented by vector $(M_v)_{\forall a \in V}$, where v denotes the level of expression of an entity like "a". According to this definition M is the Cartesian product of the sets of abstract expressions of all entities. A qualitative state represents a configuration of all the elements of a BRN at any instant of time. The number of activators of a particular variable at a given level of expression are represented by its set of resources (see the definition of resources given below)".

Definition 4 (Resources). "The set of resources R_{v_a} of a variable $a \in V$ at a level v is defined as $R_{v_a} = \{b \in D^-(a) | v_b \geq \sigma_{ba}$ and $\psi_{ba} = +)$ or $(v_b < \sigma_{ba}$ and $\psi_{ba} = -)\}$. The dynamic behaviours of BRN depends on logical parameters. The set of these logical parameters is defined as $K(D) = \{K_a(R_{v_a}) \in Z_a \forall a \in V\}$.

The parameter $K_a(R_{v_a})$ (at a level v of a) gives the information about the evolution of a. There are three cases: 1) if $v_a < K_a(R_{v_a})$ then v_a increases by one unit 2) if $v_a > K_a(R_{v_a})$ then v_a decreases

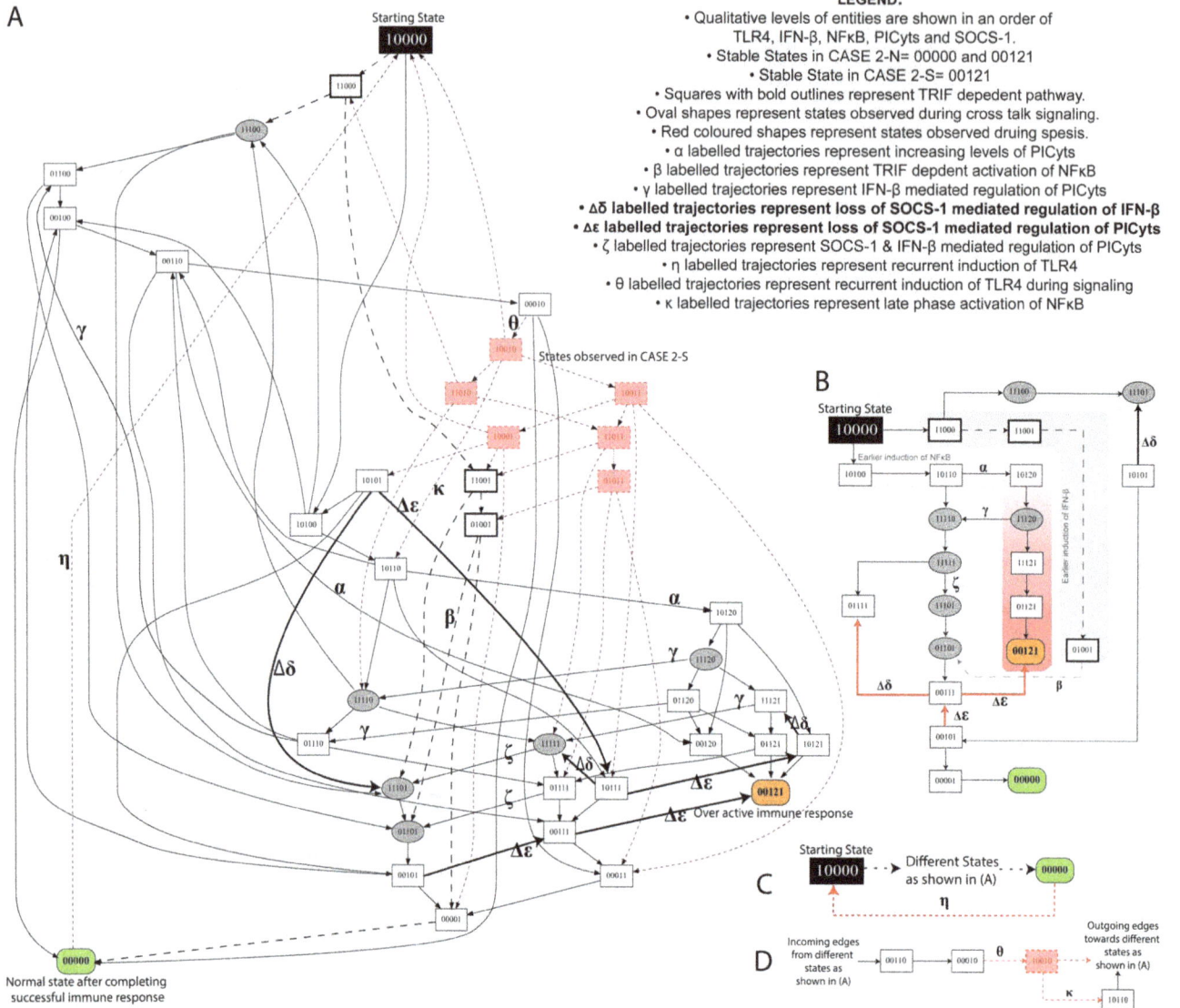

Figure 5. State graph of CASE 2-N and 2-S. (A) Each node represents a particular state observed during signalling associated with CASE 2-N and CASE 2-S. Integers "0", "1" and "2" within the nodes represent qualitative levels of proteins in the order of TLR4, IFN-β, NFκB, PICyts and SOCS-1. Inactive entities are represented by integer "0" whereas active and overactive entities are represented by integers "1" and "2", respectively. Nodes and trajectories, which were specifically observed during signalling dynamics associated with CASE 2-S, are shown in red, whereas common nodes and trajectories found in both CASES are shown in black. Trajectories start from state "10000", representing the activation of TLR4 and ultimately lead towards "00000" and "00121", which are stable states in CASE 2-N. On the other hand, only one stable state "00121" was observed during signalling dynamics associated with CASE 2-S and a trajectory labelled with "η" from state "00000" to starting state "10000" results in cyclic path. Trajectories associated with loss of SOCS-1 mediated downregulation of PICyts in CASE 2-N and CASE 2-S are presented as bold arrows labelled with symbol "Δε" whereas loss of SOCS-1 mediated downregulation of IFN-β are labelled with symbol "Δδ". MyD88 and TRIF dependent signalling are shown as black lines and dashed arrows, respectively. Nodes, which represent crosstalk of both signalling pathways i.e. IFN-β and NFκB with qualitative level "1" are presented in oval shapes. Arrows labelled with Greek small letters are used to represent trajectories associated with different signalling events (see legend in the figure). The conditions necessary to produce a state graph shown in the figure are given in Table 3. (B–D) specific states and trajectories which can possibly represent the complete state graph given in (A).

by one unit and 3) if $v_a = K_a(R_{v_a})$ then v_a cannot evolve from its current level.

It is convenient to describe the evolution from one level to another by an evolution operator "$\uparrow$" [68], which is defined in terms of entity "a" as follows:

$$v_a \uparrow K_a(R_{v_a}) = \begin{cases} v_a + 1 & if\ v_a < K_a(R_{v_a}); \\ v_a - 1 & if\ v_a > K_a(R_{v_a}); \\ v_a & if\ v_a = K_a(R_{v_a}). \end{cases}$$

Where v_a and $K_a(R_{v_a}) \in \mathbb{Z}_{\geq 0}$".

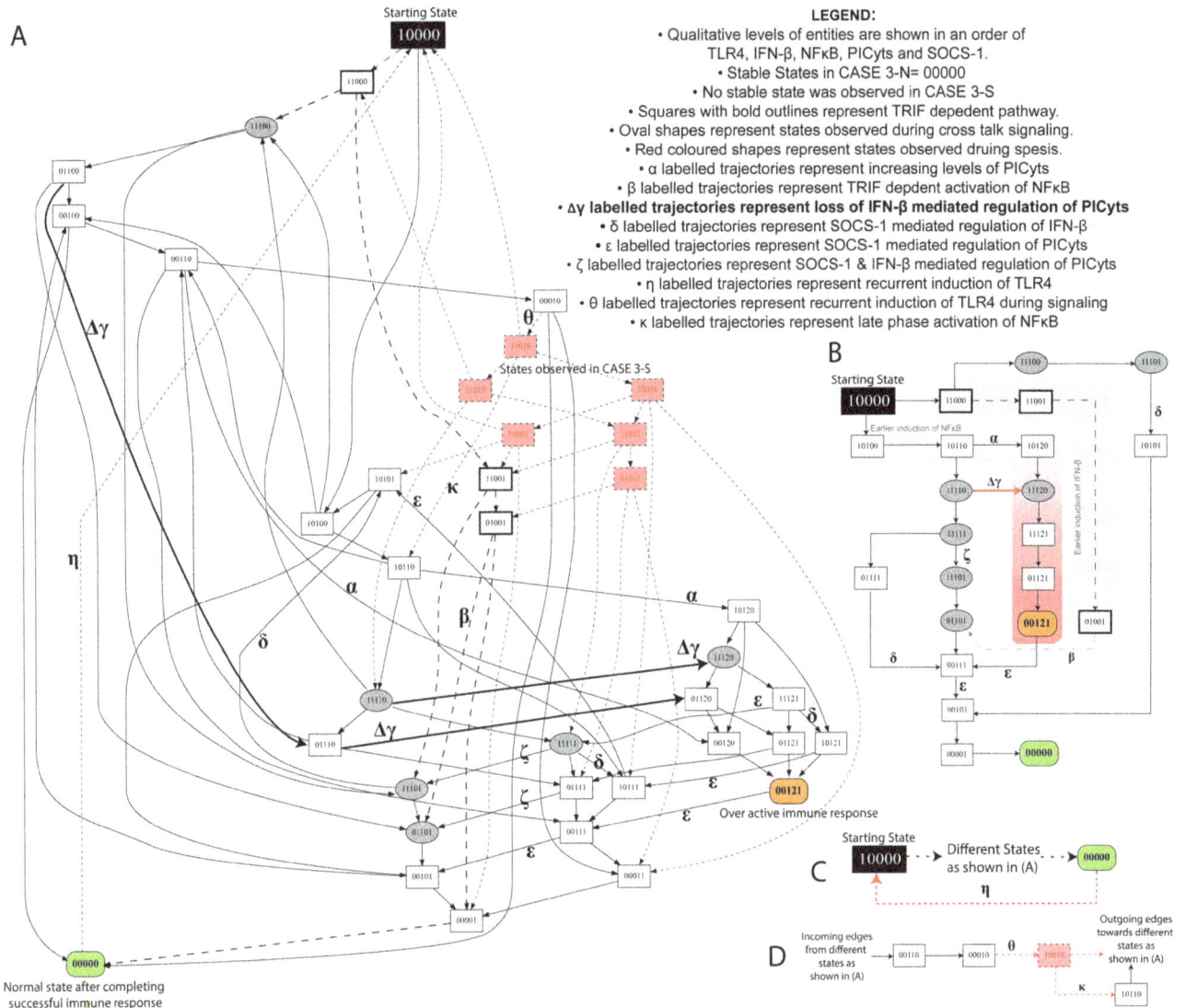

Figure 6. State graph of CASE 3-N and 3-S. (A) Each node represents a particular state observed during signalling associated with CASE 3-N and CASE 3-S. Integers "0", "1" and "2" within the nodes represent qualitative levels of proteins in the order of TLR4, IFN-β, NFκB, PICyts and SOCS-1. Inactive entities are represented by integer "0" whereas active and overactive entities are represented by integers "1" and "2", respectively. Nodes and trajectories, which were specifically observed during signalling dynamics associated with CASE 3-S, are shown in red, whereas common nodes and trajectories found in both CASES are shown in black. Trajectories start from state "10000", representing the activation of TLR4, ultimately, lead towards "00000", which is the stable state in CASE 3-N. On the other hand, a trajectory labelled with "η" from state "00000" to starting state "10000" results in a cyclic path during signalling dynamics associated with CASE 3-S. Trajectories associated with loss of IFN-β mediated downregulation of PICyts in CASE 3-N and CASE 3-S are presented as bold arrows labelled with symbol "Δγ". MyD88 and TRIF dependent signalling are shown as black lines and dashed arrows, respectively. Nodes, which represent crosstalk of both signalling pathways i.e. IFN-β and NFκB with qualitative level "1" are presented in oval shapes. Arrows labelled with Greek small letters are used to represent trajectories associated with different signalling events (see legend in the figure). The conditions necessary to produce a state graph shown in the figure are given in Table 3. (B–D) specific states and trajectories which can possibly represent the complete state graph given in (A).

Definition 5 (State Graph). "Let D be the BRN and v_a represents the expression level of an entity e.g. "a" in a state $s \in M$. Then the state graph of the BRN will be the directed graph $G = (S, T)$, where S is set of states and $T \subseteq S \times S$ represents a relation between states, called the transition relation, such that $s \to s' \in T$ if and only if:

- $\exists$ a unique $a \in V$ such that $s_{v_a} \neq s_{v_a}'$ and $s_{v_a}' = s_{v_a} \vec{\Gamma} K_a(R_{v_a})$ and
- $\forall b \in V \setminus \{a\} s_{v_b}' = s_{v_b}$"

According to this definition states evolve asynchronously, thus, in a successor state only one entity changes its level.

Reduction of the BRN

One of the limitations of the kinetic logic approach is that it has been designed to analyse relatively small BRNs because of its scalability limitations [55]. For example, the TLR4 and JAK/STAT pathway as given in Figure 1 has 22 entities and on simulation its state graph would be composed of 6291456 states as compared to less than 50 states (Figures 3–8) generated by the reduced BRN (Figure 2).

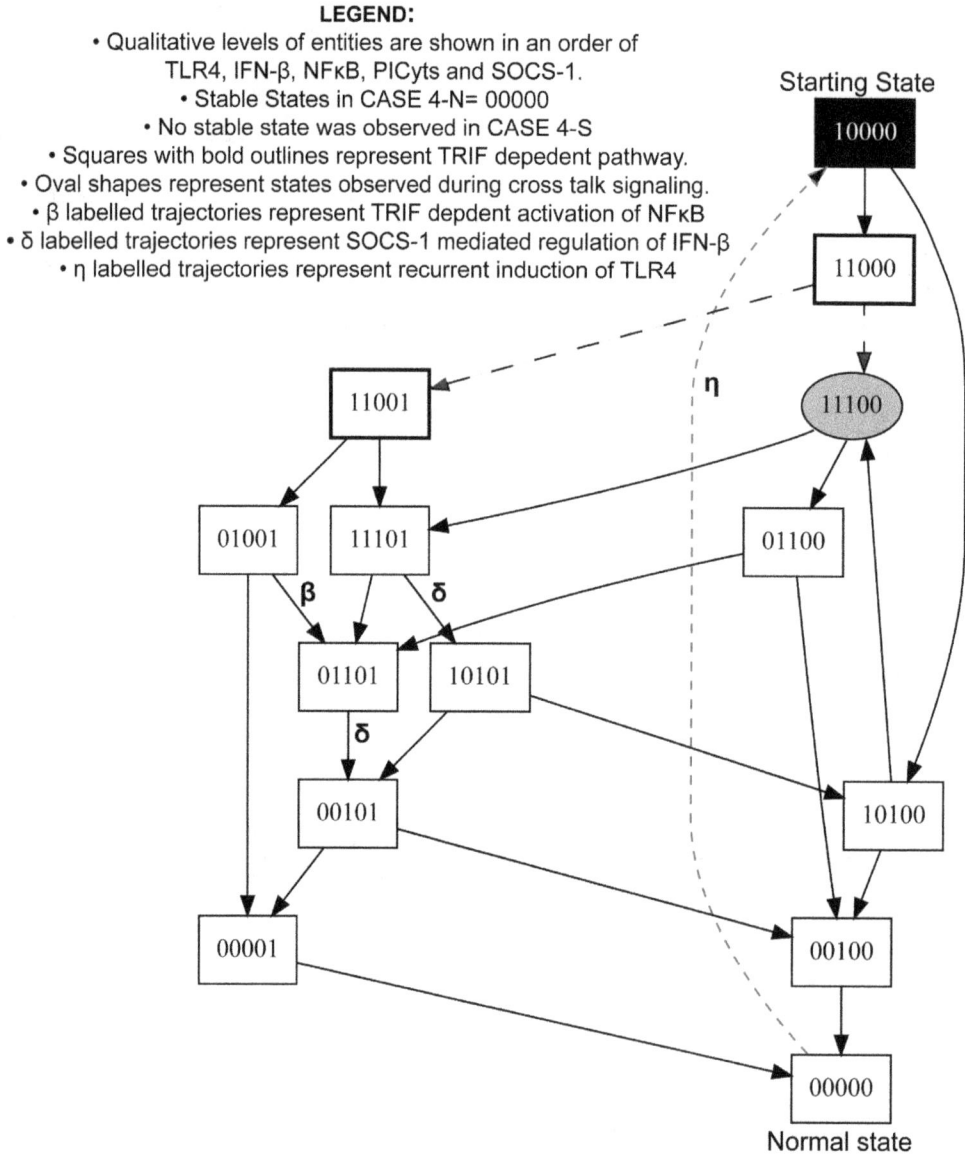

Figure 7. State graph of CASE 4-N and 4-S. Each node represents a particular state observed during signalling associated with CASE 4-N and CASE 4-S. Values "0" and "1" within the nodes represent qualitative levels of proteins in the order of TLR4, IFN-β, NFκB, PICyts and SOCS-1. Inactive entities are represented by integer "0" whereas active entities are represented by integer "1". Trajectories, which were specifically observed during signalling dynamics associated with CASE 4-S, are shown in red, whereas common states and trajectories found in both CASES are shown in black. Trajectories start from state "10000", representing the activation of TLR4, ultimately, lead towards "00000", which is a stable state in CASE 4-N. On the other hand, a trajectory labelled with "η" from state "00000" to starting state "10000" results in a cyclic path during signalling dynamics associated with CASE 4-S. State "00121" which represents the immune response was absent in state graph and not shown in this figure. MyD88 and TRIF dependent signalling are shown as black lines and dashed arrows, respectively. Nodes, which represent crosstalk of both signalling pathways i.e. IFN-β and NFκB with qualitative level "1" are presented in oval shapes. Arrows labelled with Greek small letters are used to represent trajectories associated with different signalling events (see legend in the figure). The conditions necessary to produce a state graph shown in the figure are given in Table 3.

The complexity of TLR4 and JAK/STAT pathways was reduced to make the BRN (shown in Figure 2) and resultant state graphs (Shown in Figures 3–8) tractable. Starting with the complete signalling pathways of TLR4 and JAK/STAT, adopted from previous experimental studies and databases associated with biological signalling [28–33], the BRN was reduced iteratively by following the strategies of Naldi *et. al.* [69] and Assieh *et. al.* [70]. Briefly, one such example is if an entity X1 activates another entity X2, which in turn activates X3 such that X3 inhibits X1, then we can omit X2 and represent this relation as a simple feedback loop

where X1 activates X3 and X3 inhibits X1. In the process of reduction, the behaviour of the removed entity X2 was preserved implicitly in the activation of X3 by X1 to account for the related interactions and their effects on the target nodes. Another example is given in the Figure 3.3 of the study by Assieh *et al.* [70], where a network of 13 proteins (Figure 3.3a) is reduced to 3 proteins (Figure 3.3b) using the reduction rules. Similarly in the study of Naldi *et.al.* [69], Figure 2 is presenting another example of the BRN reduction.

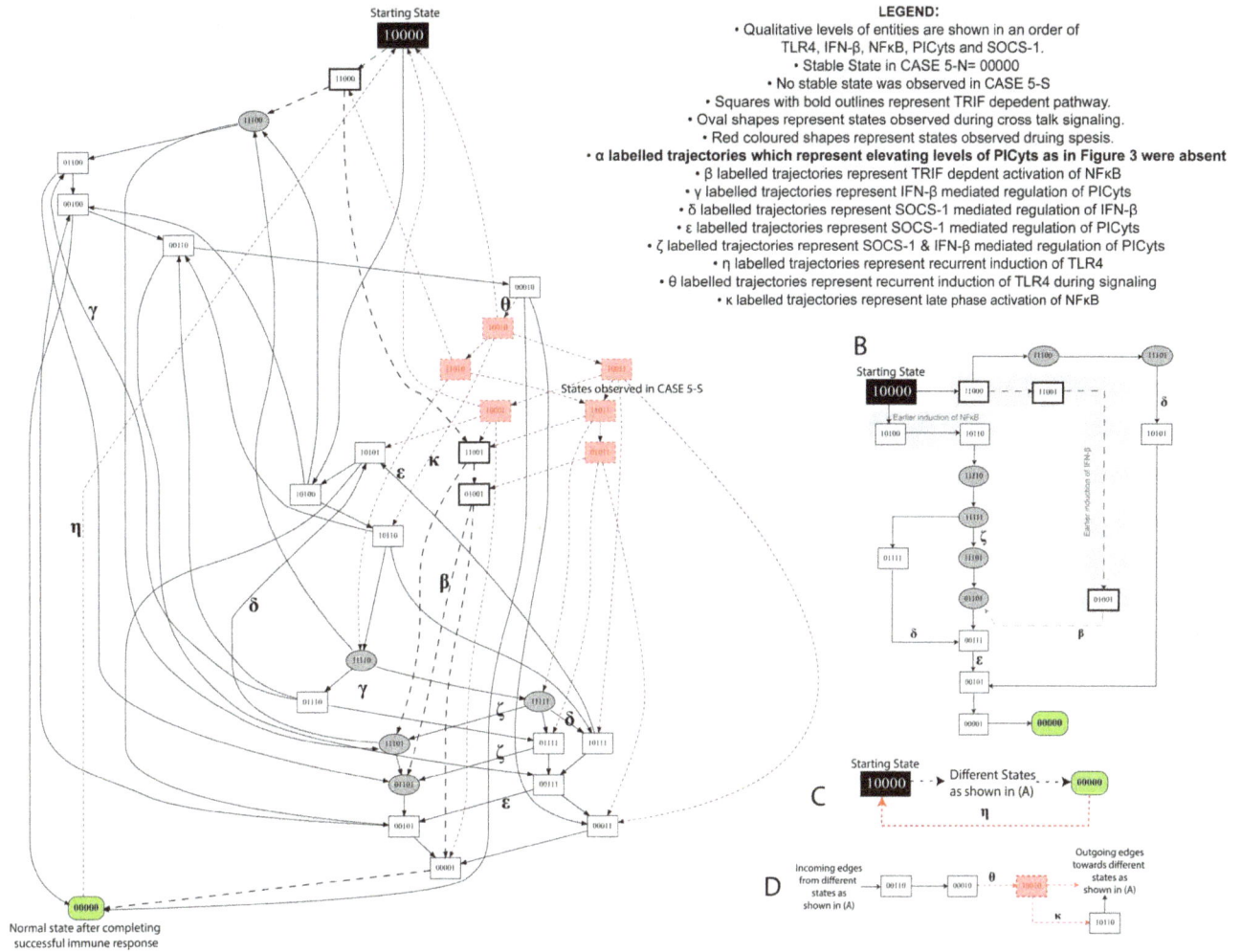

Figure 8. State graph of CASE 5-N and 5-S. (A) Each node represents a particular state observed during signalling associated with CASE 5-N and CASE 5-S. Integers "0" and "1" within the nodes represent qualitative levels of proteins in the order of TLR4, IFN-β, NFκB, PICyts and SOCS-1. Inactive entities are represented by integer "0" whereas active entities are represented by integer "1". Nodes and trajectories, which were specifically observed during signalling dynamics associated with CASE 5-S, are shown in red, whereas common nodes and trajectories found in both CASES are shown in black. Trajectories start from state "10000", representing the activation of TLR4, ultimately, lead towards "00000", which is a stable state in CASE 5-N. On the other hand, a trajectory labelled with "η" from state "00000" to starting state "10000" results in a cyclic path during signalling dynamics associated with CASE 5-S. MyD88 and TRIF dependent signalling are shown as black lines and dashed arrows, respectively. Nodes, which represent crosstalk of both signalling pathways i.e. IFN-β and NFκB with qualitative level "1" are presented in oval shapes. Arrows labelled with Greek small letters are used to represent trajectories associated with different signalling events (see legend in the figure). The conditions necessary to produce a state graph shown in the figure are given in Table 3. (B–D) specific states and trajectories which can possibly represent the complete state graph given in (A).

Discrete Modelling of the BRN

GENOTECH (provided at http://code.google.com/p/genotech/downloads/list. Steps necessary to model a BRN in GENOTECH have been described in [57]) and GINSIM (documentation and software for modelling BRNs in GINSIM are available at www.ginsim.org) [71] facilitated the construction of qualitative model of BRN (Figure 2) according to Thomas' formalism. Modelling of the BRN was performed by inserting the required entities as nodes and drawing the corresponding interactions as edges. Threshold levels and logical parameters for each entity were adjusted as discussed below. Using asynchronous strategy, the results were produced in the form of state graphs composed of states and trajectories consisting of cycling paths and paths diverging towards stable states. These state graphs were used to study the dynamics of the BRN. GENOTECH files and

equivalents in GINSIM format have been provided as Files S1–S24, for each condition discussed in results.

Threshold values of each entity in the BRN

According to the Definition 2, the threshold level "σ" is a positive integer, which represents the minimum qualitative level of an entity necessary to activate or inhibit its target entities. In contrast to the Boolean logic, kinetic logic (multivalued) permits the use of threshold level ≥ 1 [61,72]. The threshold values, which can be used, depend upon the outgoing edges from any entity. These values range from "1" to the number of outgoing edges from an entity. The reason for multivalued formalism is that a particular entity can activate or inhibit its target entities at different activation levels and thus require more than one threshold level to perform its role as an activator or inhibitor.

Table 1. Logical parameters used for each entity in modelling of non-septic TLR4 and JAK/STAT signalling using the BRN shown in Figure 2.

S.No.	Logical Parameters
1	$K_{TLR4}(\{\}) = 0$
2	$K_{TLR4}(\{NF\kappa B\}) = 0$
3	$K_{TLR4}(\{SOCS\text{-}1\}) = 0$
4	$K_{TLR4}(\{SOCS\text{-}1, NF\kappa B\}) = 0$
5	$K_{NF\kappa B\text{-}JAK/STAT}(\{\}) = 0$
6	$K_{NF\kappa B\text{-}JAK/STAT}(\{TLR4\}) = 1$
7	$K_{NF\kappa B\text{-}JAK/STAT}(\{IFN\text{-}\beta\}) = 1$
8	$K_{NF\kappa B\text{-}JAK/STAT}(\{PICyts\}) = 1$
9	$K_{NF\kappa B\text{-}JAK/STAT}(\{TLR4, IFN\text{-}\beta\}) = 1$
10	$K_{NF\kappa B\text{-}JAK/STAT}(\{TLR4, PICyts\}) = 1$
11	$K_{NF\kappa B\text{-}JAK/STAT}(\{IFN\text{-}\beta, PICyts\}) = 1$
12	$K_{NF\kappa B\text{-}JAK/STAT}(\{TLR4, PICyts, IFN\text{-}\beta\}) = 1$
13	$K_{NF\kappa B\text{-}JAK/STAT}(\{TLR4, SOCS\text{-}1\}) = 1$
14	$K_{NF\kappa B\text{-}JAK/STAT}(\{IFN\text{-}\beta, SOCS\text{-}1\}) = 1$
15	$K_{NF\kappa B\text{-}JAK/STAT}(\{PICyts, SOCS\text{-}1\}) = 1$
16	$K_{NF\kappa B\text{-}JAK/STAT}(\{TLR4, IFN\text{-}\beta, SOCS\text{-}1\}) = 1$
17	$K_{NF\kappa B\text{-}JAK/STAT}(\{TLR4, PICyts, SOCS\text{-}1\}) = 1$
18	$K_{NF\kappa B\text{-}JAK/STAT}(\{PICyts, IFN\text{-}\beta, SOCS\text{-}1\}) = 1$
19	$K_{NF\kappa B\text{-}JAK/STAT}(\{SOCS\text{-}1\}) = 0$
20	$K_{NF\kappa B\text{-}JAK/STAT}(\{SOCS\text{-}1, TLR4, IFN\text{-}\beta, PICyts\}) = 1$
21	$K_{PICyts}(\{\}) = 0$
22	$K_{PICyts}(\{NF\kappa B\}) = 0$
23	$K_{PICyts}(\{IFN\text{-}\beta\}) = 0$
24	$K_{PICyts}(\{SOCS\text{-}1\}) = 0$
25	$K_{PICyts}(\{NF\kappa B, IFN\text{-}\beta\}) = 0$
26	$K_{PICyts}(\{NF\kappa B, SOCS\text{-}1\}) = 0$
27	$K_{PICyts}(\{IFN\text{-}\beta, SOCS\text{-}1\}) = 0$
28	$K_{PICyts}(\{NF\kappa B, IFN\text{-}\beta, SOCS\text{-}1\}) = 2$
29	$K_{SOCS\text{-}1}(\{\}) = 0$
30	$K_{SOCS\text{-}1}(\{PICyts\}) = 1$
31	$K_{SOCS\text{-}1}(\{IFN\text{-}\beta\}) = 1$
32	$K_{SOCS\text{-}1}(\{PICyts, IFN\text{-}\beta\}) = 1$
33	$K_{IFN\text{-}\beta}(\{\}) = 0$
34	$K_{IFN\text{-}\beta}(\{TLR4\}) = 0$
35	$K_{IFN\text{-}\beta}(\{SOCS\text{-}1\}) = 0$
36	$K_{IFN\text{-}\beta}(\{NF\kappa B\}) = 0$
37	$K_{IFN\text{-}\beta}(\{TLR4, SOCS\text{-}1\}) = 1$
38	$K_{IFN\text{-}\beta}(\{TLR4, NF\kappa B\}) = 1$
39	$K_{IFN\text{-}\beta}(\{SOCS\text{-}1, NF\kappa B\}) = 0$
40	$K_{IFN\text{-}\beta}(\{TLR4, SOCS\text{-}1, NF\kappa B\}) = 1$

Each logical parameter has been discussed in detail in File S26.

For example SOCS-1 has been implicated for its inhibitory role in TLR4, NFκB, IFN-β and PICyts mediated signalling [48] but the specific expression levels of SOCS-1 which are necessary to inhibit all of these four entities in the presence of other resources (activators or inhibitors) are not reported. Therefore, according to Thomas' formalism, the threshold levels of SOCS-1 for its interaction with these four entities can be within the range $\{1-4\}$. In order to keep the model simple, the threshold levels of SOCS-1 were set at level "1". Similarly, for other entities, including TLR4, IFN-β and NFκB, the threshold levels were set at "1". Only PICyts mediated activation of NFκB-JAK/STAT was set at "2". Therefore, PICyts was supposed to activate SOCS-1 at the activation level "1" and NFκB-JAK/STAT at activation level "2". Threshold level "2" was used in speculation that PICyts activate the products of NFκB-JAK/STAT signalling pathway after reaching a certain qualitative threshold level, which may differ from its other actions such as activation of SOCS-1 [73–75].

Types of interaction

The entities in a BRN may represent proteins or genes, which can interact with each other. Depending upon the threshold levels, entities can either activate or inhibit other entities termed as evolving or target entities (see Definition 2 where $\psi = +$ for activators and $\psi = -$ for inhibitors). As shown in the BRN (Figure 2), TLR4, IFN-β, NFκB and PICyts are the entities, which can either activate each other or SOCS-1 depending upon their threshold levels. According to formalism, whenever the activation of these entities will reach to their threshold levels, generally taken as "1", then successors of these entities will also be activated. This relationship can be depicted by sigmoidal graph presented as Figure 5A in our previous study [57]. It can be seen that an activator below a threshold level (σ) slightly affects the activation level of its target entity. However, as soon as the activator achieves its threshold level, then the target entity also reaches to active state where it can perform its further interactions. In other words, whenever entity has threshold level $<\sigma$ then it cannot activate its target entities but when threshold level of an entity $\geq\sigma$ then it can activate its target entities. In this scenario, the entities are termed as positive regulators or activators when they activate other entities during the dynamics of the BRN shown as state graphs.

On the other hand, IFN-β, NFκB and SOCS-1 can inhibit either each other or TLR4 and PICyts. These entities are termed as negative regulators or inhibitors and process is termed as downregulation or inactivation. Entities which can inhibit evolving entities also depend upon their threshold levels. The effect of inactivation is also of sigmoidal nature and is shown as Figure 5B in our previous study [57].

Logical parameters of each entity in the BRN

Logical parameters have been described by using the relation $K_{\text{target entity}}(\{\text{resources}\}) = n$ where $n \in \{0,1,2,...\}$. Where resources are those entities of BRN, which are connected with evolving or target entity. These resources can be either activators or inhibitors depending upon their presence or absence, respectively, during a particular state. Activators were taken as resources when they were present in a particular state. On the other hand, inhibitors were taken as resources only when they were absent during a particular state.

According to the formalism, the possible number of logical parameters, which we have to define for each evolving entity depends upon the number of resources. If the number of resource

is one, then the possible number of logical parameters, which we have to define, will be two. This relation can be shown as a power set of the set of regulators (set of activators and inhibitors) of an entity. Therefore, each logical parameter corresponds to one element of the power set. In accordance with the René Thomas' formalism, the total number of logical parameters for TLR4, IFN-β, NFκB, PICyts and SOCS-1 are 4, 8, 16, 8 and 4, respectively (Table 1).

The value n for each logical parameter was unknown a priori, and was computed using the Selection of Models of Biological Networks (SMBioNet) tool [76–78]. Briefly, this tool is based on the kinetic logic formalism of René Thomas that takes a BRN with unspecified parameters and Computational Tree Logic (CTL) [79] formulae of the form $\Phi = \Phi_1 \rightarrow \{A/E\}\{G/F/X\}\Phi_2$ representing a specific biological behaviour (observation). In the formula Φ, the path quantifier A or E governs if a specific property should hold in all trajectories (A) originating from a current state or in at least one trajectory (E). Whereas, the state quantifiers G, F and X govern if a property should hold in all states (G), in a future state (F), or in the immediate successor state (X) in a trajectory (path); and finally Φ_1 and Φ_2 represent the Boolean logic formulae representing the initial expression levels and the observed expression levels of the entities, respectively. In the formula Φ, the symbol "$\rightarrow$" represents the Boolean implication operator. For example, the formula $\Phi = ((\text{TLR4} = 1 \text{ AND IFN-β} = 0 \text{ AND NFκB} = 0 \text{ AND PICyts} = 0$ AND SOCS-1 = 0) $\rightarrow EF(\text{NFκB} = 1))$ is a CTL formula where $\Phi_1 = (\text{TLR4} = 1 \text{ AND IFN-β} = 0 \text{ AND NFκB} = 0 \text{ AND PI-Cyts} = 0 \text{ AND SOCS-1} = 0)$ representing the initial expression levels of entities (TLR4 is currently active and others are inactive), and $EF(\Phi_2)$ with $\Phi_2 = (\text{NFκB} = 1)$ represents the observation that NFκB eventually activates. In this example, AND is the Boolean conjunction operator. The CTL encoded observed biological behaviours from the literature pertaining to the TLR4 and JAK/STAT pathway are given in Table 2. The input and output of the SMBioNet are provided in File S25.

Value "0" represents that evolving entity deactivates in the presence of its resources, whereas a value "1" represents activation of an entity. However, the logical parameter $K_{PICyts}(\{NF\kappa B, IFN-\beta, SOCS-1\})$ was with a value "2" depending upon the threshold level of PICyts for the induction of JAK-STAT pathway as discussed earlier. The values of these computed logical parameters were validated by previous literature. An informal description of the logical parameters with relevant evidences has been provided as File S26 that form the basis for using a specific value for each logical parameter given in Table 1.

These logical parameters were further validated by the proved conjectures [a positive feedback circuit (respectively negative feedback circuit) is a necessary condition for multistationarity

Table 2. Biological observations and concerned references from previous literature which were used to generate the CTL formula as given as input to SMBioNet.

S#	Biological observations	CTL formula in SMBioNet
1	Once TLR4 gets activated, it will then activate the downstream signaling in response to infection, which eventually leads to the induction of NFκB and IFN-β [103,112–116].	((TLR4 = 1&IFNb = 0&NFκB = 1&PICyts = 0&SOCS1 = 0)->EF(TLR4 = 1&IFNb = 1&NFκB = 1))
2	After a successful immune response or clearance of infection, all the entities will be downregulated [20,25,117].	((TLR4 = 1&IFNb = 0&NFκB = 0&PICyts = 0&SOCS1 = 0)-> EF(AG(TLR4 = 0&IFNb = 0&NFκB = 0&PICyts = 0&SOCS1 = 0)))

(respectively homeostasis). In a BRN a positive feedback circuit (respectively negative feedback circuit) is the one which contains even (respectively odd) number of negative interactions] of René Thomas [55] and biologically observed stable states. Logical parameters given in Table 1 were finally used to study the dynamics of the BRN (Figure 2) in the form of state graphs. These parameters have also been shown as tendency graphs in Figures S9–S13 using sigmoidal graphs among evolving entities and their resources.

Modelling of interventions

Models with interventions were derived by removing one or more of the interactions of IFN-β, SOCS-1, NFκB and PICyts present in the BRN (Figure 2). Associated logical parameters were also changed or removed to maintain the integrity of each model (Table 3). These interventions (discussed as CASES) were used to observe their impact on the signalling events (effects on the cyclic paths and stable states during signalling modelled for septic and non-septic) and for comparison with non-intervened or intact models. All the models which are discussed in this study have been provided as files in GENTOCH (Files S1–S12) and GINSIM (Files S13–S24) formats.

Results

Different perspectives of the TLR4 and JAK/STAT signalling were studied by simulating septic and non-septic conditions, both in the presence and absence of specific interactions among entities. The devised logical parameters for all entities (Table 1) were used to model non-septic dynamics of TLR4 and JAK/STAT signalling shown as BRN in Figure 2. Changes in specific logical parameters by removing respective edges or interactions between the entities as given in Figure 2 were used to model septic and intervened signalling (Table 3). State graphs shown in Figures 3–8 represent signalling events or dynamics of different perspectives of BRN discussed in detail below. Qualitative levels (0, 1 or 2) of TLR4, IFN-β, NFκB, PICyts and SOCS-1 represent qualitative states, which are shown as nodes, whereas trajectories represent possible progress or evolution paths of entities depending upon the logical parameters and qualitative threshold levels (Figures 3–8). In each state graph, state "10000" represents the starting state (activation of TLR4 as first signal) whereas states of "00000" and "00121" represents the downregulated and overactive immune responses, respectively.

Signalling in non-septic case

All the logical parameters used in modelling the non-septic signalling are defined in Table 1 and shown as dummy tendency graphs in Figures S9–S13. Model related to non-septic condition has been provided as File S1. Logical parameters devised for each entity were based on the experimental findings, but the incorporation of several experimental findings as a single rule for evolving entity were devised as discussed in the methods. Logical parameters were devised in such a way that after the production of overactive immune response (state "00121"), the dynamics of the BRN should reach to a stable state "00000" representing the downregulation of immune response. Simulation of non-septic model led to the generation of a state graph shown in Figure 3.

Complete TLR4 mediated induction of TRIF and MyD88 adaptor proteins are represented by the induction of IFN-β (10000→11000) and NFκB (10000→10100o), respectively. According to the previous experimental studies, MyD88 dependent pathway is induced in preference to the TRIF dependent pathway [80,81]. In the state graph, it can be noticed that the induction of

PICyt was achieved only in those trajectories in which NFκB mediated signalling was activated in preference to IFN-β. On the other hand, chances for the induction of PICyt were found comparatively lower in the presence of earlier induced IFN-β. Probably, this may create a platform for immediately required immune response against the pathogen. States, which represent a crosstalk mechanism of MyD88 and TRIF dependent signalling, are shown within the oval shapes. Downstream to these states, the presence of SOCS-1 and/or IFN-β compelled the system towards immunocompromised states (states with level "0" or "1" of PICyts). Most of the crosstalk states were observed during the activated TLR4. However, in the absence of TLR4, TRIF induced activation of NFκB (shown as 01001→01101) can be specifically observed in trajectories labelled with "β" in Figure 3. Correlated with previous experimental study, this transition was produced nearly at the end of dynamics and triggered the late phase induction of NFκB mediated proinflammatory immune responses [36].

During dynamics of the BRN, trajectories (labelled with "α" in Figure 3) were found most important for the over activation of PICyts which include (10110→10120) and (00110→00120). Both of these trajectories were associated with the absence of SOCS-1 and IFN-β along with elevated levels of PICyts (shown by level "2"). Moreover, both of these trajectories may represent the importance of TLR4 and JAK/STAT mediated induction of inflammatory responses.

The presence of IFN-β and/or SOCS-1 at different levels in the state graph were found necessary to downregulate the levels of PICyts. After the expression of PICyts, recursive action of IFN-β and then SOCS-1 maintained the homeostasis of the immune system by downregulating the levels of PICyts. After achieving the hyperinflammatory state "00121", dynamics of the BRN were led towards stable state "00000", which represents the downregulation of the immune system. Trajectories labelled with "γ" in Figure 3 highlights the role of IFN-β mediated downregulation of PICyts. The presence of IFN-β reduced the chances for induction of PICyts (trajectories downstream of state "11100") and delayed effective immune response. However, in the absence of IFN-β, fate of system was shifted towards NFκB mediated induction of PICyts.

Trajectories labelled with "δ" and "ε" in Figure 3 represent SOCS-1 mediated downregulation of IFN-β and PICyts, respectively. Generally, the behaviour of SOCS-1 was found to downregulate the levels of IFN-β in preference to PICyts. Indirectly, SOCS-1 allowed PICyts to higher expression levels in the system and then regulated the same. Some of the trajectories (labelled with "ζ" in Figure 3) in the state graph infer the combination of SOCS-1 and IFN-β mediated downregulation of PICyts and observed mostly during crosstalk of MyD88 and TRIF dependent pathways, which led the dynamics towards downregulated immune response. In this setting, it can be assumed that SOCS-1 may allow extra time for the induction of PICyts so that the immune system can cope up with the pathogens. However, subsequent SOCS-1 mediated inhibition of PICyts may implicate the decrease in damage to the host by its exacerbating immune response.

The presence of cyclic paths, termed as strongly connected components (SCC)-1 and SCC-2, in the state graph can be seen in Figure S1 and S2, respectively. SCC-1 highlights the importance of states "10100" and "10101" (Figure S1). The cyclic path between these two states represent the recurrent activation of PICyts in non-septic TLR4 signalling with subsequent downregulation. Due to the presence of IFN-β and SOCS-1, system cycled through trajectory "10100→11100→11101→10101" and produced sustained immunosuppression. On the other hand, SCC-2

Table 3. Intervened signalling.

CASE	Evolving Entity	Target entity/ies	Removed parameters	Changed parameters	Removed edge/s in Figure 2.	Produced Stable states
1-N	SOCS-1	PICyts	$K_{PICyts}(\{SOCS\text{-}1\}) = 0$, $K_{PICyts}(\{NF\kappa B, SOCS\text{-}1\}) = 0$, $K_{PICyts}(\{NF\kappa B, IFN\text{-}\beta, SOCS\text{-}1\}) = 0$	$K_{PICyts}(\{NF\kappa B, IFN\text{-}\beta\}) = 2$	SOCS-1 mediated downregulation of PICyts	00000 & 00121
1-S	SOCS-1	PICyts	$K_{PICyts}(\{SOCS\text{-}1\}) = 0$, $K_{PICyts}(\{NF\kappa B, SOCS\text{-}1\}) = 0$, $K_{PICyts}(\{NF\kappa B, IFN\text{-}\beta, SOCS\text{-}1\}) = 0$	$K_{PICyts}(\{NF\kappa B, IFN\text{-}\beta\}) = 2$, $K_{TLR4}(\{SOCS\text{-}1, NF\kappa B\}) = 1$	SOCS-1 mediated downregulation of PICyts during recurrent TLR4 signalling	00121
2-N	SOCS-1	PICyts & IFN-β	$K_{PICyts}(\{SOCS\text{-}1\}) = 0$, $K_{PICyts}(\{NF\kappa B, SOCS\text{-}1\}) = 0$, $K_{PICyts}(\{NF\kappa B, IFN\text{-}\beta, SOCS\text{-}1\}) = 0$, $K_{IFN\text{-}\beta}(\{SOCS\text{-}1\}) = 0$, $K_{IFN\text{-}\beta}(\{TLR4, SOCS\text{-}1\}) = 1$, $K_{IFN\text{-}\beta}(\{SOCS\text{-}1, NF\kappa B\}) = 0$, $K_{IFN\text{-}\beta}(\{TLR4, SOCS\text{-}1, NF\kappa B\}) = 1$	$K_{PICyts}(\{NF\kappa B, IFN\text{-}\beta\}) = 2$	SOCS-1 mediated downregulation of IFN-β and PICyts	00000 & 00121
2-S	SOCS-1	PICyts & IFN-β	$K_{PICyts}(\{SOCS\text{-}1\}) = 0$, $K_{PICyts}(\{NF\kappa B, SOCS\text{-}1\}) = 0$, $K_{PICyts}(\{NF\kappa B, IFN\text{-}\beta, SOCS\text{-}1\}) = 0$, $K_{IFN\text{-}\beta}(\{SOCS\text{-}1\}) = 0$, $K_{IFN\text{-}\beta}(\{TLR4, SOCS\text{-}1\}) = 1$, $K_{IFN\text{-}\beta}(\{SOCS\text{-}1, NF\kappa B\}) = 0$, $K_{IFN\text{-}\beta}(\{TLR4, SOCS\text{-}1, NF\kappa B\}) = 1$	$K_{PICyts}(\{NF\kappa B, IFN\text{-}\beta\}) = 2$, $K_{TLR4}(\{SOCS\text{-}1, NF\kappa B\}) = 1$	SOCS-1 mediated downregulation of IFN-β and PICyts during recurrent TLR4 signalling	00121
3-N	IFN-β	PICyts	$K_{PICyts}(\{IFN\text{-}\beta\}) = 0$, $K_{PICyts}(\{IFN\text{-}\beta, NF\kappa B\}) = 0$, $K_{PICyts}(\{IFN\text{-}\beta, SOCS\text{-}1\}) = 0$, $K_{PICyts}(\{NF\kappa B, IFN\text{-}\beta, SOCS\text{-}1\}) = 2$	$K_{PICyts}(\{NF\kappa B, SOCS\text{-}1\}) = 2$	IFN-β mediated downregulation of PICyts	00000
3-S	IFN-β	PICyts & SOCS-1	$K_{PICyts}(\{IFN\text{-}\beta\}) = 0$, $K_{PICyts}(\{IFN\text{-}\beta, NF\kappa B\}) = 0$, $K_{PICyts}(\{IFN\text{-}\beta, SOCS\text{-}1\}) = 0$, $K_{PICyts}(\{NF\kappa B, IFN\text{-}\beta, SOCS\text{-}1\}) = 2$	$K_{PICyts}(\{NF\kappa B, SOCS\text{-}1\}) = 2$, $K_{TLR4}(\{SOCS\text{-}1, NF\kappa B\}) = 1$	IFN-β mediated downregulation PICyts during recurrent TLR4 signalling	00000
4-N	NFκB	PICyts	$K_{PICyts}(\{NF\kappa B\}) = 0$, $K_{PICyts}(\{NF\kappa B, IFN\text{-}\beta\}) = 0$, $K_{PICyts}(\{NF\kappa B, SOCS\text{-}1\}) = 0$, $K_{PICyts}(\{NF\kappa B, IFN\text{-}\beta, SOCS\text{-}1\}) = 2$	-	NFκB mediated induction of PICyts	00000
4-S	NFκB	PICyts	$K_{PICyts}(\{NF\kappa B\}) = 0$, $K_{PICyts}(\{NF\kappa B, IFN\text{-}\beta\}) = 0$, $K_{PICyts}(\{NF\kappa B, SOCS\text{-}1\}) = 0$, $K_{PICyts}(\{NF\kappa B, IFN\text{-}\beta, SOCS\text{-}1\}) = 2$	$K_{TLR4}(\{SOCS\text{-}1, NF\kappa B\}) = 1$	NFκB mediated induction of PICyts during recurrent TLR4 signalling	00000
5-N	PICyts	NFκB-JAK/STAT	$K_{NF\kappa B\text{-}JAK/STAT}(\{PICyts\}) = 1$, $K_{NF\kappa B\text{-}JAK/STAT}(\{TLR4, PICyts\}) = 1$, $K_{NF\kappa B\text{-}JAK/STAT}(\{IFN\text{-}\beta, PICyts\}) = 1$, $K_{NF\kappa B\text{-}JAK/STAT}(\{TLR4, PICyts, IFN\text{-}\beta\}) = 1$, $K_{NF\kappa B\text{-}JAK/STAT}(\{PICyts, SOCS\text{-}1\}) = 1$, $K_{NF\kappa B\text{-}JAK/STAT}(\{TLR4, PICyts, SOCS\text{-}1\}) = 1$, $K_{NF\kappa B\text{-}JAK/STAT}(\{PICyts, IFN\text{-}\beta, SOCS\text{-}1\}) = 1$, $K_{NF\kappa B\text{-}JAK/STAT}(\{SOCS\text{-}1, TLR4, IFN\text{-}\beta, PICyts\}) = 1$	-	PICyts mediated induction of JAK/STAT signalling	00000
5-S	PICyts	NFκB-JAK/STAT	$K_{NF\kappa B\text{-}JAK/STAT}(\{PICyts\}) = 1$, $K_{NF\kappa B\text{-}JAK/STAT}(\{TLR4, PICyts\}) = 1$, $K_{NF\kappa B\text{-}JAK/STAT}(\{IFN\text{-}\beta, PICyts\}) = 1$, $K_{NF\kappa B\text{-}JAK/STAT}(\{TLR4, PICyts, IFN\text{-}\beta\}) = 1$, $K_{NF\kappa B\text{-}JAK/STAT}(\{PICyts, SOCS\text{-}1\}) = 1$, $K_{NF\kappa B\text{-}JAK/STAT}(\{TLR4, PICyts, SOCS\text{-}1\}) = 1$, $K_{NF\kappa B\text{-}JAK/STAT}(\{PICyts, IFN\text{-}\beta, SOCS\text{-}1\}) = 1$, $K_{NF\kappa B\text{-}JAK/STAT}(\{SOCS\text{-}1, TLR4, IFN\text{-}\beta, PICyts\}) = 1$	$K_{TLR4}(\{SOCS\text{-}1, NF\kappa B\}) = 1$	Loss of PICyts mediated induction of JAK/STAT signalling during recurrent TLR4 induction.	00000

Different CASES have been presented with respective changes in parameters. Changes presented here in each CASE accompanied other logical parameters described in Table 1 to model each CASE.

is a representation of the cycle among states produced after the induction of JAK/STAT pathway (Figure S2). During this cycle, only SOCS-1 mediated downregulation of PICyts can be seen in absence of IFN-β.

Signalling in sepsis

The continuous presence of pathogens or recurrent infections can ignite rigorous immune responses in the host's body [82]. Previous experimental studies suggested the role of recurrent induction of TLRs in persistent infections and sepsis [83,84]. In this study, continuous induction of TLR4 was the only difference between the set of logical parameters used for model septic and non-septic signalling. Therefore, recurrent induction of TLR4, represented by logical parameter $(K_{TLR4}(\{SOCS-1, NF\kappa B\}) = 1)$, was used with other logical parameters of entities given in Table 1 to model the sepsis related signalling. Model related to sepsis has been provided as File S2. Dynamics of the BRN were studied in the form of a state graph, which was merged in Figure 3 for the purpose of comparison. In Figure 3, red highlighted states in squares and dotted trajectories represent the additional states and trajectories produced during septic signalling whereas common states and trajectories both in non-septic and septic systems are shown in black.

Unlike non-septic TLR4 and JAK/STAT signalling, new events of recurrent TLR4 induction (trajectories 00000→10000, labelled with "η" and 00010→10010, labelled with "θ") and the absence of stable state "00000" were observed as characteristics of sepsis. Overall, two phases of signalling were observed in the state graph shown in Figure 3. The first phase of signalling was comparable to non-septic signalling whereas the second phase of signalling represented a late phase of signalling dynamics produced due to repetitive TLR4 induction. In this phase, TLR4 was re-induced during pre-existing levels of PICyts (trajectory 00010→10010 labelled with "θ"). Later to which, influence of IFN-β or SOCS-1 tolerated the levels of PICyts with subsequent degradation of PICyts. Comparatively, most of the states in the late phase of dynamics represented immunosuppression due to the presence of both IFN-β and SOCS-1.

Induction of NFκB as in the trajectory (10010→10110 labelled with "κ" in Figure 3) was the only trajectory, which strengthened the levels of PICyts and led the system to overactive immune response (state "00121") in the late phase of signalling. However, all the trajectories ultimately led the system towards downregulated immune response (state "00000"). Subsequent activation of the new round of TLR4 mediated signalling after the state "00000" represented the recurrent induction of TLR4 (transition labelled with "η") in absence of any other downstream proteins. In summary, the phenomenon of oscillation was present representing activation and inactivation of PICyts during complete dynamics related to the condition of sepsis along with the suppressed expression levels of PICyts in late phase of signalling dynamics of the BRN.

Interventions in signalling

Mutations and/or therapeutic interventions can change the role of resources with subsequent changes in the dynamics of the BRN (see Definition 4 in methods section). Interventions were modelled by removing one or more interactions associated with any entity present in the BRN (Figure 2) to reproduce mutations or therapeutic interventions. The effects of interventions in IFN-β, SOCS-1, NFκB and PICyts mediated signalling were compared both in septic and non-septic signalling to elaborate their importance in the dynamics of the BRN. These interventions are discussed as "CASES" and changes in logical parameters are mentioned in Table 3. Other possible interventions, given in

Table S1, were also analysed to observe their overall effects on the system in terms of stable states produced by each type of intervention.

CASE 1 (Intervention in SOCS-1 mediated downregulation of PICyts). Intervention in SOCS-1 mediated downregulation of PICyts during non-septic signalling is discussed as CASE 1-N whereas in case of sepsis, it is discussed as CASE 1-S. Modelling of CASE 1-N was performed using the logical parameters given in Table 1 except with some changes as given in Table 3. The model is provided as File S3. Figure 4 represents the state graph produced due to the simulation of CASE 1-N. In this case, two stable states were observed including downregulated or normal (state "00000") and overactive PICyt levels (state "00121"). The overall dynamics of the system were found comparable to the non-septic signalling (as shown in Figure 3) but some trajectories involving SOCS-1 mediated inhibition of PICyts were different (trajectories labelled with "Δε" in Figure 4). In those trajectories, SOCS-1 mediated inhibition of PICyts was suppressed and permitted continuous activation of PICyts with subsequent induction of JAK/STAT pathway (stable state "00121"). These trajectories were also found opposite in directions from those observed in non-septic signalling (trajectories labelled with "ε" in Figure 3); where SOCS-1 mediated downregulation of PICyts led the system towards stable state "00000". IFN-β mediated downregulation of PICyts in CASE 1-N was found ineffective to reduce the levels of PICyts because IFN-β performed its inhibitory role in the earlier part of the dynamics (trajectories labelled with "γ" in Figure 4). Moreover, PICyts was capable enough to induce SOCS-1 mediated inhibition of IFN-β which results in its continuous inactivated state during later stages of the signalling. Thus higher levels of PICyts led the system to overactive immune response (trajectories labelled with "δ" in Figure 4).

It was observed that the system evolved mostly towards stable state "00000" in absence of activated TLR4. This condition was true except for those states in which NFκB and PICyts were present simultaneously in the system (downstream signalling dynamics after states 10111,00110,00111 and 10120 labelled with stars in Figure 4). All of these states had a higher probability to produce overactive immune state (stable state "00121") in the system. The presence of homeostasis in the state graph was found comparable to SCC-1 (Figure S1) whereas SOCS-1 mediated downregulation and homeostasis in PICyts levels was absent.

States and trajectories related to CASE 1-S were incorporated in Figure 4. Model of CASE 1-S is provided as File S4. Overall, dynamics of the BRN in CASE 1-S were found similar to the CASE 1-N but some of the trajectories involving re-activation of TLR4 were found different (trajectory labelled with "η" in Figure 4). Instead of two stable states as seen in CASE 1-N, only one stable state "00121" was found in CASE 1-S. New events of recurrent TLR4 induction (trajectories 00000→10000, labelled with "η" and 00010→10010, labelled with "θ") were comparable to signalling in sepsis without any intervention as shown in Figure 3. Unlike signalling in sepsis without any interventions, SOCS-1 did not play its part in late phase signalling dynamics. Induction of IFN-β in the late phase of septic signalling was also found ineffective to attenuate the overactive immune responses in the absence of SOCS-1.

CASE 2 (Intervention in SOCS-1 mediated downregulation of IFN-β and PICyts). One of the important effects on the dynamics of the BRN would be the complete loss of SOCS-1 mediated inhibition of IFN-β and PICyts so that their levels could be elevated. To evaluate this, intervention in SOCS-1 mediated inhibition of IFN-β and PICyts was executed. Intervention in non-septic state is discussed as CASE 2-N, whereas this intervention in case of sepsis is discussed as CASE 2-S. Dynamics of the BRN in these CASES are shown as a state graph in Figure 5. Modelling was performed using the logical parameters given in Table 1 along with certain modifications (Table 3). Moreover, respective edges, which represent SOCS-1 mediated inhibition of IFN-β and PICyts in Figure 2, were also removed.

Model of CASE 2-N is provided as File S5. The dynamics of the BRN produced in CASE 2-N were found comparable to non-septic case (Figure 3) except those trajectories which reflected SOCS-1 mediated inhibition of IFN-β and PICyts (trajectories labelled with "Δδ" and "Δε", respectively in Figure 5). Trajectories labelled with "Δδ" and "Δε" were found opposite in the direction as compared to their counterparts in non-septic signalling (Figure 3). Stable states "00000" and "00121" were comparable to those found in CASE 1-N. Similar to other state graphs discussed above, the simultaneous presence of NFκB-JAK/STAT and PICyts led the trajectories mostly towards elevated levels of PICyts even in the absence of SOCS-1 mediated inhibition of IFN-β. Homeostatic downregulation was seen comparable to SCC-1 (Figure S1), whereas another homeostasis produced during non-intervened signalling (SCC-2) was abolished.

Signalling in CASE 2-S was incorporated into the Figure 5 and its model is provided as File S6. In this CASE, most of the states and trajectories associated with sepsis were found comparable to those in CASE 2-N. Only one stable state "00121" was found in CASE 2-S, whereas another stable state "00000" led the dynamics of the BRN towards recurrent induction of TLR4 like other sepsis related dynamics in this study. New events of recurrent TLR4 induction (trajectories 00000→10000, labelled with "η" and 00010→10010, labelled with "θ") were similar to the sepsis related non-intervened dynamics of the BRN (Figure 3). However, in this CASE, SOCS-1 could not play its inhibitory role in late phase signalling dynamics. Moreover, interventions in SOCS-1 mediated inhibition of IFN-β produced similar results as seen in CASE 1-S due to the activated levels of TLR4.

CASE 3 (Intervention in IFN-β mediated downregulation of PICyts). Intervention in IFN-β mediated inhibition of PICyts during non-septic and septic conditions are discussed as CASE 3-N and CASE 3-S, respectively. These CASES were used to evaluate the dynamics of the BRN and consequential immune responses in the absence of IFN-β mediated inhibition of PICyts. Intervention was derived by removing the inhibitory edge from IFN-β to PICyts as given in Figure 2. Modelling was performed using the logical parameters given in Table 1 with some exceptions given in Table 3 for CASE 3-N and CASE 3-S. Models of CASE 3-N and CASE 3-S are also provided as File S7 and File S8, respectively). A state graph of CASE 3-N is shown in Figure 6.

Only one stable state "00000" was observed during the dynamics of the BRN associated with CASE 3-N. It was observed that IFN-β mediated inhibition of PICyts during earlier phase of signalling was abolished from the system (trajectories labelled with "Δγ" in Figure 6). This interaction was speculated to resist the elevated levels of PICyts as seen above in Figures 3–5. However, the elevated levels of PICyts were downregulated by SOCS-1 when IFN-β was unable to inhibit PICyts.

Homeostatic signalling in CASE 3-N (SCC-3) was similar to that produced during the dynamics of non-septic model (SCC-1), however, trajectories were slightly shifted towards elevated levels of PICyts (Figure S3). Homeostasis during overactive PICyts (state "00121") was observed in the presence of SOCS-1 (SCC-4 and SCC-5 shown in Figure S4 and Figure S5, respectively), which represents that even in the absence of IFN-β, SOCS-1 cater the inhibition of PICyts.

Signalling in CASE 3-S was integrated in the state graph produced by CASE 3-N (Figure 6). Most of the trajectories and nodes were found common except those which involved re-activation of TLR4, as discussed above. Late phase IFN-β mediated downregulation of PICyts during septic signalling was not found.

CASE 4 (intervention in NFκB mediated induction of PICyts). NFκB mediated induction of PICyts has been targeted in various experimental studies [85,86]. This targeting was performed either by degrading the complex of NFκB or by compromising the resultant gene transcription pathway. The model was evaluated for this intervention by removing the NFκB mediated induction of PICyts as given in Figure 2. To model this intervention, logical parameters given in Table 1 were used with some exceptions given in Table 3. This intervention in non-septic and septic signalling are discussed as CASE 4-N and CASE 4-S, respectively. The models of CASE 4-N and CASE 4-S have been provided as File S9 and File S10, respectively. Simulation of CASE 4-N resulted in a single normal stable state (00000) with the absence of PICyts throughout the system (Figure 7). Homeostasis (SCC-6) was seen only between IFN-β and SOCS-1 (Figure S6).

Dynamics of the BRN produced in CASE 4-N and CASE 4-S were comparable except the recurrent induction of TLR4, as discussed above. The results implicate that an immune response could neglect the elevated endotoxemia and allow the pathogen to infect within the immunocompromised host due to the complete absence of PICyts.

CASE 5 (intervention in PICyts mediated induction of NFκB and JAK/STAT pathway). Intervention in PICyts mediated induction of NFκB and JAK/STAT pathway during non-septic signalling is discussed as CASE 5-N whereas in case of sepsis, it is discussed as CASE 5-S. Modelling of CASE 5-N and CASE 5-S were performed using the logical parameters given in Table 1 with exceptions given in Table 3. Moreover, the edge from PICyts towards NFκB-JAK/STAT, as shown in Figure 2, was also removed. The models of CASE 5-N and CASE 5-S have been provided as File S11 and File S12, respectively. The dynamics of both CASES are shown in Figure 8. Events during the simulation of CASE 5-N were slightly different from non-septic signalling (shown in Figure 3), in terms of loss of PICyts mediated induction of JAK/STAT pathway. Moreover, the higher levels of PICyts were not observed throughout the state graph, however, normal levels of PICyts were present. Stable state "00000" was present in CASE 5-N, however, in CASE 5-S, this state led towards recurrent induction of TLR4 (trajectories 00000→10000, labelled with "η"). Homeostasis due to the cyclic paths SCC-7 and SCC-8 in CASE 5-N were found comparable to SCC-1 and SCC-2 (Figures S7 and Figure S8) except that elevated levels of PICyts were not observed within any cycle.

Discussion

Methods of high throughput gene expression profiling facilitate the description of complex cellular regulatory networks and present pictures of valuable information about the signalling networks [87,88]. Regardless of the enormous amount of data associated with molecular and cellular processes produced in various settings, the dynamicity of biological networks in the presence of several interconnected factors still need to be further explored [89]. "Computational systems biology" is a discipline, which is concerned with modelling of experimentally determined values to improve our understanding about BRNs [90]. Computational modelling of BRNs provide useful information about dynamics of various signalling pathways, including control of differentiation process in helper T cells, control of organ differentiation in Arabidopsis thaliana flowers, segmentation during embryogenesis in *Drosophila melanogaster* and TLRs mediated signalling [51–53].

Sepsis is a complex pathological state of the body, which involves heterogeneous immune responses of exacerbated inflammation and immunosuppression [82]. Pathophysiology of the sepsis has been associated with pro- or anti-inflammatory responses in different scientific studies, which led to the inconsistency of the overall findings, and failure in its treatment [4]. Some studies associated the deaths in the early phase of sepsis with unrestricted and irrational SIRS in the host [91] and impelled anti-inflammatory treatments [92,93]. On the other hand, it has also been hypothesized that SIRS is followed by CARS [4,94,95]. Moreover, concomitant production of pro- and anti-inflammatory responses have also been demonstrated in polymicrobial infectious challenges, which support the continuous, highly mixed anti-inflammatory response (MARS) and implicated that both pro- and anti- inflammatory cytokines are integral parts of sepsis [96,97].

TLR4 is a central mediator of LPS induced TH1 or proinflammatory responses, whereas induction of inhibitory mediators can lead the system towards downregulated levels of PICyts [98]. Moreover, binding of cytokines to JAK/STAT receptors induce changes in gene expression levels of various other co-factors necessary for the downregulation of immune response [30]. In order to study the mechanism of sepsis at cellular level, we evaluated the qualitative roles of TLR4 and JAK/STAT signalling with their negative and positive feedback loops necessary to produce effective immune response.

TLR4 and JAK/STAT mediated signalling was designed in the current study by incorporating previous experimental studies associated with interaction of entities and their overall effect in case of sepsis (Figure 1). Reduction of the model was performed to reduce the possible states and trajectories produced during qualitative modelling (Figure 2). In this process, roles of resources in logical parameters were carefully devised so that useful information about the role of any entity present in the model should not be lost. The model was further used with different sets of logical parameters to produce non-septic, septic and intervened signalling to produce dynamics in the form of state graphs. The results of non-septic signalling (Figure 3) were used to compare any interpretations present in this study.

State graphs produced in non-septic signalling were found different from signalling during sepsis in terms of recurring signalling and activation of IFN-β and SOCS-1 in the late phase, which may reflect the immunosuppressive state of the septic patient in the later stages of sepsis. In non-septic signalling, induction of TLR4 and subsequent JAK/STAT signalling mount a successful immune response, which ultimately culminates in downregulated immune response. However, during sepsis, absence of stable state "00000" and recursive signalling through state "00121" can be correlated with the phenomenon of SIRS.

Induction of TLR4 mediated MyD88 and TRIF dependent signalling produced different responses. MyD88 dependent signalling was associated with early induction of PICyts whereas TRIF dependent signalling was associated with late induction of PICyts through Myd88 independent mechanism. This type of early PICyts and delayed IFN-β inductions have been suggested in previous experimental studies associating the time of their onsets in response to pathogen induced immune reaction [99]. Delayed activation from previous experimental studies suggested that IFN-β was produced 24 hours later to *Listeria monocytogenes* infection [100]. Moreover, IFN-β has been observed to attenuate the late hyperinflammatory responses in septic peritonitis [27]. Our study

implicates that induction of IFN-β may be present in two stages of septic signalling. In the first stage, IFN-β regulates the levels of PICyts before the induction of SOCS-1, whereas in second stage IFN-β can be induced and downregulate PICyts in late phases of sepsis. Chances for the induction of IFN-β and SOCS-1 were found equal in the late phase of the dynamics of the BRN associated with sepsis and due to this in late phase dynamics of sepsis, there are fewer chances for activation of PICyts to higher levels.

Sequential production and then downregulation of PICyts was observed as one of the interesting phenomenon. The swing in the expression levels of PICyts has already been reported which revealed the pro-inflammation with subsequent immunosuppression [13]. In our study, proinflammatory state can be correlated with those states which had higher activation levels of PICyts (qualitative level "2") whereas immunosuppression can be correlated with lower levels of PICyts (qualitative level "0 or 1"). SOCS-1 mediated inhibition of PICyts through inactivation of JAK/STAT signalling was found intriguing in the management of immunosuppression. While, inactivation of TLR4 and NFκB mediated induction of PICyts was associated with management of hyperinflammatory responses. This may suggest that therapeutic strategies during the course of sepsis should be devised according to the immune responses and expression levels of SOCS-1 and IFN-β as discussed in other studies for their role in sepsis [31,47,82].

In vitro studies suggested that recurrent induction of TLR4 through LPS challenge result in the decreased immune response known as LPS tolerance [101]. Our study suggests, that late phase induction of both SOCS-1 and IFN-β may play their roles in LPS tolerance and can produce immunosuppression. Moreover, tolerance may be related with complete absence of PICyts levels even in the continuous signalling through TLR4.

Intervened signalling presented some of the interesting assumptions produced during this study. Mutations or therapeutic intervention of SOCS-1 mediated inhibition of JAK/STAT signalling may result in the non-reversible hyperinflammatory process compared to any other intervention studied here. Moreover, the presence of SOCS-1 can balance the levels of PICyts even during incapable IFN-β mediated inhibition. On the other hand, if non-reversible immunosuppression is required, then intervention of NFκB mediated PICyts expression would produce competitive results.

The overall dynamics of the BRN have been given in Figure 9-A to show the pattern of activation and inactivation of entities. It can be seen that starting from the activation of TLR4, the dynamics actually proceed greatly towards the activation of IFN-β and then SOCS-1 during normal signalling. However, in the case of recurrent signalling, the activation of IFN-β and SOCS-1 at the same time inhibit the activation of PICyts. Based on these predictions, we hypothesize that in normal infections, which do not often lead to sepsis, the phases of regulatory signalling are somewhat different from those seen in case of sepsis as shown in Figure 9 (B–C). This is supported by previous experimental studies in which the continuous presence of pathogens repeatedly induce immune responses and produce oscillatory levels of PICyts [102]. Recurrent infections, which can lead to sepsis, have the capability to induce innate immune responses repeatedly. During this state, PICyts are inhibited to a greater extent which can lead the immune system of the host towards the temporary immunocompromised state. Inhibition may be due to the prior presence of negative regulatory factors such as SOCS-1 and IFN-β in the system, which may be induced in some earlier phase of infection or because of a co-infection. Due to this reason, innate immune

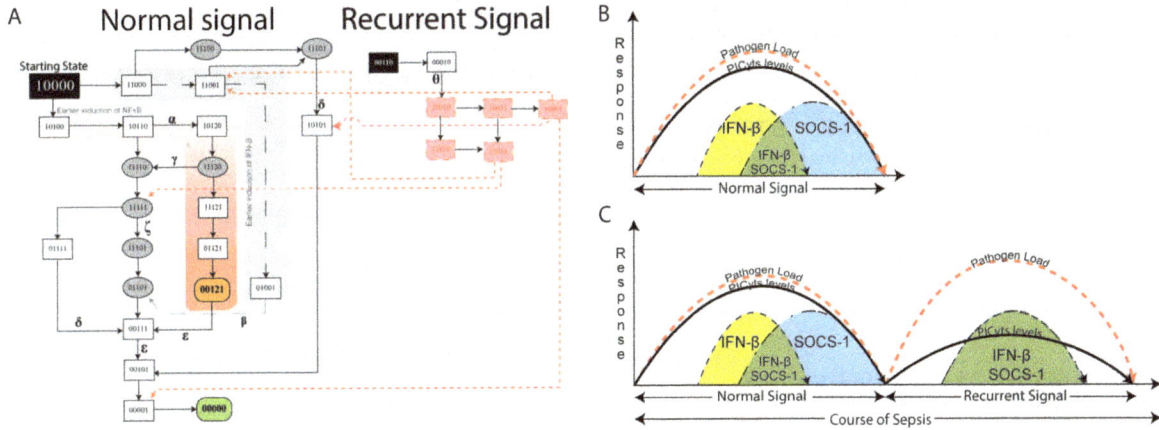

Figure 9. Implication of the study. (A) Edges labelled with Greek small letters and states as nodes are used to represent trajectories associated with different signalling events observed in this study (see legend in Figure 3). Specific states and trajectories of normal and recurrent signalling shown in Figures 3–8 were used to draw the hypothesis shown in (B–C). Possible effects of TLR4 and JAK/STAT signalling on pathogen load, induction pattern of PICyts, IFN-β and SOCS-1 mediated downregulation of PICyts are shown for non-septic (B) and septic (C) cases. During non-septic case, the pattern of IFN-β and then SOCS-1 limits the qualitative levels of PICyts along with the successful reduction of pathogen load. On the other hand, during sepsis, it has been proposed that changed expression pattern of IFN-β and SOCS-1 inhibit the PICyts with resultant increase in the pathogen load.

response may not efficiently generate an effective PICyts burst to manage the pathogen load. Moreover, the expression pattern of negative regulators such as SOCS-1 and IFN-β can be detrimental in case of sepsis. In normal infections, the pattern of IFN-β and SOCS-1 is sequential, whereas in case of sepsis, this sequential pattern of IFN-β and SOCS-1 may be changed and system becomes more vulnerable towards higher levels of pathogen load due to compromised levels of PICyts.

Conclusion

In summary, logical modelling of TLR4 and JAK/STAT dependent signalling pathways indicated specifically designed crosstalk mechanism which can induce a successful pathogenic response along with management of hyperinflammation. If entities present in these pathways lose a specific pattern of activation and/ or inactivation, then signalling can lead towards diverse outcomes. Using computer-aided qualitative approach, we have tried to highlight these patterns of entities necessary to maintain a balance in a successful immune response. Qualitative results implicated that TLR4 and JAK/STAT pathways induced elevated levels of PICyts with subsequent downregulation. This pattern of activation and then inactivation of PICyts produced homeostasis in the system while changes in the inhibitory role of SOCS-1 created overactive immune responses. The inhibitory role of IFN-β was observed during the initial stages of dynamics, but it is tempting to speculate that SOCS-1 possibly inhibit the role of IFN-β during sepsis but has the ability to manage the hyperinflammatory condition. Overall, this study suggests that intervention in SOCS-1 mediated PICyts inhibition may produce useful results in case of immunocompromised septic patients. On the other hand, intervening the TLR4 or PICyts mediated induction of NFκB-JAK/STAT pathways may be used for the management of hyperinflammatory immune responses. This computational study highlighted many questions with provision of possible answers, which need further experimental investigations. In the future, we will perform *in vitro* experiments to further investigate our predictions and produce explicit insights into the diagnosis and treatment of sepsis by involving IFN-β and SOCS-1.

Supporting Information

Figure S1   SCC-1. This cyclic graph represents the homeostatic regulation of PICyts during physiological signalling dynamics.

Figure S2   SCC-2. This cyclic graph represents the homeostasis by SOCS-1 mediated downregulation of PICyts during physiological signalling dynamics.

Figure S3   SCC-3. This cyclic graph represents the homeostasis by IFN-β mediated downregulation of PICyts during CASE 3.

Figure S4   SCC-4. This cyclic graph represents the homeostasis by SOCS-1 mediated downregulation of PICyts during CASE 3.

Figure S5   SCC-5. This cyclic graph represents the homeostasis by SOCS-1 mediated downregulation of PICyts during NFκB downstream signalling in CASE 3.

Figure S6   SCC-6. This cyclic graph represents the homeostasis between IFN-β and SOCS-1 during CASE 4.

Figure S7   SCC-7. This cyclic graph represents the homeostasis between IFN-β and SOCS-1 during CASE 5.

Figure S8   SCC-8. This cyclic graph represents the homeostasis due to SOCS-1 during CASE 5.

Figure S9   Dummy tendency graphs of TLR4 representing the associated logical parameters used in the modelling of non-septic condition.

Figure S10   Dummy tendency graphs of IFN-β representing the associated logical parameters used in the modelling of non-septic condition.

**Figure S11 Dummy tendency graphs of NFκB repre-
senting the associated logical parameters used in the
modelling of non-septic condition.**

**Figure S12 Dummy tendency graphs of PICyts repre-
senting the associated logical parameters used in the
modelling of non-septic condition.**

**Figure S13 Dummy tendency graphs of SOCS-1 repre-
senting the associated logical parameters used in the
modelling of non-septic condition.**

Table S1 Other intervention studies. Other CASES of
intervention in signalling were derived by removing specific
interactions in Figure 2 along with their logical parameters to
observe the possible stable states produced due to each condition.

File S1   Model of non-sepsis.xml.

File S2   Model of sepsis.xml.

File S3   Model of CASE 1-N.xml.

File S4   Model of CASE 1-S.xml.

File S5   Model of CASE 2-N.xml.

File S6   Model of CASE 2-S.xml.

File S7   Model of CASE 3-N.xml.

File S8   Model of CASE 3-S.xml.

File S9   Model of CASE 4-N.xml.

File S10   Model of CASE 4-S.xml.

File S11   Model of CASE 5-N.xml.

File S12   Model of CASE 5-S.xml.

File S13   Model of non-sepsis.ginml.

File S14   Model of sepsis.ginml.

File S15   Model of CASE 1-N.ginml.

File S16   Model of CASE 1-S.ginml.

File S17   Model of CASE 2-N.ginml.

File S18   Model of CASE 2-S.ginml.

File S19   Model of CASE 3-N.ginml.

File S20   Model of CASE 3-S.ginml.

File S21   Model of CASE 4-N.ginml.

File S22   Model of CASE 4-S.ginml.

File S23   Model of CASE 5-N.ginml.

File S24   Model of CASE 5-S.ginml.

**File S25   Input and output of SMBioNet for the compu-
tation of values for logical parameters given in Table 1.**

**File S26   An informal description of the logical param-
eters with relevant evidences based on previous experimental studies that forms the basis for selection of a
specific value for each logical parameter.**

Acknowledgments

The authors would like to thank the anonymous reviewers, Maria
Mukaram, Taseer Ahmad, Farzana Zenab, Reem Altaf and Rahat-ul-
Ain for their constructive comments and suggestions to improve the quality
of the paper.

Author Contributions

Conceived and designed the experiments: RZP UN JA. Performed the
experiments: RZP UN JA AA ST BA. Analyzed the data: RZP AA RH
UN JA ST BA. Contributed reagents/materials/analysis tools: JA. Wrote
the paper: RZP AA RH UN JA ST BA.

References

1. Bone R, Sibbald W, Sprung C (1992) The ACCP-SCCM consensus conference
   on sepsis and organ failure. CHEST Journal 101: 1481–1483.
2. Wheeler AP, Bernard GR (1999) Treating patients with severe sepsis. New
   England Journal of Medicine 340: 207–214.
3. Lever A, Mackenzie I (2007) Sepsis: definition, epidemiology, and diagnosis.
   BMJ: British Medical Journal 335: 879.
4. Hotchkiss RS, Karl IE (2003) The pathophysiology and treatment of sepsis.
   New England Journal of Medicine 348: 138–150.
5. Stone R (1994) Search for sepsis drugs goes on despite past failures. Science
   (New York, NY) 264: 365.
6. Wenzel RP (1992) Anti-Endotoxin Monoclonal Antibodies – A Second Look.
   New England Journal of Medicine 326: 1151–1153.
7. Angus DC, Linde-Zwirble WT, Lidicker J, Clermont G, Carcillo J, et al. (2001)
   Epidemiology of severe sepsis in the United States: analysis of incidence,
   outcome, and associated costs of care. Critical care medicine 29: 1303–1310.
8. Dombrovskiy VY, Martin AA, Sunderram J, Paz HL (2007) Rapid increase in
   hospitalization and mortality rates for severe sepsis in the United States: A
   trend analysis from 1993 to 2003*. Critical Care Medicine 35: 1244–1250.
9. Lagu T, Rothberg MB, Shieh M-S, Pekow PS, Steingrub JS, et al. (2012)
   Hospitalizations, costs, and outcomes of severe sepsis in the United States 2003
   to 2007. Critical Care Medicine 40: 754–761.
10. Dinarello CA (2000) Proinflammatory cytokines. CHEST Journal 118: 503–
    508.
11. Opal SM, DePalo VA (2000) Anti-inflammatory cytokines. CHEST Journal
    117: 1162–1172.
12. Walley KR, Lukacs NW, Standiford TJ, Strieter RM, Kunkel SL (1996)
    Balance of inflammatory cytokines related to severity and mortality of murine
    sepsis. Infection and immunity 64: 4733–4738.
13. Gogos CA, Drosou E, Bassaris HP, Skoutelis A (2000) Pro-versus anti-
    inflammatory cytokine profile in patients with severe sepsis: a marker for

prognosis and future therapeutic options. Journal of Infectious Diseases 181: 176–180.

14. Loisa P, Rinne T, Laine S, Hurme M, Kaukinen S (2003) Anti-inflammatory cytokine response and the development of multiple organ failure in severe sepsis. Acta anaesthesiologica scandinavica 47: 319–325.

15. Harris MC, D'Angio CT, Gallagher PR, Kaufman D, Evans J, et al. (2005) Cytokine elaboration in critically ill infants with bacterial sepsis, necrotizing enterocolitis, or sepsis syndrome: correlation with clinical parameters of inflammation and mortality. The Journal of pediatrics 147: 462–468.

16. Ashare A, Powers LS, Butler NS, Doerschug KC, Monick MM, et al. (2005) Anti-inflammatory response is associated with mortality and severity of infection in sepsis. American Journal of Physiology-Lung Cellular and Molecular Physiology 288: L633–L640.

17. Ward NS, Casserly B, Ayala A (2008) The Compensatory Anti-inflammatory Response Syndrome (CARS) in Critically Ill Patients. Clinics in Chest Medicine 29: 617–625.

18. Iskander KN, Osuchowski MF, Stearns-Kurosawa DJ, Kurosawa S, Stepien D, et al. (2013) Sepsis: multiple abnormalities, heterogeneous responses, and evolving understanding. Physiological reviews 93: 1247–1288.

19. Hotchkiss RS, Monneret G, Payen D (2013) Immunosuppression in sepsis: a novel understanding of the disorder and a new therapeutic approach. The Lancet infectious diseases 13: 260–268.

20. Takeda K, Akira S (2005) Toll-like receptors in innate immunity. International Immunology 17: 1–14.

21. Wittebole X, Coyle S, Kumar A, Goshima M, Lowry S, et al. (2005) Expression of tumour necrosis factor receptor and Toll-like receptor 2 and 4 on peripheral blood leucocytes of human volunteers after endotoxin challenge: a comparison of flow cytometric light scatter and immunofluorescence gating. Clinical & Experimental Immunology 141: 99–106.

22. Härter L, Mica L, Stocker R, Trentz O, Keel M (2004) Increased expression of toll-like receptor-2 and-4 on leukocytes from patients with sepsis. Shock 22: 403–409.

23. Brandl K, Gluck T, Huber C, Salzberger B, Falk W, et al. (2005) TLR-4 surface display on human monocytes is increased in septic patients. European journal of medical research 10: 319.

24. Hoebe K, Janssen E, Beutler B (2004) The interface between innate and adaptive immunity. Nature Immunology 5: 971–974.

25. Kawai T, Akira S (2010) The role of pattern-recognition receptors in innate immunity: update on Toll-like receptors. Nature immunology 11: 373–384.

26. Kendrick SF, Jones DE (2008) Mechanisms of Innate Immunity in Sepsis. Sepsis: Springer. 5–10.

27. Weighardt H, Kaiser-Moore S, Schlautkötter S, Rossmann-Bloeck T, Schleicher U, et al. (2006) Type I IFN modulates host defense and late hyperinflammation in septic peritonitis. The Journal of Immunology 177: 5623–5630.

28. Jones BW, Means TK, Heldwein KA, Keen MA, Hill PJ, et al. (2001) Different Toll-like receptor agonists induce distinct macrophage responses. Journal of Leukocyte Biology 69: 1036–1044.

29. Kawai T, Akira S (2011) Toll-like receptors and their crosstalk with other innate receptors in infection and immunity. Immunity 34: 637.

30. Schindler C, Levy DE, Decker T (2007) JAK-STAT signaling: from interferons to cytokines. Journal of Biological Chemistry 282: 20059–20063.

31. Scott MJ, Godshall CJ, Cheadle WG (2002) Jaks, STATs, Cytokines, and Sepsis. Clinical and Diagnostic Laboratory Immunology 9: 1153–1159.

32. Mi H, Thomas P (2009) PANTHER pathway: an ontology-based pathway database coupled with data analysis tools. Protein Networks and Pathway Analysis: Springer. 123–140.

33. Kanehisa M, Araki M, Goto S, Hattori M, Hirakawa M, et al. (2008) KEGG for linking genomes to life and the environment. Nucleic acids research 36: D480–D484.

34. Croft D, O'Kelly G, Wu G, Haw R, Gillespie M, et al. (2010) Reactome: a database of reactions, pathways and biological processes. Nucleic acids research: gkq1018.

35. Kawai T, Adachi O, Ogawa T, Takeda K, Akira S (1999) Unresponsiveness of MyD88-deficient mice to endotoxin. Immunity 11: 115–122.

36. Yamamoto M, Sato S, Hemmi H, Hoshino K, Kaisho T, et al. (2003) Role of adaptor TRIF in the MyD88-independent toll-like receptor signaling pathway. Science 301: 640–643.

37. Yamamoto M, Sato S, Hemmi H, Hoshino K, Kaisho T, et al. (2003) Role of Adaptor TRIF in the MyD88-Independent Toll-Like Receptor Signaling Pathway. Science 301: 640–643.

38. Yamamoto M, Sato S, Hemmi H, Uematsu S, Hoshino K, et al. (2003) TRAM is specifically involved in the Toll-like receptor 4–mediated MyD88-independent signaling pathway. Nature immunology 4: 1144–1150.

39. Kisseleva T, Bhattacharya S, Braunstein J, Schindler C (2002) Signaling through the JAK/STAT pathway, recent advances and future challenges. Gene 285: 1–24.

40. Liew FY, Xu D, Brint EK, O'Neill LA (2005) Negative regulation of toll-like receptor-mediated immune responses. Nature Reviews Immunology 5: 446–458.

41. Yang Q, Calvano SE, Lowry SF, Androulakis IP (2011) A dual negative regulation model of Toll-like receptor 4 signaling for endotoxin preconditioning in human endotoxemia. Mathematical Biosciences 232: 151–163.

42. Yoshimura A, Naka T, Kubo M (2007) SOCS proteins, cytokine signalling and immune regulation. Nature Reviews Immunology 7: 454–465.

43. Boone DL, Turer EE, Lee EG, Ahmad RC, Wheeler MT, et al. (2004) The ubiquitin-modifying enzyme A20 is required for termination of Toll-like receptor responses. Nature Immunology 5: 1052–1060.

44. Carty M, Goodbody R, Schröder M, Stack J, Moynagh PN, et al. (2006) The human adaptor SARM negatively regulates adaptor protein TRIF–dependent Toll-like receptor signaling. Nature Immunology 7: 1074–1081.

45. Šega S, Wraber B, Mesec A, Horvat A, Ihan A (2004) IFN-β1a and IFN-β1b have different patterns of influence on cytokines. Clinical neurology and neurosurgery 106: 255–258.

46. Belardelli F (1995) Role of interferons and other cytokines in the regulation of the immune response. APMIS 103: 161–179.

47. Mahieu T, Libert C (2007) Should we inhibit type I interferons in sepsis? Infection and immunity 75: 22–29.

48. Baetz A, Frey M, Heeg K, Dalpke AH (2004) Suppressor of Cytokine Signaling (SOCS) Proteins Indirectly Regulate Toll-like Receptor Signaling in Innate Immune Cells. Journal of Biological Chemistry 279: 54708–54715.

49. Johnston JA (2004) Are SOCS suppressors, regulators, and degraders? Journal of Leukocyte Biology 75: 743–748.

50. Prêle CM, Woodward EA, Bisley J, Keith-Magee A, Nicholson SE, et al. (2008) SOCS1 regulates the IFN but not NFκB pathway in TLR-stimulated human monocytes and macrophages. The Journal of Immunology 181: 8018–8026.

51. Mendoza L (2006) A network model for the control of the differentiation process in Th cells. Biosystems 84: 101–114.

52. Mendoza L, Thieffry D, Alvarez-Buylla ER (1999) Genetic control of flower morphogenesis in Arabidopsis thaliana: a logical analysis. Bioinformatics 15: 593–606.

53. Sanchez L, Thieffry D (2003) Segmenting the fly embryo::: a logical analysis of the pair-rule cross-regulatory module. Journal of Theoretical Biology 224: 517–537.

54. Samaga R, Klamt S (2013) Modeling approaches for qualitative and semi-quantitative analysis of cellular signaling networks. Cell Communication and Signaling 11: 43.

55. Thomas R, d'Ari R (1990) Biological feedback: CRC.

56. Ahmad J, Bernot G, Comet J-P, Lime D, Roux O (2007) Hybrid modelling and dynamical analysis of gene regulatory networks with delays. ComPlexUs 3: 231–251.

57. Ahmad J, Niazi U, Mansoor S, Siddique U, Bibby J (2012) Formal Modeling and Analysis of the MAL-Associated Biological Regulatory Network: Insight into Cerebral Malaria. PloS one 7: e33532.

58. De Jong H (2002) Modeling and simulation of genetic regulatory systems: a literature review. Journal of computational biology 9: 67–103.

59. Thomas R (1979) Kinetic logic: a Boolean approach to the analysis of complex regulatory systems. Lecture Notes in Biomathematics 29: 507.

60. Thomas R (1978) Logical analysis of systems comprising feedback loops. Journal of Theoretical Biology 73: 631–656.

61. Thomas R (1991) Regulatory networks seen as asynchronous automata: a logical description. Journal of Theoretical Biology 153: 1–23.

62. Snoussi EH, Thomas R (1993) Logical identification of all steady states: the concept of feedback loop characteristic states. Bulletin of Mathematical Biology 55: 973–991.

63. Thomas R, Thieffry D, Kaufman M (1995) Dynamical behaviour of biological regulatory networks–I. Biological role of feedback loops and practical use of the concept of the loop-characteristic state. Bulletin of mathematical biology 57: 247–276.

64. Thomas R (1998) Laws for the dynamics of regulatory networks. International Journal of Developmental Biology 42: 479–485.

65. Demongeot J, Kaufman M, Thomas R (2000) Positive feedback circuits and memory. Comptes Rendus de l'Académie des Sciences-Series III-Sciences de la Vie 323: 69–79.

66. Thomas R, Kaufman M (2001) Multistationarity, the basis of cell differentiation and memory. II. Logical analysis of regulatory networks in terms of feedback circuits. Chaos: An Interdisciplinary Journal of Nonlinear Science 11: 180–195.

67. Gagneur J, Casari G (2005) From molecular networks to qualitative cell behavior. FEBS letters 579: 1867–1871.

68. Bernot G, Cassez F, Comet J-P, Delaplace F, Müller C, et al. (2007) Semantics of biological regulatory networks. Electronic Notes in Theoretical Computer Science 180: 3–14.

69. Naldi A, Remy E, Thieffry D, Chaouiya C. A reduction of logical regulatory graphs preserving essential dynamical properties; 2009. Springer. 266–280.

70. Saadatpour A, Albert R, Reluga TC (2013) A reduction method for Boolean network models proven to conserve attractors. SIAM Journal on Applied Dynamical Systems 12: 1997–2011.

71. Chaouiya C, Naldi A, Thieffry D (2012) Logical modelling of gene regulatory networks with GINsim. Bacterial Molecular Networks: Springer. 463–479.

72. Tyson JJ, Chen K, Novak B (2001) Network dynamics and cell physiology. Nature Reviews Molecular Cell Biology 2: 908–916.

73. Murray PJ (2007) The JAK-STAT signaling pathway: input and output integration. The Journal of Immunology 178: 2623–2629.

74. O'Shea JJ, Gadina M, Schreiber RD (2002) Cytokine Signaling in 2002: New Surprises in the Jak/Stat Pathway. Cell 109: S121–S131.

75. Cooney RN (2002) Suppressors of cytokine signaling (SOCS): inhibitors of the JAK/STAT pathway. Shock 17: 83–90.

76. Khalis Z, Comet J-P, Richard A, Bernot G (2009) The SMBioNet method for discovering models of gene regulatory networks. Genes, Genomes and Genomics 3: 15–22.

77. Richard A, Comet J, Bernot G SMBioNet: Selection of Models of Biological Networks.

78. Bernot G, Comet J-P, Richard A, Guespin J (2004) Application of formal methods to biological regulatory networks: extending Thomas' asynchronous logical approach with temporal logic. Journal of theoretical biology 229: 339–347.

79. Huth M, Ryan M (2004) Logic in Computer Science: Modelling and reasoning about systems: Cambridge University Press.

80. Covert MW, Leung TH, Gaston JE, Baltimore D (2005) Achieving stability of lipopolysaccharide-induced NF-κB activation. Science 309: 1854–1857.

81. Clark K, Takeuchi O, Akira S, Cohen P (2011) The TRAF-associated protein TANK facilitates cross-talk within the IκB kinase family during Toll-like receptor signaling. Proceedings of the National Academy of Sciences 108: 17093–17098.

82. Remick DG (2007) Pathophysiology of sepsis. The American journal of pathology 170: 1435–1444.

83. Weighardt H, Holzmann B (2008) Role of Toll-like receptor responses for sepsis pathogenesis. Immunobiology 212: 715–722.

84. Netea MG, Van der Meer JW, Kullberg B-J (2004) Toll-like receptors as an escape mechanism from the host defense. Trends in microbiology 12: 484–488.

85. Shi C, Zhao X, Lagergren A, Sigvardsson M, Wang X, et al. (2006) Immune status and inflammatory response differ locally and systemically in severe acute pancreatitis. Scandinavian journal of gastroenterology 41: 472–480.

86. Baeuerle PA, Henkel T (1994) Function and activation of NF-kappaB in the immune system. Annual review of immunology 12: 141–179.

87. Hughes TR, Marton MJ, Jones AR, Roberts CJ, Stoughton R, et al. (2000) Functional discovery via a compendium of expression profiles. Cell 102: 109–126.

88. Kholodenko BN (2006) Cell-signalling dynamics in time and space. Nature Reviews Molecular Cell Biology 7: 165–176.

89. Kriete A, Eils R (2005) Computational systems biology: Access Online via Elsevier.

90. Kitano H (2002) Systems biology: a brief overview. Science 295: 1662–1664.

91. Bone RC (1992) Toward an epidemiology and natural history of SIRS (systemic inflammatory response syndrome). JAMA: the journal of the American Medical Association 268: 3452–3455.

92. Angus DC (2011) The Search for Effective Therapy for Sepsis. JAMA: The Journal of the American Medical Association 306: 2614–2615.

93. Remick DG (2003) Cytokine therapeutics for the treatment of sepsis: why has nothing worked? Current pharmaceutical design 9: 75–82.

94. Rittirsch D, Flierl MA, Ward PA (2008) Harmful molecular mechanisms in sepsis. Nature Reviews Immunology 8: 776–787.

95. Oberholzer A, Oberholzer C, Moldawer LL (2001) Sepsis syndromes: understanding the role of innate and acquired immunity. Shock 16: 83–96.

96. Novotny AR, Reim D, Assfalg V, Altmayr F, Friess HM, et al. (2012) Mixed antagonist response and sepsis severity-dependent dysbalance of pro-and anti-inflammatory responses at the onset of postoperative sepsis. Immunobiology 217: 616–621.

97. Tamayo E, Fernández A, Almansa R, Carrasco E, Heredia M, et al. (2011) Pro-and anti-inflammatory responses are regulated simultaneously from the first moments of septic shock. European cytokine network 22: 82–87.

98. Stoll LL, Denning GM, Weintraub NL (2006) Endotoxin, TLR4 signaling and vascular inflammation: potential therapeutic targets in cardiovascular disease. Current pharmaceutical design 12: 4229–4245.

99. Solodova E, Jablonska J, Weiss S, Lienenklaus S (2011) Production of IFN-β during *Listeria monocytogenes* Infection Is Restricted to Monocyte/Macrophage Lineage. PLoS One 6: e18543.

100. Pontiroli F, Dussurget O, Zanoni I, Urbano M, Beretta O, et al. (2012) The Timing of IFNβ Production Affects Early Innate Responses to Listeria monocytogenes and Determines the Overall Outcome of Lethal Infection. PloS one 7: e43455.

101. Fan H, Cook JA (2004) Review: Molecular mechanisms of endotoxin tolerance. Journal of endotoxin research 10: 71–84.

102. Netea MG, van der Meer JW, van Deuren M, Jan Kullberg B (2003) Proinflammatory cytokines and sepsis syndrome: not enough, or too much of a good thing? Trends in immunology 24: 254–258.

103. Fitzgerald KA, Rowe DC, Barnes BJ, Caffrey DR, Visintin A, et al. (2003) LPS-TLR4 Signaling to IRF-3/7 and NF-κB Involves the Toll Adapters TRAM and TRIF. The Journal of experimental medicine 198: 1043–1055.

104. Kim TW, Staschke K, Bulek K, Yao J, Peters K, et al. (2007) A critical role for IRAK4 kinase activity in Toll-like receptor–mediated innate immunity. The Journal of experimental medicine 204: 1025–1036.

105. Kobayashi T, Walsh MC, Choi Y (2004) The role of TRAF6 in signal transduction and the immune response. Microbes and infection 6: 1333–1338.

106. Sato S, Sanjo H, Takeda K, Ninomiya-Tsuji J, Yamamoto M, et al. (2005) Essential function for the kinase TAK1 in innate and adaptive immune responses. Nature immunology 6: 1087–1095.

107. Caamano J, Hunter CA (2002) NF-κB family of transcription factors: central regulators of innate and adaptive immune functions. Clinical microbiology reviews 15: 414–429.

108. Heyninck K, Beyaert R (1999) The cytokine-inducible zinc finger protein A20 inhibits IL-1-induced NF-[kappa] B activation at the level of TRAF6. FEBS Letters 442: 147–150.

109. Vallabhapurapu S, Karin M (2009) Regulation and function of NF-κB transcription factors in the immune system. Annual review of immunology 27: 693–733.

110. Hanada T, Yoshimura A (2002) Regulation of cytokine signaling and inflammation. Cytokine & growth factor reviews 13: 413–421.

111. Cusson-Hermance N, Khurana S, Lee TH, Fitzgerald KA, Kelliher MA (2005) Rip1 mediates the Trif-dependent toll-like receptor 3-and 4-induced NF-κB activation but does not contribute to interferon regulatory factor 3 activation. Journal of Biological Chemistry 280: 36560–36566.

112. Lu Y-C, Yeh W-C, Ohashi PS (2008) LPS/TLR4 signal transduction pathway. Cytokine 42: 145–151.

113. Nagpal K, Plantinga TS, Wong J, Monks BG, Gay NJ, et al. (2009) A TIR domain variant of MyD88 adapter-like (Mal)/TIRAP results in loss of MyD88 binding and reduced TLR2/TLR4 signaling. Journal of Biological Chemistry 284: 25742–25748.

114. Takeuchi O, Hoshino K, Kawai T, Sanjo H, Takada H, et al. (1999) Differential roles of TLR2 and TLR4 in recognition of gram-negative and gram-positive bacterial cell wall components. Immunity 11: 443–451.

115. Toshchakov V, Jones BW, Perera P-Y, Thomas K, Cody MJ, et al. (2002) TLR4, but not TLR2, mediates IFN-[beta]-induced STAT1[alpha]/[beta]-dependent gene expression in macrophages. Nat Immunol 3: 392–398.

116. Zughaier SM, Zimmer SM, Datta A, Carlson RW, Stephens DS (2005) Differential induction of the toll-like receptor 4-MyD88-dependent and-independent signaling pathways by endotoxins. Infection and immunity 73: 2940–2950.

117. Akira S, Uematsu S, Takeuchi O (2006) Pathogen recognition and innate immunity. Cell 124: 783–801.

4

Serum Levels of Caspase-Cleaved Cytokeratin-18 and Mortality Are Associated in Severe Septic Patients

Leonardo Lorente[1]*, **María M. Martín**[2], **Agustín F. González-Rivero**[3], **José Ferreres**[4], **Jordi Solé-Violán**[5], **Lorenzo Labarta**[6], **César Díaz**[7], **Alejandro Jiménez**[8], **Juan M. Borreguero-León**[3]

1 Intensive Care Unit, Hospital Universitario de Canarias, La Laguna, Tenerife, Spain, 2 Intensive Care Unit, Hospital Universitario Nuestra Señora Candelaria, Santa Cruz Tenerife, Spain, 3 Laboratory Department, Hospital Universitario de Canarias, La Laguna, Tenerife, Spain, 4 Intensive Care Unit, Hospital Clínico Universitario de Valencia, Valencia, Spain, 5 Intensive Care Unit, Hospital Universitario Dr. Negrín, Las Palmas de Gran Canaria, Spain, 6 Intensive Care Unit, Hospital San Jorge, Huesca, Spain, 7 Intensive Care Unit, Hospital Insular, Las Palmas de Gran Canaria, Spain, 8 Research Unit, Hospital Universitario de Canarias, La Laguna, Tenerife, Spain

Abstract

Objective: Apoptosis is increased in sepsis. Cytokeratin 18 (CK-18), a protein of the intermediate filament group present in most epithelial and parenchymal cells, is cleaved by the action of caspases and released into the blood as caspase-cleaved CK (CCCK)-18 during apoptosis. Circulating levels of CCCK-18 have scarcely been explored in septic patients. In one study with 101 severe septic patients, the authors reported higher serum CCCK-18 levels in non-survivors than in survivors; however, the sample size was too small to demonstrate an association between serum CCCK-18 levels and early mortality and whether they could be used as a biomarker to predict outcomes in septic patients. Thus, these were the objectives of this study with a large series of patients.

Methods: We performed a prospective, multicenter, observational study in six Spanish Intensive Care Units with 224 severe septic patients. Blood samples were collected at the time that severe sepsis was diagnosed to determine serum levels of CCCK-18, tumor necrosis factor (TNF)-alpha, interleukin (IL)-6 and IL-10. The end point was 30-day mortality.

Results: Non-surviving patients (n = 80) showed higher serum CCCK-18 levels ($P<0.001$) than survivors (n = 144). Multiple logistic regression analysis showed that serum CCCK-18 levels>391 u/L were associated with 30-day survival (Odds ratio = 2.687; 95% confidence interval = 1.449–4.983; $P = 0.002$), controlling for SOFA score, serum lactic acid levels and age. Kaplan-Meier survival analysis showed that the risk of death in septic patients with serum CCCK-18 levels >391 u/L was higher than in patients with lower values (Hazard Ratio = 3.1; 95% CI = 1.96–4.84; $P<0.001$). Serum CCCK-18 levels were positively associated with serum levels of IL-6 and lactic acid, and with SOFA and APACHE scores.

Conclusions: The major novel finding of our study, the largest cohort of septic patients providing data on circulating CCCK-18 levels, was that serum CCCK-18 levels are associated with mortality in severe septic patients.

Editor: Cordula M. Stover, University of Leicester, United Kingdom

Funding: This study was supported in part by grants from Instituto de Salud Carlos III (FIS-PI-10-01572, I3SNS-INT-11-063, and I3SNS-INT-12-087) (Madrid, Spain) and co-financed by Fondo Europeo de Desarrollo Regional (FEDER). The funders had no role in study design, data collection and analysis, decision to publish, or preparation of the manuscript.

Competing Interests: The authors have declared that no competing interests exist.

* Email: lorentemartin@msn.com

Introduction

Severe sepsis is a common, expensive, and frequently fatal condition [1,2]. The apoptotic process is one in which cells are actively eliminated via a programmed pathway during morpho-genesis, tissue remodeling, and the resolution of the immune response. Apoptosis is increased in sepsis and could contribute to multiple organ failure and death of septic patients [3–6].

Cytokeratin 18 (CK-18) is a protein of the intermediate filament group present in most epithelial and parenchymal cells [7]. During apoptosis CK-18 is cleaved at various sites by the action of caspases, and the resulting fragments are released into the blood

[8]. Full-length CK-18 is released into the blood plasma during necrosis, and CK-18 fragments are released during apoptosis. Determination of CK-18 fragments can be carried out by using a monoclonal antibody (M30) that recognizes caspase-cleaved CK-18 fragments, containing the CK-18 Asp 396 neoepitope, without detecting native or intact CK-18 [9,10].

Circulating levels of caspase-cleaved CK (CCCK)-18 has been studied in patients with liver [11–14], tumoral [15,16] and graft-versus-host [17] diseases. However, it has scarcely been explored in septic patients [18–20]. These studies found higher blood CCCK- 18 levels in septic patients than in healthy controls

[18–20]. In one study with 101 severe septic patients, higher serum CCCK-18 levels were found in non-survivors than in survivors [20]; however, the sample size was too small to demonstrate an association between serum CCCK-18 levels and early mortality and whether they could be used as a biomarker to predict outcomes in septic patients. Thus, the objective of this study was to determine whether there is an association between serum CCCK-18 levels and mortality and whether they could be used as a biomarker to predict outcomes in a large series of patients.

Methods

Design and Subjects

A prospective, multicenter, observational study was carried out in six Spanish Intensive Care Units between 2008–2009. The study was approved by the Institutional Ethic Review Boards of the six participating hospitals: Hospital Universitario de Canarias (La Laguna. Tenerife. Spain), Hospital Universitario Nuestra Señora de Candelaria (Santa Cruz de Tenerife. Spain), Hospital Universitario Dr. Negrín (Las Palmas de Gran Canaria. Spain), Hospital Clínico Universitario de Valencia (Valencia. Spain), Hospital San Jorge (Huesca. Spain) and Hospital Insular (Las Palmas de Gran Canaria. Spain). Written informed consent from the patients or from their family members was obtained.

A total of 224 patients with severe sepsis were included. The inclusion criteria used for severe sepsis were those defined by the International Sepsis Definitions Conference [21]. The exclusion criteria were: age <18 years, pregnancy, lactation, human immunodeficiency virus (HIV), white blood cell count <1,000/μl, solid or hematological tumor, or immunosuppressive, steroid or radiation therapy.

Variables recorded

The following variables were recorded for each patient: sex, age, diabetes mellitus, chronic renal failure defined as glomerular filtration rate (GFR) <60 ml/min per 1.73 m^2, chronic obstructive pulmonary disease (COPD), site of infection, microorganism responsible, bloodstream infection, empiric antimicrobial treatment, pressure of arterial oxygen/fraction inspired of oxygen (PaO$_2$/FIO$_2$), creatinine, bilirubin, leukocytes, lactic acid, platelets, international normalized ratio (INR), activated partial thromboplastin time (aPTT), Acute Physiology and Chronic Health Evaluation II (APACHE II) score [22] and Sepsis-related Organ Failure Assessment [SOFA] score [23].

End-point

The end-point of the study was 30-day mortality.

Blood samples

Blood samples from 224 patients were collected at the time severe sepsis was diagnosed. Serum was allowed to clot for 10 minutes at room temperature, then centrifuged at 1000 × g for 15 minutes and the supernatant was immediately stored in aliquot at −80°C to the end of the recruitment process. All determinations were performed by laboratory technicians blinded to all clinical data. Assays were performed at the Laboratory Department of the Hospital Universitario de Canarias (La Laguna, Santa Cruz de Tenerife, Spain).

Serum CCCK-18 analysis

CCCK-18 levels were measured in serum by enzyme-linked immunosorbent assay (ELISA) using M30 Apoptosense ELISA, PEVIVA AB (Bromma, Sweden), lot PE-0133. The M30 antibody recognises a neo-epitope exposed after caspase cleavage of K18 after the aspartic acid residue 396. M30 Apoptosense ELISA measures detects soluble caspase-cleaved K18 (ccK18) fragments containing the K18Asp396 neo-epitope. M30-antigen levels are expressed as U/l. The intra- and inter-assay coefficients of variation (CV) were <10%. The detection limit for the assay was 25 U/L.

Serum levels of tumor necrosis factor (TNF)-alpha, interleukin (IL)-6 and IL-10 analysis

TNF-alpha, IL-6 and IL-10 were measured in serum by solid-phase chemiluminescent immunometric assays (Immulite, Siemens Healthcare Diagnostics Products, Llanberis, United Kingdom). The intra-assay CV were 3.6%, 6.2%, and 9.9%, respectively. The interassay CV were 6.5%, 7.5%, and 9.9%, respectively. The detection limits for the assays were 1.7 pg/ml, 2.0 pg/ml and 1 pg/ml respectively.

Statistical Methods

Continuous variables are reported as medians and interquartile ranges. Categorical variables are reported as frequencies and percentages. Comparisons of continuous variables between groups were carried out using Mann-Whitney U test. Comparisons between groups for categorical variables were carried out with chi-square test. We plotted a receiver operating characteristic (ROC) curve using survival at 30 days as the classification variable, and serum CCCK-18 levels as the prognostic variable. Analysis of survival at 30 days with Kaplan-Meier method curve and comparisons by log-rank test were carried out using serum CCCK-18 levels lower/higher than 391 u/L as the independent variable, and survival at 30 days as the dependent variable. We used dot-plot to represent serum caspase-cleaved citokeratin (CCCK)-18 levels in 30-day surviving and non-surviving septic patients. Multiple logistic regression analysis was carried out to test the independent contribution of serum CCCK-18 levels higher than 391 u/L on the prediction of 30-day mortality, controlling for SOFA score, lactic acid levels and age. Odds ratio and 95% confidence intervals (CI) were calculated as measures of the clinical impact of the predictor variables. Wald test was calculated for each variable included in the regression model. We used Spearman's rank correlation coefficient to determine the association between continuous variables. A P value of less than 0.05 was considered statistically significant. Statistical analyses were performed with SPSS 17.0 (SPSS Inc., Chicago, IL, USA) and NCSS 2000 (Kaysville, Utah).

Results

Table 1 shows the comparison of demographic and clinical parameters between surviving (n = 144) and non-surviving (n = 80) septic patients. We found that non-surviving septic patients showed higher age, creatinine, lactic acid, INR, aPTT, SOFA and APACHE-II scores, and lower platelet count than surviving patients. In addition, non-surviving septic patients showed higher serum levels of CCCK-18 (P<0.001), IL-6 (P = 0.001) and IL-10 (P = 0.002) than survivors. No differences were observed regarding sex, diabetes mellitus, chronic renal failure, COPD, ischemic heart disease, site of infection, microorganism responsible, bloodstream infection, antimicrobial treatment and serum levels of TNF-α.

Multiple logistic regression analysis showed that serum CCCK-18 levels>391 u/L were associated with 30-day survival (Odds ratio = 2.687; 95% CI = 1.449–4.983; P = 0.002), controlling for SOFA score, serum lactic acid levels and age (Table 2).

Table 1. Patients'demographic and clinical characteristics.

	Survival (n = 144)	Non-survival (n = 80)	p-value
Sex male – n (%)	93 (64.6)	54 (67.5)	0.77
Age - median years (p 25–75)	55 (44–66)	64 (56–74)	<0.001
Diabetes mellitus – n (%)	40 (27.8)	31 (38.8)	0.10
Chronic renal failure – n (%)	8 (5.6)	8 (10.0)	0.28
COPD – n (%)	15 (10.4)	12 (15.0)	0.39
Ischemic heart disease - n (%)	13 (9.0)	5 (6.3)	0.61
Site of infection			0.68
Respiratory - n (%)	81 (56.3)	48 (60.0)	
Abdominal - n (%)	38 (26.4)	21 (26.3)	
Neurological	3 (2.1)	0	
Urinary - n (%)	8 (5.6)	4 (5.0)	
Skin - n (%)	8 (5.6)	3 (3.8)	
Endocarditis - n (%)	6 (4.2)	4 (5.0)	
Microorganism responsibles			
Unknwon - n (%	75 (52.1)	43 (53.8)	0.89
Gram-positive- n (%)	33 (22.9)	21 (26.3)	0.63
Gram-negative- n (%)	35 (24.3)	16 (20.0)	0.51
Fungii- n (%)	4 (2.8)	4 (5.0)	0.46
Anaerobe- n (%)	1 (0.7)	1 (1.3)	0.99
Bloodstream infection - n (%)	22 (15.3)	11 (13.8)	0.85
Empiric antimicrobial treatment adequate			0.96
Unknown due to negative cultures- n (%)	75 (52.1)	43 (53.8)	
Adequate - n (%)	58 (40.3)	30 (37.5)	
Unknown due to antigenuria diagnosis-n(%)	4 (2.8)	3 (3.8)	
Inadequate- n (%)	7 (4.9)	4 (5.0)	
Betalactamic plus aminoglycoside - n (%) (%)aminoglycoside- n (%)	29 (20.1)	20 (25.0)	0.40
Betalactamic plus quinolone - n (%)	79 (54.9)	43 (53.8)	0.89
PaO$_2$/FIO$_2$ ratio - median (p 25–75)	170 (113–262)	180 (100–244)	0.38
Creatinine (mg/dl) - median (p 25–75)	1.20 (0.80–1.95)	1.50 (0.90–2.75)	0.02
Bilirubin (mg/dl) - median (p 25–75)	0.90 (0.44–1.53)	1.00 (0.47–2.44)	0.60
Leukocytes (cells/mm^3) - median*10^3 (p 25–75)	15.2 (10.0–20.7)	15.3 (9.4–21.3)	0.88
Lactic acid (mmol/L) - median (p 25–75)	1.80 (1.05–3.50)	3.50 (1.45–5.95)	<0.001
Platelets (cells/mm^3) - median*10^3 (p 25–75)	192 (130–273)	124 (76–222)	<0.001
INR - median (p 25–75)	1.27 (1.10–1.53)	1.42 (1.16–1.90)	0.01
aPTT (seconds) - median (p 25–75)	32 (28–42)	38 (29–46)	0.01
SOFA score - median (p 25–75)	9 (7–11)	11 (9–15)	<0.001
APACHE-II score - median (p 25–75)	18 (14–22)	23 (18–28)	<0.001
CCCK-18 (U/l) - median (p 25–75)	311 (230–443)	453 (311–711)	<0.001
TNF-alpha - median pg/ml (percentile 25–75)	31.8 (20.0–51.2)	39.4 (18.7–76.8)	0.29
Interleukin-6 - median pg/ml (percentile 25–75)	104 (42–578)	504 (58–1000)	0.001
Interleukin-10 median pg/ml (percentile 25–75)	10.4 (5.7–38.0)	52.0 (8.4–162.5)	0.002

COPD = Chronic Obstructive Pulmonary Disease; PaO$_2$/FIO$_2$ = pressure of arterial oxygen/fraction inspired oxygen; aPTT = Activated partial thromboplastin time; INR = International normalized ratio; Acute Physiology and Chronic Health Evaluation (APACHE)-II score; SOFA = Sepsis-related Organ Failure Assessment; CCCK = caspase-cleaved citokeratin; TNF = tumor necrosis factor (TNF)-alpha; data are presented as number (percentage) or median (interquartile range).

Receiver Operating Characteristic (ROC) analysis showed that the area under curve of serum CCCK-18 levels to predict 30-day survival was 0.71 (95% CI = 0.64–0.76; $P<0.001$) (Figure 1).

Kaplan-Meier survival analysis showed that the risk of death in septic patients with serum CCCK-18 levels above 391 u/L was higher than in patients with lower values (Hazard Ratio = 3.1; 95% CI = 1.96–4.84; $P<0.001$) (Figure 2).

Table 2. Multiple logistic regression analyses to predict survival at 30 days.

	Wald test	Odds Ratio	95% Confidence Interval	P-value
Serum CCCK-18 levels>391 u/L	9.83	2.687	1.449–4.983	0.002
SOFA score	6.45	1.125	1.027–1.232	0.01
Serum lactic acid levels (mmol/L)	2.98	1.108	0.986–1.246	0.08
Age (years)	5.61	1.027	1.005–1.050	0.02

CCCK = caspase-cleaved citokeratin; SOFA = Sepsis-related Organ Failure Assessment.

We ploted serum caspase-cleaved citokeratin (CCCK)-18 levels in 30-day surviving and non-surviving septic patients (Figure 3).

We found that survival patients at 30 days with serum CCCK-18 levels above 391 u/L at the time that severe sepsis was diagnosed showed higher ICU stay that patients with lower values [24 (12–46) vs 15 (7–31) days; p = 0.04].

Serum CCCK-18 levels were positively associated with serum levels of IL-6 and lactic acid, and with SOFA and APACHE scores (Table 3).

We found that patients with liver dysfunction showed higher serum CCCK-18 levels than patients without it [413 (278–626) vs 327 (251–500) U/l; p = 0.01], and that patients with kidney dysfunction showed higher serum CCCK-18 levels than patients without it [398 (280–628) vs 318 (237–450) U/l; p<0.001].

Discussion

To our knowledge, this study includes the largest series providing data on circulating CCCK-18 levels in septic patients. The major novel findings of our study were that serum CCCK-18 levels are associated with mortality and could be used as a biomarker to predict outcomes in septic patients.

We found higher serum CCCK-18 levels in non-surviving septic patients than in survivors. These findings are in consonance with those of a study by Hofer et al. with 101 severe septic [20]; however, the sample size in that study was too small to demonstrate whether serum CCCK-18 levels are associated with mortality. The greater sample size of our study enabled us to carry out multiple regression analysis and showed, for the first time, that serum CK-18 levels are associated with mortality in septic patients. The advantage of measuring serum CCCK-18 levels to predict

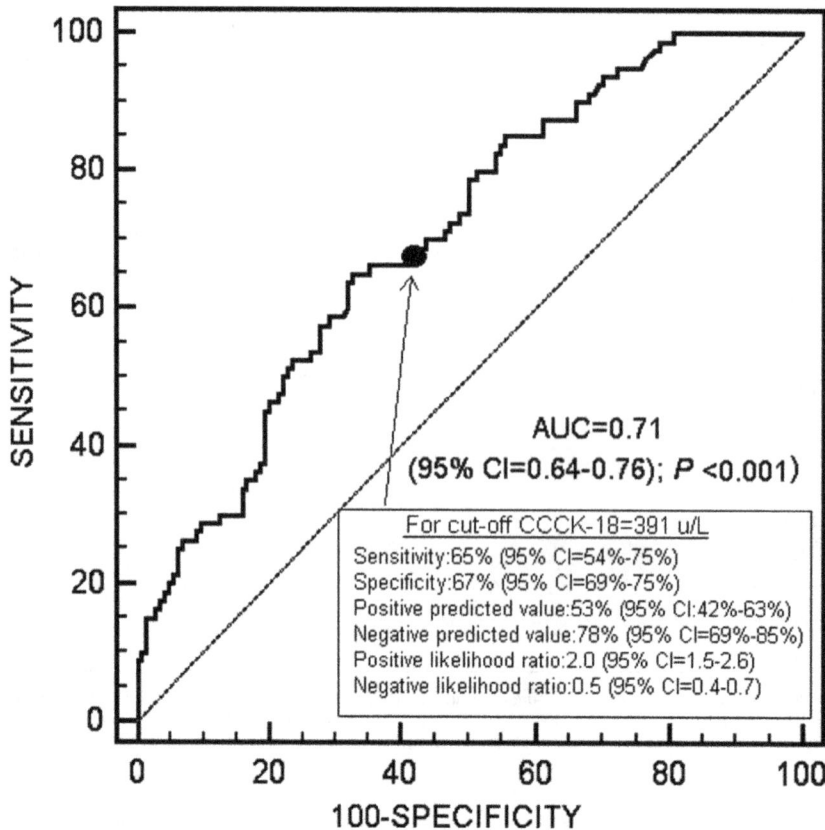

Figure 1. Receiver operation characteristic analysis using serum caspase-cleaved cytokeratin (CCCK)-18 levels as predictor of mortality at 30 days.

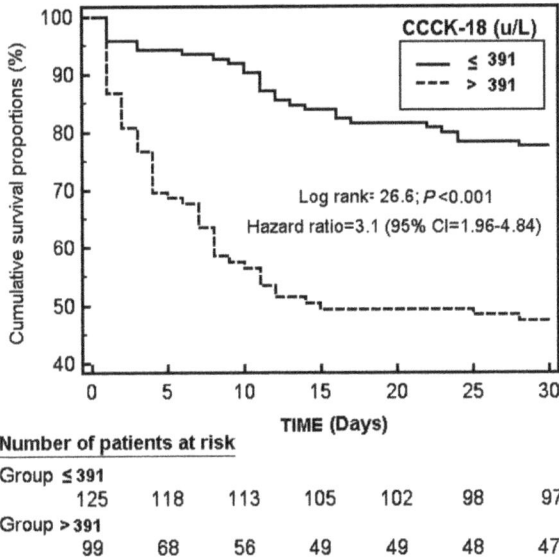

Figure 2. Survival curves at 30 days using serum caspase-cleaved citokeratin (CCCK)-18 levels higher or lower than 391 u/L.

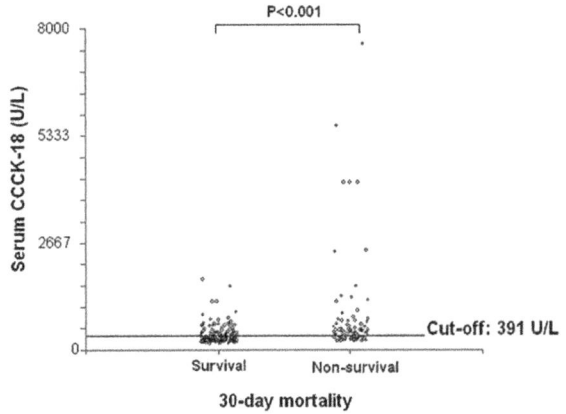

Figure 3. Dot-plot of serum caspase-cleaved citokeratin (CCCK)-18 levels in 30-day surviving and non-surviving septic patients.

survival at 30 days compared with SOFA score underlies in a higher predictive value measured with the Wald test.

Another interesting new finding of our study, according to the results of ROC curve analysis, was that serum CK-18 levels could be used as a biomarker to predict outcomes in septic patients.

Hofer et al. found an association between serum CCCK-18 and lactate levels [20]. In our study, we also found this association. In addition, we found an association between serum CCCK-18 levels and other measures of sepsis severity, such as SOFA and APACHE-II scores for the first time.

Taken together, these results indicate that serum CCCK-18 levels may be of great pathophysiological significance in septic patients and that apoptosis could contribute to multiple organ failure and death of septic patients. Apoptotic cell death occurs primarily through three different pathways: the extrinsic death receptor pathway (type I cells), the intrinsic (mitochondrial) pathway (type II cells) and the endoplasmic reticulum or stress-induced pathway [3–6]. In type I cells, apoptosis is initiated by the activation of a surface death receptor of tumor necrosis factor receptor superfamily (TNFRSF) by its cognate death ligand (TNFSF). In type II cells, the initiation of apoptosis can be activated by cytokines such as interleukin (IL)-1 and IL-6, oxygen free radicals and nitric oxide (NO); and could be reduced by the activation of anti-apoptotic members of the Bcl-2 family by means of IL-10. The death signal is transduced, then a cascade of caspases leads to cell death. During this caspase activation, CK-18 is cleaved and CCCK-18 is released into the blood. In our study, we found an association between serum CCCK-18 and Il-6 levels; however, we did not find an association between serum CCCK-18 and TNF-alpha and IL-10 levels.

From a therapeutic perspective, the development of modulators of apoptotic activity could be used as a new class of drugs for the treatment of severe sepsis. In septic rats, the administration of modulators of apoptotic activity has been found to reduce apoptosis and increase survival rates [24–26].

The strengths of our study are that it was a multicenter study (which increases the external applicability of results to other similar units) and the large sample size (which allowed us to carry

out multiple logistic regression analysis to determine the association between serum CCCK-18 levels and mortality). However, some limitations of our study should be recognized. First, no analysis of serum CCCK-18 levels during follow-up was performed. Second, measuring other inducers of apoptosis and compounds of apoptosis would be desirable in order to better evaluate the relationship with these aspects. Third, we did not determine serum CCCK-18 levels in control groups, such as patients with non-infectious systemic inflammatory response syndrome, and this would have been interesting to assess whether CCCK-18 measurements might be useful for early diagnosis of sepsis. Four, the determination of total serum CCCK-18 levels by M65 ELISA or M65 EpiDeath ELISA would have been interesting in order to quantify the leading mode of cell death (apoptosis or necrosis).

Conclusions

The major novel finding of our study, the largest cohort of septic patients providing data on circulating CCCK-18 levels, was that serum CCCK-18 levels are associated with mortality in severe septic patients.

Table 3. Correlation of serum caspase-cleaved citokeratin (CCCK)-18 levels with serum levels of TNF-α, interleukin-6, interleukin-10, and lactic acid, and with SOFA and APACHE-II scores.

	rho	P-value
TNF-α	0.09	0.31
Interleukin-6	0.15	0.03
Interleukin-10	0.11	0.21
Lactic acid (mmol/L)	0.20	0.003
SOFA score	0.27	<0.001
APACHE score	0.30	<0.001

TNF = tumor necrosis factor; SOFA = Sepsis-related Organ Failure Assessment score; APACHE = Acute Physiology and Chronic Health Evaluation (APACHE)-II score; rho = Spearman's rank correlation coefficient.

Author Contributions

Conceived and designed the experiments: L. Lorente. Performed the experiments: L. Lorente MMM JF JSV L. Labarta CD AFGR JMBL.

Analyzed the data: L. Lorente AJ. Contributed reagents/materials/analysis tools: AFGR JMBL. Contributed to the writing of the manuscript: L. Lorente.

References

1. Vincent JL, Sakr Y, Sprung CL, Ranieri VM, Reinhart K, et al. (2006) Sepsis in European intensive care units: results of the SOAP study. Crit Care Med 34: 344–353.
2. Angus DC, Linde-Zwirble WT, Lidicker J, Clermont G, Carcillo J, et al. (2001) Epidemiology of severe sepsis in the United States: analysis of incidence, outcome, and associated costs of care. Crit Care Med 29: 1303–1310.
3. Fischer U, Schulze-Osthoff K (2005) Apoptosis-based therapies and drug targets. Cell Death Differ 12 Suppl 1: 942–961.
4. Wesche-Soldato DE, Swan RZ, Chung CS, Ayala A (2007) The apoptotic pathway as a therapeutic target in sepsis. Curr Drug Targets 8: 493–500.
5. Huttunen R, Aittoniemi J (2011) New concepts in the pathogenesis, diagnosis and treatment of bacteremia and sepsis. J Infect 63: 407–419.
6. Harjai M, Bogra J, Kohli M, Pant AB (2013) Is suppression of apoptosis a new therapeutic target in sepsis? Anaesth Intensive Care 41: 175–183.
7. Chu PG, Weiss LM (2002) Keratin expression in human tissues and neoplasms. Histopathology 40: 403–439.
8. Caulín C, Salvesen GS, Oshima RG (1997) Caspase cleavage of keratin 18 and reorganization of intermediate filaments during epithelial cell apoptosis. J Cell Biol 138: 1379–1394.
9. Leers MP, Kölgen W, Björklund V, Bergman T, Tribbick G, et al. (1999) Immunocytochemical detection and mapping of a cytokeratin 18 neo-epitope exposed during early apoptosis. J Pathol 187: 567–572.
10. Hägg M, Bivén K, Ueno T, Rydlander L, Björklund P, et al. (2002) A novel high-through-put assay for screening of pro-apoptotic drugs. Invest New Drugs 20: 253–259.
11. Bantel H, Lügering A, Heidemann J, Volkmann X, Poremba C, et al. (2004) Detection of apoptotic caspase activation in sera from patients with chronic HCV infection is associated with fibrotic liver injury. Hepatology 40: 1078–1087.
12. Sgier C, Müllhaupt B, Gerlach T, Moradpour D, Negro F, et al. (2010) Effect of antiviral therapy on circulating cytokeratin-18 fragments in patients with chronic hepatitis C. J Viral Hepat 17: 845–850.
13. Sumer S, Aktug Demir N, Kölgelier S, Cagkan Inkaya A, Arpaci A, et al. (2013) The Clinical Significance of Serum Apoptotic Cytokeratin 18 Neoepitope M30 (CK-18 M30) and Matrix Metalloproteinase 2 (MMP-2) Levels in Chronic Hepatitis B Patients with Cirrhosis. Hepat Mon 13: e10106.
14. Parfieniuk-Kowerda A, Lapinski TW, Rogalska-Plonska M, Swiderska M, Panasiuk A, et al. (2014) Serum cytochrome c and m30-neoepitope of cytokeratin-18 in chronic hepatitis C. Liver Int 34: 544–550.
15. Ueno T, Toi M, Bivén K, Bando H, Ogawa T, et al. (2003) Measurement of an apoptotic product in the sera of breast cancer patients. Eur J Cancer 39: 769–774.
16. Greystoke A, O'Connor JP, Linton K, Taylor MB, Cummings J, et al. (2011) Assessment of circulating biomarkers for potential pharmacodynamic utility in patients with lymphoma. Br J Cancer 104: 719–725.
17. Luft T, Conzelmann M, Benner A, Rieger M, Hess M, et al. (2007) Serum cytokeratin-18 fragments as quantitative markers of epithelial apoptosis in liver and intestinal graft-versus-host disease. Blood 110: 4535–4542.
18. Roth GA, Krenn C, Brunner M, Moser B, Ploder M, et al. (2004) Elevated serum levels of epithelial cell apoptosis-specific cytokeratin 18 neoepitope m30 in critically ill patients. Shock 22: 218–220.
19. Moore DJ, Greystoke A, Butt F, Wurthner J, Growcott J, et al. (2012) A pilot study assessing the prognostic value of CK18 and nDNA biomarkers in severe sepsis patients. Clin Drug Investig 32: 179–187.
20. Hofer S, Brenner T, Bopp C, Steppan J, Lichtenstern C, et al. (2009) Cell death serum biomarkers are early predictors for survival in severe septic patients with hepatic dysfunction. Crit Care 13: R93.
21. Levy MM, Fink MP, Marshall JC, Abraham E, Angus D, et al. (2003) International Sepsis Definitions Conference: 2001 SCCM/ESICM/ACCP/ATS/SIS International Sepsis Definitions Conference. Intensive Care Med 29: 530–538.
22. Knaus WA, Draper EA, Wagner DP, Zimmerman JE (1985) APACHE II: a severity of disease classification system. Crit Care Med 13: 818–829.
23. Vincent JL, Moreno R, Takala J, Willatts S, De Mendonça A, et al. for the Working Group on Sepsis-related Problems of the European Society of Intensive Care Medicine (1996) The Sepsis-related Organ Failure Assessment (SOFA) score to describe organ dysfunction/failure. Intensive Care Med 22: 707–710.
24. Hotchkiss RS, Chang KC, Swanson PE, Tinsley KW, Hui JJ, et al. (2000) Caspase inhibitors improve survival in sepsis: a critical role of the lymphocyte. Nat Immunol 1: 496–501.
25. Chung CS, Song GY, Lomas J, Simms HH, Chaudry IH, et al. (2003) Inhibition of Fas/Fas ligand signaling improves septic survival: differential effects on macrophage apoptotic and functional capacity. J Leukoc Biol 74: 344–351.
26. Wesche-Soldato DE, Chung CS, Lomas-Neira J, Doughty LA, Gregory SH, et al. (2005) In vivo delivery of caspase-8 or Fas siRNA improves the survival of septic mice. Blood 106: 2295–2301.

5

An Increase in CD3+CD4+CD25+ Regulatory T Cells after Administration of Umbilical Cord-Derived Mesenchymal Stem Cells during Sepsis

Yu-Hua Chao[1,2,3], Han-Ping Wu[4,5♋], Kang-Hsi Wu[6,7♋], Yi-Giien Tsai[3,8,9], Ching-Tien Peng[6,7,10], Kuan-Chia Lin[11,12], Wan-Ru Chao[1,3,13], Maw-Sheng Lee[1,14]*, Yun-Ching Fu[15,16]*

1 Institute of Medicine, Chung Shan Medical University, Taichung, Taiwan, 2 Department of Pediatrics, Chung Shan Medical University Hospital, Taichung, Taiwan, 3 School of Medicine, Chung Shan Medical University, Taichung, Taiwan, 4 Department of Pediatrics, Taichung Tzuchi Hospital, the Buddhist Medical Foundation, Taichung, Taiwan, 5 Department of Medicine, Tzu Chi University, Hualien, Taiwan, 6 School of Chinese Medicine, China Medical University, Taichung, Taiwan, 7 Department of Hemato-oncology, Children's Hospital, China Medical University Hospital, China Medical University, Taichung, Taiwan, 8 Departments of Pediatrics, Changhua Christian Hospital, Changhua, Taiwan, 9 School of Medicine, Kaohsiung Medical University, Kaohsiung, Taiwan, 10 Department of Biotechnology and Bioinformatics, Asia University, Taichung, Taiwan, 11 School of Nursing, National Taipei University of Nursing and Health Sciences, Taipei, Taiwan, 12 Life-Course Epidemiology and Human Development Research Group, National Taipei University of Nursing and Health Sciences, Taipei, Taiwan, 13 Department of Pathology, Chung Shan Medical University Hospital, Taichung, Taiwan, 14 Department of Obstetrics and Gynecology, Chung Shan Medical University Hospital, Taichung, Taiwan, 15 Institute of Clinical Medicine, National Yang-Ming University, Taipei, Taiwan, 16 Department of Pediatrics, Taichung Veterans General Hospital, Taichung, Taiwan

Abstract

Sepsis remains an important cause of death worldwide, and vigorous immune responses during sepsis could be beneficial for bacterial clearance but at the price of collateral damage to self tissues. Mesenchymal stem cells (MSCs) have been found to modulate the immune system and attenuate sepsis. In the present study, MSCs derived from bone marrow and umbilical cord were used and compared. With a cecal ligation and puncture (CLP) model, the mechanisms of MSC-mediated immunoregulation during sepsis were studied by determining the changes of circulating inflammation-associated cytokine profiles and peripheral blood mononuclear cells 18 hours after CLP-induced sepsis. In vitro, bone marrow-derived MSCs (BMMSCs) and umbilical cord-derived MSCs (UCMSCs) showed a similar morphology and surface marker expression. UCMSCs had stronger potential for osteogenesis but lower for adipogenesis than BMMSCs. Compared with rats receiving PBS only after CLP, the percentage of circulating CD3+CD4+CD25+ regulatory T (Treg) cells and the ratio of Treg cells/T cells were elevated significantly in rats receiving MSCs. Further experiment regarding Treg cell function demonstrated that the immunosuppressive capacity of Treg cells from rats with CLP-induced sepsis was decreased, but could be restored by administration of MSCs. Compared with rats receiving PBS only after CLP, serum levels of interleukin-6 and tumor necrosis factor-α were significantly lower in rats receiving MSCs after CLP. There were no differences between BMMSCs and UCMSCs. In summary, this work provides the first in vivo evidence that administering BMMSCs or UCMSCs to rats with CLP-induced sepsis could increase circulating CD3+CD4+CD25+ Treg cells and Treg cells/T cells ratio, enhance Treg cell suppressive function, and decrease serum levels of interleukin-6 and tumor necrosis factor-α, suggesting the immunomodulatory association of Treg cells and MSCs during sepsis.

Editor: Jacques Zimmer, Centre de Recherche Public de la Santé (CRP-Santé), Luxembourg

Funding: The study was supported by the Chung Shan Medical University Hospital (CSH-2014-C-029), the China Medical University Hospital (DMR-103-037), the Research Laboratory of Pediatrics, Children's Hospital, China Medical University, and the Taiwan Ministry of Health and Welfare Clinical Trial and Research Center of Excellence (MOHW103-TDU-B-212-113002). The funders had no role in study design, data collection and analysis, decision to publish, or preparation of the manuscript.

Competing Interests: The authors declare that they have no conflicts of interest.

* Email: kso579@hotmail.com.tw (MSL); 8850ar@hotmail.com.tw (YCF)

♋ These authors contributed equally to this work.

Introduction

Even with standard therapeutic approaches, sepsis remains an important cause of mortality worldwide [1]. Under such conditions, vigorous immune responses could be beneficial for bacterial clearance. However, the hyperactive and out-of-balance network of cytokines may lead to tissue damage, multiple organ dysfunction and even death. Therefore, it is important to examine innovative and efficacious strategies to bring the immune responses back into balance to ultimately improve outcomes.

Mesenchymal stem cells (MSCs) have been a promising platform for cell-based therapy over the last decade. Apart from their capacity to differentiate into a variety of cell lineages and their clinical interest in tissue repair [2], MSCs have emerged as potent immune regulators [3–8]. Being receptive to excessive inflammation, MSCs would orchestrate the pathogen clearance through promotion of immune cell survival and function followed by suppression of the immune responses in the resolution of inflammation. Several studies demonstrated the beneficial effects of MSCs in septic animals [9–12], but the mechanisms of MSC-mediated regulation during sepsis are not fully elucidated.

In the present study, the immunomodulatory properties of MSCs were investigated using a well-established cecal ligation and puncture (CLP) murine model of polymicrobial sepsis. The mechanisms were studied by determining the changes of circulating inflammation-associated cytokine profiles and peripheral blood mononuclear cells after MSC administration during sepsis. Due to the limited data available regarding umbilical cord-derived MSCs (UCMSCs) for sepsis, MSCs derived from bone marrow and umbilical cord were used and compared.

Materials and Methods

Isolation of MSCs from bone marrow

The study was approved by the institutional review board of the Chung Shan Medical University Hospital (CSMUH No: CS13157). Bone marrow cells were obtained from iliac crest aspirates of healthy donors with written informed consents. Bone marrow-derived MSCs (BMMSCs) were isolated and cultured as our previous reports [13,14]. In brief, mononuclear cells were isolated by Ficoll-Paque density gradient centrifugation (1.077 g/ml; Amersham Biosciences, Uppsala, Sweden), and then seeded in low-glucose DMEM (Gibco, Gaithersburg, MD) supplemented with 10% fetal bovine serum (FBS; Gibco, Gaithersburg, MD) and 1% antibiotic-antimycotic (Gibco, Gaithersburg, MD). Cells were incubated at 37°C with 5% CO_2 in a humidified atmosphere. After 48 hours, non-adherent cells were washed out, and culture medium was changed twice per week thereafter.

Isolation of MSCs from umbilical cords

UCMSCs were collected and isolated as our previous reports [14–16]. Briefly, umbilical cord was obtained from full-term infants immediately after birth with written informed consents from the parents. The cord blood vessels were carefully removed to retain Wharton's jelly. Wharton's jelly was digested in 1 mg/ml collagenase (Sigma, St. Louis, MO), and then placed in α-MEM (Gibco, Carlsbad, CA) supplemented with FBS and antibiotic-antimycotic. After culture for 48 hours, medium with suspension of non-adherent cells was discarded and medium was replaced twice a week thereafter.

Identification of MSCs

When reaching 80–90% confluence, cultured cells were detached with trypsin-EDTA (Gibco, Carlsbad, CA) and replated at a density of 6×10^3 cells/cm^2 for subculture. MSCs, either BMMSCs or UCMSCs, of passage 5 were used for further studies.

To evaluate the expression of surface markers, cultured MSCs were detached, washed, and resuspended in phosphate-buffered saline (PBS; Gibco, Gaithersburg, MD). After fixing and blocking, the cells were immunolabeled with FITC or PE conjugated mouse antihuman antibodies specific to CD34, CD45, CD14, CD29, CD44, CD73, CD90, CD105, HLA-A, HLA-B, HLA-C or HLA-DR. The nonspecific mouse IgG served as isotype control. All reagents were purchased from BD Biosciences. Data were analyzed by flow cytometry (FACSCalibur; BD Biosciences, San Jose, CA) with CellQuest software.

To evaluate differentiation potential, cultured MSCs were detached from culture dishes and replated in 60-mm dishes. For induction of osteogenesis, MSCs were grown in DMEM with 10% FBS, 10 mM β-glycerophosphate (Sigma, St Louis, MO), 0.1 μM dexamethasone (Sigma, St Louis, MO), and 0.2 mM ascorbic acid

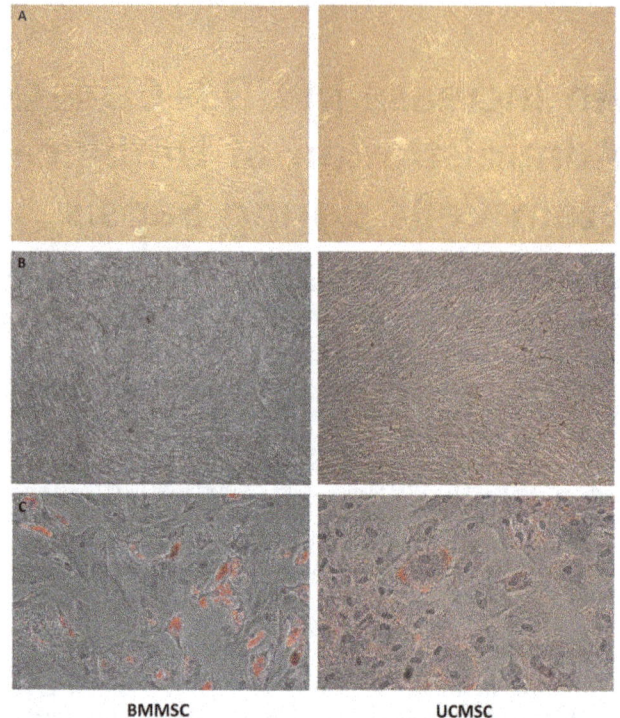

Figure 1. Comparison of BMMSCs and UCMSCs. (A) In vitro culture, BMMSCs and UCMSCs showed a similar spindle-shaped morphology (100×). **(B)** UCMSCs had stronger potential for osteogenesis than BMMSCs after 2-week induction (von Kossa staining, 100×). **(C)** UCMSCs had lower potential for adipogenesis than BMMSCs after 2-week adipogenic induction (Oil red O staining, 200×).

(Sigma, St Louis, MO). After 2 weeks, osteogenic differentiation was demonstrated by mineralized deposits stainable with von Kossa stain (Cedarlane, Ontario, Canada). To promote adipogenesis, MSCs were incubated in DMEM with 10% FBS, 1 μM dexamethasone, 0.5 mM 3-isobutyl-1-methylxanthine (Sigma, St Louis, MO), 0.1 mM indomethacin (Sigma, St Louis, MO), and 10 μg/ml insulin (Novo Nordisk A/S, Bagsværd, Denmark). After 2 weeks, adipogenic differentiation was demonstrated by intracellular accumulation of lipid droplets stainable with oil red O (Sigma, St Louis, MO).

CLP Model of polymicrobial sepsis in rats

The experimental protocol was approved by the Institutional Animal Care and Use Committee of the Chung Shan Medical University Experimental Animal Center (No: 1430). Male immune competent Wistar rats weighing 250 to 300 g were provided by the National Science Council. CLP, a well-established murine model of polymicrobial sepsis, leads to a focal inflammation and subsequently becomes systemic rapidly as a consequence of continuous dissemination of endogenous intestinal bacteria. This model closely resembles the septic process in humans [17,18], and thus was employed in our study. Briefly, rats were anesthetized by intramuscular injection of 75 mg/kg ketamine and 5 mg/kg xylazine. After laparotomy, the distal one half of the cecum was ligated with a 4–0 silk tie. A single through-and-through perforation was made in the ligated segment with a 18-gauge needle and a 1 mm column of fecal material was extruded through the puncture site. Then the cecum was replaced into abdomen and the abdominal incision was closed in two layers with 3–0 silk

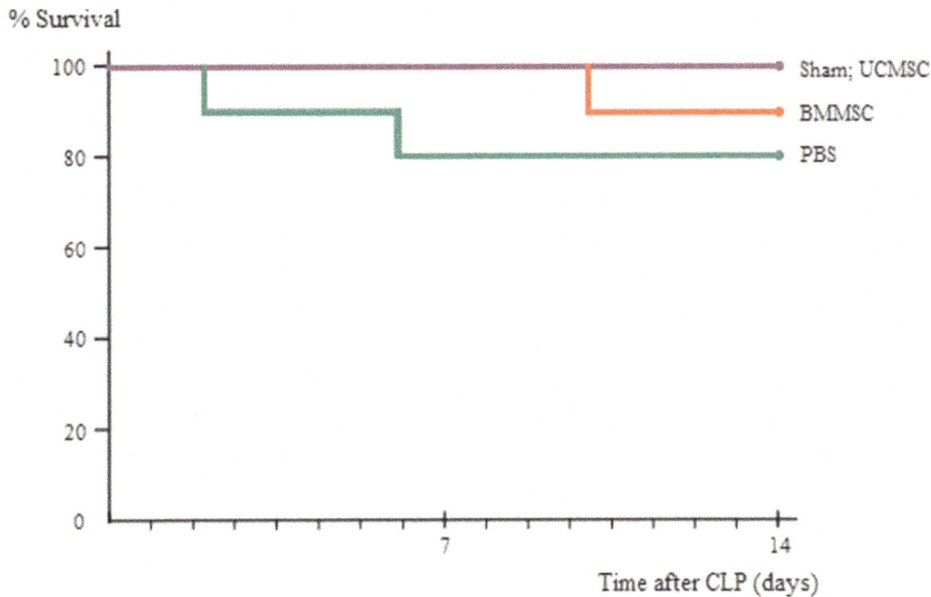

Figure 2. The beneficial effects from MSC administration on survival in rats with CLP-induced sepsis. Survival was evaluated for 14 days. Although no statistical significance, it appeared that rats receiving UCMSCs or BMMSCs after CLP had lower mortality rates than rats receiving PBS only after CLP. n = 10 rats/group.

sutures. Sham-operated rats underwent the same procedure, including opening the peritoneum and exposing the bowel, but without ligation and needle perforation of the cecum.

Administration of MSCs after CLP

To assess the effects of MSC administration after CLP-induced polymicrobial sepsis, rats of BMMSC and UCMSC groups received five millions BMMSCs and UCMSCs in 0.3 ml sterile PBS via the tail vein 4 hours after CLP, respectively. In vitro cultured BMMSCs and UCMSCs of passage 5 were used in this study. In PBS group and sham control group, sterile PBS in a volume of 0.3 ml with no cells was administered at the same time point. Depending on the experiment, rats were either euthanized at 18 hours after surgery to harvest blood and organs, or were observed every 6 hours for 14 days to determine survival.

Determination of serum cytokine levels

After sacrificed at 18 hours after CLP or sham operation, blood was collected and then serum was separated by centrifugation at 10,000 g for 10 min at 4°C, aliquoted, and stored at −80°C until assayed. For determination of circulating cytokine levels, the concentrations of granulocyte-macrophage colony-stimulating factor (GM-CSF), monocyte chemotactic protein (MCP)-1, interleukin (IL)-1, IL-6, tumor necrosis factor-α (TNF-α), and IL-10 were measured using bead-based multiplex immunoassays with flow cytometry (eBioscience FlowCytomix; Bender MedSystems, Vienna, Austria), according to the manufacturer's instructions.

Analysis of peripheral blood mononuclear cells

After sacrificed, one part of blood collected in a EDTA-containing tube was used for analysis of peripheral blood mononuclear cells by their cell surface markers. Flow cytometry was performed on FACSCalibur with CellQuest software following the manufacturer's instructions. FITC, PE, or APC conjugated monoclonal antibodies specific to rat CD3, CD4, CD8a, CD11b, CD11b/c, CD25, Gran, CD45RA, or CD161a were employed

with appropriate isotype matched controls. All reagents were purchased from BD Biosciences.

Assessment of regulatory T (Treg) cell function

Spleens were harvested after sacrificed at 18 hours after CLP or sham operation. They were cut into pieces, milled with tissue grinder, and filtered. Red blood cells were removed, and splenocytes were isolated by Ficoll-Paque gradient centrifugation (GE Healthcare, Uppsala, Sweden). CD4+CD25+ and CD4+CD25- cells were isolated using CD4+CD25+ Treg cell isolation kits (Miltenyi Biotec, Bergisch Gladbach, Germany). The purity of the CD4+CD25+ T cell population analyzed by flow cytometry was greater than 95%. To evaluate the suppressive capacity of Treg cells, carboxyfluorescein succinimidyl ester (CFSE; Invitrogen, Carlsbad, CA)-labeled CD4+CD25- cells were stimulated by a IL-2 (1000 U/ml)/CD3 (3.75 µg/ml)/CD28 (3 µg/ml) mixture (BD Pharmigen, San Diego, CA) at the density of 1×10^6 cells/well in 24-well plates for 3 days. Then isolated CD4+CD25+ Treg cells (1×10^5 cells/well) were added into the well and cocultured for 3 days. Proliferation of CFSE-labeled CD4+CD25- cells were rated using flow cytometry (FC500, Beckman Coulter, Fullerton, CA), as previous described [19].

Detection of the transferred human MSCs in recipient rats

For detection of the transferred human MSCs in the peripheral blood of the recipient rat, one part of blood was collected in a tube containing EDTA immediately after sacrificed. Red blood cells were lysed by RBC Lysis Solution (Qiagen, Foster, CA), and cells were collected as a pellet after centrifugation. The cells were washed and resuspended in PBS, and then immunolabeled with purified mouse antihuman APC-conjugated CD44 or PE-conjugated CD105 monoclonal antibody (BD Pharmigen, San Diego, CA). Data were analyzed by flow cytometry following the manufacturer's instruction.

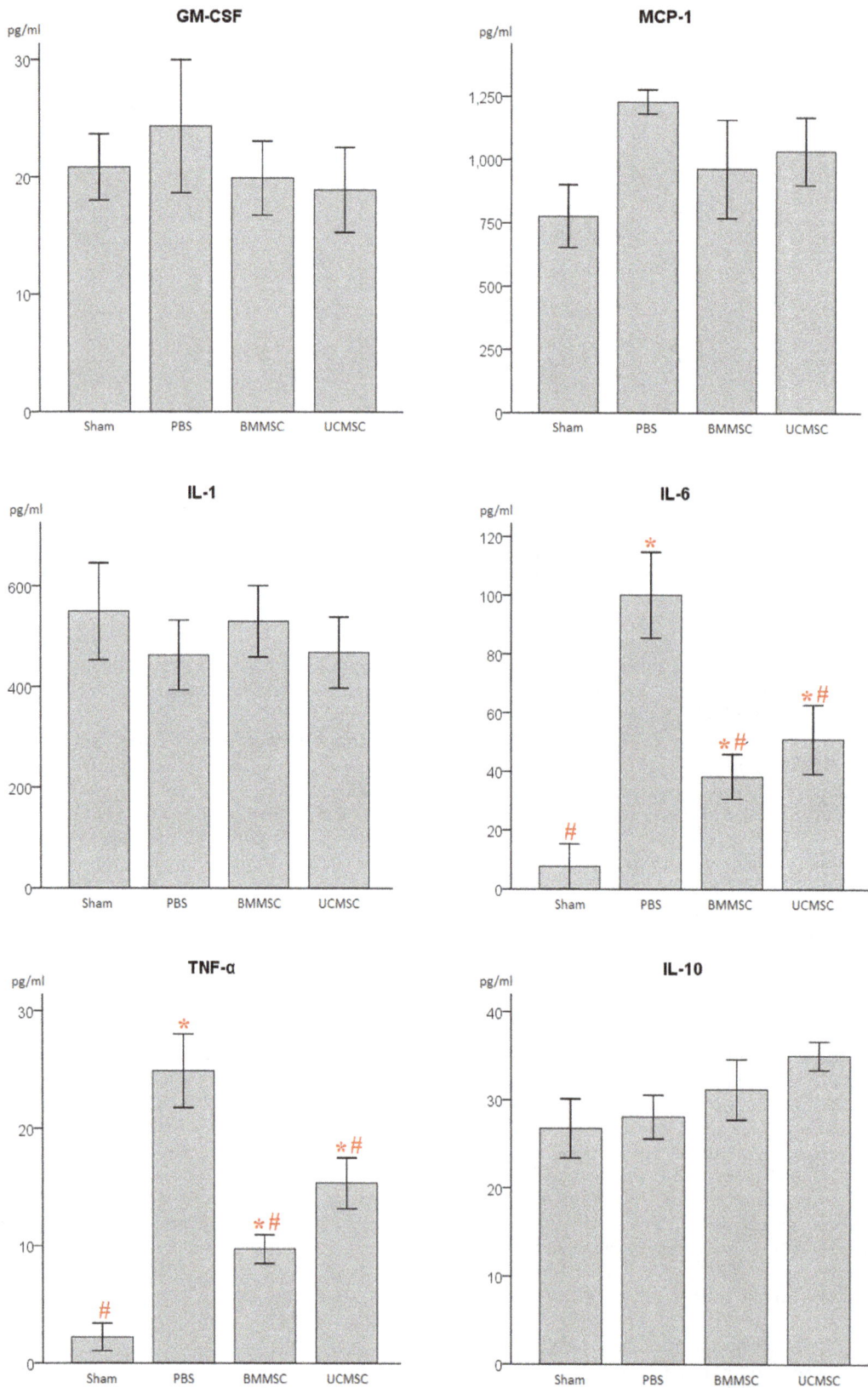

Figure 3. Changes of circulating inflammation-associated cytokine profiles in rats 18 hours after CLP. Compared with sham-operated rats, serum levels of IL-6 and TNF-α were elevated in rats undergoing CLP (i.e. BMMSC, UCMSC and PBS groups). Compared with rats receiving PBS only after CLP, the levels of IL-6 and TNF-α were significantly lower in rats receiving MSCs, either BMMSCs or UCMSCs. There were no significant

differences in these two parameters between rats receiving BMMSCs and UCMSCs. There were no significant differences in serum levels of GM-CSF, MCP-1, IL-1 and IL-10 among sham control, BMMSC, UCMSC and PBS groups. Data are presented as mean ± SEM. n = 6–9 rats/group. *$p < 0.05$ versus sham control group. # $p < 0.05$ versus PBS group.

For detection of the transferred MSCs in the lung of the recipient rat, the lung tissue was fixed in 10% neutral buffered formalin and then embedded in paraffin. Thin sections of 5 μm thickness were obtained for immunohistochemical staining specific to human CD44 and CD105 (GeneTex, Irvine, CA), according to the manufacturer's protocol.

Statistical analysis

Data analysis was performed using SPSS 16.0 for Windows. Survival was analyzed with Kaplan-Meier survival curves. For continuous variables, Kruskal-Wallis test was used to compare groups and Games-Howell test was as post-hoc test. Statistical value of $p < 0.05$ was considered to be significant.

Results

Characteristics of MSCs

In vitro culture, BMMSCs and UCMSCs showed a similar spindle-shaped morphology (Figure 1A). Both revealed a consistent immunophenotypic profile which was negative for CD34, CD45, CD14, and HLA-DR, and positive for CD29, CD44, CD73, CD90, CD105, HLA-A, HLA-B, and HLA-C. There was no significant difference in the expression level of any single surface marker between BMMSCs and UCMSCs. Under respective induction conditions, both BMMSCs and UCMSCs can achieve osteogenic and adipogenic differentiation. It is interesting to note that UCMSCs had significantly stronger potential for osteogenesis but lower for adipogenesis, as shown by more intense von Kossa stain (Figure 1B) and less intense Oil red O stain (Figure 1C).

Survival study

Figure 2 shows the beneficial effects from MSC administration on survival after CLP-induced sepsis in rats. In the absence of antibiotics therapy, the mortality rates in rats receiving UCMSCs or BMMSCs after CLP were reduced compared with rats receiving PBS only after CLP although no statistical significance.

Changes of cytokine profiles in rats with sepsis after MSC administration

To assess the changes of inflammation-associated cytokine profiles after MSC administration during sepsis, serum concentrations of GM-CSF, MCP-1, IL-1, IL-6, TNF-α, and IL-10 were measured 18 hours after CLP or sham operation (Figure 3). Compared with sham-operated rats, serum levels of IL-6 and TNF-α were elevated significantly in rats undergoing CLP, whether receiving MSCs or not. It is worth noting that serum IL-6 and TNF-α levels were significantly lower in rats receiving BMMSCs or UCMSCs than rats receiving PBS only after CLP. These results may implicate that MSCs could rescue rats from the exacerbated inflammatory status after CLP-induced sepsis. There was no significant difference in the serum level of any measured cytokine between rats receiving BMMSCs and UCMSCs after CLP.

Changes of peripheral blood mononuclear cells in rats with sepsis after MSC administration

To evaluate the activation of the immune system during the inflammatory process induced by CLP, a panel of peripheral blood mononuclear cells, which may participate in the innate or adaptive immune network, were measured 18 hours after CLP or sham

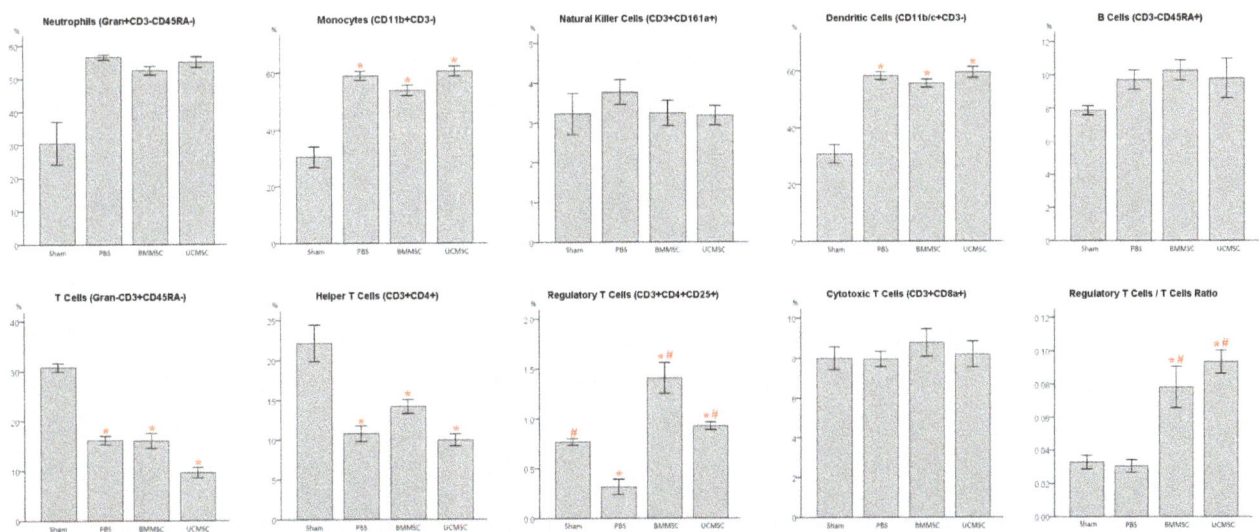

Figure 4. Analysis of peripheral blood mononulcear cells in rats 18 hours after CLP. Compared with sham-operated rats, the percentages of circulating CD11b+CD3- monocytes and CD11b/c+CD3- dendritic cells were elevated in rats undergoing CLP (i.e. BMMSC, UCMSC and PBS groups). Compared with rats receiving PBS only after CLP, the percentage of circulating CD3+CD4+CD25+ Treg cells was significantly higher in rats receiving BMMSCs or UCMSCs after CLP, and so was the ratio of Treg cells/T cells. There were no significant differences in these two parameters between rats of BMMSC and UCMSC groups. Data are presented as mean ± SEM. n = 6–9 rats/group. *$p < 0.05$ versus sham control group. #$p < 0.05$ versus PBS group.

A

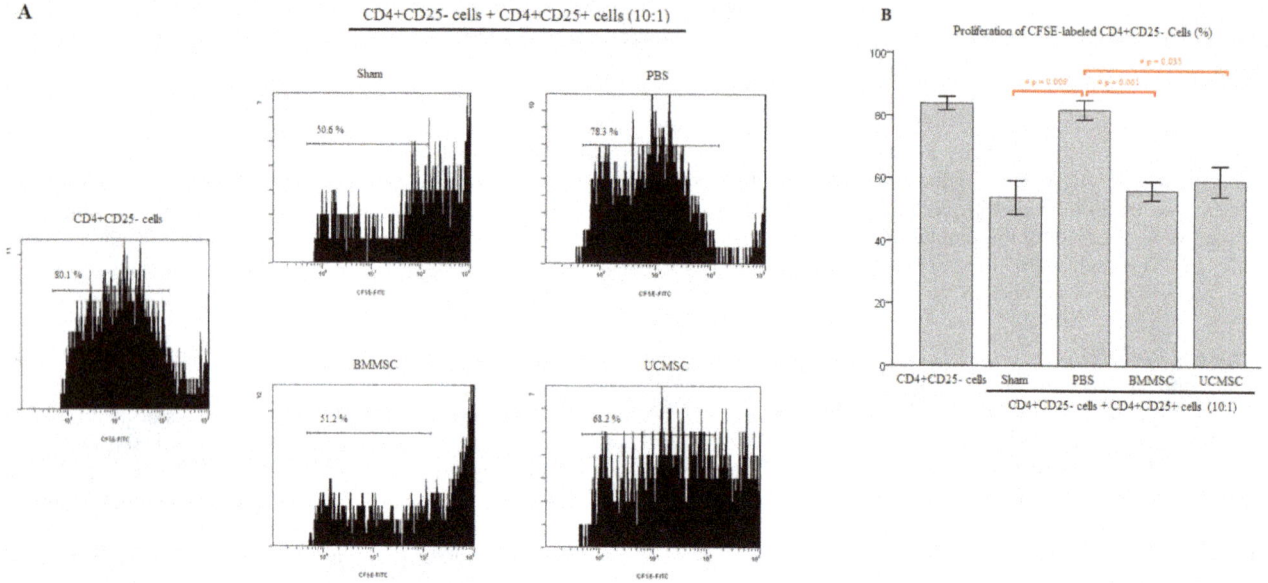

B

Figure 5. Treg cell suppressive function in rats 18 hours after CLP. (A) Analysis of CFSE-labeled CD4+CD25- cell proliferation by flow cytometry after pre-treatment with a IL-2/CD3/CD28 mixture was shown. (B) Proliferation of CFSE-labeled CD4+CD25- cells was decreased when cocultured with CD4+CD25+ Treg cells from rats of Sham, BMMSC, and UCMSC groups. The suppressive capacity of CD4+CD25+ cells from rats receiving PBS only after CLP nearly disappeared. Data are presented as mean ± SEM. n=6–9 rats/group. #p<0.05 versus PBS group.

operation by their specific surface markers (Figure 4). Compared with sham-operated rats, the percentages of circulating CD11b+ CD3- monocytes and CD11b/c+CD3- dendritic cells were elevated significantly in rats undergoing CLP, indicating the activation of the innate immune system after CLP-induced inflammation. Of importance, the percentage of circulating CD3+CD4+CD25+ Treg cells and the ratio of Treg cells/T cells were significantly higher in rats receiving BMMSCs or UCMSCs than rats receiving PBS only after CLP, suggesting that the actions of MSCs may be associated with CD3+CD4+CD25+ Treg cells in this model. There was no significant difference in any peripheral blood mononuclear cells between BMMSC and UCMSC groups.

Restoration of Treg cell suppressive function in rats with sepsis after MSC administration

In addition to an increase in the percentage of circulating CD3+ CD4+CD25+ Treg cells in the peripheral blood, we further demonstrated the restoration of Treg cell suppressive function in rats with sepsis after MSC administration. As shown in Figure 5, proliferation of CFSE-labeled CD4+CD25- cells was suppressed when cocultured with isolated CD4+CD25+ Treg cells from rats receiving BMMSCs or UCMSCs after CLP. In contrast, the suppressive capacity of CD4+CD25+ Treg cells from rats receiving PBS only after CLP was significantly decreased. These results implicated that immunosuppressive function of Treg cells could be restored by administration of MSCs. Our study provides the first evidence for the increase in Treg cell suppressive function after MSC administration in a septic animal model.

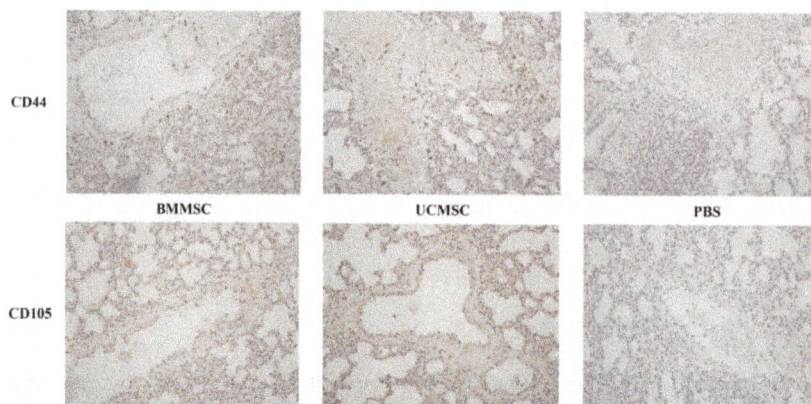

Figure 6. Evaluation of lung immunohistochemistry in rats 18 hours after CLP. Positive cells for CD44 or CD105 which represented the transferred human MSCs can be found in the perivascular interstitial area 14 hours after administration of BMMSCs or UCMSCs (200×).

Detection of the transferred human MSCs in recipient rats

Further, we tried to find where the transferred human MSCs homed to. At 14 hours after administering BMMSCs or UCMSCs to rats, no cells with CD44 or CD105 expression which represented the transferred human MSCs can be detected by flow cytometry in the peripheral blood. While positive cells for CD44 or CD105 were found in the perivascular interstitial area of the lung sections from rats 14 hours after MSC administration (Figure 6).

Discussion and Conclusion

Dysregulation of a variety of immune cells in response to sepsis, which is associated with increased rates of morbidity and mortality in septic patients, has been demonstrated [20,21]. MSCs have been found to modulate immune functions [3–8]. In our previous study, we found that UCMSCs could effectively treat severe graft versus host disease after hematopoietic stem cell transplantation, which is a paradigm of immune-mediated host tissue damage [16]. Administering MSCs to mice after CLP was reported to improve survival and organ function [9–12], implicating that MSCs may bring immune responses back into balance and attenuate self-tissue damage during sepsis. Regarding how MSCs exert their immunoregulation during sepsis, most investigations focused on the effects of MSCs on neutrophil or monocyte/macrophage function [9–12]. Compared with rats receiving PBS only after CLP, the present study showed that the percentage of circulating Treg cells and the ratio of Treg cells/T cells were elevated significantly in rats receiving MSCs after CLP. Further study regarding Treg cell function demonstrated that the immunosuppressive capacity of Treg cells from rats with CLP-induced sepsis was diminished, but could be restored by administration of MSCs. Consistent with the previous reports that Treg cells can control the production of pro-inflammatory cytokines during infection [9,22–24], we found that levels of serum IL-6 and TNF-α decreased in rats receiving MSCs compared with rats receiving PBS only after CLP. This work provides support for the involvement of Treg cells in the immunoregulatory effects of MSCs during sepsis.

Treg cells play an important role in the regulation of immune responses. During infectious processes, Treg cells can suppress the activation of naive autoreactive CD4 helper and CD8 cytotoxic T cells which have the potential to attack the body's health tissues, and control the production of pro-inflammatory cytokines [22,23,25]. And thus minimize the collateral tissue damage. In CLP-induced septic mice, adoptive transfer of in vitro-stimulated Treg cells had positive effects on bacterial clearance and survival [26], and the suppressive capacity of Treg cells was prerequisite for the recovery from severe sepsis [27]. The complex interactions between MSCs and Treg cells, two important components of peripheral tolerance in the immune system, have been investigated. MSCs were demonstrated to generate Treg cells and regulate their function [28–34], but it has not been reported whether MSCs also can exert their immunomodulatory capacity via Treg cells during sepsis. In the present study, administration of BMMSCs or UCMSCs to septic rats could increase the percentage of circulating Treg cells, the ratio of Treg cells/T cells, and the suppressive function of Treg cells. Thus, levels of serum IL-6 and TNF-α, indices of acute inflammation, decreased. Here, we first reported the alterations in number and function of Treg cells after MSC administration during sepsis in an animal model. And this work provides valuable evidence for the association of Treg cells and MSC-mediated immunomodulation during sepsis.

A broad spectrum of factors produced by MSCs have been reported to affect cell performance, including insulin-like growth factor, hepatocyte growth factor, epidermal growth factor, vascular endothelial growth factor, stromal cell-derived factor-1, IL-10, IL-8, IL-6, prostaglandin E2, etc [35–37]. Although cross-species effects have been demonstrated from administration of xenogeneic MSCs, the mechanisms by which MSCs exert their cross-species activity remain unclear. Additionally, there is substantial evidence that infused MSCs have higher engraftment efficiencies within sites of inflammation or injury [38]. In the absence of tissue damage, a large number of systemically administered MSCs was found to lodge in the pulmonary vascular bed [39]. In the present study, the transferred MSCs cannot be detected in the peripheral blood 14 hours after administration but they were found in the pulmonary perivascular interstitium. MSC homing soon to the lung in the recipient rat after systemic administration may be important for amelioration of lung injury. It remains difficult to determine how long the transferred MSCs survive in the recipients. Although no evidence of donor MSCs in the majority of patients 6 months after MSC administration, MSC chimerism still can be demonstrated in several patients at such a long time after administration [40,41].

For clinical use, a key factor is the origin of MSCs to be expanded in vitro. Bone marrow is considered as the traditional source, but MSCs can also be isolated from other tissues. In our previous studies, we found that UCMSCs can promote hematopoietic engraftment after hematopoietic stem cell transplantation [15,42] and treat refractory graft-versus-host disease effectively [16]. While the properties of UCMSCs may be similar to their bone marrow counterparts, their characteristics and functional importance in sepsis also need to be investigated. In the present study, BMMSCs and UCMSCs showed a similar in vitro-cultured morphology and surface marker expression. It is of interest that UCMSCs exhibited stronger potential for osteogenesis but lower for adipogenesis than BMMSCs. In CLP-induced septic rats, UCMSCs appeared to have similar effects as BMMSCs. As to be easily harvested and efficiently cultured, umbilical cord might represent a feasible source of MSCs for clinical application.

The ability of MSCs to fine-tune immune responses has led to the idea that MSCs could be attractive candidates of cell-based therapy for infection control and immune regulation. Much still remains to be discovered and further works are warranted.

Author Contributions

Conceived and designed the experiments: YHC HPW. Performed the experiments: YGT CTP KCL WRC. Analyzed the data: YHC MSL YCF. Contributed reagents/materials/analysis tools: KHW. Wrote the paper: YHC HPW KHW.

References

1. Angus DC, Linde-Zwirble WT, Lidicker J, Clermont G, Carcillo J, et al. (2001) Epidemiology of severe sepsis in the United States: analysis of incidence, outcome, and associated costs of care. Crit Care Med 29: 1303–1310.

2. Caplan AI (2007) Adult mesenchymal stem cells for tissue engineering versus regenerative medicine. J Cell Physiol 213: 341–347.

3. Nauta AJ, Fibbe WE (2007) Immunomodulatory properties of mesenchymal stromal cells. Blood 110: 3499–3506.

4. English K (2013) Mechanisms of mesenchymal stromal cell immunomodulation. Immunol Cell Biol 91: 19–26.

5. Chao YH, Wu HP, Chan CK, Tsai C, Peng CT, et al. (2012) Umbilical cord-derived mesenchymal stem cells for hematopoietic stem cell transplantation. J Biomed Biotechnol 2012: 759503.

6. Yagi H, Soto-Gutierrez A, Parekkadan B, Kitagawa Y, Tompkins RG, et al. (2010) Mesenchymal stem cells: Mechanisms of immunomodulation and homing. Cell Transplant 19: 667–679.

7. Rasmusson I (2006) Immune modulation by mesenchymal stem cells. Exp Cell Res 312: 2169–2179.

8. Wu KH, Wu HP, Chan CK, Hwang SM, Peng CT, et al. (2013) The role of mesenchymal stem cells in hematopoietic stem cell transplantation: from bench to bedsides. Cell Transplant 22: 723–729.

9. Nemeth K, Leelahavanichkul A, Yuen PS, Mayer B, Parmelee A, et al. (2009) Bone marrow stromal cells attenuate sepsis via prostaglandin E(2)-dependent reprogramming of host macrophages to increase their interleukin-10 production. Nat Med 15: 42–49.

10. Mei SHJ, Haitsma JJ, Dos Santos CC, Deng Y, Lai PFH, et al. (2010) Mesenchymal stem cells reduce inflammation while enhancing bacterial clearance and improving survival in sepsis. Am J Resp Crit Care 182: 1047–1057.

11. Hall SRR, Tsoyi K, Ith B, Padera RF Jr, Lederer JA, et al. (2013) Mesenchymal stromal cells improve survival during sepsis in the absence of heme oxygenase-1: the importance of neutrophils. Stem Cells 31: 397–407.

12. Krasnodembskaya A, Samarani G, Song Y, Zhuo H, Su X, et al. (2012) Human mesenchymal stem cells reduce mortality and bacteremia in gram-negative sepsis in mice in part by enhancing the phagocytic activity of blood monocytes. Am J Physiol-Lung C 302: L1003–1013.

13. Chao YH, Peng CT, Harn HJ, Chan CK, Wu KH (2010) Poor potential of proliferation and differentiation in bone marrow mesenchymal stem cells derived from children with severe aplastic anemia. Ann Hematol 89: 715–723.

14. Chan CK, Wu KH, Lee YS, Hwang SM, Lee MS, et al. (2012) The Comparison of Interleukin 6-Associated Immunosuppressive Effects of Human ESCs, Fetal-Type MSCs, and Adult-Type MSCs. Transplantation 94: 132–138.

15. Wu KH, Sheu JN, Wu HP, Tsai C, Sieber M, et al. (2013) Cotransplantation of Umbilical Cord-Derived Mesenchymal Stem Cells Promote Hematopoietic Engraftment in Cord Blood Transplantation: A Pilot Study. Transplantation 95: 773–777.

16. Wu KH, Chan CK, Tsai C, Chang YH, Sieber M, et al. (2011) Effective treatment of severe steroid-resistant acute graft-versus-host disease with umbilical cord-derived mesenchymal stem cells. Transplantation 91: 1412–1416.

17. Wu HP, Yang WC, Wu KH, Chen CY, Fu YC (2012) Diagnosing appendicitis at different time points in children with right lower quadrant pain: comparison between Pediatric Appendicitis Score and the Alvarado score. World J Surg 36: 216–221.

18. Lee WI, Huang JL, Jaing TH, Shyur SD, Yang KD, et al. (2011) Distribution, clinical features and treatment in Taiwanese patients with symptomatic primary immunodeficiency diseases (PIDs) in a nationwide population-based study during 1985–2010. Immunobiology 216: 1286–1294.

19. Tsai YG, Yang KD, Niu DM, Chien JW, Lin CY (2010) TLR2 agonists enhance CD8+Foxp3+ regulatory T cells and suppress Th2 immune responses during allergen immunotherapy. J Immunol 184: 7229–7237.

20. Wisnoski N, Chung C-S, Chen Y, Huang X, Ayala A (2007) The contribution of CD4+ CD25+ T-regulatory-cells to immune suppression in sepsis. Shock 27: 251–257.

21. Fry DE (2012) Sepsis, systemic inflammatory response, and multiple organ dysfunction: the mystery continues. Am Surgeon 78: 1–8.

22. Cambos M, Belanger B, Jacques A, Roulet A, Scorza T (2008) Natural regulatory (CD4+CD25+FOXP+) T cells control the production of pro-inflammatory cytokines during Plasmodium chabaudi adami infection and do not contribute to immune evasion. Int J Parasitol 38: 229–238.

23. Sun J, Han ZB, Liao W, Yang SG, Yang Z, et al. (2011) Intrapulmonary delivery of human umbilical cord mesenchymal stem cells attenuates acute lung injury by expanding CD4+CD25+ Forkhead Boxp3 (FOXP3)+ regulatory T cells and balancing anti- and pro-inflammatory factors. Cellular Physiology & Biochemistry 27: 587–596.

24. Gonzalez-Rey E, Anderson P, Gonzalez MA, Rico L, Buscher D, et al. (2009) Human adult stem cells derived from adipose tissue protect against experimental colitis and sepsis. Gut 58: 929–939.

25. Belkaid Y, Rouse BT (2005) Natural regulatory T cells in infectious disease. Nat Immunol 6: 353–360.

26. Heuer JG, Zhang T, Zhao J, Ding C, Cramer M, et al. (2005) Adoptive transfer of in vitro-stimulated CD4+CD25+ regulatory T cells increases bacterial clearance and improves survival in polymicrobial sepsis. J Immunol 174: 7141–7146.

27. Kuhlhorn F, Rath M, Schmoeckel K, Cziupka K, Nguyen HH, et al. (2013) Foxp3+ regulatory T cells are required for recovery from severe sepsis. Plos One 8: e65109.

28. Casiraghi F, Azzollini N, Cassis P, Imberti B, Morigi M, et al. (2008) Pretransplant infusion of mesenchymal stem cells prolongs the survival of a semiallogeneic heart transplant through the generation of regulatory T cells. J Immunol 181: 3933–3946.

29. Kavanagh H, Mahon BP (2011) Allogeneic mesenchymal stem cells prevent allergic airway inflammation by inducing murine regulatory T cells. Allergy 66: 523–531.

30. Ge W, Jiang J, Arp J, Liu W, Garcia B, et al. (2010) Regulatory T-cell generation and kidney allograft tolerance induced by mesenchymal stem cells associated with indoleamine 2,3-dioxygenase expression. Transplantation 90: 1312–1320.

31. Gonzalez MA, Gonzalez-Rey E, Rico L, Buscher D, Delgado M (2009) Adipose-derived mesenchymal stem cells alleviate experimental colitis by inhibiting inflammatory and autoimmune responses. Gastroenterology 136: 978–989.

32. Perico N, Casiraghi F, Introna M, Gotti E, Todeschini M, et al. (2011) Autologous mesenchymal stromal cells and kidney transplantation: a pilot study of safety and clinical feasibility. Clin J Am Soc Nephro 6: 412–422.

33. Engela AU, Hoogduijn MJ, Boer K, Litjens NHR, Betjes MGH, et al. (2013) Human adipose-tissue derived mesenchymal stem cells induce functional de-novo regulatory T cells with methylated FOXP3 gene DNA. Clin Exp Immunol 173: 343–354.

34. English K, Ryan JM, Tobin L, Murphy MJ, Barry FP, et al. (2009) Cell contact, prostaglandin E(2) and transforming growth factor beta 1 play non-redundant roles in human mesenchymal stem cell induction of CD4+CD25(High) forkhead box P3+ regulatory T cells. Clin Exp Immunol 156: 149–160.

35. Moghadasali R, Mutsaers HA, Azarnia M, Aghdami N, Baharvand H, et al. (2013) Mesenchymal stem cell-conditioned medium accelerates regeneration of human renal proximal tubule epithelial cells after gentamicin toxicity. Exp Toxicol Pathol 65: 595–600.

36. Sze SK, de Kleijn DP, Lai RC, Khia Way Tan E, Zhao H, et al. (2007) Elucidating the secretion proteome of human embryonic stem cell-derived mesenchymal stem cells. Mol Cell Proteomics 6: 1680–1689.

37. Ivanova-Todorova E, Bochev I, Dimitrov R, Belemezova K, Mourdjeva M, et al. (2012) Conditioned medium from adipose tissue-derived mesenchymal stem cells induces CD4+FOXP3+ cells and increases IL-10 secretion. J Biomed Biotechnol: 295167.

38. Karp JM, Leng Teo GS (2009) Mesenchymal stem cell homing: the devil is in the details. Cell Stem Cell 4: 206–216.

39. Kyriakou C, Rabin N, Pizzey A, Nathwani A, Yong K (2008) Factors that influence short-term homing of human bone marrow-derived mesenchymal stem cells in a xenogeneic animal model. Haematologica 93: 1457–1465.

40. Ball LM, Bernardo ME, Roelofs H, Lankester A, Cometa A, et al. (2007) Cotransplantation of ex vivo expanded mesenchymal stem cells accelerates lymphocyte recovery and may reduce the risk of graft failure in haploidentical hematopoietic stem-cell transplantation. Blood 110: 2764–2767.

41. Lazarus HM, Koc ON, Devine SM, Curtin P, Maziarz RT, et al. (2005) Cotransplantation of HLA-identical sibling culture-expanded mesenchymal stem cells and hematopoietic stem cells in hematologic malignancy patients. Biol Blood Marrow Transplant 11: 389–398.

42. Chao YH, Tsai C, Peng CT, Wu HP, Chan CK, et al. (2011) Cotransplantation of umbilical cord MSCs to enhance engraftment of hematopoietic stem cells in patients with severe aplastic anemia. Bone Marrow Transplant 46: 1391–1392.

6

Loss of the Endothelial Glucocorticoid Receptor Prevents the Therapeutic Protection Afforded by Dexamethasone after LPS

Julie E. Goodwin[1]*, Yan Feng[1], Heino Velazquez[2], Han Zhou[1], William C. Sessa[3,4]

1 Department of Pediatrics, Yale University School of Medicine, New Haven, Connecticut, United States of America, 2 Department of Internal Medicine, Veterans Affairs Hospital, West Haven, Connecticut, United States of America, 3 Vascular Biology and Therapeutics Program, Yale University School of Medicine, New Haven, Connecticut, United States of America, 4 Department of Pharmacology, Yale University School of Medicine, New Haven, Connecticut, United States of America

Abstract

Glucocorticoids are normally regarded as anti-inflammatory therapy for a wide variety of conditions and have been used with some success in treating sepsis and sepsis-like syndromes. We previously demonstrated that mice lacking the glucocorticoid receptor in the endothelium (GR $^{EC\ KO}$ mice) are extremely sensitive to low-dose LPS and demonstrate prolonged activation and up regulation of NF-κB. In this study we pre-treated these GR $^{EC\ KO}$ mice with dexamethasone and assessed their response to an identical dose of LPS. Surprisingly, the GR $^{EC\ KO}$ mice fared even worse than when given LPS alone demonstrating increased mortality, increased levels of the inflammatory cytokines TNF-α and IL-6 and increased nitric oxide release after the dexamethasone pre-treatment. As expected, control animals pre-treated with dexamethasone showed improvement in all parameters assayed. Mechanistically we demonstrate that GR $^{EC\ KO}$ mice show increased iNOS production and NF-κB activation despite treatment with dexamethasone.

Editor: Jose Carlos Alves-Filho, University of São Paulo, Brazil

Funding: This work was supported by an NIH Mentored Clinical Scientist Research Award (K08-DK078623), a Bartner Research Discovery Scholar Award to JG and HL64793, HL61371, HL081190, HL096670 and PO1 HL107205 from the National Institutes of Health to WS. The authors also acknowledge the Yale Mouse Metabolic Phenotyping Core: U24 DK59635 and the George M. O'Brien Kidney Center at Yale: NIH grant P30 DK079310. The funders had no role in study design, data collection and analysis, decision to publish or preparation of the manuscript.

Competing Interests: The authors have declared that no competing interests exist.

* Email: julie.goodwin@yale.edu

Introduction

Exogenous glucocorticoids (GCs), such as dexamethasone, are anti-inflammatory compounds which are used to treat a variety of chronic inflammatory conditions as well as acute septic shock and sepsis-like syndromes. Dexamethasone (DEX) exerts its effects through the glucocorticoid receptor (GR), a nuclear hormone receptor that is ubiquitously expressed in most cells of the body and widely conserved across species [1]. Previous studies in animal models have demonstrated that prophylaxis with DEX prior to the onset of sepsis can decrease production of inflammatory cytokines, such as TNF-α, and reduce morbidity and mortality [2,3]. In human trials, steroids have been used with considerably less success in this setting for many decades, as the mechanisms by which they confer their anti-inflammatory effects are still not clear [4,5]. Recent studies have also suggested that rodent models may not be ideal systems in which to recapitulate human sepsis [6,7] and thus the role of steroids in these systems is not clear.

Previous studies have shown clearly that GR has cell specific roles. For example, deletion of GR in the central nervous system results in mice with profoundly altered hypothalamic-pituitary-adrenal (HPA) axes and tenfold elevated circulating corticosterone levels as well as reduced anxiety-related behavior [8]. We recently showed that mice with tissue-specific deletion of GR in the endothelium were almost completely protected from steroid-induced hypertension [9], yet had increased mortality and hemodynamic instability in response to relatively low-dose LPS [10]. Given the dramatic phenotype we observed when these mice were treated with LPS, here we studied the role of endothelial GR in the setting of DEX pre-treatment before the administration of an identical dose of LPS. We hypothesized that the absence of endothelial GR would be a critical mediator of DEX effectiveness in this model of LPS-induced sepsis.

In this study we show that the presence of endothelial GR is required for DEX to rescue the animals from LPS-induce morbidity and mortality, and furthermore that in most parameters studied, DEX and LPS together result in worse outcomes than LPS alone in mice lacking the receptor in the endothelium. We further show that administration of DEX and LPS in the absence of endothelial GR results in increased levels of TNF-α, and iNOS and increased activation of NF-κB. Thus, though DEX is administered systemically, the presence of endothelial GR is required to mediate its protective effects in this setting. These data potentially have direct applicability to the approach to sepsis in human patients.

Materials and Methods

Mice

Male mice, age 8–12 weeks, with average weights of 20–25 grams, with tissue specific excision of the endothelial glucocorticoid receptor, designated GR $^{EC\ KO}$ mice and littermate controls, designated GR fl/fl were used for experimentation as described [9]. These mice are fully congenic, having been back-crossed for more than 20 generations. Mice used in these experiments were treatment-naïve and housed in standard mouse cages with a maximum of 5 animals/cage. They were maintained in a standard environment with 12-hour light/dark cycles and with free access to food and water throughout.

GR $^{EC\ KO}$ mice and littermate controls were pretreated with DEX via intraperitoneal (IP) injection and then injected IP 2 hours later with a single dose of LPS. DEX injections were performed between 8 and 9 AM and then LPS was administered between 10 and 11 AM. The two mouse genotypes were treated simultaneously. All experiments were performed according to a protocol approved by the Institutional Animal Care and Use Committee at the Yale University School of Medicine, and were consistent with the NIH Guidelines for the Care of Laboratory Animals. Pain and suffering were minimized as much as possible.

For this survival study, to assess the degree of impairment and/or pain which resulted from this injection the following parameters were used: loss of mobility, failure to groom, and presence of diarrhea. If an animal was found to have 1 or more of these symptoms for more than 8 hours it was euthanized by an overdose of ether and cervical dislocation. Half lives of LPS are estimated to be anywhere from 60–120 min [11], so 8 hours would represent a minimum of 4 half lives when <10% of the LPS would still be predicted to be present. If the mouse was symptomatic at this time, it was deemed unlikely to recover spontaneously. Mice were monitored 3 times/day for 3 days after injection. Mice were kept in their original cages throughout the experiment.

Drug injections

LPS from E. Coli strain O55: B5 (VWR) was dissolved in PBS and prepared fresh prior to each experiment. A dose of 12.5 mg/kg was used according to several previously published studies [12,13]. Dexamethasone phosphate (MP Biomedicals) was dissolved in PBS and prepared fresh prior to each experiment.

Serum measurements

Corticosterone measurement was performed by ELISA (Assay Designs) according to the manufacturer's instructions. Nitric Oxide was measured by the Total Nitric Oxide Assay Kit (Assay Designs) according to the manufacturer's instructions. Mouse IL-6 and TNF-alpha levels were measured by ELISAs from Pierce Biotechnology.

Apoptosis determination

Tissue sections were mounted on glass slides and TUNEL staining was performed using the ApopTag Peroxidase In Situ Apoptosis Detection Kit (Chemicon International). Five fields from each slide were analyzed and quantified by Image J software. On other slides CD68 (Serotec) staining was performed to identify macrophages and images were also analyzed by ImageJ software. The same gray scale threshold was used for all images and the area of each tissue occupied by macrophages was calculated for 3 sections per sample and averaged.

Blood pressure measurement

Male mice, 10–12 weeks old, were maintained under 1.75% (vol/vol) isoflurane anesthesia. The carotid artery was catheterized and both a bladder catheter and peripheral IV line for intermittent saline injections were placed. After a 30 to 60 minute equilibration period dexamethasone 2 mg/kg was administered IV followed 2 hours later by LPS 5 mg/kg IV. Mice were monitored continuously by oscillometric blood pressure measurement for 4–6 hours after injection.

Western blot

Tissues were snap frozen in liquid nitrogen, pulverized, and resuspended in lysis buffer (50 mM Tris-HCl pH 7.4, 0.1 mM EDTA, 0.1 mM EGTA, 1% NP-40, 0.1% sodium deoxycholate, 0.1% sodium dodecyl sulfate (SDS), 100 mM NaCl, 10 mM NaF, 1 mM sodium pyrophosphate, 1 mM sodium orthovanadate, 1 mM Pefabloc SC, and 2 mg/ml protease inhibitor cocktail (Roche Diagnostics)). Cells were lysed on ice with lysis buffer. Protein concentrations were determined with the DC Protein assay kit (Bio-Rad Laboratories). Lysates were analyzed by SDS-polyacrylamide gel electrophoresis (PAGE) and immunoblotting. Primary antibodies used include the following: iNOS (Cayman) and GAPDH (Affinity Bioreagents). Secondary antibodies were fluorescence-labeled antibodies (LI-COR Biotechnology). Bands were visualized with the Odyssey Infrared Licor system

NF-κB activation

NF-κB Activation was measured by the TransAM NF-κB p65 kit (Active Motif) according to the manufacturer's instructions.

Cell culture

Mouse lung endothelial cells (MLEC) were isolated as described [14]. Mouse-specific control or GR siRNA (Qiagen) was used at a concentration of 50 nM to effectively knock down GR. Cells were either (1) untreated, (2) treated with DEX alone (1 μM) for 24 hours, (3) treated with TNF-α alone (10 ng/ml) for 24 hours or (4) simultaneously treated with both DEX and TNF-α for 24 hours.

Quantitative PCR

Total RNA was isolated from cells using the RNeasy mini kit (Qiagen) according to the manufacturer's instructions. RNA was revere transcribed using the Taqman Reverse Transcriptase kit (Applied Biosystems). qPCR was performed on a Bio-Rad iQ5 machine using the resultant cDNA, $2 \times$ SA Biosciences RT^2 qPCR Master mix and gene specific primers. Primers used for the detection of mouse GRα were: 5′ AAAGAGCTAGGAAAAGC-CATTGTC 3′ and 5′ TCAGCTAACATCTCTGGGAATTCA 3′ and for mouse GRβ were: 5′ AAAGAGCTAGGAAAAGC-CATTGTC 3′ and 5′ CTGTCTTTGGGCTTTTGAGATAGG 3′. A common forward primer was used as described [15]. Gene expression was normalized to the housekeeping gene 18 s.

Statistical analysis

Data are presented as mean ± SEM. Survival statistics were calculated by the Mantel-Cox test. Serum parameters, tissue macrophage expression levels, and apoptosis levels were evaluated by one-way ANOVA with Bonferroni's posttest. Blood pressure and hemodynamic data was evaluated by repeated measures ANOVA with Bonferroni's posttest. Statistical significance was set at a p value <0.05.

Results

GR $^{EC\ KO}$ mice are not rescued by dexamethasone after induction of sepsis by LPS

Endothelial GR deficient mice (GR $^{EC\ KO}$) were generated as previously described [10].

GR $^{EC\ KO}$ mice and Cre- GR fl/fl mice were pretreated with dexamethasone (DEX) (2 mg/kg IP) 2 hours before challenge with LPS (12.5 mg/kg IP) and survival was monitored over a period of 96 hours. We have previously shown that this dose of LPS resulted in greater than 50% mortality in GR $^{EC\ KO}$ mice, while produced very little mortality in controls [10]. We reproduced those experiments here again demonstrating that LPS-treated GR $^{EC\ KO}$ mice (n = 5) have 60% mortality while control animals (n = 8) show 12.5% mortality after an identical dose of LPS (Figure 1A). After pre-treatment with DEX, GR $^{EC\ KO}$ mice (n = 9) exhibited only 22% survival at the conclusion of the observation period compared to 100% of controls (n = 8) (p = 0.0031, Figure 1B). We have also previously demonstrated that this dose of DEX could rescue control animals treated with 80 mg/kg LPS [10]. GR $^{EC\ KO}$ mice demonstrated a more severe phenotype during the monitoring period which included decreased activity, decreased oral intake, shivering, diarrhea, and conjunctivitis.

Dexamethasone does not stabilize BP in GR $^{EC\ KO}$ mice after acute LPS injection

To investigate the early hemodynamics in mice given DEX and LPS, continuous blood pressure monitoring was performed in anesthetized GR $^{EC\ KO}$ and control mice (n = 5/group) through indwelling carotid artery catheters. After a one-hour period of acclimation, DEX (2 mg/kg, IV) was administered and then LPS (5 mg/kg, IV) followed 2 hours later. As was previously observed in other experiments [9], there was a strong trend towards baseline mean arterial pressure (MAP) being slightly elevated in GR $^{EC\ KO}$ mice compared to controls (78.4±0.73 mm Hg vs. 73.1±1.91 mm Hg, p = 0.05). Three hours after LPS injection MAP in GR $^{EC\ KO}$ mice had fallen to 58.0±7.18 mm Hg while that of controls was relatively unchanged at 71.7±2.07 mm Hg (p = 0.03), and 4 hours after LPS injection MAP in GR $^{EC\ KO}$ mice was quite low at 42.9±6.17 mm Hg while controls were able to maintain their MAP at 71.4±2.07 mm Hg (p<0.01) (Figure 1C). These data show that loss of GR in the endothelium prevents hemodynamic stabilization by DEX.

Dexamethasone is unable to suppress inflammation or nitric oxide release in GR $^{EC\ KO}$ mice

In order to further investigate the increased mortality and hemodynamic collapse observed in the GR $^{EC\ KO}$ mice, corticosterone levels, nitric oxide levels and markers of inflammation were measured. All measurements were made in 4–6 mice/group. Endogenous corticosterone was measured at baseline and 8 hours after LPS treatment in mice that had been treated with LPS only and also those pre-treated with DEX and then given LPS. There was no difference in baseline levels; after LPS only, corticosterone levels were 622.1±108.2 ng/ml in control animals and 645.4±20.9 ng/ml in GR $^{EC\ KO}$ mice (p = NS). After DEX+ LPS corticosterone levels were 743.6±37 ng/ml in controls and 619.2±54 ng/ml in GR $^{EC\ KO}$ mice (p = NS) demonstrating that the hypothalamic-pituitary-adrenal axis was functioning appropriately and release of corticosterone was similar in both groups under all conditions tested (Figure 2A).

Whole blood NOx (the sum of nitrite and nitrate) in plasma was measured in both groups either 8 hours after administration of

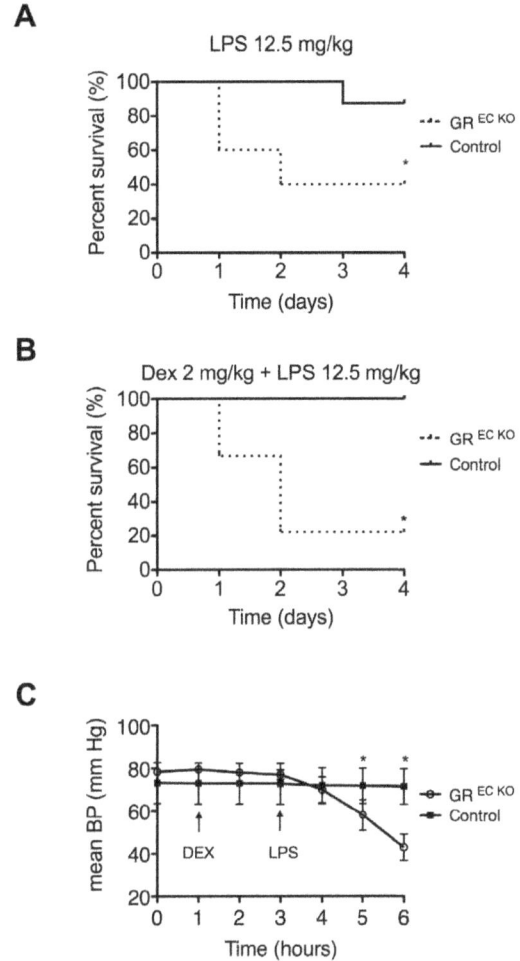

A

LPS 12.5 mg/kg

GR $^{EC\ KO}$
Control

B

Dex 2 mg/kg + LPS 12.5 mg/kg

GR $^{EC\ KO}$
Control

C

GR $^{EC\ KO}$
Control

Figure 1. Impaired survival in GR $^{EC\ KO}$ mice after DEX. (A) GR $^{EC\ KO}$ mice show increased mortality after LPS treatment. (B) Mortality in GR $^{EC\ KO}$ mice is further increased in GR $^{EC\ KO}$ mice following DEX pre-treatment while controls are fully rescued following DEX+LPS. (C) Continuous blood pressure monitoring demonstrates hemodynamic instability in GR $^{EC\ KO}$ mice following pre-treatment with DEX while blood pressure is completely stabilized in control mice. *p<0.05

LPS alone or 8 hours after LPS in those mice pre-treated for 2 hours with DEX. There were no differences in NOx levels at baseline. After LPS alone, control animals demonstrated a level of 29.4±6.7 μM while GR $^{EC\ KO}$ mice showed levels of 25±4.8 μM (p = NS). After DEX+ LPS, control mice demonstrated levels close to baseline at 12.0±0.9 μM, while GR $^{EC\ KO}$ mice showed markedly elevated levels at 43.5±9.2 μM (p = 0.015) (Figure 2B). It is important to note these levels exceed those in the GR $^{EC\ KO}$ mice treated with LPS alone.

We also measured levels of the inflammatory cytokines TNF-α and IL-6 at the same time point (Figure 2C, 2D) and observed a similar pattern. Both cytokines were able to be suppressed to near normal/undetectable levels in control animals pre-treated with DEX, while GR $^{EC\ KO}$ mice demonstrated levels that were significantly higher than those in mice treated with LPS alone, highlighting the fact that DEX is unable to suppress inflammation in GR $^{EC\ KO}$ mice challenged with LPS.

A

B

C

D

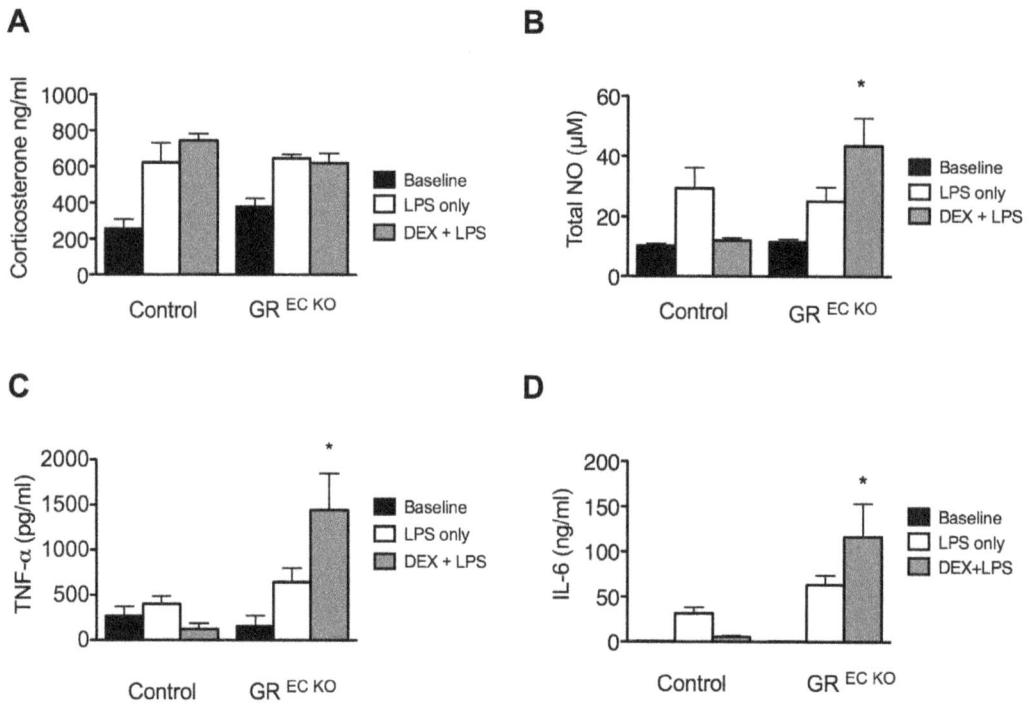

Figure 2. Heightened inflammation in GR $^{EC\ KO}$ mice following DEX pre-treatment. (A) No differences in corticosterone level were observed between GR $^{EC\ KO}$ mice and controls for any of the conditions tested. (B) Total nitric oxide levels in GR $^{EC\ KO}$ mice are increased following DEX+LPS. (C) TNF-α and (D) IL-6 levels are significantly increased in GR $^{EC\ KO}$ mice following DEX+LPS treatment while they are nearly unchanged from baseline in controls. All blood samples were collected 8 hours after LPS treatment (and 10 hours after DEX pre-treatment, if applicable). *$p < 0.05$ compared to similarly treated controls.

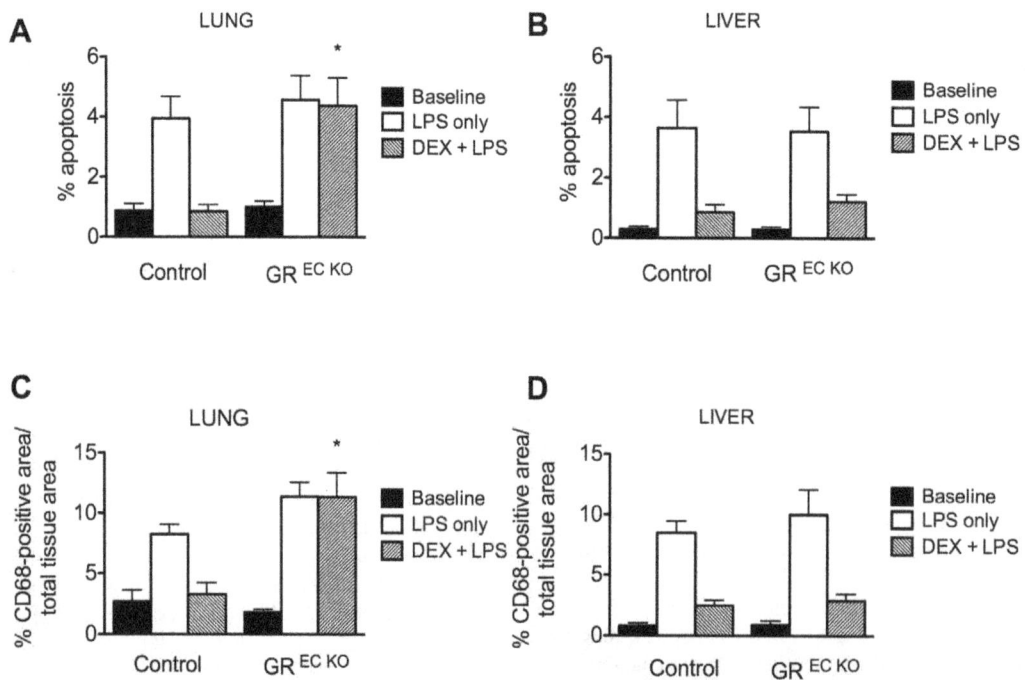

A

B

C

D

Figure 3. Lung apopotosis (A) and macrophage infiltration (C) are not improved by DEX in GR $^{EC\ KO}$ mice. Both GR $^{EC\ KO}$ mice and controls show an improvement in liver apoptosis (B) and macrophage infiltration (D) following DEX. *$p < 0.05$ compared to similarly treated controls.

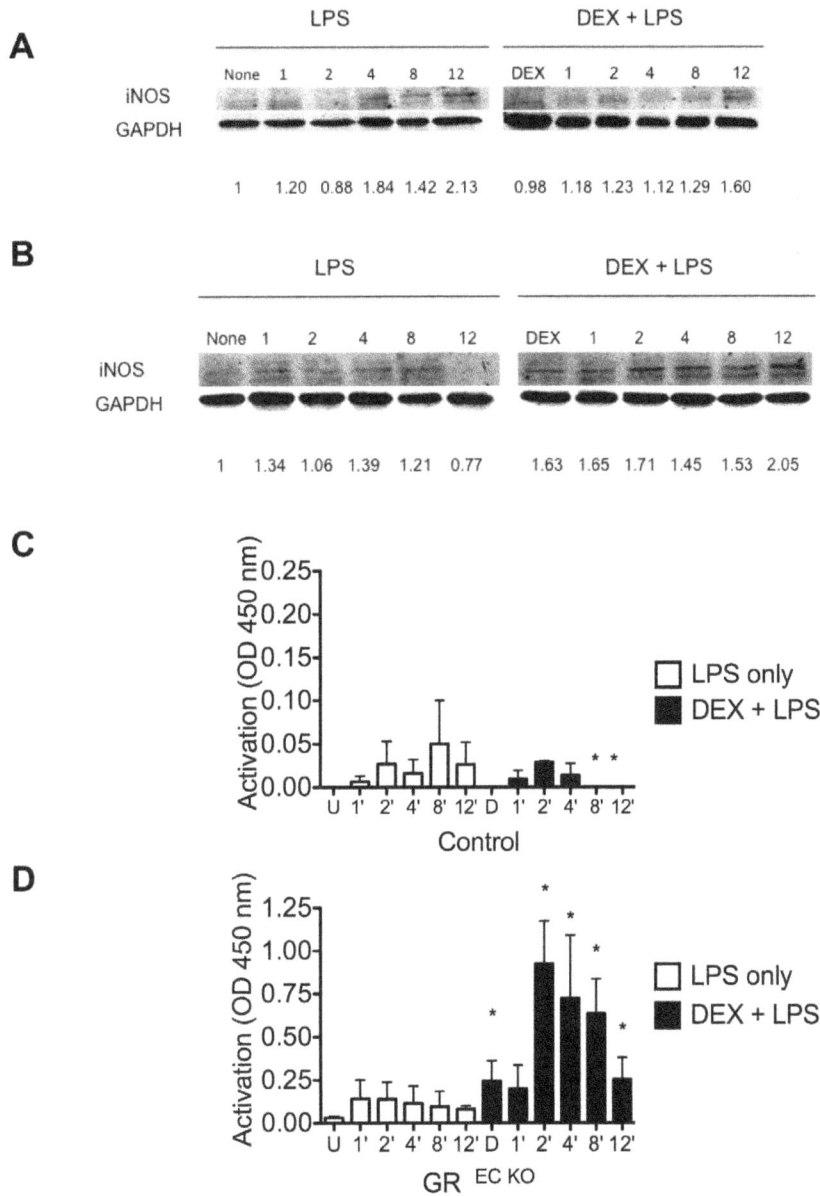

Figure 4. Increased iNOS expression and NF-κB activation in GR $^{EC\ KO}$ mice. Western blot of aortic homogenates from controls and GR $^{EC\ KO}$ mice treated with LPS alone or DEX+LPS and harvested at the indicated timepoints. Densitometry values are indicated below each lane. Activation of NF-κB was assayed in the same homogenates. (A) Control mice show decreased expression of iNOS when given DEX+LPS as compared to LPS alone and while (B) GR $^{EC\ KO}$ mice show increased iNOS levels following DEX+LPS as compared to LPS alone. (C) Activation of NF-κB is suppressed following DEX pre-treatment in control animals while in (D) GR $^{EC\ KO}$ mice increased activation of NF-κB is shown at every time point. *p<0.05 compared to similarly treated control. U = untreated, D = dexamethasone.

Dexamethasone reduces apoptosis and macrophage recruitment in the liver, but not the lungs of GR $^{EC\ KO}$ mice

To examine the effects of DEX+LPS on specific tissues, apoptosis and macrophage recruitment were assessed by TUNEL staining and CD68 staining, respectively in the liver and lung of GR $^{EC\ KO}$ and control mice (n = 4/group). Organs were harvested 8 hours after LPS injection. In the lung, DEX was able to suppress apoptosis and lessen macrophage recruitment to near baseline levels in control animals but was ineffective in both regards in GR $^{EC\ KO}$ mice (Figure 3A, 3C). In contrast, DEX was effective in reducing apoptosis and macrophage recruitment in the livers of

both GR $^{EC\ KO}$ and control mice (Figure 3B, 3D) implying that endothelial GR is not essential for hepatic protection by DEX.

Dexamethasone increases iNOS expression and NF- κB activation in GR $^{EC\ KO}$ mice after LPS

We previously showed that GR $^{EC\ KO}$ mice have increased iNOS expression after LPS [10]. To determine if pre-treatment with DEX affected the vascular control of iNOS, we pre-treated control and GR $^{EC\ KO}$ mice with DEX (2 mg/kg, IP) followed 2 hours later by LPS (12.5 mg/kg, IP) and harvested aortas over a range of time points to quantify iNOS protein levels. In control animals, LPS alone increased iNOS levels and pre-treatment with

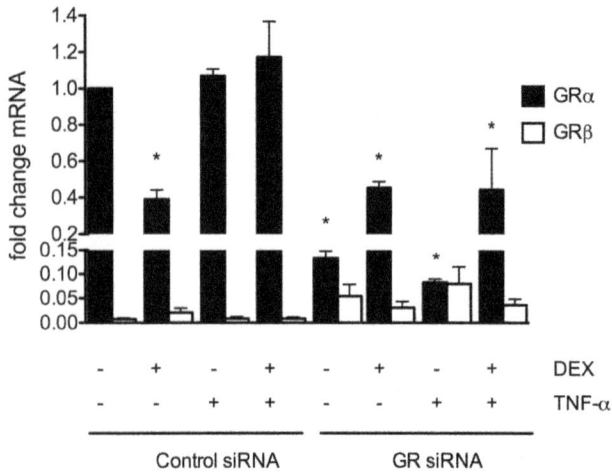

Figure 5. Expression profile of GRα and GRβ mRNA in endothelial cells. Real time PCR analysis was performed on mouse lung endothelial cells treated as described. Values were normalized to untreated control siRNA GRα levels and represent mean ± SEM for 3 independent samples. Cells were isolated from C57/BL6 mice. *p <0.05 compared to untreated control siRNA GRα levels.

DEX reduced iNOS as shown by Western blotting at the time points examined (Figure 4A). In contrast, DEX increased iNOS protein levels in GR $^{EC KO}$ mice at all time points even up until 12 hours after LPS injection (Figure 4B). To determine if the increased iNOS expression was a result of enhanced NF-κB activation, we assayed the activity of the p65 subunit of NF-κB, which is accessible only when NF-κB is activated and bound to its target DNA. As shown in Figure 4C, pre-treatment with DEX was able to suppress NF-κB activation by 8 hours after LPS administration in the control animals, while in the GR $^{EC KO}$ mice DEX pre-treatment resulted in heightened activation of NF-κB at almost all time points tested (Figure 4D).

Low expression of GRβ in endothelial cells

The existence of mouse GRβ was only recently confirmed in 2010 and little is known about its role in physiology [15]. In humans there is evidence that GRβ can inhibit GRα resulting in glucocorticoid resistance. To assess whether up regulation of GRβ in endothelial cells could play a role in the poor response to DEX observed in our mutant mice, we measured GRα and GRβ mRNA by qPCR in mouse lung endothelial cells at baseline and after treatment with DEX only, TNF-α only, or a combination of both. As shown in Figure 5, GRα mRNA was significantly decreased in GR siRNA-treated endothelial cells as expected and was significantly decreased in DEX treated cells, also as expected. The GRβ isoform was present in very low abundance in all conditions tested (~1–5%). There was a trend towards increased expression of GRβ after GR siRNA and DEX treatment though this did not reach statistical significance.

Discussion

The major finding of this study is that selective elimination of endothelial GR prevents the therapeutic protection by DEX in the setting of LPS induced sepsis syndrome. Mechanistically this occurs by increased activation of NF-κB resulting in increased expression of iNOS, hemodynamic instability, and increased levels of inflammatory cytokines such as IL-6 and TNF-α. While our previous work has demonstrated that presence of endothelial GR

is necessary for appropriate suppression of NF-κB [10], this study shows that absence of the receptor essentially mitigates and reverses the expected beneficial effects of DEX, which has been shown to prevent LPS-induced sepsis in several animal models [16–18]. Our study is particularly striking given that the expression of GR in all other cell types is unchanged, including in many immunologic cells germane to these studies such as macrophages, lymphocytes and neutrophils.

It is well known that glucocorticoids are effective therapy for many conditions mediated by NF-κB, a rapid response transcription factor involved in a host of immune and inflammatory conditions [19]. However, in our model the exogenous glucocorticoid not only is ineffective in rescuing GR $^{EC KO}$ mice following LPS but actually serves to worsen the phenotype. It should be re-iterated that GR $^{EC KO}$ mice demonstrate extreme sensitivity to LPS even in the absence of DEX, [10], a fact that highlights the importance of the endothelial GR since mice are traditionally viewed as an LPS-resistant species [20].

In trying to elcudiate how DEX promotes inflammation under our experimental conditions, it is important to consider the main mechanisms of how DEX is thought to suppress inflammation. Two hypothesis currently exist in this regard: (i) through direct protein interactions of GR with NF-κB and (ii) though interactions of GR with IκB, an inhibitory protein [19]. Our previous work has shown that elimination of endothelial GR results in prolonged activation of endothelial NF-κB in response to LPS [10]. Recent work has also suggested that the presence of the β isoform of the glucocorticoid receptor may be responsible for glucocorticoid resistance under some conditions, including in human septic shock [21,22].

Hinds et al. discovered the existence of the β isoform of the glucocorticoid receptor in mice in 2010. As in humans, this isoform is unresponsive to the glucocortioid agonist DEX and is able to inhibit GRα under some conditions [15]. Though little characterization of this isoform has yet been performed in mouse, the relative abundance of the β isoform seems to vary with the tissue/cell type investigated, ranging from ~30% of GRα in mouse embryonic fibroblasts and spleen to less than 5% in liver [15]. These results are in good agreement with human studies [23,24] and the predominance in the spleen is consistent with the known dominant effect of GRβ in lymphoid tissue [25]. Haim et al. recently showed that LPS affects the levels of GR isoforms in bone marrow-derived macrophages, a cell type that is of great import in sepsis models [26]. These authors showed that incubation of these cells with 1 μM DEX resulted in a substantial decrease in the expression of both GRα and GRβ isoforms. Interestingly, in this study, treatment with LPS alone resulted in significant upregulation of both isoforms while treatment with DEX + LPS caused upregulation of GRβ and downregulation of GRα [26]. Endothelial cells have not previously been characterized though, based on our results, GRβ exists at very low levels in this cell type. Though there was a trend toward increased expression of GRβ with DEX and TNFα treatments in the GR siRNA-treated cells, it did not reach statistical significance. Of note, there was also a trend towards increased expression of GRα in the DEX-treated GR siRNA cells, which supports the ineffectiveness of DEX in suppressing inflammation observed *in vivo* in the knockout phenotype, though it is not clear if this may be cause or effect.

A number of recent publications have begun to report potentially deleterious effects of DEX in situations where they would normally be expected to be beneficial, raising the question of whether up regulation of GRβ under certain conditions may be playing a role. A recent study in the cancer literature notes that steroids unexpectedly promote cancer cell survival and induce chemotherapy-resistance in breast cancer [27], potentially analogous to the worsening septic phenotype we observe in the GR ^{EC} ^{KO} mice treated with DEX+LPS. These authors speculate that GR could interact with different NF-κB subunits which would result in regulation of genes through different NF-κB signaling pathways. A similar deleterious effect has been found in acute brain injury, whereby administration of steroids has been found to augment inflammation [28]. Interestingly one of the mouse models used in these studies was an endothelial GR knockout (using Tie-2 Cre) which clearly showed pro-inflammatory effects of steroids on the blood-brain barrier mediated through endothelial GR. However, in this study the expression of the GRβ isoform was not assessed. New data suggests that perhaps the anti-inflammatory actions of GR cannot be explained by a unifying mechanism but that characteristics of target genes and transcriptional state may provide situation-specific repression [29].

Finally it has been shown in *in vivo* models in both rats and mice that NF-κB activation can follow a biphasic response with early activation (6–24 hours) being associated with iNOS expression and pro-inflammatory cytokines and the late phase (> 48 hours) being associated with absence of iNOS protein expression and paradoxical prolongation of inflammation [30]. Importantly, the NF-κB inhibitors used in this study were pharmacologic and not steroid-based. Though our experiments were performed during the 'early phase' and seem consistent with the pro-inflammatory response including iNOS activation, it is possible that the effects of DEX on NF-κB may include some dimerization that has not yet been characterized. Determining why DEX pre-treatment results in such a dramatic worsening of the phenotype in the GR $^{EC KO}$ mice will clearly require further study; however, it highlights that fact that mechanism of steroids' presumed ubiquitous anti-inflammatory action is clearly not well-understood despite their widespread clinical usage.

Supporting Information

Checklist S1 ARRIVE checklist.

Author Contributions

Conceived and designed the experiments: JG WS. Performed the experiments: JG YF HV HZ. Analyzed the data: JG HV. Contributed reagents/materials/analysis tools: JG HV WS. Wrote the paper: JG WS.

References

1. Stolte EH, van Kemenade BM, Savelkoul HF, Flik G (2006) Evolution of glucocorticoid receptors with different glucocorticoid sensitivity. J Endocrinol 190: 17–28.
2. Berry LJ, Smythe DS (1964) Effects of Bacterial Endotoxins on Metabolism. Vii. Enzyme Induction and Cortisone Protection. J Exp Med 120: 721–732.
3. Spink WW, Anderson D (1954) Experimental studies on the significance of endotoxin in the pathogenesis of brucellosis. J Clin Invest 33: 540–548.
4. Rhen T, Cidlowski JA (2005) Antiinflammatory action of glucocorticoids–new mechanisms for old drugs. N Engl J Med 353: 1711–1723.
5. Saklatvala J (2002) Glucocorticoids: do we know how they work? Arthritis Res 4: 146–150.
6. Osuchowski MF, Remick DG, Lederer JA, Lang CH, Aasen AO, et al. (2014) Abandon the mouse research ship? Not just yet! Shock 41: 463–475.
7. Seok J, Warren HS, Cuenca AG, Mindrinos MN, Baker HV, et al. (2013) Genomic responses in mouse models poorly mimic human inflammatory diseases. Proc Natl Acad Sci U S A 110: 3507–3512.
8. Tronche F, Kellendonk C, Reichardt HM, Schutz G (1998) Genetic dissection of glucocorticoid receptor function in mice. Curr Opin Genet Dev 8: 532–538.
9. Goodwin JE, Zhang J, Gonzalez D, Albinsson S, Geller DS (2011) Knockout of the vascular endothelial glucocorticoid receptor abrogates dexamethasone-induced hypertension. J Hypertens 29: 1347–1356.
10. Goodwin JE, Feng Y, Velazquez H, Sessa WC (2013) Endothelial glucocorticoid receptor is required for protection against sepsis. Proc Natl Acad Sci U S A 110: 306–311.
11. Langklotz S, Schakermann M, Narberhaus F (2011) Control of lipopolysaccharide biosynthesis by FtsH-mediated proteolysis of LpxC is conserved in enterobacteria but not in all gram-negative bacteria. J Bacteriol 193: 1090–1097.
12. Chauhan SD, Seggara G, Vo PA, Macallister RJ, Hobbs AJ, et al. (2003) Protection against lipopolysaccharide-induced endothelial dysfunction in resistance and conduit vasculature of iNOS knockout mice. FASEB J 17: 773–775.
13. Laubach VE, Foley PL, Shockey KS, Tribble CG, Kron IL (1998) Protective roles of nitric oxide and testosterone in endotoxemia: evidence from NOS-2-deficient mice. Am J Physiol 275: H2211–2218.
14. Fernandez-Hernando C, Ackah E, Yu J, Suarez Y, Murata T, et al. (2007) Loss of Akt1 leads to severe atherosclerosis and occlusive coronary artery disease. Cell Metab 6: 446–457.
15. Hinds TD Jr, Ramakrishnan S, Cash HA, Stechschulte LA, Heinrich G, et al. (2010) Discovery of glucocorticoid receptor-beta in mice with a role in metabolism. Mol Endocrinol 24: 1715–1727.
16. Figlewicz DP, Filkins JP (1978) Dexamethasone antagonism of glucose dyshomeostasis in endotoxin shock. Circ Shock 5: 317–323.
17. Kaddoura S, Curzen NP, Evans TW, Firth JD, Poole-Wilson PA (1996) Tissue expression of endothelin-1 mRNA in endotoxaemia. Biochem Biophys Res Commun 218: 641–647.
18. Wang X, Nelin LD, Kuhlman JR, Meng X, Welty SE, et al. (2008) The role of MAP kinase phosphatase-1 in the protective mechanism of dexamethasone against endotoxemia. Life Sci 83: 671–680.
19. Lee JI, Burckart GJ (1998) Nuclear factor kappa B: important transcription factor and therapeutic target. J Clin Pharmacol 38: 981–993.
20. Bonin CP, Baccarin RY, Nostell K, Nahum LA, Fossum C, et al. (2013) Lipopolysaccharide-induced inhibition of transcription of tlr4 in vitro is reversed by dexamethasone and correlates with presence of conserved NFkappaB binding sites. Biochem Biophys Res Commun 432: 256–261.
21. Guerrero J, Gatica HA, Rodriguez M, Estay R, Goecke IA (2013) Septic serum induces glucocorticoid resistance and modifies the expression of glucocorticoid isoforms receptors: a prospective cohort study and in vitro experimental assay. Crit Care 17: R107.
22. Taniguchi Y, Iwasaki Y, Tsugita M, Nishiyama M, Taguchi T, et al. (2010) Glucocorticoid receptor-beta and receptor-gamma exert dominant negative effect on gene repression but not on gene induction. Endocrinology 151: 3204–3213.
23. Oakley RH, Sar M, Cidlowski JA (1996) The human glucocorticoid receptor beta isoform. Expression, biochemical properties, and putative function. J Biol Chem 271: 9550–9559.
24. Webster JC, Oakley RH, Jewell CM, Cidlowski JA (2001) Proinflammatory cytokines regulate human glucocorticoid receptor gene expression and lead to the accumulation of the dominant negative beta isoform: a mechanism for the generation of glucocorticoid resistance. Proc Natl Acad Sci U S A 98: 6865–6870.
25. Oakley RH, Webster JC, Sar M, Parker CR Jr, Cidlowski JA (1997) Expression and subcellular distribution of the beta-isoform of the human glucocorticoid receptor. Endocrinology 138: 5028–5038.
26. Haim YO, Unger ND, Souroujon MC, Mittelman M, Neumann D (2014) Resistance of LPS-activated bone marrow derived macrophages to apoptosis mediated by dexamethasone. Sci Rep 4: 4323.
27. Ling J, Kumar R (2012) Crosstalk between NFkB and glucocorticoid signaling: a potential target for breast cancer therapy. Cancer Lett 322: 119–126.
28. Sorrells SF, Caso JR, Munhoz CD, Hu CK, Tran KV, et al. (2013) Glucocorticoid signaling in myeloid cells worsens acute CNS injury and inflammation. J Neurosci 33: 7877–7889.
29. Gupte R, Muse GW, Chinenov Y, Adelman K, Rogatsky I (2013) Glucocorticoid receptor represses proinflammatory genes at distinct steps of the transcription cycle. Proc Natl Acad Sci U S A 110: 14616–14621.
30. Lawrence T, Gilroy DW, Colville-Nash PR, Willoughby DA (2001) Possible new role for NF-kappaB in the resolution of inflammation. Nat Med 7: 1291–1297.

7

Bacteriology and Changes in Antibiotic Susceptibility in Adults with Community-Acquired Perforated Appendicitis

Hong Gil Jeon[1], Hyeong Uk Ju[1], Gyu Yeol Kim[2], Joseph Jeong[3], Min-Ho Kim[4], Jae-Bum Jun[1]*

1 Department of Internal Medicine, Ulsan University Hospital, University of Ulsan College of Medicine, Ulsan, Republic of Korea, **2** Department of Surgery, Ulsan University Hospital, University of Ulsan College of Medicine, Ulsan, Republic of Korea, **3** Department of Laboratory Medicine, Ulsan University Hospital, University of Ulsan College of Medicine, Ulsan, Republic of Korea, **4** Biomedical Research Center, Ulsan University Hospital, University of Ulsan College of Medicine, Ulsan, Republic of Korea

Abstract

This study evaluated bacterial etiology and antibiotic susceptibility in patients diagnosed with community-acquired perforated appendicitis over a 12-year-period. We retrospectively reviewed records of adult patients diagnosed with perforated appendicitis at an 800-bed teaching hospital between January 2000 and December 2011. In total, 415 culture-positive perforated appendicitis cases were analyzed. *Escherichia coli* was the most common pathogen (277/415, 66.7%), followed by *Streptococcus* species (61/415, 14.7%). The susceptibility of *E. coli* to ampicillin, piperacillin/tazobactam, ceftriaxone, cefepime, amikacin, gentamicin, and imipenem was 35.1%, 97.1%, 97.0%, 98.2%, 98.9%, 81.8%, and 100%, respectively. The overall susceptibility of *E. coli* to quinolones (ciprofloxacin or levofloxacin) was 78.7%. During the study period, univariate logistic regression analysis showed a significant decrease in *E. coli* susceptibility to quinolones (OR = 0.91, 95% CI 0.84–0.99, $P = 0.040$). We therefore do not recommend quinolones as empirical therapy for community-acquired perforated appendicitis.

Editor: D William Cameron, University of Ottawa, Canada

Funding: The authors have no support or funding to report.

Competing Interests: The authors have declared that no competing interests exist.

* Email: uvgotletter@hanmail.net

Introduction

Acute appendicitis is one of the most common abdominal surgical emergencies; it is also typically a community-acquired infection. Despite the generally favorable outcome, complicated appendicitis, such as perforated appendicitis, is associated with increased morbidity compared with simple acute appendicitis [1,2]. Because *Escherichia coli* and *Bacteroides fragilis* are most commonly associated with appendicitis, antibiotic therapies are generally selected to target these bacteria [3,4].

For adult patients with community-acquired complicated intra-abdominal infections of mild-to moderate severity, the use of ticarcillin-clavulanate, cefoxitin, ertapenem, moxifloxacin, or tigecycline as single-agent therapy or combinations of metronidazole with cefazolin, cefuroxime, ceftriaxone, cefotaxime, levofloxacin, or ciprofloxacin are recommended by Infectious Diseases Society of America (IDSA) guidelines [5]. However, with increased *E. coli* resistance to quinolones, investigation of local microbiologic findings had been proposed when selecting empirical therapies [5].

Because previous literature has reported a proportionally greater ratio of extended-spectrum β-lactamase (ESBL) and quinolone-resistant *E. coli* among bacteria responsible for community-acquired abdominal infections in Asia compared to other regions, careful selection of empirical antibiotics is particularly important in Asia [6–8]. We therefore conducted a study of the local microbiological profile and changes in antibiotic resistance in community-acquired perforated appendicitis over the past 12 years. These results may help us to inform selection of empirical antibiotic treatments for community-acquired complicated appendicitis.

Materials and Methods

Patient selection and data collection

We retrospectively reviewed the records of adult patients (age ≥ 18 years) who were diagnosed to have perforated appendicitis at Ulsan University Hospital, an 800-bed teaching hospital, between January 2000 to December 2011. Hospital charts and follow-up records were reviewed.

Definitions

Perforated appendicitis was defined as either gross or microscopic evidence of appendiceal perforation. The appendix was not considered to be ruptured by the mere presence of suppurative peritoneal fluid or gangrenous appendicitis without microscopic evidence of perforation.

Community-acquired appendicitis was defined as appendicitis that occurred within 48 hours of hospital admission. Patients were excluded from the study if they had at least 1 of the following health care risk factors: 1) presence of an invasive device at time of admission, 2) history of MRSA infection or colonization, 3) history of surgery, hospitalization, dialysis, or residence in a long-term care facility in the 12 months preceding the culture date [5].

Systemic inflammatory response syndrome (SIRS), sepsis, severe sepsis, and septic shock were defined as described elsewhere [9].

Specimen culture, species identification, and susceptibility testing

Specimens were obtained by swabbing the suppurative peritoneal fluid or periappendiceal abscess. In some cases, specimens were obtained by swabbing the lumen of appendix or by retrieving the suppurative peritoneal fluid via syringe aspiration. The swab specimens were transported to the laboratory in a transport medium (Amies transport medium without Charcoal; Asan Pharmaceuticals Co., Ltd., Hwasung, Korea). The specimens were either dispatched to the microbiology laboratory directly or stored in the operating room until the next day if collected after the working hours. The specimens were inoculated on blood agar, chocolate agar, and MacConkey agar plates. Samples were not inoculated into anaerobic culture. An automated VITEK 2 system (bioMerieux, Inc. Durham, NC, USA) was used to identify pathogens and perform ESBL susceptibility testing. The Vitek 2 ESBL test has 6 wells containing cefepime at 1 μg/mL, cefotaxime at 0.5 μg/mL, and ceftazidime at 0.5 μg/mL alone and in combination with clavulanic acid (10 μg/mL, 4 μg/mL, and 4 μg/mL, respectively); growth rate in each well is quantitatively assessed with an optical scanner. The proportional growth reduction (over 50%) in wells containing cephalosporin plus clavulanic acid compared with those containing cephalosporin alone was considered evidence of ESBL production. Susceptibility testing results were interpreted according to the National Committee for Clinical Laboratory Standards (CLSI) guidelines published in 2009 [10]. However, cephalosporin susceptibility results of ESBL-positive strains were interpreted on the basis of the strains' respective minimal inhibitory concentration (MIC) breakpoints.

Ethics statement

This retrospective study was approved by the Institutional Review Board (IRB) committee of Ulsan University Hospital. Written consent given by the patients was waived by the approving IRB.

Statistical analysis

Statistical analyses were performed by using IBM SPSS Statistics for Windows, version 21 (IBM Corp., Armonk, NY, USA). The Chi-squared test was used to compare frequencies. A univariate logistic regression model was used to calculate odds ratios (OR), 95% confidence intervals, and p-values. The significance level was set at 0.05.

Results

Study population and clinical characteristics

Of 3,379 patients, 567 (16.7%) who received appendectomies during the study period were diagnosed with perforated appendicitis. Of these, we discarded 4 cases of health care-associated infection, 6 without confirmatory cultures, and 142 culture-negative cases; in total, we analyzed 415 culture-positive perforated appendicitis cases. The average length of hospitalization was 9.1±5.1 days. Patient ages ranged between 20 years and 94 years (mean 48.6±17.0 years), with 51.1% (212/415) men (Table 1). A majority of patients (404, 97.3%) underwent open appendectomy via a McBurney incision; laparotomy with a low midline incision was performed in 9 patients (2.2%) and

laparoscopic appendectomy was performed in 2 patients (0.5%). The most common underlying disease was hypertension, reported in 56 patients (13.5%). Severe sepsis or septic shock was observed in 70 patients (16.8%), while 1 patient (0.2%) died of sepsis after mechanical ileus. Post-operative complications included wound infection in 18 patients (4.3%), abdominal abscesses or peritonitis in 7 patients (1.6%), and mechanical ileus in 6 patients (1.4%). A combination therapy comprising cephalosporin and metronidazole was the most frequent empirical antibiotic treatment.

Microbiological features

The most commonly isolated bacteria was *E. coli* (277 isolates, 66.7%), followed by *Streptococcus* spp. (61, 14.7%), *Enterococcus* spp. (32, 7.7%), *Klebsiella* spp. (25, 6.0%), and *Pseudomonas aeruginosa* (24, 5.8%) (Table 2). More than 2 organisms were isolated in 75 cases (18.0%).

Antibiotic susceptibilities of isolated organisms

Data on antibiotic susceptibilities of isolated organisms showed that *E. coli* had 78.7% susceptibility to quinolones (ciprofloxacin or levofloxacin). Susceptibilities to ampicillin, aztreonam, ampicillin/sulbactam, amoxicillin/clavulanic acid, piperacillin/tazobactam, cefazolin, cefoxitin, ceftriaxone, cefepime, trimethoprim/sulfamethoxazole, amikacin, gentamicin, tobramycin, and imipenem were 35.1%, 95.2%, 41.4%, 83.5%, 97.1%, 89.8%, 97.7%, 97.0%, 98.2%, 65.6%, 98.9%, 81.8%, 83.4%, and 100%, respectively (Table 3). ESBL-producing strains accounted for 3.9% of *E. coli* species. *Streptococcus* species showed 68.9% susceptibility to penicillin, and 100% susceptibility to ceftriaxone. *Enterococcus* species were 71.9% susceptible to penicillin. The susceptibilities of *P. aeruginosa* to piperacillin/tazobactam, cefepime, quinolones, amikacin, and imipenem were 95.2%, 100%, 87.5%, 100%, and 95.8%, respectively.

Comparisons of bacterial species and *E. coli* isolate antibiotic susceptibilities by clinical severity

We compared the bacterial species and antibiotic susceptibilities of *E. coli* isolates according to the clinically indicated severity (Table 4). The cases were redistributed into two major groups: "sepsis" and "severe sepsis." Infected patients without SIRS and the patients with sepsis were grouped together in the "sepsis" group, whereas the patients with severe sepsis and septic shock were grouped together in the "severe sepsis" group. A total of 345 patients (83.1%) were included in the sepsis group and 70 (16.9%) were included in the severe sepsis group. *E. coli* isolates were found more frequently in the severe sepsis group (74.3%) than in the sepsis group (65.2%), but the difference was not statistically significant. The isolation rates of the other species were also not significantly different between groups. There were no statistically significant differences in *E. coli* susceptibility to all antibiotics between groups.

Changes in *E. coli* antimicrobial susceptibility according to the year

Yearly changes in *E. coli* antimicrobial susceptibility during the study period were examined (Fig. 1). Univariate logistic regression analysis showed that *E. coli* susceptibility to quinolones significantly decreased, with annual susceptibility rates of 89.4%, 83.3%, 89.2%, 84.2%, 66.6%, 74.0%, 82.6%, 69.2%, 80.0%, 61.9%, 65.0%, and 85.0%, during the period of 2000 to 2011 (OR = 0.91, 95% CI 0.84–0.99, $P = 0.040$). In particular, *E. coli* susceptibility to cefoxitin ($P = 0.052$) and ceftriaxone ($P = 0.054$) decreased during the study period, but the change was not statistically

Table 1. Baseline characteristics of patients with perforated appendicitis.

Characteristics	Number (%)
Number of culture positive patients	415
Hospital day (Mean ± SD)	9.1±5.1
Age (Mean ± SD)	48.6±17.0
Sex	
male	212 (51.1)
female	203 (48.9)
Operation method	
laparoscopic	2 (0.5)
McBurney	404 (97.3)
laparotomy	9 (2.2)
Underlying disease	
hypertension	56 (13.5)
diabetes mellitus	26 (6.3)
hepatitis B virus	16 (3.9)
solid cancer	12 (2.9)
Initial manifestation	
infection without SIRS	73 (17.6)
sepsis	272 (65.7)
severe sepsis	67 (16.1)
septic shock	3 (0.7)
In-hospital mortality	
alive	414 (99.8)
death	1 (0.2)
Infectious complication	
wound infection	18 (4.3)
intra-abdominal abscess or peritonitis	7 (1.6)
mechanical ileus	6 (1.4)
Antibiotics	
1st (or 2nd) generation cephalosporin + metronidazole	215 (51.8)
3rd generation cephalosporin + metronidazole	193 (46.5)
ciprofloxacin + metronidazole	4 (1.0)
piperacillin/tazobactam	3 (0.7)

SIRS = systemic inflammatory response syndrome.

significant. Nor were any statistically significant changes observed in *E. coli* susceptibility to other antibiotics such as ampicillin ($P = 0.235$), aztreonam ($P = 0.168$), piperacillin/tazobactam ($P = 0.645$), cefazolin ($P = 0.126$), cefepime ($P = 0.393$), trimethoprim/sulfamethoxazole ($P = 0.732$), amikacin ($P = 0.835$), gentamicin ($P = 0.389$), and tobramycin ($P = 0.645$).

Discussion

This study evaluated microbiological profiles and antibiotic susceptibilities of pathogens isolated from cases of perforated appendicitis. The flora detected in complicated intra-abdominal infection differs between community-acquired and nosocomial infections. We considered appendicitis suitable for studying community-acquired bacterial infections since this illness is largely community-acquired. In fact, only 4 patients discarded from analysis owing to health care-associated infections. *P. aeruginosa*

isolates in this study showed overall high levels of antibiotic susceptibility with no multidrug-resistant strains, supporting the idea that appendicitis is more commonly a community-acquired rather than nosocomial infection [11].

E. coli was the most common pathogen identified in this study (66.7% of all isolates), similar to findings in previous appendicitis literature [3,12]. Similarly, *Streptococcus* and *Enterococcus* species were the most frequently isolated gram-positive organisms [12,13]. The ratio of ESBL-producing *E. coli* was 3.9%, within previously reported ranges of 3.5–15.4% [8,14]. The isolation rate of *E. coli* was greater in the severe sepsis group, although this difference was not statistically significant. Some studies have reported that *P. aeruginosa* is a commonly isolated strain in appendicitis, with an isolation rate of 19–32%; however, this was not the case in the current study [12,15].

Although *E. coli* showed a high susceptibility rate of 97% to second- and third-generation cephalosporins that are most

Table 2. Distribution of bacterial species.

	Species	Number (%)[f]
Gram negative organism	Escherichia coli	277 (66.7)
	Klebsiella species[a]	25 (6.0)
	Pseudomonas aeruginosa	24 (5.8)
	Other gram negative organism[b]	45 (10.8)
Gram positive organism	Streptococcus species[c]	61 (14.7)
	Enterococcus species[d]	32 (7.7)
	Staphylococcus aureus	6 (1.4)
	Other gram positive organism[e]	23 (5.5)

[a]Includes: K. pneumoniae, K. oxytoca.
[b]Includes: Achromobacter xylosoxidans, Acinetobacter lwoffii, Aeromonas hydrophila, Comamonas testosteroni, Hafnia alvei, Proteus mirabilis, Raoultella planticola, Serratia species, Enterobacter cloacae.
[c]Includes: S. alactolyticus, S. anginosus, S. cristatus, S. constellatus, S. gordonii, S. intermedius, S. mitis, S. salivarius, S. sanguinis, Viridans Streptococci.
[d]Includes: E. avium, E. faecalis, E. faecium, E. gallinarum, E. hirae, E. raffinosus.
[e]Includes: Gemella morbillorum, Lactococcus garvieae, Leuconostoc mesenteroides, Pediococcus pentosaceus.
[f]Polymicrobial infection: 75 cases (18.0%).

Table 3. Antibiotic susceptibilities of isolated organisms that caused perforated appendicitis.

Antibiotic	E. coli (total) (n = 277)	E. coli (non-ESBL) (n = 266)	E. coli (ESBL) (n = 11)	Streptococcus species (n = 61)	Enterococcus species (n = 32)	P. aeruginosa (n = 24)
Penicillin				42/61 (68.9)	23/32 (71.9)	
Ampicillin	97/276 (35.1)	97/265 (36.6)	0/11 (0)		24/27 (88.8)	
Aztreonam	220/231 (95.2)	217/220 (98.6)	3/11 (27.2)			
Ampicillin/sulbactam	84/203 (41.4)	84/200 (42.0)	0/3 (0)			
Amoxicillin/clavulanic acid	61/73 (83.5)	55/65 (84.6)	6/8 (75.0)			
Piperacillin/tazobactam	240/247 (97.1)	229/236 (97.0)	11/11 (100)			20/21 (95.2)
Cefazolin	248/276 (89.8)	248/265 (93.5)	0/11 (0)			
Cefoxitin	264/270 (97.7)	254/259 (98.0)	10/11 (90.9)			
Ceftriaxone	267/275 (97.0)	262/264 (99.2)	5/11 (45.4)	39/39 (100)		2/24 (8.3)
Cefepime	227/231 (98.2)	220/220 (100)	7/11 (63.6)			22/22 (100)
Quinolone	218/277 (78.7)	215/266 (80.8)	3/11 (27.2)		25/28 (89.2)	21/24 (87.5)
Trimethoprim/sulfamethoxazole	181/276 (65.6)	177/265 (66.7)	4/11 (36.3)	34/47 (72.3)	11/17 (64.7)	1/24 (4.1)
Amikacin	274/277 (98.9)	264/266 (99.2)	10/11 (90.9)			24/24 (100)
Gentamicin	226/276 (81.8)	221/265 (83.4)	5/11 (45.4)			24/24 (100)
Tobramycin	231/277 (83.4)	227/266 (85.3)	4/11 (36.3)			24/24 (100)
Vancomycin				60/61 (98.3)	30/32 (93.7)	
Imipenem	276/276 (100)	265/265 (100)	11/11 (100)	11/11 (100)	23/26 (88.5)	23/24 (95.8)

Table 4. Comparisons of bacterial species and antibiotic susceptibilities of *E. coli* between the sepsis group and the severe sepsis group.

	Sepsis[a] (%)	Severe sepsis[b] (%)	*P*-value
Species			
E. coli	225/345 (65.2)	52/70 (74.3)	0.142
P. aeruginosa	20/345 (5.8)	4/70 (5.7)	0.978
Streptococcus species	52/345 (15.1)	9/70 (12.9)	0.633
Enterococcus species	25/345 (7.3)	7/70 (10.0)	0.431
Antibiotics susceptibilities of *E. coli*			
Piperacillin/tazobactam	197/202 (97.5)	43/45 (95.6)	0.472
Cefoxitin	214/220 (97.3)	50/50 (100)	0.238
Ceftriaxone	215/223 (96.4)	52/52 (100)	0.166
Cefepime	184/187 (98.4)	43/44 (97.7)	0.760
Ciprofloxacin or levofloxacin	176/225 (78.2)	42/52 (80.8)	0.686

[a]Infection without SIRS (systemic inflammatory response syndrome) & sepsis.
[b]Severe sepsis & septic shock.

commonly used for empirical antibiotic treatment, the susceptibility decreased during the study period, albeit without statistical significance ($P = 0.052$ and $P = 0.054$, respectively). The susceptibility to quinolones was 78.7%, with a statistically significant ($P = 0.040$) decrease during the study period. Previous studies by Bochicchio et al (2006) and Rob et al (2013) reported that the susceptibility rate of *E. coli*, isolated from appendicitis samples, to quinolones was 71.4–85.6% [6,8]. The *E. coli* susceptibility to quinolones and cephalosporins reported by Rob et al (2013) was lower than that reported by Bochicchio et al (2006). This may be attributable to *E. coli*'s increased resistance to the antibiotics or the lowered MIC breakpoint for cephalosporins set by the CLSI guidelines. For most antibiotics, *E. coli* susceptibility rates observed in this study were similar to those reported by Bochicchio

et al (2006), with the susceptibility rate to quinolones being slightly lower. Both previous studies found high susceptibilities to carbapenem, amikacin, and piperacillin/tazobactam; in this study, ESBL-producing organisms were particularly sensitive to piperacillin/tazobactam (12/12, 100%). The susceptibility of *Streptococcus* species to penicillin was 68.9%, and all strains were susceptible to ceftriaxone. *P. aeruginosa* isolated in this study was highly susceptible to amikacin, cefepime, piperacillin/tazobactam, and carbapenem, but was slightly less susceptible to quinolones (87.5%).

All patients undergoing operation for appendicitis should receive antimicrobial therapy [16]. Appropriate antimicrobial therapy includes agents effective against facultative and aerobic gram-negative organisms and anaerobic organisms. There are

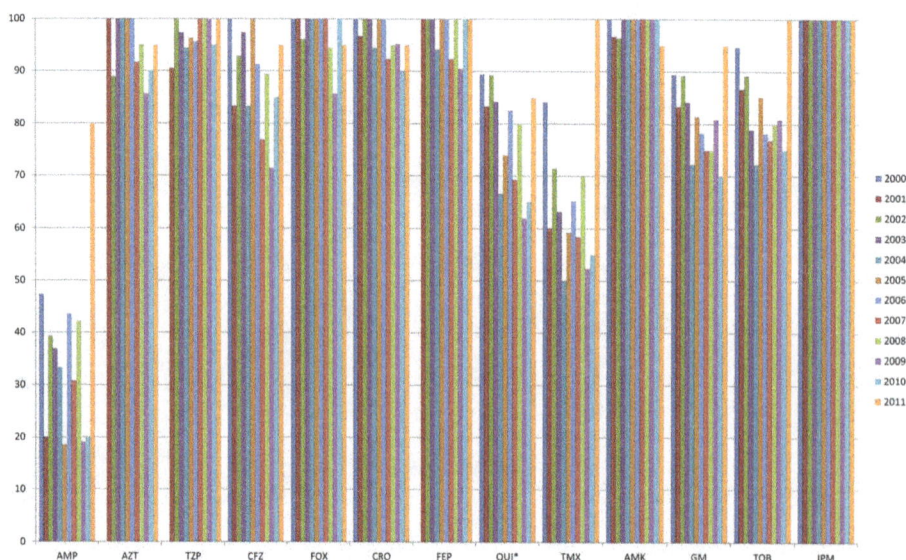

Figure 1. Change of antimicrobial susceptibility among *E. coli* during the 12-year-period. AMP, ampicillin; AZT, aztreonam; TZP, piperacillin/tazobactam; CFZ, cefazolin; FOX, cefoxitin; CRO, ceftriaxone; FEP, cefepime; QUI, quinolone; TMX, trimethoprim/sulfamethoxazole; AMK, amikacin; GM, gentamicin; TOB, tobramycin; IPM, imipenem. * During the study period, there was a significant decrease in antimicrobial susceptibility on univariate logistic regression analysis ($P = 0.040$).

data that inadequate empiric antibiotic therapy results in increased morbidity or treatment failure in complicated appendicitis [17,18]. If resistance to a given antibiotic is present in 10%–20% or more of isolates of a common intra-abdominal pathogen in the community, use of that agent should be avoided [5]. A report in Taiwan proposed that a quinolone be used to treat community-acquired complicated intra-abdominal infections, as *E. coli* was found to be 82–85% susceptible to ciprofloxacin and levofloxacin [19]. In this study, however, the resistance rate of *E. coli* to quinolones is >20%; therefore, its use as an empirical antibiotic is not advisable in Korea. Second- and third-generation cephalosporins appeared to be an appropriate treatment for this application according to our results. Although third-generation cephalosporins might be a better treatment choice because that *Streptococcus* species showed 100% susceptibility to ceftriaxone, further studies are needed to thoroughly trace variations in susceptibility, given that the decrease in *E. coli* susceptibility, observed during the study period, was not statistically significant. Piperacillin/tazobactam and carbapenem might be considered to treat *P. aeruginosa* or ESBL-producing organisms in patients with signs of severe sepsis such as organ dysfunction. However, these species were not frequently isolated in all patient groups including the severe sepsis group of the current study, and spectrum of these antibiotics may be too broad. *E. coli* also showed high susceptibility to amikacin, but concerns remain regarding use of aminoglycoside antibiotics owing to their nephrotoxicity and ototoxicity. Considering the high resistance of *E. coli* to ampicillin and ampicillin/sulbactam–and the questionable significance of enterococci as pathogens in complicated intra-abdominal infections–these antibiotics are not recommended for treating perforated appendicitis.

On the basis of evidence that culture testing of intraoperative specimens does not affect the prognosis of patients with perforated appendicitis, many institutions may not perform routine culture testing [20,21]. However, considering the current reality of increasing antibiotic resistance, routine culture testing might be useful to identify changes in susceptibility and to select appropriate antibiotics [5]. Anaerobic cultures are not necessary for patients with community-acquired intra-abdominal infection if empiric antimicrobial therapy active against common anaerobic pathogens is provide [5]. Although anaerobic bacteria culturing was not performed in this study, previous reports on anaerobic culture showed that *Bacteroides fragilis*, along with *E. coli*, was the most commonly isolated pathogen in appendicitis [14,20]. In past studies of appendicitis that conducted anaerobic susceptibility testing, *B. fragilis* was found to be more than 95% susceptible to metronidazole [4,14,22]. Anaerobic bacteria culturing could be considered for future studies if an increase in anaerobic bacterial resistance to metronidazole is observed.

The retrospective nature of the present study might have resulted in intrinsic bias and the data may not represent the entire population because data was collected from a single institution. However, considering that the quinolone resistance rate we observed was similar to that reported in previous studies conducted in Korea [23,24]–which involved community-acquired *E. coli* bacteremia originated from various infections including intra-abdominal infection–we speculated that quinolone resistance rate among *E. coli* causing intra-abdominal infection in Korea should be similar to the one determined in this study.

In conclusion, *E. coli* was the most commonly identified pathogen in patients with perforated appendicitis. The quinolone resistance rate was >20% in *E. coli* isolated from community-acquired perforated appendicitis. The isolates were decreasingly susceptible to quinolones during the study period. We advise against the use of quinolones as a first line antibiotic therapy in community-acquired perforated appendicitis in Korea.

Author Contributions

Conceived and designed the experiments: J-BJ. Performed the experiments: HGJ HUJ. Analyzed the data: GYK JJ M-HK. Contributed to the writing of the manuscript: J-BJ.

References

1. Lau WY, Wong SH (1981) Randomized, prospective trial of topical hydrogen peroxide in appendectomy wound infection. High risk factors. Am J Surg 142: 393–397.
2. Schmit PJ, Hiyama DT, Swisher SG, Bennion RS, Thompson JE Jr (1994) Analysis of risk factors of postappendectomy intra-abdominal abscess. J Am Coll Surg 179: 721–726.
3. Bennion RS, Baron EJ, Thompson JE Jr, Downes J, Summanen P, et al. (1990) The bacteriology of gangrenous and perforated appendicitis–revisited. Ann Surg 211: 165–171.
4. Lau WY, Teoh-Chan CH, Fan ST, Yam WC, Lau KF, et al. (1984) The bacteriology and septic complication of patients with appendicitis. Ann Surg 200: 576–581.
5. Solomkin JS, Mazuski JE, Bradley JS, Rodvold KA, Goldstein EJ, et al. (2010) Diagnosis and management of complicated intra-abdominal infection in adults and children: guidelines by the Surgical Infection Society and the Infectious Diseases Society of America. Clin Infect Dis 50: 133–164.
6. Bochicchio GV, Baquero F, Hsueh PR, Paterson DL, Rossi F, et al. (2006) In vitro susceptibilities of Escherichia coli isolated from patients with intra-abdominal infections worldwide in 2002–2004: results from SMART (Study for Monitoring Antimicrobial Resistance Trends). Surg Infect (Larchmt) 7: 537–545.
7. Paterson DL, Rossi F, Baquero F, Hsueh PR, Woods GL, et al. (2005) In vitro susceptibilities of aerobic and facultative Gram-negative bacilli isolated from patients with intra-abdominal infections worldwide: the 2003 Study for Monitoring Antimicrobial Resistance Trends (SMART). J Antimicrob Chemother 55: 965–973.
8. Lob SH, Badal RE, Bouchillon SK, Hawser SP, Hackel MA, et al. (2013) Epidemiology and susceptibility of Gram-negative appendicitis pathogens: SMART 2008–2010. Surg Infect (Larchmt) 14: 203–208.
9. Bone RC, Sibbald WJ, Sprung CL (1992) The ACCP-SCCM consensus conference on sepsis and organ failure. Chest 101: 1481–1483.
10. Clinical and Laboratory Standards Institute (2009) Performance standards for antimicrobial susceptibility testing. Nineteenth informational supplement. Document M100–S19. Wayne, PA: CLSI.
11. Montravers P, Lepape A, Dubreuil L, Gauzit R, Pean Y, et al. (2009) Clinical and microbiological profiles of community-acquired and nosocomial intra-abdominal infections: results of the French prospective, observational EBIIA study. J Antimicrob Chemother 63: 785–794.
12. Guillet-Caruba C, Cheikhelard A, Guillet M, Bille E, Descamps P, et al. (2011) Bacteriologic epidemiology and empirical treatment of pediatric complicated appendicitis. Diagn Microbiol Infect Dis 69: 376–381.
13. Chen CY, Chen YC, Pu HN, Tsai CH, Chen WT, et al. (2012) Bacteriology of acute appendicitis and its implication for the use of prophylactic antibiotics. Surg Infect (Larchmt) 13: 383–390.
14. Chan KW, Lee KH, Mou JW, Cheung ST, Sihoe JD, et al. (2010) Evidence-based adjustment of antibiotic in pediatric complicated appendicitis in the era of antibiotic resistance. Pediatr Surg Int 26: 157–160.
15. Fallon SC, Hassan SF, Larimer EL, Rodriguez JR, Brandt ML, et al. (2013) Modification of an evidence-based protocol for advanced appendicitis in children. J Surg Res 185: 273–277.
16. Andersen BR, Kallehave FL, Andersen HK (2001) Antibiotics versus placebo for prevention of postoperative infection after appendectomy. Cochrane Database Syst Rev: CD001439.
17. Yellin AE, Heseltine PN, Berne TV, Appleman MD, Gill MA, et al. (1985) The role of Pseudomonas species in patients treated with ampicillin and Sulbactam for gangrenous and perforated appendicitis. Surg Gynecol Obstet 161: 303–307.
18. Berne TV, Yellin AW, Appleman MD, Heseltine PN (1982) Antibiotic management of surgically treated gangrenous or perforated appendicitis. Comparison of gentamicin and clindamycin versus cefamandole versus cefoperazone. Am J Surg 144: 8–13.
19. Lau YJ, Chen YH, Huang CT, Lee WS, Liu CY, et al. (2012) Role of moxifloxacin for the treatment of community-acquired [corrected] complicated intra-abdominal infections in Taiwan. J Microbiol Immunol Infect 45: 1–6.

20. Kokoska ER, Silen ML, Tracy TF Jr, Dillon PA, Kennedy DJ, et al. (1999) The impact of intraoperative culture on treatment and outcome in children with perforated appendicitis. J Pediatr Surg 34: 749–753.
21. Foo FJ, Beckingham IJ, Ahmed I (2008) Intra-operative culture swabs in acute appendicitis: a waste of resources. Surgeon 6: 278–281.
22. Wojcik-Stojek B, Bulanda M, Martirosian G, Heczko P, Meisel-Mikolajczyk F (2000) In vitro antibiotic susceptibility of Bacteroides fragilis strains isolated from excised appendix of patients with phlegmonous or gangrenous appendicitis. Acta Microbiol Pol 49: 171–175.
23. Lee S, Han SW, Kim KW, Song do Y, Kwon KT (2014) Third-generation cephalosporin resistance of community-onset Escherichia coli and Klebsiella pneumoniae bacteremia in a secondary hospital. Korean J Intern Med 29: 49–56.
24. Park S, Park J, Lee S (2005) Analysis on the etiology and prognostic factors of community-acquired bacteremia in a community-based tertiary hospital. Infect Chemother 37: 255–264.

8

A Biomarker Panel (Bioscore) Incorporating Monocytic Surface and Soluble TREM-1 Has High Discriminative Value for Ventilator-Associated Pneumonia: A Prospective Observational Study

Vimal Grover[1,2,3], Panagiotis Pantelidis[2,4], Neil Soni[1,3], Masao Takata[3], Pallav L. Shah[5,6], Athol U. Wells[6], Don C. Henderson[2,4], Peter Kelleher[2,4], Suveer Singh[1,3,5]*

1 Magill Department of Anaesthesia, Critical Care and Pain, Chelsea and Westminster Hospital National Health Service Foundation Trust, London, United Kingdom, 2 Immunology Section, Department of Medicine, Imperial College, London, United Kingdom, 3 Department of Surgery and Cancer, Imperial College, London, United Kingdom, 4 Department of Immunology, Imperial College Healthcare National Health Service Trust, London, United Kingdom, 5 Department of Respiratory Medicine, Chelsea and Westminster Hospital National Health Service Foundation Trust, London, United Kingdom, 6 Department of Respiratory Medicine, Royal Brompton & Harefield Hospitals National Health Service Foundation Trust, London, United Kingdom

Abstract

Introduction: Ventilator-associated pneumonia (VAP) increases mortality in critical illness. However, clinical diagnostic uncertainty persists. We hypothesised that measuring cell-surface and soluble inflammatory markers, incorporating Triggering Receptor Expressed by Myeloid cells (TREM)-1, would improve diagnostic accuracy.

Methods: A single centre prospective observational study, set in a University Hospital medical-surgical intensive Care unit, recruited 91 patients into 3 groups: 27 patients with VAP, 33 ventilated controls without evidence of pulmonary sepsis (non-VAP), and 31 non-ventilated controls (NVC), without clinical infection, attending for bronchoscopy. Paired samples of Bronchiolo-alveolar lavage fluid (BALF) and blood from each subject were analysed for putative biomarkers of infection: Cellular (TREM-1, CD11b and CD62L) and soluble (IL-1β, IL-6, IL-8, sTREM-1, Procalcitonin). Expression of cellular markers on monocytes and neutrophils were measured by flow cytometry. Soluble inflammatory markers were determined by ELISA. A biomarker panel ('Bioscore'), was constructed, tested and validated, using Fisher's discriminant function analysis, to assess its value in distinguishing VAP from non VAP.

Results: The expression of TREM-1 on monocytes (mTREM-1) and neutrophils (nTREM-1) and concentrations of IL-1β, IL-8, and sTREM-1 in BALF were significantly higher in VAP compared with non-VAP and NVC ($p < 0.001$). The BALF/blood mTREM-1 was significantly higher in VAP patients compared to non-VAP and NVC (0.8 v 0.4 v 0.3 $p < 0.001$). A seven marker Bioscore (BALF/blood ratio mTREM-1 and mCD11b, BALF sTREM-1, IL-8 and IL-1β, and serum CRP and IL-6) correctly identified 88.9% of VAP cases and 100% of non-VAP cases.

Conclusion: A 7-marker bioscore, incorporating cellular and soluble TREM-1, accurately discriminates VAP from non-pulmonary infection.

Editor: Charles Dela Cruz, Yale University, United States of America

Funding: This work was supported by Chelsea and Westminster Health Charity (http://www.cwhc.org.uk/), Westminster Medical School Research Trust (JRC 09/10 SG006), and National Institute of Academic Anaesthesia, UK (http://www.niaa.org.uk/). The funders had no role in study design, data collection and analysis, decision to publish, or preparation of the manuscript.

Competing Interests: The authors have declared that no competing interests exist.

* Email: suveer.singh@imperial.ac.uk

Introduction

Ventilator-associated pneumonia (VAP) remains a common complication of critical illness, affecting over 10% of intubated patients, prolonging ICU stay, with an estimated attributable mortality of 13% [1–3]. This is despite the introduction of health improvement strategies such as Ventilator care bundles, which have apparently reduced the incidence [4,5], even though antibiotic prescriptions remain high for pulmonary sepsis in ICU [5]. Standardisation of diagnostic criteria for VAP is important for benchmarking, but no single best definition exists [6]. This in part has led to proposals for simplifying definitions into infective and non-infective ventilator associated complications [7].

Confirmatory diagnosis by microbiological culture is often too slow for clinical need, whilst even quantitative microbiological analysis is subject to the variations in the sampling site, or elusive despite other criteria being fulfilled [8]. Biomarkers may facilitate clinical confirmation and aid differentiation of pulmonary from non-pulmonary sepsis. This would allow earlier, targeted antibiotic intervention, direct clinicians' decision-making for 'antibiotic de-escalation' regimens and potentially reduce selective pressure for multi-resistant bacteria [9,10]. The role of inflammatory biomarkers including TREM-1 (Triggering Receptor Expressed on Myeloid Cells-1), IL-1, IL-6, IL-8, Procalcitonin (PCT) and more traditional indices, i.e. white cell count and CRP remains unclear. Only some show clinical diagnostic utility for VAP [11–14]. Differences in definitions of VAP patient populations, severity of disease, and assay techniques account for much of the conflicting data reported [15,16]. Furthermore, failure of many studies to consider the dynamic relationships between soluble and cell surface inflammatory proteins (e.g.TREM-1), differential expression of inflammatory markers by neutrophils and monocytes, and compartmentalization of inflammatory immune responses at the site of tissue infection in reference to blood, are likely contributory factors.

The aim of this study was to determine if, and which combination of paired blood and bronchoalveolar lavage fluid (BALF) inflammatory biomarkers (soluble and cell surface based, including TREM-1), could correctly classify patients with VAP from ventilated patients without evidence of pulmonary sepsis.

Materials and Methods

Study participants

Informed, witnessed and written assent was obtained from a relative or designated carer for all ventilated patients. Written consent was obtained from all day case bronchoscopy patients. Ethical permission was obtained from the local institutional board (Barking and Havering Local Research Ethics Committee, Ilford, Essex, UK), through the National Research Ethics Service (NRES) of the United Kingdom 08/H0702/61.

The study sample was selected from patients hospitalized between Feb 2009 and Aug 2011 in the Intensive Care unit, and Lady Kilmarnock bronchoscopy suite of the Chelsea and Westminster Hospital NHS Foundation Trust, London, United Kingdom. Adult patients (>18 years) were recruited into the following 3 groups; ventilator associated pneumonia, ventilated controls without evidence of pulmonary sepsis or with non-pulmonary sepsis (non-VAP), and non-ventilated non-infected controls (NVC).

In accordance with the 2005 guidelines of the American Thoracic Society/Infectious Diseases Society of America, the criteria for diagnosis of VAP were evidence of new infiltrates on chest radiographs after 48 hours of endotracheal intubation and presence of at least 2 of the following: fever (temperature >38°C or higher than basal temperature), abnormal white cell count (≥10 000/μL or <4000/μL), and purulent respiratory tract secretions [2]. As per recommendations, BALF samples were collected via directed bronchoscopy, semi-quantitatively reported (SQ) and cultured for microorganisms [17].

The clinical pulmonary infection score (CPIS) defined VAP and non-VAP [17,18]. Thus, VAP was predefined as CPIS >5 and positive BALF microbiology. Non-VAP was predefined as CPIS score <6 and negative microbiology. This was a modification of the original CPIS, by additionally incorporating SQ microbiological data. The patient cohorts comprised non-infected ventilated patients, or individuals with non-pulmonary infection (i.e. intra-abdominal, indwelling devices) confirmed on clinical, radiological and microbiological grounds. To control for the effects of mechanical ventilation on pulmonary inflammation, BALF and

blood samples were obtained from a cohort of non-ventilated control patients (NVC) undergoing day case bronchoscopy for non-infective respiratory disorders (i.e., chronic obstructive pulmonary disease, COPD, interstitial lung disease, ILD, or solitary pulmonary nodules).

Comparison of CPIS with the European Hospitals in Europe Link for Infection Control through Surveillance programme (HELICS) criteria (PN4) revealed excellent concordance using the Cohen kappa statistic (0.95) [15,19]. Two patients with VAP would have been classified as non-VAP using HELICS and one patient with non-VAP could possibly have been placed into the VAP cohort. Initial chest radiographic interpretation was that of the clinical investigators, with all radiographs being independently confirmed by a radiologist.

Data on exclusion criteria, and description of procedures for obtaining informed consent and for sampling, processing of BALF and blood and group classification are provided in an online supplement.

Laboratory studies

Twenty two individual inflammatory markers were measured. In blood these consisted of six cell surface [3 monocytic and 3 neutrophilic (TREM-1, CD11b and CD62L)] and five soluble proteins sTREM-1, IL-6, PCT, CRP and the white cell count (WCC). In BALF, the same six cell surface markers were measured and five soluble proteins above the limit of detection for ELISA were sTREM-1, IL-1β, IL-6, IL-8 and PCT. Nine BALF/blood marker ratios were calculated.

Immunophenotypic analysis was performed on peripheral blood and BALF cell suspensions using 5-colour flow cytometry (Cytomics FC500 Beckman Coulter, Beckman-Coulter, Villepinte, France). Blood and BALF cells were isolated following standard centrifugation procedures, and washed in phosphate buffered saline/1% fetal calf serum (FCS). 100 μl aliquot cell suspensions were then stained with monoclonal antibodies for 30 minutes. Further details on monoclonal antibodies used, on instrumentation and software analysis are provided in an on line supplement. CD45 staining and side scatter properties were initially used to select CD14 and CD16 positive cells as markers of monocytes and neutrophils respectively. Isotype controls were used to delineate specific protein expression on the cell surface of inflammatory cells. Geometric mean fluorescent intensity (MFI) was used as an index of protein concentration expressed by a particular blood or BALF cell population. Details on measurement of cytokines and inflammatory mediators (sTREM-1, IL-1β, IL-6 and IL-8) and PCT are provided in an online supplement. Urea was determined by ELISA (Abcam, Cambridge, UK) and was used to correct for dilutional effects in BALF [20].

Statistical Analysis

Anthropometric data was reported as medians and interquartile ranges. Differences between the groups for individual biomarkers were determined using the Kruskal-Wallis test followed by the Mann-Whitney U test with Dunn's post-hoc correction for multiple analyses when there were any statistical differences between individual groups.

Fisher's discriminant function analysis (FDA) was used to determine the optimal combination of biomarkers that could discriminate between VAP and non-VAP patient groups. A variable was entered into the "model" if the significance level of its F-value was <0.05 and was removed if the significance level was ≥0.05. The model was then used to classify each of the 91 cases into a diagnostic group. In order to check that the result of the biomarker model was not skewed by the presence of outlier data the model was internally validated by means of the leave-one-out method, which involves omitting a single observation from the original sample, and then using the remaining observations to assign the omitted case either to the VAP or non-VAP patient group.

The model was cross-validated by repeat random sub-sampling - by repeatedly (10 times) randomly assigning original cases into a training cohort (60% of original cases) to obtain new classification function coefficients for the analytes derived from the original model. The new function coefficients obtained were applied to a test cohort that consisted of the remaining cases (40%), to confirm the reliability of the model [21–24]. Further statistical information is available in an online supplement. All analysis was conducted using the SPSS v19 software package (SPSS, Chicago, IL, USA) and GraphPad Prism software (California, USA). Independent statistical analysis was performed.

Results

Study participants

Ninety one patients were recruited consecutively. There were 27 VAP, 33 non-VAP and 31 NVC patients (Table 1). There were no statistically significant differences between the groups with respect to age, sex, history of cigarette smoking, presence of chest x-ray infiltrates and APACHE II score. Twenty eight-day mortality was 3 deaths in the VAP group, 4 in the non-VAP group (none in the NVC). The majority of patients in the VAP and non-VAP groups were receiving antibiotics at the time of sampling. Thirty percent of ventilated patients received steroids for sepsis. The distribution of steroids between VAP and non-VAP groups were not statistically significant. Nine VAP and 13 non-VAP patients were post-operative cases. Within the NVC group, 7 patients had lung cancer, 9 COPD, 2 pulmonary sarcoidosis, 1 lung fibrosis, 6 with benign lung nodules and 7 with normal findings.

The following organisms were isolated (patients): Serratia marcescens (2), Klebsiella spp (4), Pseudomonas spp (9), methicillin sensitive staphylococcal aureus, MSSA, (4), methicillin resistant staphylococcal aureus, MRSA (3), Escherischia coli, (5), Acinetobacter baumanii (5), Stenotrophomonas (2) and Proteus mirabilis (2). Twenty eight organisms were isolated from VAP patients and the remaining eight bacteria were found in non-VAP patients (non-pulmonary infection).

The CRP was significantly elevated in VAP and non-VAP compared to NVC group (p<0.001). White cell count was significantly higher in VAP than NVC (p<0.001). Neither CRP nor WCC distinguished VAP from non-VAP.

Cellular and soluble inflammatory mediators in blood

In blood, there was no significant difference in the expression of cellular and soluble biomarkers between VAP and non-VAP (Table 2). However, the concentration of sTREM-1, IL-6, PCT and expression of CD62L on CD14 gated monocytes were significantly higher in VAP and non-VAP groups compared with NVC (Table 2). This suggests blood based biomarker activation resulting from ventilation, but that it is not discriminatory between VAP and non-VAP patients.

Cellular and soluble inflammatory mediators in BALF

By contrast, analysis of BALF showed significantly increased expression of cellular mTREM-1 and nTREM-1, and increased concentration of soluble IL-1β in VAP compared with non-VAP and NVC groups (p<0.001) (Table 2). Furthermore, whilst the increased expression of mTREM-1 from BALF in VAP was significant (p<0.001) (Figure 1a), this difference between VAP and the other two groups was greater when the compartmentalization ratio BALF/blood mTREM-1 was used (Figure 1b). This was not the case for BALF/Blood nTREM-1. The BALF/Blood ratios of CD11b on monocytes and sTREM-1 were also significantly higher

Table 1. Characteristics of patients recruited to study.

	VAP	Non-VAP	NVC
Number of patients	27	33	31
Age	68 (23–84)	62 (18–89)	59 (18–84)
Sex (% male/% female)	70/30	52/48	61/39
CPIS	7 (6–9)	3 (0–5)	N/A
Microbiology (% +ve)	100	12	0
APACHE II score	18 (5–45)	15 (2–24)	N/A
Smoking (% current/ex/none)	44/15/40	30/21/49	35/13/52
Antibiotics (% pre-BALF)	89	70	32
CXR (% with shadowing)	96	55	81
Steroids (%)	30	30	6
28-day mortality (%)	11	12	0
Post-surgical (%)	37	39	0
Burns injury (% of cases)	15	15	0
WCC (x10⁹/l)	15 (4–24)	9 (3–27)	7 (3–18)*
CRP (mg/L)	84 (7–320)	102(2–341)†	6 (1–296)*

The median and range (lowest-highest) is shown for each group. APACHE II and CPIS are only applicable to the ventilated patients. Some variables are presented as percentages. Statistically significant differences between the groups were determined using the Mann-Whitney U test with post-hoc Dunn correction and are indicated as follows: VAP versus NVC (p<0.001)* and non-VAP versus NVC (p<0.001)†. CPIS = Clinical Pulmonary Infection Score. APACHE II = Acute Physiology and Chronic Health Evaluation II score. VAP = ventilator-associated pneumonia. NVC = non-ventilated control. Non-VAP = ventilated non-pulmonary infected control. CXR = Chest X-ray. WCC = White cell count. CRP = C-reactive protein.

Table 2. Expression of cell-surface and soluble proteins in study participants with VAP, non-VAP and NVC.

	VAP	Non-VAP	NVC
Blood			
mTREM-1	5.1 (3.2–8.6)	4.6 (3.1–6.1)	6.5 (4.3–10.9)
nTREM-1	4.7 (2.6–7.3)	3.8 (2.3–6.1)	4.5 (3.1–7.4)
mCD11b	47.2 (30.0–70.0)	43.3 (27.6–52.3)	39.2(21.7–51.8)
nCD11b	44.0 (33.4–91.9)	59.8 (43.4–82.9)	49.0 (38.0–81.0)
mCD62L	9.4 (7.3–15.1)	9.5 (7.4–13.2)	5.4 (3.9–9.4)*
nCD62L	9.6 (6.0–17.0)	8.3 (6.0–10.5)	8.6 (6.8–10.5)
sTREM-1 (μg/ml)	0.18 (0.01–0.03)	0.15 (0.08–0.30)	0.09 (0.06–0.15)[†,‡]
IL-1β (μg/ml)	N/A	N/A	N/A
IL-6 (μg/ml)	0.09 (0.03–0.21)	0.08 (0.03–0.17)	0.008 (0.005–0.02)*
IL-8 (μg/ml)	N/A	N/A	N/A
PCT (ng/ml)	1.3 (0.3–5.3)	2.9 (0.6–8.3)	N/A*
Corrected BALF			
mTREM-1	3.9 (2.5–5.4)	1.6 (1.1–2.3)	1.8 (1.2–2.9)[§]
nTREM-1	2.0 (1.7–3.3)	1.5 (1.2–2.2)**	1.7 (1.3–3.0)
mCD11b	25.2 (9.0–81.2)	18.6 (13.7–31.2)	21.0 (6.9–47.3)
nCD11b	47.0 (15.1–86.0)	32.9 (20.3–62.5)	24.0 (6.0–73.5)
mCD62L	1.2 (1.0–1.5)	1.1 (1.0–1.3)	1.2 (1.0–1.4)
nCD62L	1.4 (1.0–2.1)	1.1 (1.0–1.4)	1.2 (1.0–1.7)
sTREM-1 (μg/ml)	20.14 (9.45–43.94)	5.19 (2.83–10.96)[††]	7.61 (3.05–18.32)
IL-1β (μg/ml)	3.02 (1.47–8.59)	0.79 (0.36–1.51)	0.53 (0.19–2.79)[§]
IL-6 (μg/ml)	3.80 (1.32–17.71)	2.08 (1.23–5.75)	1.45 (0.52–2.52)[‡‡]
IL-8 (μg/ml)	48.60 (20.78–101.10)	12.16(5.71–17.3)[§§]	16.33 (3.12–67.15)
PCT (ng/ml)	16.8 (9.7–51.7)	12.5(6.8–27.4)	9.6(4.1–18.2)
Corrected BALF/blood ratio			
mTREM-1	0.8(0.5–1.0)	0.4(0.2–0.5)	0.3(0.2–0.4)[§]
nTREM-1	0.6(0.2–0.8)	0.4(0.3–0.8)	0.4(0.2–1.1)
mCD11b	0.53(0.4–2.3)	0.4(0.2–0.7)[§§]	0.5(0.2–1.3)
nCD11b	0.7(0.5–2.0)	0.5(0.2–0.9)	0.5(0.1–1.4)
mCD62L	0.2(0.1–0.5)	0.1(0.1–0.2)	0.2(0.1–0.3)
nCD62L	0.2(0.1–0.3)	0.2(0.1–0.2)	0.2(0.1–0.2)
sTREM-1	190(70–337)	30(11–85)[§§]	84(26–228)[‖]
IL-1β	N/A	N/A	N/A
IL-6	77(20–145)	43(41–230)	134(230–355)
IL-8	N/A	N/A	N/A
PCT	29(3–55)	4(2–23)	N/A

The median and interquartile range for each patient group is reported. Statistically significant differences between groups were determined using the Mann-Whitney U and post hoc Dunn correction as follows: VAP and non-VAP versus NVC (p<0.001)*, VAP versus NVC (p<0.001)[†] and non-VAP versus NVC (p<0.05)[‡], VAP versus non-VAP and NVC (p<0.001)[§], VAP versus non-VAP (p<0.01)**, VAP versus non-VAP (p<0.001)[††], VAP versus NVC (p<0.01)[‡‡], VAP versus non-VAP (p<0.001)[§§] and NVC> non-VAP (p<0.01)[‖]. The lower limits of detection for the sTREM-1, IL-1β, IL-6, IL-8 and PCT assays were 0.01 μg/ml, 0.001 μg/ml, 0.0007 μg/ml, 0.004 μg/ml and 0.05 ng/ml respectively. N/A indicates below assay detection limit. BALF levels were corrected for dilution occurring with bronchoscopy using urea analysis. BALF/blood ratios were only calculable if BALF and blood measurements were obtained. VAP = ventilator-associated pneumonia. Non-VAP = ventilated patients with no evidence of pulmonary infection. NVC = non-ventilated non-infected patients.

in VAP group compared to non-VAP, but not when compared to NVC (Table 2). The expression of cellular mTREM-1, nTREM-1, and CD11b was lower in BALF than blood (Table 2), although the reductions seen were notably less in patients with VAP, as compared with non-VAP and NVC groups, hence the higher BALF/blood ratio (Table 2). Other soluble markers IL-1β, IL-8 and sTREM-1 were significantly raised in the VAP compared with non-VAP groups. IL-6 was similar in VAP and non-VAP groups but higher than NVC (Figure 2). None of the individual markers in blood, BALF or BALF/blood ratios had sufficient accuracy in distinguishing VAP from non-VAP (data not shown).

Classification of individual cases within each study group using a biomarker panel

To determine whether a biomarker panel might have better discriminating ability than individual markers, and to separate the

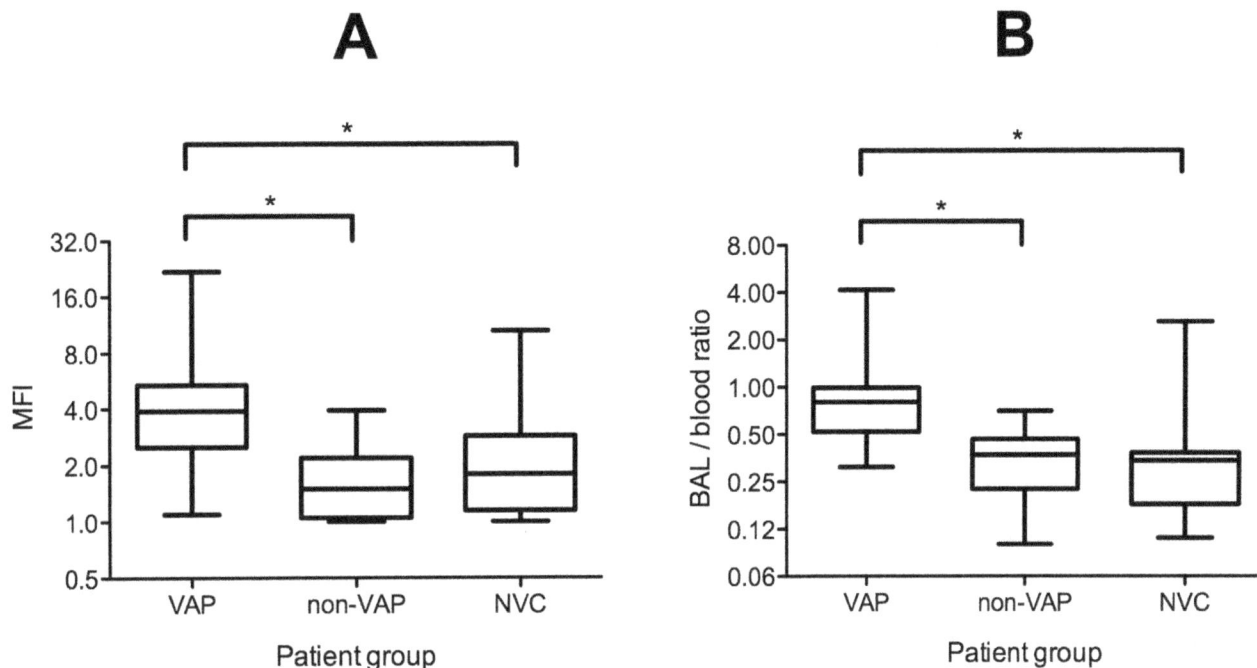

Figure 1. BALF levels and BALF/blood ratios of monocytic TREM-1. Box (interquartile) and whisker (range) plots showing expression of TREM-1 by CD14+ monocytes in BALF (Figure 1a) and the BALF/blood ratio of TREM-1 expression by monocytes in blood and BALF (Figure 1b) from patients with VAP, non-VAP (ventilated non-pulmonary infected control) and NVC (non-ventilated control). BALF levels were corrected for dilution occurring with bronchoscopy using urea measurement. Statistically significant differences between groups were determined using the Mann-Whitney U and post hoc Dunn correction as follows: monocyte TREM-1 levels for VAP versus non-VAP and NVC (p<0.001)* and BALF/blood monocytic TREM-1 ratio VAP versus non-VAP and NVC (p<0.001)*. MFI = mean fluorescence intensity.

effects of ventilation from infection, Fisher Discriminant Analysis (FDA) was performed to build a 'model' that could best predict to which group (VAP and non-VAP) a study participant belonged on the basis of the biological measurements alone. To build the model we used all the VAP and non-VAP cases in the study and the 22 different markers and their compartmentalized ratios. A seven marker Bioscore consisting of BALF/blood cell expression ratio for monocyte mTREM-1 and mCD11b, BALF levels of sTREM-1, IL-8 and IL-1β, blood levels of CRP and IL-6 was shown to discriminate between VAP and non-VAP patients.

The 7 marker-bioscore produced 100% correct classification of the non-VAP patients and 88.9% correct classification of VAP patients. The NVC group which was treated as an unknown was defined as non-VAP in 90.7% of the cases using this model. In order to control for the possibility that the findings of the biomarker panel might be skewed by results obtained from any particular patient, we performed a leave one out cross validation analysis which produced the same level of accuracy with the original model (100% for non-VAP, 88.9% for VAP).

In order to assess the robustness of the model further, individual cases were then randomly assigned into a training cohort (60% of original cases) to obtain new classification function coefficients for the 7 analytes and the remaining 40% were used as unknowns for classification. In this cross-validation model the average predictive accuracies for the patients in the testing cohort were 71.0% for VAP and 98.5% for non-VAP. The reduction in classification for VAP was largely driven by the model attributing a number of NVC as VAP and to the limited power of the testing cohort analysed.

Discussion

This study demonstrates that a combination of cell surface and soluble markers of inflammation, in particular TREM-1, sampled in blood and BALF simultaneously, can accurately discriminate VAP from ventilated patients without pulmonary sepsis. The use of a compartmentalization ratio, as a measure of site-specific immune response, results in a further improvement in diagnostic classification. These data have implications for the accurate diagnosis [25], antibiotic usage and management of VAP [26]. The results also address a potential weakness of previous studies which have measured only soluble mediators, often in one compartment. These may not fully account for the dynamic interaction between cell surface receptors and their soluble counterparts (e.g. mTREM-1 and sTREM-1 respectively), and site specific flux between the alveolar lung space and blood [27].

The findings suggest that monocytic surface receptor mTREM-1 and its neutrophilic counterpart nTREM-1 are compartmentalized within the lung, with increased expression in VAP. Although the expression of TREM-1 on pulmonary inflammatory cells has not to our knowledge previously been assessed in patients with VAP, the results are consistent with increased mTREM-1 reported in patients with community acquired pneumonia [28]. Soluble TREM-1 levels in BALF were significantly elevated and discriminatory in patients with VAP compared to non-VAP, in keeping with some, [12,14,29,30] but not all studies, [13,31,32]. The BALF/blood ratio of mTREM-1, mCD11b and sTREM-1 were significantly higher in patients with VAP compared to those without VAP suggesting site-specific utility. Pulmonary infection may be distinguished from abdominal infection by combining BALF sTREM-1 and blood Procalcitonin measurement, although with lesser discrimination than our use of combined cell surface/

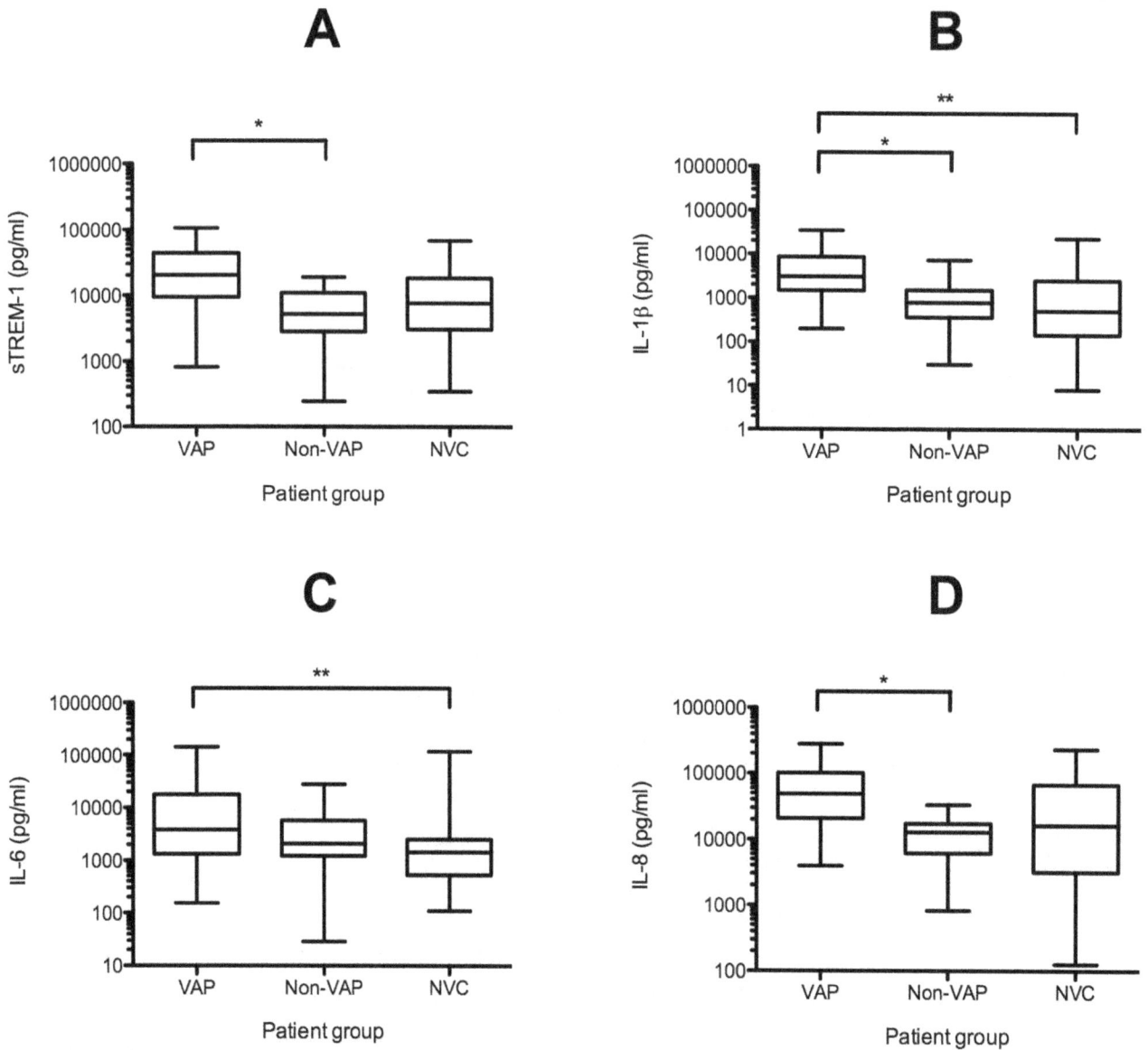

Figure 2. Soluble cytokine levels in BALF. Box (interquartile) and whisker (range) plots showing (a) sTREM-1, (b) IL-1β, (c) IL-6 and (d) IL-8 levels in BALF of patients with VAP, non-VAP (ventilated non-pulmonary infected control) and NVC (non-ventilated control). The BALF levels were corrected for dilution occurring with bronchoscopy using urea measurement. The concentration of BALF sTREM-1, IL-1β and IL-8 were significantly higher in VAP than non-VAP (p<0.001)*. BALF IL-1β and IL-6 were higher in the VAP compared with the NVC patient group (p<0.001)**.

soluble markers [12]. Ramirez et al reported the discriminative ability of site-sampled sTREM-1 for identifying pulmonary from abdominal infection in a critically ill cohort [33]. Thus, analysis of site-specific inflammatory markers may be useful in distinguishing infective sites, although measurement of cell surface markers over soluble proteins will not be influenced by dilutional variance from BALF.

The BALF/blood ratios of neutrophil-based nTREM-1 and nCD11b were not raised in VAP, unlike their monocytic counterparts. This difference is consistent with data from patients in septic shock, in whom blood mTREM-1 but not nTREM-1 levels increased compared with controls [34]. Expression of TREM-1 on neutrophils initially falls over minutes and then increases following in vitro LPS stimulation. In contrast TREM-1 levels on monocytes steadily increase over hours. It is possible that

the recruitment timescale for VAP misses early neutrophilic changes [35]. Indeed, expression of TREM-1 by neutrophils may have passed its peak before time definitions of VAP allow measurement. Sampling individuals with suspected VAP at earlier time points may clarify differential kinetics of TREM-1 expression.

Surface TREM-1 may act as a link in the pathway from infective organism, to upregulation of the inflammatory cytokines. That said, it is unlikely to be specific for infection as opposed to inflammation. Experimentally, mTREM-1 activation in conjunction with lipopolysaccharide (LPS) increases IL-8 and IL-1β release, with amplification seen in septic shock, as in our study, [36,37]. Such changes in IL-8 and IL-1β are in accordance with Conway-Morris et al, who have demonstrated high area under the curve (AUC) for them in suspected VAP [13]. Others have found elevated BALF IL-1β and IL-6 levels in VAP, when using a lung to blood ratio like in this study [38]. The BALF/blood ratios of soluble cytokines were non-discriminatory in this study, perhaps due to significant compartmentalization by the time of sampling, producing very low blood levels.

The difference in expression of mTREM-1 in VAP from non-VAP was more notable in BALF than blood, although the MFI were lower in BALF (Table 2). This may be due to increased shedding of up-regulated BALF mTREM-1 within the lung, as evidenced by the significantly greater increase in soluble sTREM-1 compared with blood. A potential mechanism is suggested to involve the balance between bacterial induced metalloproteinase (MMP) mediated cleavage of TREM-1 from surface of monocytes and action of specific MMP inhibitors [39]. Moreover, neutrophil derived MMP production is seen to increase markedly in BALF as compared to plasma from patients with hospital acquired pneumonia, whereas the specific tissue inhibitors of MMP (TIMP) were increased in plasma compared to BALF [40].

The limitations of this study are addressed here. First, no gold standard for VAP diagnosis exists. We included patients, who based on the CPIS scoring system, plus semi-quantitative microbiological testing were highly likely to have the presence or absence of VAP in order to test putative biomarkers. CPIS has been criticized by some for its potentially low diagnostic accuracy based upon clinico-radiological criteria. However, all current definitions of VAP remain subject to limitations. We acknowledge that semi-quantitative microbiology is less specific than Quantitative, but as sensitive for identifying pulmonary infection [41]. However, even the use of quantitative microbiology from directed BALF will potentially miss an important group of VAP patients (defined by standard clinic-patho-radiological criteria), if not meeting the predefined cutoff values of colony forming units/ml (cfu/ml). The arbitrary 48 h requirement for mechanical ventilation in most definitions of VAP provides important standardization but will also miss some pulmonary sepsis in ventilated patients developing prior to that timepoint. In order to mitigate against these concerns, we redefined the VAP and non VAP patients by other well established validated international criteria. Thus, the diagnostic definitions used were highly concordant when the HELICS criteria for pneumonia were used [15]. Reassuringly, from a biological perspective, the raised BALF IL-1β and IL-8 levels in VAP from our study concur with a group utilizing different diagnostic methodology, implying the validity to such approaches [13]. Therefore, the type of diagnostic criteria, particularly quantitative microbiology, used were not a major influence on the bioscore's discriminability.

Second, this study did not encompass the whole range of infective aetiologies. For instance, no patients had mycoplasma, Legionella or proven respiratory viral pneumonias, and few had bilateral lung infiltrates. The management of viral pneumonias in particular, would benefit from early diagnostic biomarkers. Third, the absence of patients with ARDS does not allow us to comment on how the bioscore might perform in discriminating severe pulmonary inflammation from pulmonary infection. Fourth, and from a practical consideration, flow cytometry is a specialized technique. It requires samples with sufficient numbers of cells, which mandates adequate directed BALF samples, likely targeted bronchoscopy and makes serial biomarker analysis challenging.

However, BALF samples are the current standard of care a microbiological diagnosis of VAP [16]. Fifth, a number of patients were receiving antibiotics and steroids at the time of sampling, with potential immunomodulatory activity. Given the prevalence of these key standard interventions in critically ill patients, we believe this pragmatic approach enhances the applicability of the findings. Sixth, the immune response to infecting pathogens in VAP, as in sepsis, is likely to involve neutrophils, monocytes and lymphocytes, [42]. As such we have not necessarily looked at all potentially relevant phagocytic or T cell markers. That said, the value of biomarker panels that include sTREM-1, PCT and CD64 on neutrophils has recently demonstrated the ability to predict sepsis in the setting of unselected critical illness, confirming the need to pursue such discriminatory panels in VAP, as in other disease states [42,43]. Finally, we acknowledge that these results require validation in an external cohort of patients with suspected VAP, to see whether the bioscore 7 panel retains its discriminatory accuracy. Moreover, such a study is needed to see how the biomarker components, particularly mTREM-1, sTREM-1, IL1 and IL8, will perform and whether the BALF/blood ratio offers improved accuracy.

In conclusion, a 7 biomarker panel comprising soluble and cell-surface inflammatory markers including TREM-1 in combination with BALF/blood ratio differentiates VAP from non-pulmonary infection with good diagnostic accuracy. Such an approach, that incorporates these practically relevant and easily measurable biomarkers, to confirm or refute suspected VAP, requires confirmation.

Supporting Information

Table S1 BALF bacterial growth in patient groups. The table shows the BALF microbiological results with patients of CPIS >6, CPIS <6 and CPIS = 6. CPIS = Clinical pulmonary infection score. VAP = Ventilator-associated pneumonia

Materials and Methods S1 Supporting information on study participants, biomarker measurement, biomarker panel construction and validation.

Acknowledgments

We would like to acknowledge the valuable assistance received by the Staff of the Intensive Care Unit, Operating Theatres, Bronchoscopy unit, and the Chelsea and Westminster Hospital ICU Patient's forum. We thank Dr Berge Azadian, clinical Microbiologist for his help comments. We thank Professor Athol Wells, internationally recognised in the respiratory field for his statistical knowledge and the use of complex data analysis, for providing independent statistical advice. He was not involved in study design, data collection or initial analysis.

Author Contributions

Conceived and designed the experiments: VG PP NS DCH PK SS. Performed the experiments: VG PLS SS. Analyzed the data: VG PP NS MT PLS AUW DCH PK SS. Contributed reagents/materials/analysis tools: VG PP NS MT PLS AUW DCH PK SS. Contributed to the writing of the manuscript: VG PP NS MT PLS AUW DH PK SS.

References

1. Alberti C, Brun-Buisson C, Burchardi H, Martin C, Goodman S, et al (2002) Epidemiology of sepsis and infection in ICU patients from an international multicentre cohort study. Int Care Med 28: 108–121.

2. American Thoracic Society and Infectious Diseases Society of America (2005) Guidelines for the management of adults with hospital-acquired, ventilator-associated, and healthcare-associated pneumonia. Am J Respir Crit Care Med 171: 388–416.

3. Melsen WG, Rovers MM, Groenwold RHH, Bergmans DCJJ, Camus C, et al (2013) Attributable mortality of ventilator-associated pneumonia: a meta-analysis of individual patient data from randomised prevention studies. Lancet Infect Dis 13: 665–71.

4. Bekaert M, Timsit JF, Vansteelandt S, Depuydt P, Vesin A, et al (2011) Attributable mortality of ventilator-associated pneumonia: a reappraisal using causal analysis. Am J Respir Crit Care Med 184: 1133–9.

5. Kollef MH, Hamilton CW, Ernst FR (2012) Economic impact of ventilator-associated pneumonia in a large matched cohort. Infect Control Hosp Epidemiol 33: 250–6.

6. Klompas M (2007) Does this patient have ventilator-associated pneumonia? JAMA 297: 1583–93.

7. Kollef MH (2012) Prevention of ventilator-associated pneumonia or ventilator-associated complications: a worthy, yet challenging, goal. Crit Care Med 40: 271–7.

8. Chastre J, Trouillet JL, Combes A, Luyt CE (2010) Diagnostic techniques and procedures for establishing the microbial etiology of ventilator-associated pneumonia for clinical trials: the pros for quantitative cultures. Clin Infect Dis 51 Suppl 1: S88–92.

9. Rea-Neto A, Youssef NC, Tuche F, Brunkhorst F, Ranieri VM, et al (2008) Diagnosis of ventilator-associated pneumonia: a systematic review of the literature. Crit Care 12: R56.

10. Lisboa T, Rello J (2008) Diagnosis of ventilator-associated pneumonia: is there a gold standard and a simple approach? Curr Opin Infect Dis 21: 174–8.

11. Gibot S, Cravoisy A, Levy B, Bene MC, Faure G, et al (2004) Soluble triggering receptor expressed on myeloid cells and the diagnosis of pneumonia. N Engl J Med 350: 451–8.

12. Gibot S, Cravoisy A, Dupays R, Barraud D, Nace L, et al (2007) Combined measurement of procalcitonin and soluble TREM-1 in the diagnosis of nosocomial sepsis. Scand J Infect Dis 39: 604–8.

13. Conway Morris A, Kefala K, Wilkinson TS, Moncayo-Nieto OL, Dhaliwal K, et al (2010) Diagnostic importance of pulmonary interleukin-1 beta and interleukin-8 in ventilator-associated pneumonia. Thorax 65: 201–7.

14. Anand NJ, Zuick S, Klesney-Tait J, Kollef MH (2009) Diagnostic implications of soluble triggering receptor expressed on myeloid cells-1 in BALF fluid of patients with pulmonary infiltrates in the ICU. Chest 135: 641–7.

15. Suetens C, Savey A, Labeeuw J, Morales I (2002) The ICU-HELICS programme: towards European surveillance of hospital-acquired infections in intensive care units. Euro Surveill 7: 127–8.

16. Conway Morris A, Kefala K, Simpson AJ, Wilkinson TS, Everingham K, et al (2009) Evaluation of the effect of diagnostic methodology on the reported incidence of ventilator-associated pneumonia. Thorax 64: 516–22.

17. Pugin J, Auckenthaler R, Mili N, Janssens JP, Lew PD, et al (1991) Diagnosis of ventilator-associated pneumonia by bacteriologic analysis of bronchoscopic and nonbronchoscopic "blind" bronchoalveolar lavage fluid. Am Rev Respir Dis 143: 1121–1129.

18. Luna CM, Blanzaco D, Niederman MS, Matarucco W, Baredes NC, et al (2003) Resolution of ventilator-associated pneumonia: prospective evaluation of the Clinical Pulmonary Infection Score as an early clinical predictor of outcome. Crit Care Med 31: 676–682.

19. Cohen J (1960) A coefficient of agreement for nominal scales. Educ Psychol Meas 20: 37–46.

20. Rennard SI, Basset G, Lecossier D, O'Donnell KM, Pinkston P, et al (1986) Estimation of volume of epithelial lining fluid recovered by lavage using urea as marker of dilution. J Appl Physiol 60: 532–8.

21. Beirne P, Pantelidis P, Charles P, Wells AU, Abraham DJ, et al (2009) Multiplex immune serum biomarker profiling in sarcoidosis and systemic sclerosis. Eur Resp J 34: 1376–82.

22. Picard R, Cook D (1984) Cross-Validation of Regression Models. J Am Stat Assoc 79 : 575–583.

23. Kohavi R (1995) A study of cross-validation and bootstrap for accuracy estimation and model selection. Proc of the Fourteenth Int Joint Conf on Art Intel 2: 1137–1143.

24. Efron B, Tibshirani R (1997) Improvements on cross-validation: The.632+ Bootstrap Method. J Am Stat Assoc 92: 548–560.

25. Chastre J, Fagon JY (2002) Ventilator-associated pneumonia. Am J Respir Crit Care Med 165: 867–903.

26. Leone M, Garcin F, Bouvenot J, Boyadjec I, Visintini P, et al (2007) Ventilator-associated pneumonia: breaking the vicious circle of antibiotic overuse. Crit Care Med 35: 379–385.

27. Gibot S, Massin F, Le Renard P, Bene MC, Faure GC, et al (2005) Surface and soluble triggering receptor expressed on myeloid cells-1: expression patterns in murine sepsis. Crit Care Med 33: 1787–93.

28. Richeldi L, Mariani M, Losi M, Maselli F, Corbetta L, et al (2004) Triggering receptor expressed on myeloid cells: role in the diagnosis of lung infections. Eur Respir J 24: 247–50.

29. Huh JW, Lim CM, Koh Y, Oh YM, Shim TS, et al (2008) Diagnostic utility of the soluble triggering receptor expressed on myeloid cells-1 in bronchoalveolar lavage fluid from patients with bilateral lung infiltrates. Crit Care 12: R6.

30. Determann RM, Millo JL, Gibot S, Korevaar JC, Vroom MB, et al (2005) Serial changes in soluble triggering receptor expressed on myeloid cells in the lung during development of ventilator-associated pneumonia. Int Care Med 31: 1495–500.

31. Oudhuis GJ, Beuving J, Bergmans D, Stobberingh EE, ten Velde G, et al (2009) Soluble Triggering Receptor Expressed on Myeloid cells-1 in bronchoalveolar lavage fluid is not predictive for ventilator-associated pneumonia. Int Care Med 35: 1265–70.

32. Song Y, Lynch SV, Flanagan J, Zhuo H, Tom W, et al (2007) Increased plasminogen activator inhibitor-1 concentrations in bronchoalveolar lavage fluids are associated with increased mortality in a cohort of patients with Pseudomonas aeruginosa. Anesthesiology 106: 252–61.

33. Ramirez P, Kot P, Marti V, Gomez MD, Martinez R, et al (2011) Diagnostic implications of soluble triggering receptor expressed on myeloid cells-1 in patients with acute respiratory distress syndrome and abdominal diseases: a preliminary observational study. Crit Care 2011: R50.

34. Gibot S, Le Renard PE, Bollaert PE, Kolopp-Sarda MN, Bene MC, et al (2005) Surface triggering receptor expressed on myeloid cells 1 expression patterns in septic shock. Int Care Med 31: 594–7.

35. Knapp S, Gibot S, de Vos A, Versteeg HH, Colonna M, et al (2004) Cutting edge: expression patterns of surface and soluble triggering receptor expressed on myeloid cells-1 in human endotoxemia. J Immunol 173: 7131–4.

36. Bleharski JR, Kiessler V, Buonsanti C, Sieling PA, Stenger S, et al (2003) A role for triggering receptor expressed on myeloid cells-1 in host defense during the early-induced and adaptive phases of the immune response. J Immunol 170: 3812–8.

37. Bouchon A, Facchetti F, Weigand MA, Colonna M (2001) TREM-1 amplifies inflammation and is a crucial mediator of septic shock. Nature 410: 1103–7.

38. Millo JL, Schultz MJ, Williams C, Weverling GJ, Ringrose T et al (2004) Compartmentalisation of cytokines and cytokine inhibitors in ventilator-associated pneumonia. Int Care Med 30: 68–74.

39. Gomez-Pina V, Soares-Schanoski A, Rodriguez-Rojas A, Del Fresno C, Garcia F, et al (2007) Metalloproteinases shed TREM-1 ectodomain from lipopolysaccharide-stimulated human monocytes. J Immunol 179: 4065–73.

40. Hartog CM, Wermelt JA, Sommerfeld CO, Eichler W, Dalhoff K, et al (2003) Pulmonary matrix metalloproteinase excess in hospital-acquired pneumonia. Am J Respir Crit Care Med 167: 593–8.

41. Baselski V and Klutts JS (2013) Quantitative cultures of bronchoscopically obtained specimens should be performed for optimal management of Ventilator-Associated Pneumonia. J Clin Microbiol 51(3): 740–4.

42. Gibot S, Béné MC, Noel R, Massin F, Guy J, et al (2012) Combination biomarkers to diagnose sepsis in the critically ill patient. 186: 65–71.

43. Zethelius B, Berglund L, Sundstrom J, Ingelsson E, Basu S, et al (2008) Use of multiple biomarkers to improve the prediction of death from cardiovascular causes. N Engl J Med 358: 2107–2116.

9

Early Prediction of Intensive Care Unit–Acquired Weakness Using Easily Available Parameters: A Prospective Observational Study

Luuk Wieske[1,2,3]*, **Esther Witteveen**[1,3], **Camiel Verhamme**[2], **Daniela S. Dettling-Ihnenfeldt**[4], **Marike van der Schaaf**[4], **Marcus J. Schultz**[1,3], **Ivo N. van Schaik**[2], **Janneke Horn**[1]

1 Department of Intensive Care Medicine, Academic Medical Center, Amsterdam, the Netherlands, 2 Department of Neurology, Academic Medical Center, Amsterdam, the Netherlands, 3 Laboratory of Experimental Anesthesiology and Intensive Care (L•E•I•C•A), Academic Medical Center, Amsterdam, the Netherlands, 4 Department of Rehabilitation, Academic Medical Center, Amsterdam, the Netherlands

Abstract

Introduction: An early diagnosis of Intensive Care Unit–acquired weakness (ICU–AW) using muscle strength assessment is not possible in most critically ill patients. We hypothesized that development of ICU–AW can be predicted reliably two days after ICU admission, using patient characteristics, early available clinical parameters, laboratory results and use of medication as parameters.

Methods: Newly admitted ICU patients mechanically ventilated ≥2 days were included in this prospective observational cohort study. Manual muscle strength was measured according to the Medical Research Council (MRC) scale, when patients were awake and attentive. ICU–AW was defined as an average MRC score <4. A prediction model was developed by selecting predictors from an a-priori defined set of candidate predictors, based on known risk factors. Discriminative performance of the prediction model was evaluated, validated internally and compared to the APACHE IV and SOFA score.

Results: Of 212 included patients, 103 developed ICU–AW. Highest lactate levels, treatment with any aminoglycoside in the first two days after admission and age were selected as predictors. The area under the receiver operating characteristic curve of the prediction model was 0.71 after internal validation. The new prediction model improved discrimination compared to the APACHE IV and the SOFA score.

Conclusion: The new early prediction model for ICU–AW using a set of 3 easily available parameters has fair discriminative performance. This model needs external validation.

Editor: Jorge I. F. Salluh, D'or Institute of Research and Education, Brazil

Funding: The authors received no specific funding for this work. Dr. L. Wieske is supported by a personal grant (ZonMw–AGIKO grant [project number 40-00703-98-11636]) from the Netherlands Organization for Health Research and Development. The funders had no role in study design, data collection and analysis, decision to publish, or preparation of the manuscript.

Competing Interests: The authors of this manuscript have the following competing interests: Prof. I.N. van Schaik received departmental honoraria for serving on scientific advisory boards and a steering committee for CSL-Behring. The other authors declare that they have no competing interests.

* Email: L.Wieske@amc.uva.nl

Introduction

Intensive Care Unit–acquired weakness (ICU–AW) is a frequent and debilitating neuromuscular complication of critical illness. [1,2] Development of ICU-AW is associated with increased mortality and short- and long term morbidity. [3–5] Currently, no specific treatments for ICU-AW exist. For future treatments to be successful, timing may be of importance. The first signs of ICU-AW can be found starting from day 2 after admission when decreased excitability of muscle and nerve can be observed. [6,7] Initiation of treatment at this moment may be more effective because the observed abnormalities may still be reversible. [8,9] Such early treatment would require an early diagnosis of ICU-AW. At present, the diagnosis of ICU–AW is based on clinical examination using manual muscle strength assessment. [1] In most critically ill patients, manual muscle strength assessment is not possible early in the disease course due to impaired consciousness or attentiveness. [10] A solution to this diagnostic delay may be to quantify the risk that a patient will develop ICU-AW using a prediction model early after ICU admission.

ICU–AW is associated with several risk factors, including sepsis, the presence of multiple organ dysfunction syndrome (MODS) and severity of illness. [11] Prediction of ICU–AW on the basis of these risk factors is scarcely studied. A combination of the Acute Physiology and Chronic Health Evaluation (APACHE) score and presence of the Systemic Inflammatory Response Syndrome

(SIRS) could identify patients at high risk for development of ICU-AW, although the predictive performance was not reported. [12] A cumulative Sequential Organ Failure Assessment (SOFA) score of the first week of ICU admission also has predictive value but this approach does not allow early prediction [13].

We hypothesized that early prediction of ICU–AW is possible and reliable. To investigate this, we built a prediction model based on previously identified risk factors for ICU–AW. The predictive performance of the model was compared to those of the APACHE IV scores and the SOFA score.

Methods

Design and ethical approval

We performed a prospective observational cohort study using the STARD guidelines. [14] The institutional review board of the Academic Medical Center, Amsterdam, The Netherlands, decided (decision notice W13_080#13.17.0100) that data for this study could be collected and analyzed without written informed consent of the patient and specifically approved the use of that data for this study because no additional procedures were performed and therefore this study did not fulfill the criteria for medical research stated in the Dutch 'Law on medical research'.

Study setting

The study was performed in a 30 beds tertiary mixed medical-surgical ICU of the Academic Medical Center in the Netherlands. In this ICU, several standards of care are applied including glucose control between 90 mg/dl and 144 mg/dl. Sedation is stopped as soon possible. Norepinephrine is the first line vasopressor drug and corticosteroids (100 mg of hydrocortisone intravenously 3 times daily) are given in refractory septic shock. All patients receive early rehabilitation.

In– and exclusion criteria

Consecutive, newly admitted ICU patients, mechanically ventilated for ≥2 days, were included. We excluded patients who had a neuromuscular disorder (e.g. Guillain-Barré syndrome), stroke, out-of-hospital cardiac arrest or spinal injury as reason for ICU admission. In addition, we excluded patients with a poor pre-hospital functional status (modified Rankin scale ≥4 [15]) and patients with pre-existing spinal injury.

Strength assessment (reference standard)

Physical therapists, blinded for all other parameters, assessed muscle strength when patients were alert (Richmond Agitation and Sedation Scale between −1 and 1 [16]) and attentive (able to follow verbal commands using arms or eye-lids). When patients are alert and attentive, muscle strength can be reliably assessed using the MRC score. [17] MRC scores were assessed bilaterally in 6 pre-specified muscle groups: wrist dorsiflexors, elbow flexors, shoulder abductors, hip flexors, knee extensors and ankle dorsiflexors. MRC scores of muscle groups were summated and divided by the number of muscle groups that could be tested to obtain an average MRC score. When a muscle group could not be assessed, no value was imputed. ICU–AW was diagnosed when weakness had developed after ICU admission, was symmetric and the average MRC score was <4 [1].

Candidate predictors

Candidate predictors were based on risk factors for ICU-AW identified through a literature search (see material S1). We extracted risk factors that were easily available in the first two days after ICU admission and had a univariate association, in at least one study. To improve suitability for prediction, some of the extracted risk factors were redefined into candidate predictors with more clear definitions. Candidate predictors regarding medical history and the presence of suspected sepsis were scored during ICU admission; all others were obtained from the electronic patient record after ICU discharge. Candidate predictors were collected blinded for the reference standard.

Additional data collected

The following additional clinical characteristics were collected: the Acute Physiology and Chronic Health Evaluation IV (APACHE IV) score and the maximal Sequential Organ Failure Assessment (SOFA) score during the first two days after ICU admission. Also, data on the number of days with mechanical ventilation, length of stay in the ICU and ICU mortality were collected.

Sample size

We assumed that ICU–AW would occur in 50% of patients [11] and that 5 patients with ICU–AW needed to be included per candidate predictor. We defined a set of 20 candidate predictors, so 200 patients were needed.

Statistical analysis

Candidate predictors with right-tailed distributions were logarithmically transformed. Predictors for the model were selected from candidate predictors using two steps. First, using a bootstrapped backward selection process, candidate predictors included in ≥50% of the bootstrap samples (N:1000; p<0.5 for inclusion) were selected. [18,19] Next, the selected candidate predictors were consecutively entered in a logistic regression model and only those candidate predictors that led to a discriminatory increase in model fit were retained. Candidate predictors were entered in descending order of inclusion frequency in bootstrap samples. For every addition, the change in Akaike Information Criterion (AIC) between models was compared. [20] An AIC change >−2 between additions was interpreted as non-discriminatory and the candidate predictors included before that addition were selected as predictors.

Next, we constructed a model with these predictors. Discriminative performance was analyzed using the area under the Receiver Operating Characteristic (AUC–ROC) curve and internally validated using bootstrapping (N:1000). We defined AUC-ROC values between 0.90–1 as excellent, 0.80–0.90 as good, 0.70–0.80 as fair, 0.60–0.70 as poor and <0.60 as failed. Odds ratios were adjusted using the calibration slope after internal validation. [18] Calibration was assessed graphically and using goodness of fit (Hosmer–Lemeshow test).

Performance of the new prediction model was compared to the APACHE IV score and maximal SOFA score in the first two ICU days using continuous net reclassification improvement (cNRI), which is a measure of discrimination resembling the AUC-ROC but more sensitive to change [21].

Finally, we performed two sensitivity analyses; we investigated discrimination of the prediction model for more severe ICU-AW (ICU-AW defined using a lower cut-off, i.e. an average MRC<3). Second, we investigated the influence of missing data by repeating predictor selection and model discrimination analyses on data sets in which missing data was imputed using multivariate imputation by chained equations (10 iterations of 10 imputations). [22] For the imputation model, all 20 candidate predictors as well as the presence of ICU-AW were used. Imputed values were checked for validity.

Mean values are presented with standard deviation (±SD), median values with interquartile range (IQR) and proportions with percentages and total numbers. Differences between proportions were assessed using chi-square test. Differences between normally distributed variables were assessed using Welch's t-test; differences between non-normally distributed continuous variables were assessed using Wilcoxon rank-sum test. Analyses were done using R (version: 2.15.2).

Results

Patients

Figure 1 displays the flow chart. Patients were screened from January 2011 until December 2012. Muscle strength could be assessed in 212 patients. Of those patients, 103 patients (49%) were diagnosed with ICU–AW. Table 1 shows patient and admission characteristics.

Candidate predictors

The literature search identified two systematic reviews on risk factors for ICU-AW. [11,23] Three additional recently published cohort studies were found. [24–26] We extracted 17 risk factors (see material S1) and redefined some of the risk factors so that they were suitable as candidate predictors (see figure S1). Three extra candidate predictors that have never been investigated but are likely to be of importance in ICU-AW were added, i.e. presence of pre-existing polyneuropathy, presence of risk factors for polyneuropathy and systemic corticosteroid use prior to ICU admission. All 20 candidate predictors are displayed in table 2; table S1 displays descriptions and definitions.

Predictor selection

Table 2 gives an overview of the distributions of the different candidate predictors for patients who did or did not develop ICU–AW. Because of the low number of patients with a pre–existing polyneuropathy, this candidate predictor was excluded from predictor selection. After backward selection, highest lactate, treatment with any aminoglycoside, age and lowest ionized Ca^{2+} were included in ≥50% of bootstrap samples (table 2). After

consecutive addition of these candidate predictors into a logistic regression model, addition of lowest ionized Ca^{2+} did not result in discriminatory change in AIC (table 3). Therefore, highest lactate, treatment with any aminoglycoside and age were selected as predictors.

Prediction model

Table 3 shows the multivariate odds ratios for the 3 predictors, both unadjusted and adjusted for overfitting. The AUC–ROC of the prediction model was 0.72 (95%-CI: 0.65–0.79; panel A figure 2) and decreased to 0.71 after interval validation. The model showed good calibration (panel B of figure 2) without evidence for lack of fit. A spreadsheet calculator based on the prediction model is provided as material S2.

Comparison with APACHE IV and SOFA scores

The AUC-ROC of the maximal SOFA score in the first two ICU days for prediction of ICU-AW was 0.64 (95%-CI: 0.57–0.72); the AUC-ROC of the APACHE IV score was 0.66 (95%-CI: 0.58–0.73). Discrimination improved when using the new prediction model, both when compared to the maximal SOFA score in the first two ICU days and APACHE IV score (cNRI: 34% (95%-CI: 6 to 62) and 48% (95%-CI: 20 to 75), respectively).

Sensitivity analyses

For prediction of more severe ICU–AW (severe ICU-AW defined as an average MRC score <3; 64 of 212 patients met this definition), discriminative performance of the prediction model was not different (AUC-ROC: 0.72).

Highest lactate levels were missing in 17 patients; no other parameters had missing values. When repeating the backward selection process on data sets with missing lactate levels imputed, the same candidate predictors had a selection frequency of ≥50% and no additional candidate predictors were identified. Furthermore, based on change in AIC, addition of lowest ionized Ca^{2+} was non-discriminatory in all the imputation models. The discriminative performance of the prediction model was not different (averaged AUC–ROC after internal validation: 0.71) in the imputed data sets.

Table 1. Patient and admission characteristics.

	ICU-AW (N:103)	no ICU-AW (N:109)	p-value
age, mean ± SD	63±15	59±16	0.08
females, n (%)	52 (50)	40 (37)	0.06
reason for admission: planned surgical, n (%)	18 (17)	26 (24)	
reason for admission: emergency surgical, n (%)	28 (27)	21 (19)	0.29
reason for admission: medical, n (%)	57 (55)	62 (57)	
APACHE IV score, mean ± SD (3 missing)	89±25	74±28	<0.01
maximal SOFA score in first two days, mean ± SD	11±3	9±3	<0.01
average MRC score, median (IQR)	2.5 (1.3 to 3.2)	4.8 (4 to 5)	n.a.
day of MRC assessment after ICU admission, median (IQR)	9 (6–16)	7 (5–9)	<0.01
days with MV, median days (IQR)	13 (6 to 22)	6 (4 to 8)	<0.01
LOS ICU, median days (IQR)	16 (9 to 28)	8 (6 to 11)	<0.01
ICU mortality, n (%)	35 (34)	10 (9)	<0.01

ICU-AW: Intensive Care Unit – acquired weakness; LOS ICU: length of stay in the intensive care unit; APACHE IV: Acute Physiology and Chronic Health Evaluation IV; SOFA: Sequential Organ Failure Assessment; MV: mechanical ventilation; MRC: Medical Research Council; n.a.: not applicable.

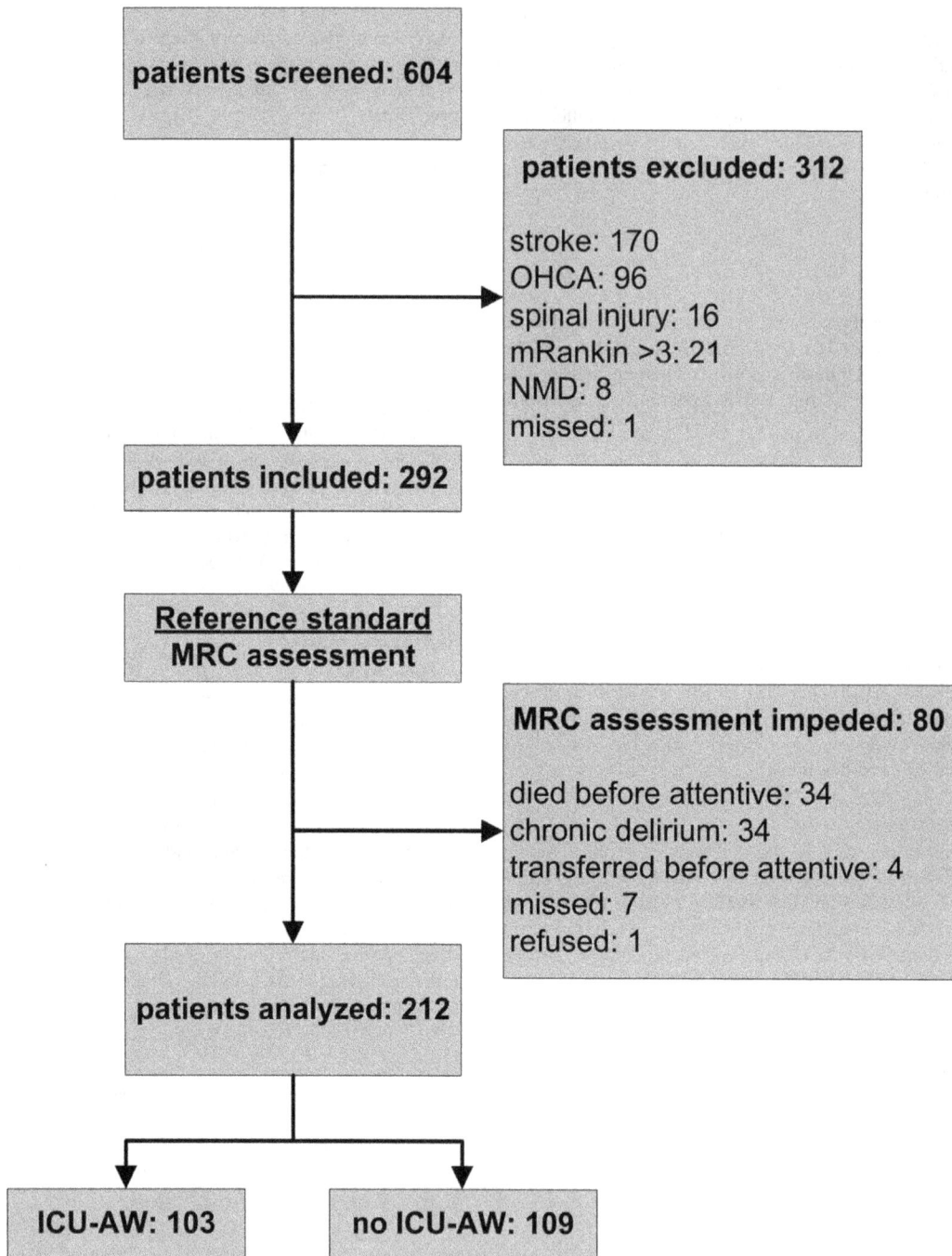

Figure 1. Study flowchart. ICU-AW: Intensive Care Unit – acquired weakness; OHCA: out-of hospital cardiac arrest; mRankin: modified Rankin score; NMD: neuromuscular disorder; MRC: muscle strength as assessed with Medical Research Council scale.

Discussion

After the first two days of stay in the ICU, development of ICU-AW can be predicted using highest lactate levels, treatment with any aminoglycoside and age as predictors. Discriminative performance of the prediction model was fair.

Comparison with previous studies

This is the first prediction model that has been developed specifically for early prediction of ICU-AW. When compared to previously identified predictors for ICU-AW, i.e. the APACHE and SOFA scores, the new prediction model had better discriminative performance [12,13].

Other, more technically demanding, methods for early prediction of ICU-AW have also been investigated. Weber-Carstens et al studied early electrophysiological testing and found a sensitivity of 83% and specificity of 89% for direct muscle stimulation. [27] This is indicative of a better discriminative performance than our prediction model, but electrophysiological studies in general, and direct muscle stimulation in particular, are technically demanding

Table 2. Candidate predictors for development of prediction model for early prediction of Intensive Care Unit – acquired weakness.

candidate predictors*	distribution		p-value	selection percentage in bootstrap samples
	ICU-AW (N:103)	no ICU-AW (N:109)		
patient characteristics				
females, n (%)	52 (50)	40 (37)	0.06	37.1
age, mean ± SD	63±15	59±16	0.08	57.6
risk factor for a polyneuropathy in medical history, n (%)	35 (34)	40 (37)	0.79	13.4
pre-existing polyneuropathy prior to ICU admission, n (%)	3 (3)	1 (1)	0.57	n.a.
systemic corticosteroid use prior to ICU admission, n (%)	7 (7)	9 (8)	0.89	10.7
clinical parameters				
suspected sepsis, n (%)	78 (76)	70 (64)	0.09	14.7
unplanned admission, n (%)	85 (83)	83 (76)	0.33	10.9
presence of shock, n (%)	75 (73)	67 (61)	0.11	24.6
RASS score, median (IQR)	−3 (−5 to −1)	−2 (−3 to 0)	<0.01	48.2
laboratory parameters				
average urine production, median ml/h (IQR)	70 (20 to 122)	102 (64 to 134)	<0.01	14.4
highest glucose, mean mg/dl ± SD	243.8±78.5	220.5±67.3	0.02	38.5
lowest glucose, mean mg/dl ± SD	85.8±22.3	89.6±25.8	0.25	22.2
lowest pH, mean ± SD	7.21±0.1	7.25±0.1	0.02	17.3
lowest P/F ratio, median (IQR)	186 (127 to 245)	178 (134 to 246)	0.98	27.9
lowest platelet count, median×10⁹/L (IQR)	103 (45 to 151)	127 (85 to 197)	0.01	21.0
highest lactate, median mmol/L (IQR; 17 missing)	4.5 (3.0 to 7.0)	2.8 (1.7 to 4.8)	<0.01	89.5‡
lowest ionized Ca²⁺, mean mmol/L ± SD	0.97±0.11	0.98±0.13	0.53	51.6
medication				
treatment with any corticosteroid, n (%)	81 (79)	63 (58)	<0.01	33.9
repeated treatment with any neuromuscular blocker§, n (%)	17 (17)	18 (17)	1.00	20.3
treatment with any aminoglycoside, n (%)	51 (50)	30 (28)	<0.01	80.4

*all clinical, laboratory and medication parameters were scored using information from the first two ICU days, except for the RASS score which was scored around two days after ICU admission;
‡logarithmically transformed;
§more than one administration of any neuromuscular blocker.
ICU-AW: Intensive Care Unit – acquired weakness; RASS: Richmond Agitation and Sedation Scale; n.a.: not applicable.
Table displaying distributions and differences between patients with and without Intensive Care Unit – acquired weakness for the candidate predictors. In the final column selection percentages of the candidate predictors in bootstrap samples based on backward selection are presented.

and are not widely available in ICUs. [1] Diagnostic potential of other methods for an early diagnosis of ICU-AW, like ultrasound or biological markers, has been scarcely studied [1,28,29].

Biological plausibility of the prediction model

Several hypotheses have been proposed that provide biological plausibility for the predictors that have been included in our model. Bolton proposed that tissue hypoxia caused by impaired microcirculation, for which lactate levels are a marker, is involved in pathogenesis of ICU-AW. [30,31] Aminoglycosides may be involved in ICU-AW because they can impair neuromuscular transmission and because of their neurotoxicity. [30,32] With aging, there is an accumulating burden of (neuromuscular) co-morbidities, a physiological loss of skeletal muscle mass and a decrease in mobility; all of which could lead to an increased susceptibility to develop ICU-AW. [33] All of these hypotheses remain speculative since none have been investigated properly.

We would like to emphasize that a good discriminatory performance of a predictor does not mean that this predictor also plays a (important) role in the pathogenesis of ICU-AW.

Table 3. Construction of prediction model.

candidate predictors	selection percentage in bootstrap samples	change in AIC	multivariate OR (95%-CI)	adjusted multivariate OR[†]
highest lactate[‡] (17 missing)	89.5	n.a.	2.18 (1.39 to 3.43)	2.08
treatment with any aminoglycoside	80.4	−5.8	2.75 (1.44 to 5.26)	2.59
age	57.6	−2.8	1.02 (1.00 to 1.04)	1.02
lowest ionized Ca^{2+}	51.6	−1.6	not included	n.a.

[‡]logarithmically transformed.
[†]adjusted for overfitting using a shrinkage factor (i.e. calibration slope) of 0.94 obtained after internal validation.
n.a.: not applicable; AIC: Akaike Information Criterion; OR: odds ratio; CI: confidence interval.
Candidate predictors that were included in ≥50% of bootstrap samples (table 2) were entered consecutively into a logistic regression model starting with the most selected candidate predictor. For every subsequent step, the change in Akaike Information Criterion (AIC) was compared and candidate predictors were only included in the prediction model if addition resulted in a change in AIC<−2. In the final columns unadjusted and adjusted multivariate odds ratio's for predictors included in the prediction model are presented.

Prediction model analyses do not require multivariate analyses to assess an independent association between a variable and the outcome, from which a causal relation may be inferred. [34] For prediction, only the discriminatory performance is important. Sepsis for example was not selected although it is a well-known risk factor for ICU-AW because it was not discriminatory in our population as it was highly prevalent in both patients with and without ICU-AW.

Strengths and limitations

Strengths of this study are the inclusion of a diagnostically relevant population and the use of easily available predictors. Our study also has limitations. First, the number of candidate predictors was larger than the general rule of thumb of 1 candidate predictor for 10 events. [34] Although our candidate predictors were based on previously identified risk factors, this does not necessarily mean that these parameters are also good predictors. We expected that not all candidate predictors would have predictive value and therefore decided to include more

candidate predictors than is recommended. To reduce the subsequent risk of overfitting, we performed a bootstrapped backward selection process, followed by an additional selection step based on model fit. The prediction model we developed and evaluated was adequately powered, with 1 predictor per 33 events and a modest degree of overfitting evident after internal validation. Second, we chose a liberal p-value for inclusion in the prediction model to prevent erroneous elimination of "true" predictors. [18] This may however increase the risk of including "noise" predictors. Finally, we chose not to include composite candidate predictors, like existing severity of illness or organ failures scores (for example APACHE or SOFA). These existing scores contain several variables that are not associated with ICU-AW or include variables that we already included. Therefore, adding these scores as a whole would have led to the inclusion of variables twice or variables with no discriminatory value. A large and inefficient dataset would have been needed to feed the model. Our goal was to only add simple candidate predictors with a unique discrim-

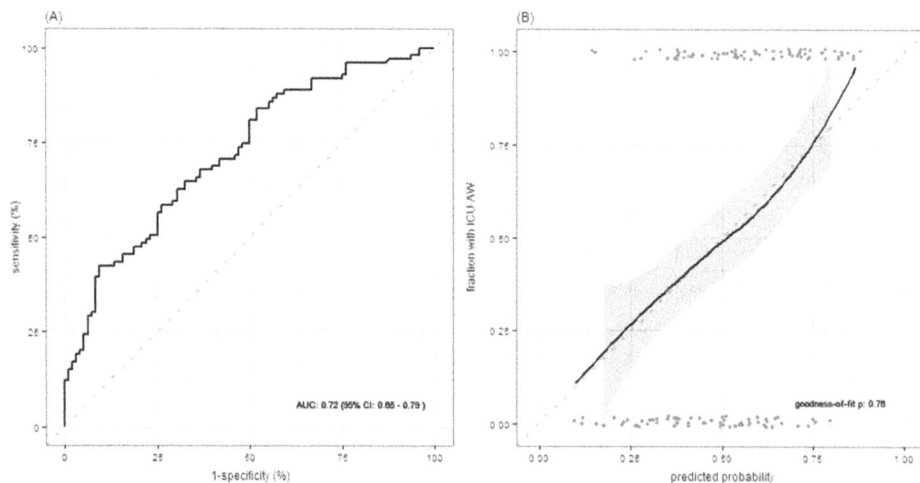

Figure 2. Model performance for early prediction of Intensive Care Unit – acquired weakness. Panel A shows the receiver operating characteristic (ROC) curve assessing discrimination of the prediction model. Panel B shows model calibration assessed with a fitted curve based on loess regression with 95% confidence interval (perfect model calibration is illustrated by the dotted line). Goodness-of-fit assessed with the Hosmer–Lemeshow test is shown. Grey points represent predicted probabilities for individual patients. AUC: area under the receiver operating characteristic curve; CI: confidence interval; ICU-AW: Intensive Care Unit – acquired weakness.

inatory value in order to keep the data set necessary as small and efficient as possible.

Framework for future studies

The ability to predict ICU-AW early after ICU admission and circumvent this limitation of muscle strength assessment as a diagnostic method can be an important step in critical care and research. Our study indicates that this prediction model, using easily available predictors, may be an option to achieve this. However, we did not investigate external validity, which is mandatory to ascertain the true discriminative performance of a prediction model. [35] It will be important to externally validate this prediction model in a multicenter setting to maximize generalizability. The discriminative performance after external validation, possibly recalibrated and updated with new predictors in future, will determine the true value of this model and whether or not it can be used in the clinic.

If the model is found to be reliable enough for clinical application it may be used to improve prognostication and to guide patient management. Also, prediction may be used to start therapies early, before structural damage to nerves and muscles has occurred, which is thought to possibly increase treatment effects. [10] Currently, no high quality evidence is available supporting an intervention for ICU-AW but some prospects exist. Early mobilization, starting when patients are still sedated, may be effective for preventing ICU-AW. [36] Early administration of intravenous immunoglobulins did not prevent ICU-AW. [37] Other pharmacological options, like melatonin, oxytocin, levetiracetam, indomethacin and leupeptin, have only been investigated in animals models. [38–40] Clinical research is needed to confirm these observations and to find new therapeutic options.

Conclusion

Early prediction of ICU–AW is possible using a set of 3 easily available predictors. Discriminative performance of the prediction model seems fair but needs external validation.

Supporting Information

Figure S1 Redefining of relevant risk factors into candidate predictors.

Table S1 Descriptions and definitions for candidate predictors.

Material S1 Supporting text concerning selection of candidate predictors.

Material S2 Spreadsheet calculator.

Material S3 Data set.

Acknowledgments

This research was performed within the framework of CTMM, the Center for Translational Molecular Medicine (www.ctmm.nl), project MARS (grant 04I-201).

Author Contributions

Conceived and designed the experiments: LW EW CV MJS INvS JH. Performed the experiments: LW EW DSD-I MvdS. Analyzed the data: LW EW CV DSD-I MvdS MJS INvS JH. Contributed to the writing of the manuscript: LW EW CV DSD-I MvdS MJS INvS JH.

References

1. Stevens RD, Marshall SA, Cornblath DR, Hoke A, Needham DM, et al. (2009) A framework for diagnosing and classifying intensive care unit-acquired weakness. Crit Care Med 37: S299–308.
2. Latronico N, Bolton CF (2011) Critical illness polyneuropathy and myopathy: a major cause of muscle weakness and paralysis. Lancet Neurol 10: 931–941.
3. Latronico N, Shehu I, Seghelini E (2005) Neuromuscular sequelae of critical illness. Curr Opin Crit Care 11: 381–390.
4. Ali NA, O'Brien JM, Hoffmann SP, Phillips G, Garland A, et al. (2008) Acquired weakness, handgrip strength, and mortality in critically ill patients. Am J Respir Crit Care Med 178: 261–268.
5. Sharshar T, Bastuji-Garin S, Stevens RD, Durand M-C, Malissin I, et al. (2009) Presence and severity of intensive care unit-acquired paresis at time of awakening are associated with increased intensive care unit and hospital mortality. Crit Care Med 37: 3047–3053.
6. Khan J, Harrison TB, Rich MM, Moss M (2006) Early development of critical illness myopathy and neuropathy in patients with severe sepsis. Neurology 67: 1421–1425.
7. Tennilä A, Salmi T, Pettilä V, Roine RO, Varpula T, et al. (2000) Early signs of critical illness polyneuropathy in ICU patients with systemic inflammatory response syndrome or sepsis. Intensive Care Med 26: 1360–1363.
8. Latronico N, Shehu I, Guarneri B (2009) Use of electrophysiologic testing. Crit Care Med 37: S316–S320.
9. Novak KR, Nardelli P, Cope TC, Filatov G, Glass JD, et al. (2009) Inactivation of sodium channels underlies reversible neuropathy during critical illness in rats. J Clin Invest 119: 1150–1158.
10. Hough CL, Lieu BK, Caldwell ES (2011) Manual muscle strength testing of critically ill patients: feasibility and interobserver agreement. Crit Care 15: R43.
11. Stevens RD, Dowdy DW, Michaels RK, Mendez-Tellez PA, Pronovost PJ, et al. (2007) Neuromuscular dysfunction acquired in critical illness: a systematic review. Intensive Care Med 33: 1876–1891.
12. De Letter MA, Schmitz PI, Visser LH, Verheul FA, Schellens RL, et al. (2001) Risk factors for the development of polyneuropathy and myopathy in critically ill patients. Crit Care Med 29: 2281–2286.
13. Bednarik J, Vondracek P, Dusek L, Moravcova E, Cundrle I (2005) Risk factors for critical illness polyneuromyopathy. J Neurol 252: 343–351.
14. Bossuyt PM, Reitsma JB, Bruns DE, Gatsonis CA, Glasziou PP, et al. (2003) The STARD statement for reporting studies of diagnostic accuracy: explanation and elaboration. The Standards for Reporting of Diagnostic Accuracy Group. Ann Intern Med 44: 639–650.
15. Van Swieten JC, Koudstaal PJ, Visser MC, Schouten HJ, van Gijn J (1988) Interobserver agreement for the assessment of handicap in stroke patients. Stroke 19: 604–607.
16. Sessler CN, Gosnell MS, Grap MJ, Brophy GM, O'Neal PV, et al. (2002) The Richmond Agitation-Sedation Scale: validity and reliability in adult intensive care unit patients. Am J Respir Crit Care Med 166: 1338–1344.
17. Vanpee G, Hermans G, Segers J, Gosselink R (2014) Assessment of limb muscle strength in critically ill patients: a systematic review. Crit Care Med 42: 701–711.
18. Steyerberg EW, Eijkemans MJ, Harrell FE, Habbema JD (2001) Prognostic modeling with logistic regression analysis: in search of a sensible strategy in small data sets. Med Decis Making 21: 45–56.
19. Brunelli A, Rocco G (2006) Internal validation of risk models in lung resection surgery: bootstrap versus training-and-test sampling. J Thorac Cardiovasc Surg 131: 1243–1247.
20. Akaike H (1974) A new look at the statistical model identification. Autom Control IEEE Trans 19: 716–723.
21. Pencina MJ, D'Agostino Ralph B S, Steyerberg EW (2010) Extensions of net reclassification improvement calculations to measure usefulness of new biomarkers. Stat Med 30: 11–21.
22. Heymans MW, van Buuren S, Knol DL, van Mechelen W, de Vet HCW (2007) Variable selection under multiple imputation using the bootstrap in a prognostic study. BMC Med Res Methodol 7: 33.
23. De Jonghe B, Cook D, Sharshar T, Lefaucheur J-P, Carlet J, et al. (1998) Acquired neuromuscular disorders in critically ill patients: a systematic review. Groupe de Reflexion et d'Etude sur les Neuromyopathies En Reanimation. Intensive Care Med 24: 1242–1250.
24. Nanas S, Kritikos K, Angelopoulos E, Siafaka A, Tsikriki S, et al. (2008) Predisposing factors for critical illness polyneuromyopathy in a multidisciplinary intensive care unit. Acta Neurol Scand 118: 175–181.

25. Weber-Carstens S, Deja M, Koch S, Spranger J, Bubser F, et al. (2010) Risk factors in critical illness myopathy during the early course of critical illness: a prospective observational study. Crit Care 14: R119.

26. Anastasopoulos D, Kefaliakos A, Michalopoulos A (2011) Is plasma calcium concentration implicated in the development of critical illness polyneuropathy and myopathy? Crit Care 15: R247.

27. Weber-Carstens S, Koch S, Spuler S, Spies CD, Bubser F, et al. (2009) Nonexcitable muscle membrane predicts intensive care unit-acquired paresis in mechanically ventilated, sedated patients. Crit Care Med 37: 2632–2637.

28. Cartwright MS, Kwayisi G, Griffin LP, Sarwal A, Walker FO, et al. (2013) Quantitative neuromuscular ultrasound in the intensive care unit. Muscle Nerve 47: 255–259.

29. Grimm A, Teschner U, Porzelius C, Ludewig K, Zielske J, et al. (2013) Muscle ultrasound for early assessment of critical illness neuromyopathy in severe sepsis. Crit Care 17: R227.

30. Bolton CF (2005) Neuromuscular manifestations of critical illness. Muscle Nerve 32: 140–163.

31. Marshall JC (2001) Inflammation, coagulopathy, and the pathogenesis of multiple organ dysfunction syndrome. Crit Care Med 29: S99–106.

32. Maramattom BV, Wijdicks EFM (2006) Acute neuromuscular weakness in the intensive care unit. Crit Care Med 34: 2835–2841.

33. Puthucheary Z, Montgomery H, Moxham J, Harridge S, Hart N (2010) Structure to function: muscle failure in critically ill patients. J Physiol 588: 4641–4648.

34. Moons KGM, Kengne AP, Woodward M, Royston P, Vergouwe Y, et al. (2012) Risk prediction models: I. Development, internal validation, and assessing the incremental value of a new (bio)marker. Heart 98: 683–690.

35. Moons KGM, Kengne AP, Grobbee DE, Royston P, Vergouwe Y, et al. (2012) Risk prediction models: II. External validation, model updating, and impact assessment. Heart 98: 691–698.

36. Hermans G, De Jonghe B, Bruyninckx F, Van den Berghe G (2014) Interventions for preventing critical illness polyneuropathy and critical illness myopathy. Cochrane database Syst Rev 1: CD006832.

37. Brunner R, Rinner W, Haberler C, Kitzberger R, Sycha T, et al. (2013) Early treatment with IgM-enriched intravenous immunoglobulin does not mitigate critical illness polyneuropathy and/or myopathy in patients with multiple organ failure and SIRS/sepsis: a prospective, randomized, placebo-controlled, double-blinded trial. Crit Care 17: R213.

38. Ruff RL, Secrist D (1984) Inhibitors of prostaglandin synthesis or cathepsin B prevent muscle wasting due to sepsis in the rat. J Clin Invest 73: 1483–1486.

39. Erbaş O, Yeniel AÖ, Akdemir A, Ergenoğlu AM, Yilmaz M, et al. (2013) The beneficial effects of levetiracetam on polyneuropathy in the early stage of sepsis in rats: electrophysiological and biochemical evidence. J Invest Surg 26: 312–318.

40. Erbaş O, Ergenoglu AM, Akdemir A, Yeniel AÖ, Taskiran D (2013) Comparison of melatonin and oxytocin in the prevention of critical illness polyneuropathy in rats with experimentally induced sepsis. J Surg Res 183: 313–320.

10

The Role of Whole Blood Impedance Aggregometry and Its Utilisation in the Diagnosis and Prognosis of Patients with Systemic Inflammatory Response Syndrome and Sepsis in Acute Critical Illness

Gareth R. Davies[2], Gavin M. Mills[1], Matthew Lawrence[1,2], Ceri Battle[1,3], Keith Morris[1,4], Karl Hawkins[1,2], Phylip Rhodri Williams[5], Simon Davidson[6], Dafydd Thomas[1,7], Phillip Adrian Evans[1,2]*

1 NISCHR Haemostasis Biomedical Research Unit (HBRU), Morriston Hospital, Swansea, Wales, United Kingdom, 2 Institute of Life Science, College of Medicine, Swansea University, Singleton Park, Swansea, Wales, United Kingdom, 3 Intensive Therapy Unit, Abertawe Bro Morgannwg University Health Board, Swansea, Wales, United Kingdom, 4 School of Applied Science, University of Wales Institute Cardiff, Cardiff, Wales, United Kingdom, 5 College of Engineering, Swansea University, Singleton Park, Swansea, Wales, United Kingdom, 6 Department of Haematology, Royal Brompton and Harefield NHS Foundation Trust, London, United Kingdom, 7 Cardiac Intensive Care Unit, Abertawe Bro Morgannwg University Health Board, Swansea, Wales, United Kingdom

Abstract

Objective: To assess the prognostic and diagnostic value of whole blood impedance aggregometry in patients with sepsis and SIRS and to compare with whole blood parameters (platelet count, haemoglobin, haematocrit and white cell count).

Methods: We performed an observational, prospective study in the acute setting. Platelet function was determined using whole blood impedance aggregometry (multiplate) on admission to the Emergency Department or Intensive Care Unit and at 6 and 24 hours post admission. Platelet count, haemoglobin, haematocrit and white cell count were also determined.

Results: 106 adult patients that met SIRS and sepsis criteria were included. Platelet aggregation was significantly reduced in patients with severe sepsis/septic shock when compared to SIRS/uncomplicated sepsis (ADP: 90.7 ± 37.6 vs 61.4 ± 40.6; $p < 0.001$, Arachadonic Acid 99.9 ± 48.3 vs 66.3 ± 50.2; $p = 0.001$, Collagen 102.6 ± 33.0 vs 79.1 ± 38.8; $p = 0.001$; SD $\pm$ mean)). Furthermore platelet aggregation was significantly reduced in the 28 day mortality group when compared with the survival group (Arachadonic Acid 58.8 ± 47.7 vs 91.1 ± 50.9; $p < 0.05$, Collagen 36.6 ± 36.6 vs 98.0 ± 35.1; $p = 0.001$; SD $\pm$ mean)). However haemoglobin, haematocrit and platelet count were more effective at distinguishing between subgroups and were equally effective indicators of prognosis. Significant positive correlations were observed between whole blood impedance aggregometry and platelet count (ADP 0.588 $p < 0.0001$, Arachadonic Acid 0.611 $p < 0.0001$, Collagen 0.599 $p < 0.0001$ (Pearson correlation)).

Conclusions: Reduced platelet aggregometry responses were not only significantly associated with morbidity and mortality in sepsis and SIRS patients, but also correlated with the different pathological groups. Whole blood aggregometry significantly correlated with platelet count, however, when we adjust for the different groups we investigated, the effect of platelet count appears to be non-significant.

Editor: Kathleen Freson, University of Leuven, Belgium

Funding: This work is part-funded by the European Social Fund (ESF) through the European Union's Convergence programme administered by the Welsh Government. The funders had no role in study design, data collection and analysis, decision to publish, or preparation of the manuscript.

Competing Interests: PAE and PRW have signed the International Committee of Medical Journal Editors (ICMJE) form for declaration of interest. All other authors declare no competing conflicts of interest.

* Email: Phillip.A.Evans@wales.nhs.uk

Introduction

Sepsis is a life threatening condition and common complication of critical illness [1]. It is characterised by a systemic inflammatory response to an ongoing infectious process and can lead to hypotension, multi organ dysfunction (MOD) and death [2]. Systemic inflammation can also have non-infectious causes such as burns, pancreatitis and ketoacidosis, and is termed systemic

Table 1. Demographics of Subject Groups.

	Healthy	SIRS	Sepsis	Severe Sepsis	Septic Shock
Number	42	21	42	17	26
Male (%)	21 (50.0)	12 (57.1)	19 (45.2)	8 (47.1)	16 (61.5)
Age (Years)	60.1±16.5	62.8±20.4	56.6±19.6	63.9±21.4	68.6±13.0
Primary Site of Infection					
Respiratory Tract (%)	-	-	27 (64.3)	10 (58.8)	10 (38.5)
Urinary Tract (%)	-	-	7 (16.7)	4 (23.5)	6 (23.1)
GI Tract (%)	-	-	3 (7.1)	0 (0)	6 (23.1)
Other (%)	-	-	5 (11.9)	3 (17.6)	4 (15.4)
Comorbidities					
Diabetes Mellitus (%)	0 (0)	12 (57.1)	4 (9.5)	4 (23.5)	9 (34.6)
COPD (%)	0 (0)	3 (14.3)	19 (45.2)	2 (11.8)	4 (15.4)
Congestive Heart Failure (%)	0 (0)	2 (9.5)	1 (2.4)	0 (0)	2 (7.7)
Active Cancer (%)	0 (0)	0 (0)	1 (2.4)	0 (0)	3 (11.5)
28 Day Mortality (%)	-	2 (9.5)	1 (2.4)	0 (0)	3 (11.5)
SOFA Score	-	3 (2, 7)	3 (1.25, 3)	5 (4, 6)	9 (6, 12)
Hospital LOS (days)	-	6 (4.5, 14.5)	5 (2, 8.5)	9 (5.5, 19)	14 (2.5, 43)

COPD = Chronic Obstructive Pulmonary Disease; SOFA = Sepsis-relates Organ Failure Assessment; LOS = Length of Stay.

inflammatory response syndrome (SIRS). Prevalence of SIRS due to sterile or infectious causes is very high, affecting up to one third of all hospital patients [3] and it remains a challenge to differentiate sepsis from sterile SIRS which is vital in guiding effective treatment.

It has been shown previously that coagulation is activated across the septic range [4,5] This activation can express itself as either a mildly increased risk of thrombosis to systemic formation of intravascular thrombi, known as disseminated intravascular coagulation (DIC). Altered coagulation contributes to the pathogenesis and outcome of sepsis. In severe sepsis microthrombi formation in the vasculature alters perfusion of blood into the organs, contributing to multiple organ dysfunction syndrome (MODS) [6]. Sepsis is also the leading cause of thrombocytopenia [7] which is related to poor outcome [8]. Studies have highlighted that the function of platelets goes beyond haemostatic regulation [9,10] and there is increasing evidence that platelets are key mediators of inflammation and the immunological response to infection [11]. Platelet aggregation is enhanced in the presence of lipopolysaccharide (LPS) in vitro [12], which has been identified to be dependent on toll-like receptor 4 pathway [13]. This suggests increased platelet aggregation measurements might be observed in patients with sepsis.

The role of platelet aggregation is very important in inflammation. In severe sepsis, platelet aggregation has been often shown to be decreased [14][15][16]; however, this has yet to be investigated in the whole sepsis spectrum. Whole blood impedance aggregometry (multiplate) is a point of care test that can be used to measure platelet aggregation in response to different agonists and has been shown to be a predictor of diagnosis and prognosis in patients with severe sepsis [15]. However, it has also been suggested that whole blood impedance aggregometry is dependent on whole blood parameters (platelet count, haematocrit, haemoglobin and white cell count) [17][18]. Of particular relevance to whole blood impedance aggregometry are platelet counts of less than 150×10^9/L [19].

The primary aim of this study was to assess the diagnostic and prognostic accuracy of whole blood aggregometry in patients who present across the septic range and to compare these results against the whole blood parameters (platelet count, white cell count, haematocrit and haemoglobin). The secondary aim of the study was to investigate the dependence of whole blood aggregometry on the whole blood parameters.

Materials and Methods

Ethical Approval

Full ethical approval was given by the South West Wales Research Ethics Committee. Informed 2-stage written consent was given by patients with capacity to do so. Assent was obtained from personal or legal representation in cases where capacity to give informed consent was lacking.

Patients

A total of 106 patients were recruited from October 2011 to November 2013 in a large teaching hospital in Wales. All patients were considered eligible as per the SIRS criteria defined in 2003 [20]. 42 healthy volunteers from a similar demographic population group and matched for gender and age were recruited as a control group. Patients with any disease that affects the coagulation profile including liver cirrhosis and renal disease were excluded. Patients that had received anticoagulant therapy were also excluded. Patient outcome was evaluated at 28 days.

Sepsis-related Organ Failure Assessment (SOFA) score [21] was determined over the first 24 hours to assess organ function. Patients were assigned to groups as follows: 1) Sterile SIRS 2) Uncomplicated sepsis 3) Severe sepsis 4) Septic shock as per the criteria defined in 2003 [20]. Assignment into groups was blinded and performed by an experienced intensive care specialist independent of the study. All platelet aggregation data was also validated independently.

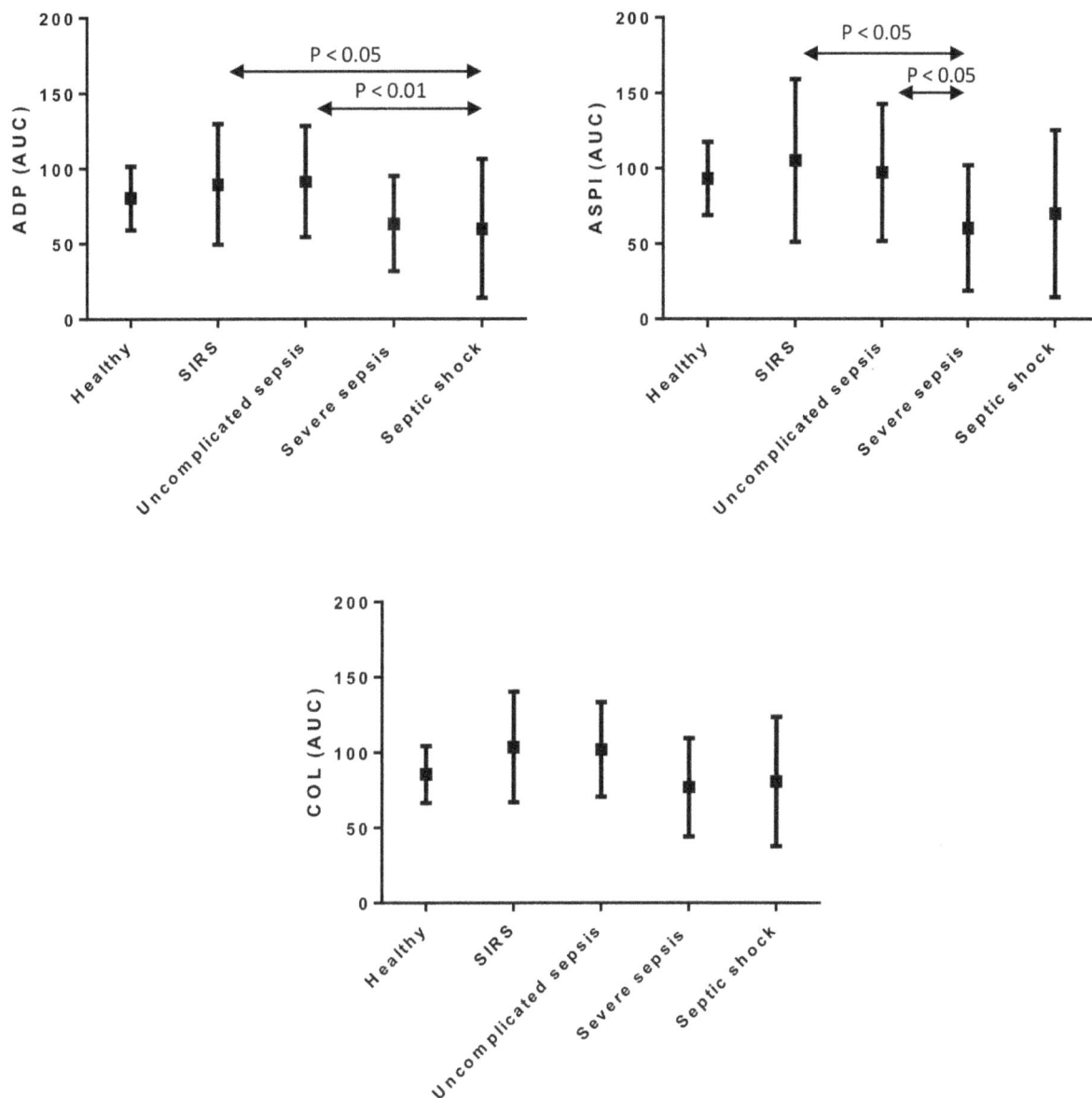

Figure 1. Comparison of platelet aggregometry measurements in different pathological groups and healthy control. Platelet aggregation measurements induced by ADP, ASPI and Collagen agonists are shown in the different pathological groups and healthy control. Aggregometry measurements are expressed as area under the curve (AUC, arbitrary units). Significant differences between the groups are indicated by p-values, as assessed by Bonferroni post-hoc analysis.

Blood Sampling

Blood was drawn at time of admission to the emergency department or intensive care unit, at 6 hours and 24 hours post admission to assess disease progression and the effect of treatment. For multiplate analysis, blood was drawn into 3mL hirudin blood tubes (Verum Diagnostica, Munich, Germany) as per manufacturers' recommendations. Testing was performed 20 minutes after the blood was drawn. A total volume of 300 μL of hirudinised blood was added to 300 μL normal saline in the multiplate test cell, which was then incubated at 37°C for 3 minutes. Blood samples were then activated using three different reagents 1) adenosine diphosphate (ADP test, Verum Diagnostica GmbH), 2) arachadonic acid test of cyclooxygenase activity (ASPI test, Verum Diagnostica GmbH) and 3) collagen (COL test, Verum Diagnostica GmbH) agonists. Aggregometry measurements were assessed via the area under the curve measurement (arbitrary units).

A 4 ml aliquot of blood was taken for full blood count (FBC) analysis to determine all the whole blood parameters. Samples were collected into plastic, full-draw dipotassium EDTA Vacuettes (Greiner Bio-One, Stonehouse, UK Ref: 454286). FBC was analysed using a Sysmex XE 2100 (Sysmex UK, Milton Keynes, UK) automated haematology analyser within 2 hrs of collection.

Statistical Analysis

All statistical analysis was carried out on GraphPad Prism version 6 (GraphPad software, La Jolla, CA, USA). Values are given as mean and standard deviation or alternatively median and quartiles. For continuous variables T-test was used to detect significant differences between normally distributed groups and

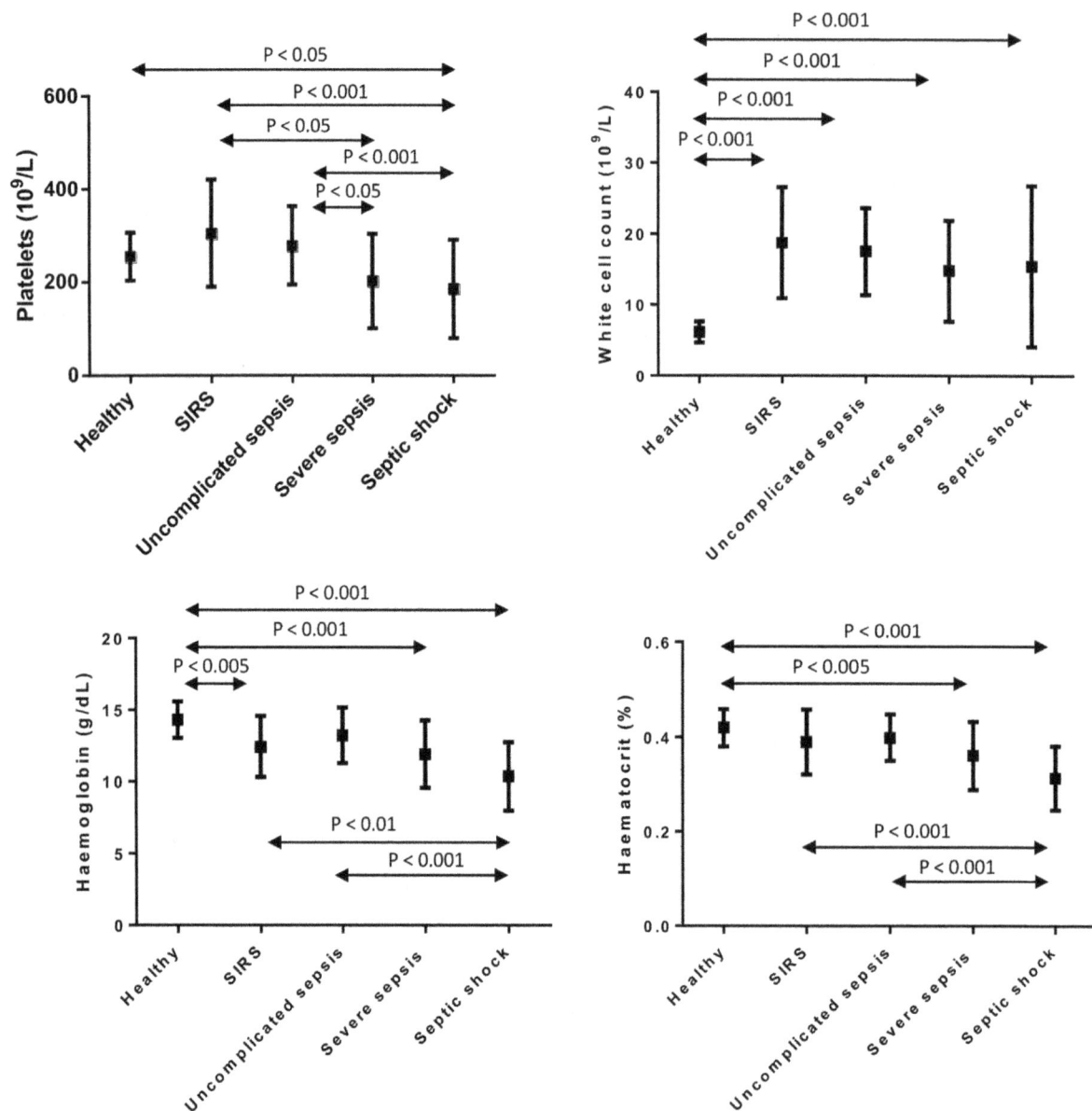

Figure 2. Comparison of whole blood parameters in different pathological groups and healthy control. Platelet count, white cell count, haemoglobin and haematocrit measurements are shown in different pathological groups and healthy control. Significant differences between the groups are indicated by p-values, as assessed by Bonferroni post-hoc analysis.

Kruskal-Wallis was used to detect differences in non-normally distributed data. Data normality was assessed using the Kolmogorov-Smirnov and Shapiro-Wilk tests using an α of 0.05. Bonferroni post hoc correction was used to assess multiple comparisons across groups. Receiver operating characteristics were determined to assess discrimination between groups. Sensitivities and specificities were determined from the optimal cut-off values, which were calculated as the point at which the Youden Index was maximised [22].

Pearson's correlation coefficient was used to investigate relationships between whole blood aggregometry and whole blood parameters. Analysis of Covariance (ANCOVA) was used to adjust for changes in platelet aggregation in the different groups investigated, with the platelet count as a covariate using the General Linear Model method.

To adjust for the effect of low platelet count on whole blood impedance aggregometry, data was reanalysed for patients with platelet counts greater than 100×10^9/L only.

Statistical significance was defined as a p-value of less than 0.05 (two-tailed).

Results

Platelet aggregometry and full blood count were assessed in a total of 106 patients that met SIRS criteria. This included 21 SIRS, 42 uncomplicated sepsis, 17 severe sepsis and 26 septic shock patients. A healthy group of 42 volunteers was also recruited. Clinical characteristics are presented in Table 1.

Table 2. Comparison of SIRS/Uncomplicated sepsis and severe sepsis/septic shock.

	Healthy (n = 42)	SIRS/Uncomplicated Sepsis (n = 62)	Severe Sepsis/Septic Shock (n = 43)	Significance value (Healthy vs SIRS/Uncomplicated)	Significance Value (SIRS/Uncomplicated vs Severe/Septic Shock
ADP (AUC)	80.4±21.1	90.7±37.6	61.4±40.6	NS	<0.001
ASPI (AUC)	93.2±24.3	99.9±48.3	66.3±50.2	NS	0.001
COL (AUC)	85.5±19.0	102.6±33.0	79.1±38.8	0.01	0.001
Platelet Count (10^9/L)	255.6±51.9	295.0±110.9	192.5±103.2	0.03	<0.001
White Cell Count (10^9/L)	6.2±1.5	17.9±6.7	15.2±9.9	<0.001	NS
Haemoglobin (g/dL)	14.3±1.3	13.0±2.0	11.0±2.5	<0.001	<0.001
Haematocrit (%)	0.42±0.04	0.39±0.06	0.33±0.07	0.01	<0.001

Platelet Aggregometry for Diagnosing Sepsis Severity

The results, shown in Figure 1, demonstrate reduced platelet aggregometry values in patients with severe sepsis and septic shock when compared to SIRS and uncomplicated sepsis when ADP and ASPI were used as the agonist, but this was not the case when Collagen was used as the agonist. Platelet aggregometry values in the patient groups were comparable to those of the healthy group.

Results for haemoglobin, haematocrit, platelet count and white cell count are presented in Figure 2. Significant progressive reductions in haemoglobin, haematocrit and platelet count were observed across the sepsis spectrum, with increasing severity. White cell count was elevated in all patient groups when compared to the healthy group.

Platelet Aggregometry for the Diagnosis of Severe Sepsis

To assess platelet aggregometry as a diagnostic marker of severe sepsis, patients were assigned to two groups: SIRS/uncomplicated sepsis and severe sepsis/septic shock. The results, displayed in Table 2, show significantly reduced platelet aggregation, haemoglobin, haematocrit and platelet count in patients with severe sepsis/septic shock when compared to SIRS/uncomplicated sepsis patients.

To further assess discrimination between SIRS/uncomplicated sepsis and severe sepsis/septic shock groups, receiver operating characteristics were analysed (Figure 3). The corresponding area under the curve and significance are shown in Table 3. All parameters except for white cell count showed significant discrimination between groups as defined by p-values of less than 0.05. This indicates that whole blood impedance aggregometry is able to distinguish between those with SIRS/uncomplicated sepsis and severe sepsis/septic shock, particularly when ADP is used as the agonist. The most significant discriminatory power, apart from SOFA score, was observed with ADP aggregometry, haematocrit and platelet count.

Optimal cut-off points were determined as described in the methods section. Sensitivity, specificity and the optimal cut-off for each parameter are displayed in Table 4.

Platelet Aggregometry for Determining Prognosis in Sepsis Patients

All patients were followed up for 28-day mortality. Characteristics of 28 day survival and mortality groups are shown in Table 5. Platelet aggregometry was significantly reduced in the 28-day mortality group using ASPI and COL agonists; however, with ADP activation this did not appear to be the case. Haemoglobin, platelet count and white cell count were all significantly reduced in

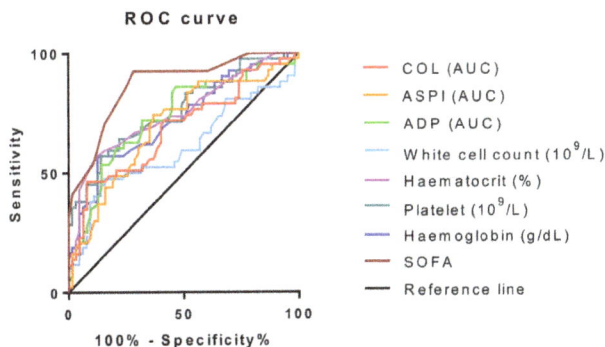

Figure 3. Receiver operating characteristics for discrimination between SIRS/Uncomplicated Sepsis and Severe Sepsis/Septic Shock groups. Receiver operating characteristics are shown for platelet aggregometry measurements, whole blood parameters and sepsis-related organ failure assessment (SOFA) score as a discriminator between patients with and without organ dysfunction.

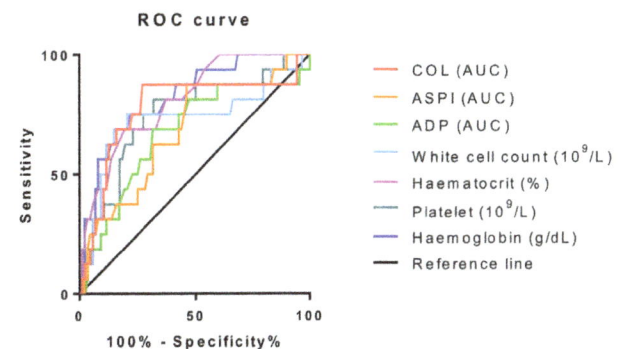

Figure 4. Receiver operating characteristics for discrimination between survivors and non-survivors at 28 days. Receiver operating characteristics are shown for platelet aggregometry measurements and whole blood parameters for the discrimination between 28-day mortality and survival.

Table 3. Receiver Operating Characteristics for the Diagnosis of Severe Sepsis.

Test Result Variable(s)	Area	Std. Error	Asymptomatic Sig.	Asymptomatic 95% Confidence Interval (Lower Bound)	Asymptomatic 95% Confidence Interval (Upper Bound)
ADP (AUC)	0.740	0.051	<0.001	0.640	0.840
ASPI (AUC)	0.697	0.054	0.001	0.592	0.802
COL (AUC)	0.689	0.055	0.001	0.582	0.796
Platelet Count (10^9/L)	0.759	0.049	<0.001	0.664	0.855
White Cell Count (10^9/L)	0.608	0.060	0.061	0.491	0.726
Haemoglobin (g/L)	0.722	0.052	<0.001	0.620	0.823
Haematocrit (%)	0.746	0.051	<0.001	0.646	0.846
SOFA	0.870	0.036	<0.001	0.799	0.942

SOFA = Sepsis-related Organ Failure Assessment score.

the 28-day mortality group. Receiver operating characteristic curves showing discrimination between survivors and non-survivors are shown in Figure 4. The AUC, significance and confidence intervals are shown in Table 6. All measured parameters showed significant discrimination between survivors and non-survivors (Asymptomatic Sig <0.05). This indicates reduced whole blood parameters and impaired platelet function are strongly related to poor outcome in sepsis patients.

Effect of Treatment on Platelet Aggregation

To assess the effect of treatment and disease progression on platelet aggregation, measurements were repeated at 6 and 24 hours post admission. The results, shown in Figure 5, demonstrate a significant reduction in ADP induced aggregation over 24 hours in the SIRS and uncomplicated sepsis groups. Haemoglobin and haematocrit were also significantly reduced over 24 hours in uncomplicated sepsis. No other significant changes were observed in any of the groups over 24 hours. Reduced platelet aggregation and whole blood parameters were observed in the more severe groups over the 24 hours; however, this was not significant.

Dependence of Platelet Aggregometry on Whole Blood Parameters

Correlation analysis was used to assess the dependence of platelet aggregometry on platelet count, haemoglobin and leukocyte count. Platelet aggregation correlated significantly with all blood count parameters (Table 7). Using correlation analysis, R2 values were 0.363, 0.420 and 0.379 (p<0.001) for ADP, ASPI and Collagen agonists respectively.

Analysis of the effect of platelet count on platelet aggregation using all three aggregating agents and using Analysis of Covariance (General Linear Model) would suggest that the platelet count significantly affects platelet aggregation, however, the change in platelet aggregation for ADP, collagen and aspirin is significantly different in the sepsis and non-sepsis groups even when we adjust for the platelet count (P<0.005, ANCOVA). Hence, this analysis would support the view that sepsis has an effect on both the platelet count together with platelet function.

Adjusting for Low Platelet Count

To correct for the potential effects low platelet count had on Multiplate readings, data was reanalysed for patients with a platelet count greater than 100×10^9/L (n = 97). Platelet aggregometry using all three agonists (ADP, ASPI and collagen) remained significant at distinguishing between SIRS/uncomplicated sepsis and severe sepsis/septic shock (ADP 68.8±39.9 vs 90.7±37.6, p<

Table 4. Sensitivity and Specificity for the Diagnosis of Severe Sepsis.

Cutoff	Sensitivity (%)	Specificity (%)
ADP <75.5	75.6	71.9
ASPI <85.5	73.2	64.9
COL <62.5	48.8	93
Platelet Count <211.5	61	80.7
White Cell Count <12.35	48.8	82.5
Haemoglobin <11.35	58.5	86
Haematocrit <0.322	53.7	91.2
SOFA>3.5	92.7	71.9

Sensitivity: Percentage of severe sepsis patients with a positive test.
Specificity: Percentage of SIRS/uncomplicated sepsis patients with a negative test.
SOFA = Sepsis-related Organ Failure Assessment score.

Table 5. Characteristics of Survivors and Non-Survivors in Relation to Platelet Aggregation and Whole Blood Parameters.

	28 Day Survival (n = 89)	28 Day Mortality (n = 16)	Significance value
ADP (AUC)	81.6±39.2	62.9±49.8	0.097
ASPI (AUC)	91.1±50.9	58.8±47.7	0.02
COL (AUC)	98.0±35.1	64.8±36.6	0.001
Platelet Count (10^9/L)	268.3±117.7	174.4±91.9	0.003
White Cell Count (10^9/L)	17.8±7.6	11.3±9.2	0.003
Haemoglobin (g/dL)	12.6±2.2	9.7±2.1	<0.001
Haematocrit (%)	0.38±0.06	0.30±0.06	<0.001

Comparisons were made using two-sample t-test.

0.05; ASPI 76.4±50.7 vs 99.9±48.3, p<0.05; COL 85.7±37.8 vs 102.6±33.0, p<0.05). All measured parameters except for ADP aggregometry remained significantly lower in the 28-day mortality group (p<0.05).

Discussion

This, to our knowledge, is the first study to assess whole blood aggregometry across the entire pathological spectrum of SIRS and sepsis. The data demonstrates that a reduction in aggregometry measurements, haemoglobin and platelet count are associated with increasing severity of sepsis. Several authors have reported and reviewed that platelet function as well as platelet count is significantly modulated during sepsis-in particular severe sepsis [4,15,23]. Our data supports these findings in that our analysis demonstrated both a significant reduction and a significant modulation of platelet aggregation mediated through all three agonists used herein. Platelets display a number of properties besides repairing damaged vascular endothelium and preventing bleeding. It is known that platelets act to induce pro-inflammatory events [24] and can engage infectious pathogens [25]. The sophisticated interplay of platelets with bacteria may culminate in sepsis that is characterized by significant progressive reductions in platelet count and platelet function with increasing severity of the sepsis. This study supports the view that significant changes in platelet count occur during sepsis. Although there was a reduction in platelet count with progression of sepsis, our findings showed that there was also a marked decrease in platelet activity.

As a marker of prognosis, haemoglobin was found to be a highly significant predictor of 28-day mortality, which has been described previously [26]. Low platelet count, white cell count and platelet aggregometry by ASPI and collagen activation were also significantly associated with mortality, but this was not the case when ADP was used as the agonist. The significant association between ADP aggregometry and severity but not mortality is interesting and could provide insight into the progression of some of the pathogenic mechanisms of sepsis. Previous studies have suggested that anti-platelet therapy could be beneficial in critically ill patients by reducing microvascular thrombi formation and hence improving perfusion [27,28]. It is possible that platelet responses to ADP could be blunted if platelets have been exposed to ADP in vivo, as previously it has been shown that platelets exposed to ADP become desensitised, and unresponsive to restimulation [29]. This is a cause for concern in patients in which there is a degree of haemolysis as ADP released from the red cells could cause platelet refractoriness to further agonist exposure. This could be an additional mechanism for the reduced ADP responses observed in the severe sepsis and septic shock groups.

Reduced platelet aggregometry measurements were observed in patients with severe sepsis and septic shock when compared to SIRS and uncomplicated sepsis. Previously it has been hypothesised that reduced platelet aggregation might be observed in severe sepsis and septic shock as consumption of platelets with increased activation occurs due to the hypercoagulable state and endothelial dysfunction [30]. This suggests that platelet aggregometry could be a biomarker of endothelial function and the level of ongoing DIC. The findings in this study support previous studies that have observed reduced platelet aggregometry in patients with severe

Table 6. Receiver Operating Characteristics for Survivors and Non-Survivors for Platelet Aggregation and Whole Blood Parameters.

Test Result Variable(s)	Area	Std. Error	Asymptomatic Sig.	Asymptomatic 95% Confidence Interval (Lower Bound)	Asymptomatic 95% Confidence nterval (Upper Bound)
ADP (AUC)	.675	.079	0.027	.521	.829
ASPI (AUC)	.686	.072	0.018	.546	.827
COL (AUC)	.777	.075	<0.001	.631	.924
Platelet Count (10^9/L)	.750	.068	0.001	.616	.884
White Cell Count (10^9/L)	.731	.083	0.003	.568	.895
Haemoglobin (g/L)	.822	.055	<0.001	.714	.930
Haematocrit (%)	.811	.053	<0.001	.707	.914

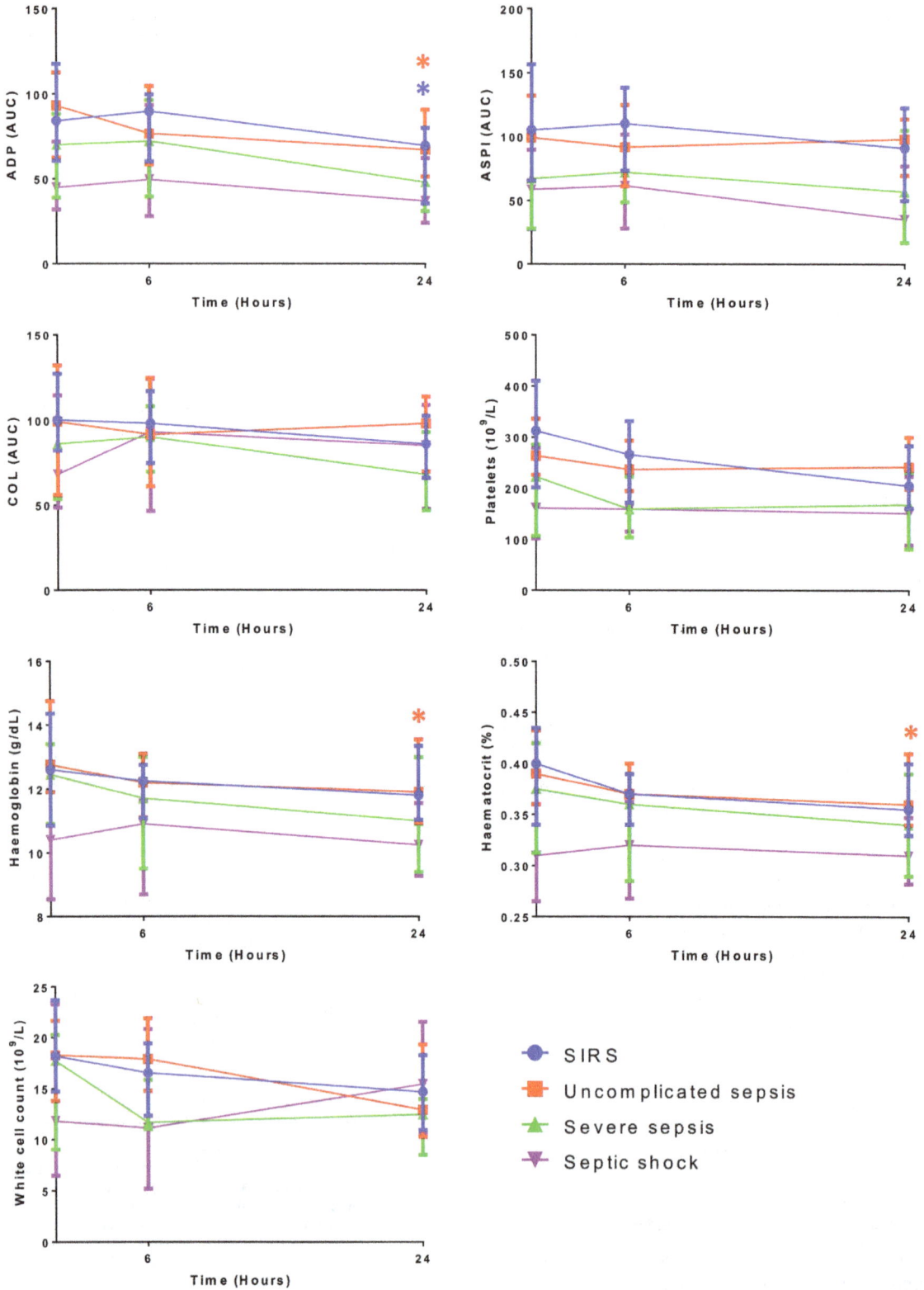

Figure 5. Effect of treatment and disease progression on platelet aggregation and whole blood parameters. Platelet aggregation and whole blood parameters were measured at baseline, 6 hours and 24 hours are shown. *Significant result (P<0.05), two-sample t-test.

sepsis [15,16]. Furthermore, this study demonstrates that platelet aggregometry measurements using collagen as the agonist were

significantly increased in patients with uncomplicated sepsis/sirs compared to healthy volunteers. However, this was not the case

Table 7. Pearson's Correlations of Whole Blood Aggregometry versus Whole Blood Parameters.

Agonist		Platelet Count (10^9/L)	White Cell Count (10^9/L)	Haemoglobin (g/dL)	Haematocrit (%)
ADP (AUC)	Pearson Correlation	0.598	0.254	0.228	0.265
	Sig (2-tailed)	<0.001	0.009	0.020	0.007
ASPI (AUC)	Pearson Correlation	0.635	0.362	0.252	0.307
	Sig (2-tailed)	<0.001	<0.001	0.010	0.001
Collagen (AUC)	Pearson Correlation	0.607	0.476	0.189	0.247
	Sig (2-tailed)	<0.001	<0.001	0.055	0.012

when using ADP or ASPI agonists. The data presented in this study suggests that platelet count and haemoglobin are equally as effective as whole blood impedance aggregometry as diagnostic and prognostic tools in patients that meet SIRS and sepsis criteria. The strong relationship between haemoglobin and sepsis severity and outcome is an interesting one. It is clear from the literature that red blood cell derangement is common occurrence in severe sepsis and this contributes to impairment of the microcirculation leading to eryptosis and reduced circulating haemoglobin [31,32]. Consequently haemoglobin measurements could be providing information on micro perfusion and hence organ dysfunction. Recent studies has also highlighted the impact low haemoglobin level have on blood CO_2 binding capacity [33]. This suggests anaemia could contribute to acidosis, and enhance coagulopathy in sepsis.

We observed that different agonists yielded different operating characteristics when assessing diagnosis and prognosis. This can be explained as each of these agonists causes activation of platelets via a different route e.g. ADP through the P2Y receptors, ASPI through COX-1 cyclooxygenase pathway and Collagen through glycoprotein VI and therefore display different strengths in their ability to activate platelets, some being more effective activators than others. In SIRS/sepsis patients, it could be the case that this variability is heightened.

When assessing the effect of platelet count on platelet aggregation, significant correlations were observed. Furthermore, when excluding subjects with a low platelet count from the analysis, platelet aggregation remained significantly reduced with relation to severity and poor outcome. Although platelet aggregation values are affected by platelet count, variability exists in both platelet count and platelet function in the healthy range and it is also possible to achieve normal aggregometry readings at low platelet counts [18]. Therefore, taking into account the limitations of the assay, there remains a trend to significantly reduced platelet function with increasing severity of disease in this study population.

Limitations

This large pilot observational study has a number of limitations. The inherent problem of this and other reported studies is the heterogeneity of the disease, treatment and comorbidities. It is also difficult to take into account differences in medication and treatment between groups, and to assess this fully, a much larger number of patients would be required. In order to overcome some of these limitations we implemented tight inclusion/exclusion criteria and excluded patients that were receiving anticoagulant therapy at baseline. Sample size could be viewed as a limitation in this study; however, the sample size was powerful enough for us to detect several significant differences between groups. Further larger prospective studies are required to build on the findings of this study.

Conclusions

This study supports the view that significant changes in platelet function occur across the sepsis spectrum, possibly due to different pathophysiological mechanisms. There remains a trend towards worsening platelet function with increasing severity in patients with SIRS and sepsis that is independent of platelet count.

Furthermore, our study demonstrates that haemoglobin and platelet count have greater diagnostic and prognostic value than whole blood impedance aggregometry measurements in patients with SIRS and sepsis. This research further highlights the importance of red blood cells and platelet count in patients with SIRS and sepsis and the potential benefits therapeutic intervention addressing red blood cell rheology and function could have. Further larger studies are now required to explore and determine how the mechanistic role of platelet activity and change across the sepsis spectrum is related to the disease process and outcome.

Acknowledgments

We thank Robert Aubrey, Nia Davies, Sharon Storton, Ahmed Sabra and Lindsay D'Silva for recruitment assistance; Sophia Stanford and Vanessa Evans for technical support; and the medical and nursing staff at Morriston Hospital Emergency Department and Intensive Therapy Unit.

Author Contributions

Conceived and designed the experiments: PAE DT. Performed the experiments: GRD GMM MJL. Analyzed the data: GRD CB KM KH SD PAE PRW. Contributed reagents/materials/analysis tools: KM. Wrote the paper: GRD PAE. Revised the manuscript critically for important intellectual content: GMM MJL CB KM KH PRW SD DT.

References

1. Vincent J-L, Sakr Y, Sprung CL, Ranieri VM, Reinhart K, et al. (2006) Sepsis in European intensive care units: Results of the SOAP study*. Crit Care Med 34: 344–353.
2. Bone R, Balk R, Cerra F, Dellinger R, Fein A, et al. (1992) Definitions for sepsis and organ failure and guidelines for the use of innovative therapies in sepsis. The ACCP/SCCM Consensus Conference Committee. American College of Chest Physicians/Society of Critical Care Medicine. Chest 101: 1644–1655.
3. Brun-Buisson C (2000) The epidemiology of the systemic inflammatory response. Intensive Care Med 26 Suppl 1: S64–S74.
4. Mavrommatis AC, Theodoridis T, Orfanidou A, Roussos C, Christopoulou-Kokkinou V, et al. (2000) Coagulation system and platelets are fully activated in uncomplicated sepsis. Crit Care Med 28: 451–457.
5. Gando S, Nanzaki S, Sasaki S, Aoi K, Kemmotsu O (1998) Activation of the extrinsic coagulation pathway in patients with severe sepsis and septic shock. Crit Care Med 26: 2005–2009.

6. Dempfle C-E (2004) Coagulopathy of sepsis. Thromb Haemost 91: 213–224.

7. Thiolliere F, Serre-Sapin AF, Reignier J, Benedit M, Constantin JM, et al. (2013) Epidemiology and outcome of thrombocytopenic patients in the intensive care unit: results of a prospective multicenter study. Intensive Care Med 39: 1460–1468.

8. Gafter-Gvili A, Mansur N, Bivas A, Zemer-Wassercug N, Bishara J, et al. (2011) Thrombocytopenia in Staphylococcus aureus bacteremia: risk factors and prognostic importance. Mayo Clin Proc 86: 389–396.

9. Caudrillier A, Kessenbrock K, Gilliss BM, Nguyen JX, Marques MB, et al. (2012) Platelets induce neutrophil extracellular traps in transfusion-related acute lung injury. 122: 2661–2671.

10. Sharron M, Hoptay CE, Wiles AA, Garvin LM, Geha M, et al. (2012) Platelets induce apoptosis during sepsis in a contact-dependent manner that is inhibited by GPIIb/IIIa blockade. PLoS One 7: e41549.

11. Aslam R, Speck ER, Kim M, Crow AR, Bang KW, et al. (2006) Platelet Toll-like receptor expression modulates lipopolysaccharide-induced thrombocytopenia and tumor necrosis factor-alpha production in vivo. Blood 107: 637–641.

12. Salat A, Murabito M, Boehm D, Bodingbauer G, Pulaki S, et al. (1999) Endotoxin enhances in vitro platelet aggregability in whole blood. Thromb Res 93: 145–148.

13. Zhang G, Han J, Welch EJ, Ye RD, Voyno-Yasenetskaya TA, et al. (2009) Lipopolysaccharide stimulates platelet secretion and potentiates platelet aggregation via TLR4/MyD88 and the cGMP-dependent protein kinase pathway. J Immunol 182: 7997–8004.

14. Woth G, Varga A, Ghosh S, Krupp M, Kiss T, et al. (2011) Platelet aggregation in severe sepsis. J Thromb Thrombolysis 31: 6–12.

15. Adamzik M, Görlinger K, Peters J, Hartmann M (2012) Whole blood impedance aggregometry as a biomarker for the diagnosis and prognosis of severe sepsis. Crit Care 16: R204.

16. Brenner T, Schmidt K, Delang M, Mehrabi a, Bruckner T, et al. (2012) Viscoelastic and aggregometric point-of-care testing in patients with septic shock – cross-links between inflammation and haemostasis. Acta Anaesthesiol Scand 56: 1277–1290.

17. Würtz M, Hvas AM, Kristensen SD, Grove EL (2012) Platelet aggregation is dependent on platelet count in patients with coronary artery disease. Thromb Res 129: 56–61.

18. Hanke AA, Roberg K, Monaca E, Sellmann T, Weber CF, et al. (2010) Impact of platelet count on results obtained from multiple electrode platelet aggregometry (Multiplate). Eur J Med Res 15: 214–219.

19. Stissing T, Dridi NP, Ostrowski SR, Bochsen L, Johansson PI (2011) The influence of low platelet count on whole blood aggregometry assessed by Multiplate. Clin Appl Thromb Hemost 17: E211–7.

20. Levy MM, Fink MP, Marshall JC, Abraham E, Angus D, et al. (2003) 2001 SCCM/ESICM/ACCP/ATS/SIS International Sepsis Definitions Conference. Crit Care Med 31: 1250–1256.

21. Vincent J, Moreno R, Takala J, Willatts S, de Mendonca A, et al. (1996) The SOFA (Sepsis-related Organ Failure Assessment) score to describe organ dysfunction/failure. Intensive care Med 22: 707–710.

22. Akobeng AK (2007) Understanding diagnostic tests 3: Receiver operating characteristic curves. Acta Paediatr 96: 644–647.

23. Garraud O, Hamzeh-Cognasse H, Pozetto B, Cavaillon JM, Cognasse F (2013) Bench to bedside review: platelets and active immune functions – new clues for immunopathology? Crit Care 17: 236.

24. Henn V, Slupsky JR, Grafe M, Anagnostopoulos I, Forster R, et al. (1998) C40 ligand on activated platelets triggers an inflammatory reaction of endothelial cells. Nature 391: 591–594.

25. Fitzgerald JR, Foster TJ, Cox D (2006) The interactions of bacterial pathogens with platelets. Nat Rev Microbiol 4: 445–457.

26. Ter Avest E, de Jong M, Brümmer I, Wietasch GJ, Ter Maaten JC (2013) Outcome predictors of uncomplicated sepsis. Int J Emerg Med 6: 9.

27. Winning J, Neumann J, Kohl M, Claus RA, Reinhart K, et al. (2010) Antiplatelet drugs and outcome in mixed admissions to an intensive care unit. Crit Care Med 38: 32–37.

28. Winning J, Reichel J, Eisenhut Y, Hamacher J, Kohl M, et al. (2009) Anti-platelet drugs and outcome in severe infection: clinical impact and underlying mechanisms. Platelets 20: 50–57.

29. Baurand A, Eckly A, Bari N, Léon C, Hechler B, et al. (2000) Desensitization of the platelet aggregation response to ADP: differential down-regulation of the P2Y1 and P2cyc receptors. Thromb Haemost 84: 484–491.

30. Lundahl TH, Petersson J, Fagerberg IH, Berg S, Lindahl TL (1998) Impaired platelet function correlates with multi-organ dysfunction. A study of patients with sepsis. Platelets 9: 223–225.

31. Reggiori G, Occhipinti G, De Gasperi A, Vincent J-L, Piagnerelli M (2009) Early alterations of red blood cell rheology in critically ill patients. Crit Care Med 37: 3041–3046.

32. Kempe DS, Akel A, Lang PA, Hermle T, Biswas R, et al. (2007) Suicidal erythrocyte death in sepsis. J Mol Med (Berl) 85: 273–281.

33. Chiarla C, Giovannini I, Giuliante F, Vellone M, Ardito F, et al. (2010) Significance of hemoglobin concentration in determining blood CO2 binding capacity in critical illness. Respir Physiol Neurobiol 172: 32–36.

11

Why Children with Severe Bacterial Infection Die: A Population–Based Study of Determinants and Consequences of Suboptimal Care with a Special Emphasis on Methodological Issues

Elise Launay[1,2*S], **Christèle Gras-Le Guen**[1,3S], **Alain Martinot**[4], **Rémy Assathiany**[5], **Elise Martin**[1], **Thomas Blanchais**[1], **Catherine Deneux-Tharaux**[2], **Jean-Christophe Rozé**[6], **Martin Chalumeau**[2,7]

1 CHU Nantes, Hôpital de la Mère et de l'Enfant, Clinique médicale pédiatrique, Faculté de médecine de Nantes, Nantes, France, 2 Inserm U1153, Obstetrical, Perinatal and Pediatric Epidemiology Research Team, Research Center for Epidemiology and Biostatistics Sorbonne Paris Cité (CRESS), Paris Descartes University, Paris, France, 3 CHU Nantes, Hôpital de la Mère et de l'Enfant, Urgences pédiatriques, Faculté de médecine de Nantes, Nantes, France, 4 CHU de Lille, Hôpital R. Salengro, Unité d'urgences pédiatriques et de maladies infectieuses, Université de Lille-Nord de France, Lille, France, 5 Association pour le Recherche et l'Enseignement en Pédiatrie Générale (AREPEGE); Association Française de Pédiatrie Ambulatoire (AFPA), Cabinet de Pédiatrie, Issy-les-Moulineaux, France, 6 CHU Nantes, Hôpital de la Mère et de l'Enfant, Réanimation pédiatrique et néonatale, Faculté de médecine de Nantes, Nantes, France, 7 Hôpital Necker Enfants Malades, AP-HP, Service de pédiatrie générale, Paris Descartes University, Paris, France

Abstract

Introduction: Suboptimal care is frequent in the management of severe bacterial infection. We aimed to evaluate the consequences of suboptimal care in the early management of severe bacterial infection in children and study the determinants.

Methods: A previously reported population-based confidential enquiry included all children (3 months- 16 years) who died of severe bacterial infection in a French area during a 7-year period. Here, we compared the optimality of the management of these cases to that of pediatric patients who survived a severe bacterial infection during the same period for 6 types of care: seeking medical care by parents, evaluation of sepsis signs and detection of severe disease by a physician, timing and dosage of antibiotic therapy, and timing and dosage of saline bolus. Two independent experts blinded to outcome and final diagnosis evaluated the optimality of these care types. The effect of suboptimal care on survival was analyzed by a logistic regression adjusted on confounding factors identified by a causal diagram. Determinants of suboptimal care were analyzed by multivariate multilevel logistic regression.

Results: Suboptimal care was significantly more frequent during early management of the 21 children who died as compared with the 93 survivors: 24% vs 13% (p = 0.003). The most frequent suboptimal care types were delay to seek medical care (20%), under-evaluation of severity by the physician (20%) and delayed antibiotic therapy (24%). Young age (under 1 year) was independently associated with higher risk of suboptimal care, whereas being under the care of a paediatric emergency specialist or a mobile medical unit as compared with a general practitioner was associated with reduced risk.

Conclusions: Suboptimal care in the early management of severe bacterial infection had a global independent negative effect on survival. Suboptimal care may be avoided by better training of primary care physicians in the specifics of pediatric medicine.

Editor: Susanna Esposito, Fondazione IRCCS Ca' Granda Ospedale Maggiore Policlinico, Università degli Studi di Milano, Italy

Funding: The authors received no specific funding for this work. Inserm Unit 1153 received a grant from the Bettencourt Foundation (Coups d'élan pour la recherche française) in support of its research activities. The funders had no role in study design, data collection and analysis, decision to publish, or preparation of the manuscript.

Competing Interests: The authors have declared that no competing interests exist.

* Email: elise.launay@chu-nantes.fr

S These authors contributed equally to this work.

Introduction

Bacterial infection remains a major cause of childhood mortality in industrialised countries. [1] In 2009, Harndern et al. reviewed pediatric deaths in 5 regions of the United Kingdom and found that among the 15% of deaths related to infection, failure to recognise and manage severe bacterial infection (SBI) was the most common avoidable primary care factor. [2] In 2010, we published a population-based study evaluating optimality of care for 21 children who died due to SBI: the initial medical management was suboptimal in 76% of cases, with a delay in seeking medical care in 33%. [3] These alarming frequencies in suboptimal initial care in pediatric patients with SBI do not allow for drawing conclusions on the relationship between suboptimal care and outcomes because both studies focused on patients who died.

The consequences of suboptimal care in pediatric patients with SBI have been examined in 4 studies. [4,5,6,7] All found clinically meaningful and statistically significant associations between suboptimal care and morbidity and mortality. [4,5,6,7] However, the results were limited by methodological concerns such as selection bias related to hospital-based recruitment, [6] classification bias related to arbitrary definition of diagnosis delay as consultation more than once before hospitalisation, [5] non-independent evaluation of the optimality of care, [7] non-justified use of continuous variables in multivariable models, [4,5,7] and/or selection of non-appropriate variables for adjustment (without using a causal diagram that could help deal with co-variables that could be confounders or intermediate variables). [8,9] No study examined the determinants of this suboptimal care to inform corrective actions for parents and healthcare workers.

The aim of the present study was to evaluate the determinants and consequences of suboptimal care in the initial management of SBI in children, using appropriate methodological approaches, to evaluate the relevance of future targeted corrective actions for parents and healthcare workers.

Methods

General methodology

The present study is an extension of a previously published population-based confidential enquiry into the quality of initial care in children age from 3 months to 16 years who died of SBI from January 2000 to March 2006 in a geographic zone of France comprising two adjoining administrative districts. [3] The definition of SBI (bacterial infection leading to admission to the pediatric intensive care unit [PICU]), the strategy of identification of cases, and the assessment of exhaustiveness were described in detail in the previous publication. Pediatric care in this area was provided by one university hospital center (in Nantes), four general hospitals, pediatricians in private practice, general practitioners (GPs), and two call centers for medical emergencies that could send emergency mobile medical teams (including physicians specialized in emergency medicine) to the patient's home. For the present study, we defined a control group of pediatric patients who survived a SBI during the same period and in the same geographic region. The organization of care called for all children older than 3 months and requiring hospitalization for SBI to be transferred to the PICU of the Nantes university hospital. Thus, controls were all pediatric patients hospitalised for SBI in the PICU of the hospital during the study period. Controls were identified by discharge codes and the microbiology laboratory electronic files as described previously. [3] The initial research was approved by Institutional Review Committee (Comité de Protection des Personnes Ile de France III) and this extension was

approved by the ethics committee of the Nantes university hospital (Groupe Nantais d'Ethique dans le Domaine de la Santé), which approved a waiver of the need for consent. The results were reported according to the STROBE checklist for reporting observational studies. [10]

Data were collected as previously described from the complete patient medical file: a pre-established template reconstructed the timed and dated medical observations with blinding to final diagnosis or outcome. [3] Children whose files were too incomplete to trace the clinical history with sufficient precision were identified and excluded.

Optimality of care evaluation

Two experts (an experienced pediatrician in private practice and a pediatric intensive care specialist who supervises a pediatric emergency department), blinded to final diagnosis and outcome, independently determined the suboptimal character of the initial management as described previously. [3] These two experts were not involved in the management of any included children. Experts had to justify their final conclusion by giving details on the optimality (optimal or not optimal) of each care in terms of specific criteria selected from national and international clinical practice guidelines applicable during the study period: [11,12,13] the timing of administration of antibiotics for meningococcemia (immediate in case of extensive purpura) and the modality of administration of hemodynamic support in septic shock (bolus up to 40 mL/kg in the first hour). As in the study by Nadel et al., [6] which evaluated suboptimal care for meningococcal disease, we defined delay in seeking medical care by parents as the absence of immediate consultation in cases of fever with a purpuric rash or accompanied by other signs of severity: cyanosis, moaning, convulsions, confusion, impairment of higher functions, intense headaches, intense muscle or articular pain, marked asthenia, persistent vomiting, or cold hands or feet. We also arbitrarily considered the failure to seek medical care when a high fever lasted more than 48 hr as a delay in seeking medical care. For each child, we were then able to evaluate the optimality of 6 different key types of care: 1) seeking medical care by parents; 2) evaluation of sepsis signs and detection of severe disease by a physician, 3) timing of antibiotic therapy, 4) dosage of antibiotic therapy, 5) timing of saline bolus, and 6) dosage of saline bolus.

Analyses

We described the children studied, their demographic characteristics, and their final diagnoses, especially bacteriologic. We analyzed signs of severe disease: signs of sepsis (tachycardia, bradycardia, and tachypnea), [14] presence of tonus disorders, impaired vigilance, respiratory distress, moaning, or other signs of potential SBI, such as meningism or extensive purpura. We described the sequence of care of children (first medical contact and number of consultations before hospitalization).

We assessed the degree of agreement between the two experts for each type of care by calculating the κappa coefficient interpreted with the Landis and Koch scale. [15] In cases of disagreement, the optimal nature of the care was determined by a third expert. We analyzed the 6 categories of suboptimal care by outcome and physicians' qualification. We also analyzed risk factors for death (relation between suboptimal care and death) and determinants of suboptimal medical care (excluding seeking medical care).

We analyzed the crude and adjusted association between number of suboptimal care and death. The number of suboptimal care was the sum of the 6 above-mentioned types for each child and thus ranged from 0 to 6. To identify confounding variables,

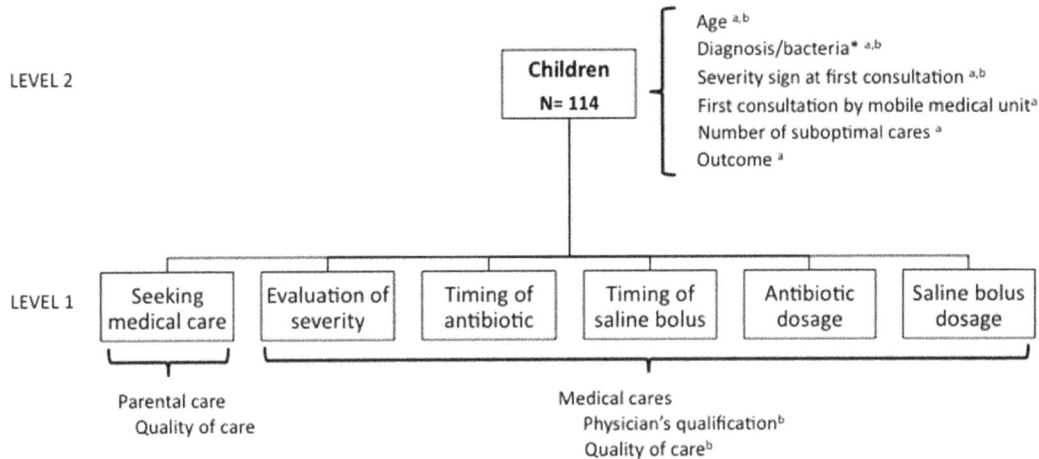

Figure 1. Structure of data. a = co-variables used in the study of the consequences of suboptimal care. b = co-variables used in the study of the determinants of medical sub-optimal care.

we built a theorical causal diagram between optimality of care and outcome (dead/alive at discharge from hospital) based on the published pathophysiological concepts of severe sepsis (Figure S1) and adapted from this a "realistic" causal diagram between optimality of initial care (before admission to a PICU) and outcome considering the available data and using DAGitty software (Figure S2). [16,17] Clinical phenotype was defined by diagnosis (meningitis versus other diagnosis) and two other variables reflecting the measurable intrinsic severity of the disease: presence of severity sign at the first consultation and first consultation by a mobile medical unit (this unit is reserved for patients with the most severe condition in France). Covariables tested on univariate analysis were age of children, diagnosis, sign of severe disease at the first consultation, and first consultation by a mobile medical unit (Figure 1). Relevant variables according to the causal diagram were included in multivariate analyses.

To evaluate the determinants of the quality of initial medical care, we considered each of the 5 medical care types by children. We used a hierarchical regression model that took into account the hierarchical structure of the data (i.e., non-independence of the variables for the 5 care types), and allowed us to include characteristics of care at the care level (level 1; i.e., quality of each care [optimal/suboptimal] and qualification of physician giving the care) and characteristics of the children at the level of the child (level 2; i.e., age of children, diagnosis, and presence of signs of severe disease at first consultation [Figure 1]). We included variables considered associated with suboptimal care (Figure S2). First, we estimated a random intercept model without any variable ("empty" model) to obtain the baseline children-level variance and to test the effect of children. Then, we included care and children characteristics and estimated the association of these variables and quality of care. We calculated the proportion of the model's variance explained by level 1 and level 2 variables defined as (variance of the model with level 1 variables – variance of the empty model)/variance of empty model and (variance of the model with level 1 and level 2 variables – variance of the empty model)/variance of empty model, respectively. Quantitative variables were tested for linearity and transformed into polynomials of the smallest degree when deviation was observed. Analyses involved use of Stata 11 (StataCorp, College Station, TX, USA).

Results

Patients and care pathway

In total, 119 patients were eligible; five (4%) were excluded because of incomplete charts, for 114 patients analysed (Figure S3). Overall, 21 children died (18%, 95% confidence interval [95% CI] 11–25) before PICU admission (n = 1) or PICU discharge (n = 20), and 93 survived. The clinical characteristics of the 21 children who died were described elsewhere. [3] The median age of the 114 included children was 2.4 years [interquartile range 0.7–6.7 years], the sex ratio was 1.3 (M/F) and one half had known serious medical conditions at the time of diagnosis (Table 1). More than a half of the children (63%) presented signs of severe disease at the first medical contact. Meningitis was the most frequent diagnosis (57%), followed by purpura fulminans (35%). Meningococcus was found in 47% of cases. The first medical contact was a GP in 66% of cases, an emergency physician in 25%, and a mobile medical unit in 9%; 60% of children were hospitalized after this first medical contact. Children whose first medical contact was the mobile medical unit were more likely to have severity signs at this first medical contact (100% versus 60%, p = 0.01).

Optimality of care

Agreement between experts was "moderate" for evaluation of the optimality of the delay to seek medical care and for saline bolus dosage, with a κ coefficient of 0.40±0.06 and 0.46±0.09, respectively (p<0.001). Agreement with the optimality of the 4 other medical care types (severity evaluation, antibiotic therapy timing and dosage, and saline bolus timing) was "substantial" or "almost perfect," with κ 0.78±0.09; 0.78±0.09; 0.67±0.09 and 0.88±0.09, respectively (p<0.001). Overall, 52% of children received at least one care type evaluated as suboptimal, and 25% received two or more suboptimal care types (Table 1). Among the 684 individual care types delivered, 104 (15%, 95% CI 12–18%) were suboptimal. Parental delay in seeking medical care and physician underestimation of severity and delayed antibiotic administration accounted for 70% of this suboptimal care (22%, 22% and 26%, respectively). The frequency of suboptimal care in the initial management did not significantly decrease over the years (19% to 15% from 2000 to 2005; p for trend>0.8) nor did the frequency of each type of care (p>0.2).

Table 1. Patient characteristics and care pathways before admission to a pediatric intensive care unit, quality of care and their association with outcome by dead and alive children and univariate and multivariate analysis.

	Total n = 114 (%)	Dead n = 21 (%)	Alive n = 93 (%)	Univariate analysis			Multivariate analysis[§]		
				OR	95% CI	p	aOR	95% CI	p
PATIENTS									
Age, yr									
Median[a] [IQR]	2.4 [0.7–6.7]	2.0 [0.9–2.8]	2.9 [0.7–7.1]	0.85	0.73–1.0	0.057	0.82	0.68–0.99	0.04
<1 yr	32 (28)	7 (33)	25 (27)						
1 to 2 yr	21 (18)	4 (19)	17 (18)			0.01			
2 to 5 yr	27 (24)	9 (43)	18 (19)						
≥5 yr	34 (30)	1 (5)	33 (36)						
Sex ratio M/F	1.28	1.33	1.27			0.92			
Underlying medical conditions, n (%)	39 (52)	7 (33)	32 (34)			0.93			
Severity signs at first medical contact[b], n (%)	72 (63)	16 (76)	56 (60)			0.17			
Final diagnosis, n (%)									
Purpura fulminans and others[c]	49 (43)	14 (67)	35 (38)	1	-	-	1	-	-
Meningitis	65 (57)	7 (33)	58 (62)	0.30	0.11–0.85	0.02	0.31	0.10–0.98	0.047
Bacteria involved, n (%)									
Streptococcus pneumoniae	31 (27)	3 (14)	28 (30)						
Neisseria meningitidis	54 (47)	12 (57)	42 (45)						
Other[d]	11 (10)	4 (19)	7 (8)			0.17			
No documentation	18 (16)	2 (10)	16 (17)						
with purpura fulminans	10 (55)	1 (50)	9 (56)						
CARE PATHWAYS									
First medical contact									
GP or emergency physician, n (%)	104 (91)	15 (71)	89 (96)	1	-	-	1	-	-
Mobile medical unit	10 (9)	6 (29)	4 (4)	8.9	2.05–38.6	<0.001	8.72	1.76–43.28	0.008
No of medical contacts, n (%)									
1	68 (60)	15 (71)	53 (57)						
2	37 (32)	6 (29)	31 (33)			0.43			
>2	9 (8)	0	9 (10)						
QUALITY OF CARES									
No. of suboptimal care, by children									
Median [IQR][a]	1 [0–1]	1 [0–2]	0 [0–1]	1.55	1.06–2.26	0.025	1.65	1.07–2.54	0.022
0	55 (48)	7 (33)	48 (52)						
1	31 (27)	5 (24)	26 (28)						
2	17 (15)	5 (24)	12 (13)						

Table 1. Cont.

	Total n=114 [%]	Dead n=21 (%)	Alive n=93 (%)	Univariate analysis			Multivariate analysis[s]		
				OR	95% CI	p	aOR	95% CI	p
3	5 (4)	1 (5)	4 (4)						
4	6 (5)	3 (14)	3 (3)						
No suboptimal care/no care, % [95% CI]	15 [12–18]	24 [16–32]	13 [10–16]			0.003			
Care types									
Parental care, n (%)									
Seeking medical care									
Suboptimal	23 (20)	6 (29)	17 (18)	1.79	0.60–5.34	0.29			
Optimal	91 (80)	15 (71)	76 (82)	1	-	-			
Medical care, n (%)									
Evaluation of severity									
Suboptimal	23 (20)	7 (33)	16 (17)	2.40	0.82–7.03	0.10			
Optimal	91 (80)	14 (67)	77 (83)	1	-	-			
Antibiotic therapy timing									
Suboptimal	27 (24)	5 (24)	22 (24)	1	0.33–3.08	0.98			
Optimal	87 (76)	16 (76)	71 (76)	1	-	-			
Saline bolus timing									
Suboptimal	14 (12)	5 (24)	9 (10)	2.92	0.84–10.1	0.08			
Optimal	100 (88)	16 (76)	84 (90)	1	-	-			
Saline bolus dosage									
Suboptimal	12 (11)	7 (33)	5 (5)	**8.80**	2.23–34.7	0.002			
Optimal	102 (89)	14 (67)	88 (95)	1	-	-			
Antibiotic therapy dosage									
Suboptimal	5 (4)	0 (0)	5 (5)	0.67	0.01–6.03	0.29			
Optimal	109 (96)	21 (100)	88 (95)	1	-	-			

aOR, adjusted odds ratio; 95% CI, 95% confidence interval; IQR, interquartile range.

[s]Logistic regression model.

[a]Age and no. of suboptimal care were treated as continuous variables (no deviation to linearity).

[b]Severity signs were hemodynamic failure, purpura, conscientiousness impairment, respiratory distress, meningism, behavioural changes or hypotonia.

[c]Others were 2 pneumonia with pleural effusion and a septic shock following pyelonephritis in a child with malformative uropathy in the deceased group, and 2 septic shock on bacterial cellulitis and a bacterial tracheitis in the survivor group.

[d]Others were, for survivors, *Haemophilus influenzae* (n = 3), Group B *Streptococcus* (n = 1), *Staphylococcus aureus* (n = 1), and for deceased children, *E.coli* (n = 1), Group A *Streptococcus* (n = 1), *Salmonella spp* (n = 1) and *Mycoplama pneumoniae* (n = 1).

Table 2. Risk factors for medical suboptimal care.

	Optimal n = 489 (%)	Suboptimal n = 81 (%)	Univariate analysis			Multivariate analysis *,**		
			OR	95% CI	p	aOR	95% CI	p
Age								
<1 yr	125 (26)	35 (43)	1			1		
1–2	95 (19)	10 (12)	0.38	0.18–0.81	0.009	0.32	0.11–0.98	0.046
2–5 yr	119 (24)	16 (20)	0.48	0.25–0.92	0.02	0.37	0.14–0.98	0.045
≥5 yr	150 (31)	20 (25)	0.48	0.26–0.87	0.01	0.24	0.09–0.64	0.004
Physician qualification, n (%)								
General practitioner	55 (11)	27 (33)	1			1		
Adult emergency	16 (3)	7 (9)	0.90	0.33–2.44	0.82	0.63	0.15–2.62	0.53
Pediatric emergency	322 (66)	37 (46)	0.23	0.13–0.42	<0.001	0.16	0.08–0.35	<0.001
Mobile medical unit	83 (17)	6 (7)	0.15	0.05–0.40	<0.001	0.09	0.03–0.31	<0.001
Pediatric ward	13 (3)	4 (5)	0.63	0.18–2.13	0.45	0.65	0.11–3.67	0.63
Severity signs at first consultation, n (%)								
No	182 (87)	28 (13)	1			1		
Yes	307 (85)	53(15)	1.12	0.68–1.84	0.6	1.3	0.59–2.90	0.51
Final diagnosis, n (%)								
Other	210 (86)	35 (14)	1			1		
Meningitis	279 (86)	46 (14)	0.99	0.62–1.59	0.9	0.73	0.34–1.59	0.43

*Multivariate analysis involved a hierarchical logistic regression model with random intercept and effects.

**Significant associations remained when age was transformed into polynomials (X = 10/[age − 2.5]), aOR for age 1.04, 95% CI 1.01–1.07, p = 0.003.

Factors associated with outcome

As compared with children who died, survivors were more frequently older than 5 years (p<0.05; Table 1) and diagnosed as having meningitis (62% vs 33%). The two groups did not differ in other demographic, clinical or bacteriologic characteristics or total number of medical contacts before admission to the ICU (p>0.1, Table 1). For children who died, the first medical contact was frequently a mobile medical unit (vs GP office or hospital emergency department): 29% vs 4% (p<0.001). The proportion of suboptimal care among all care types during the initial management was higher for children who died than survived: 24% vs 13% (95% CI of the risk difference: 9–13%). On univariate analysis, insufficient saline bolus was significantly associated with death (OR = 8.8; 95% CI: 2.23–34.7), under-evaluation of severity and delay to administer saline bolus was associated but not significantly with death (OR = 2.74; 95% CI: 0.82–7.03 and 2.92; 95% CI: 0.84–10.1 respectively) (Table 1).

After adjustment for confounders, each suboptimal care (continuous variable, no deviance to linearity) increased the odds of death by 65% (adjusted odds ratio [aOR] 1.65, 95% CI 1.08–2.54, p = 0.02) (Table 1). Each year of age (continuous variable, no deviation to linearity) decreased the odds of death (aOR 0.82, 95% CI 0.68–0.99, p = 0.04), as did having meningitis as compared with other diagnoses (aOR 0.31, 95% CI 0.10–0.98, p = 0.047). A first medical contact by the mobile medical unit was associated with an adverse outcome (aOR 8.72, 95% CI 1.76–43.28, p = 0.008) (Table 1).

Determinants of optimality of medical care

Among the 570 cares received by children during their initial management (Table 2), the repartition of suboptimal care differed by physician qualification. The proportion of suboptimal care was 33% for those provided by a GP, 30% for those in adult emergency settings, 24% for those in pediatric wards, 10% for those in pediatric emergency care and 7% for those in the mobile medical unit (p<0.001). The proportion of under-evaluation of severity was 30% for a GP, 9% for pediatric emergency care and 0% for the mobile medical unit (p = 0.001). The proportion of delayed antibiotic therapy was 50% for a GP, 20% for pediatric emergency care and 0% for the mobile medical unit (p = 0.02). The other types of care (antibiotic therapy dosage and timing and dosage of saline bolus) did not differ by physician qualification.

On univariate analysis, younger children (<1 year) were at increased risk of suboptimal care (see Table 2), and odds of suboptimal care were lower with pediatric emergency or mobile medical unit care than GP care (OR 0.23, 95% CI 0.13–0.42; and OR 0.15, 95% CI 0.05–0.40, respectively) (Table 2). We found no association between final diagnosis or presence of severity sign at first medical contact and quality of care. The optimality of care varied significantly between children (i.e., children effect, empty model, p<0.001). After adjustment in a multilevel multivariate model, the association between optimality of care and age of children (dichotomised in 4 classes or transformed in polynomials) and physician qualification remained stable (Table 2). The variance of the empty model was 1.56, that of the model with a level 1 variable (physician qualification) was 1.54 and that of the full model (level 1 and 2 variables) was 1.21. Level 1 variables explained 2% of the variance, whereas level 1 and 2 variables explained 21% of the variance.

Discussion

We found a strong association of suboptimal medical care and death for children with an SBI: each suboptimal care increased the odds of death by 65%. Some types of care, particularly the dosage of saline bolus, were associated more with death than others. The gold standard to demonstrate causality in medical research is a controlled double blind randomised trial, but such studies are obviously not ethical in the case of SBI. Observational study analysis of causal association requires being aware of the risk of bias. [18] Here, we studied the determinants and consequences of suboptimal care in the early management of SBI in pediatric patients using an adequate approach to deal with the structure and type of data, including multilevel analysis and fractional polynomials [19,20,21] while minimizing the selection bias for children who died by using a population recruitment pattern with exhaustivity checking. As recommended by methodological standards, [22] suboptimality of care was evaluated by two independent experts who were blinded to the final diagnosis and outcome, with an overall high level of agreement between experts.

The strength of the significant association between suboptimal care and death remained nearly unchanged after adjustment for potential confounders: age of children, final diagnosis and initial severity of disease (represented as having a first medical contact by a mobile medical unit). However, some variables were inaccurately measured and/or some explanatory variables were lacking in the model. Indeed, we show a gap between the number of variables in the theoretical causal diagram and the one used (Figure S1 and Figure S2). For example, we could have explained more accurately the risk of death by considering genetic susceptibility to infection or bacterial virulence. [23,24] We were also limited in the evaluation of initial severity of the infection because of the retrospective design of the study. First medical contact by a mobile medical unit is an objective and reliable evaluation of clinical severity because in France, the mobile medical unit aims to care for children with the most severe disease who could not be transported to the hospital before receiving emergency care. Nevertheless, the presence of a severity sign at the first medical examination is a more arguable reflection of intrinsic severity because of the retrospective design of the study. For example, data on vital signs at the first medical contact, which are a key point to evaluate clinical severity in children in the context of SBI, [25] were sometimes missing, which led to inaccurate evaluation of severity of the disease for statistical analysis and also difficulty for the expert to accurately assess the optimality of the severity evaluation. Experts evaluated only misinterpretation of vital signs when they were mentioned. Here, we demonstrated the significant and independent global effect of suboptimal care on outcome, but we cannot affirm that suboptimal care in the early management was directly responsible for death because suboptimal care in the PICU was not assessed. Moreover, we analyzed only six types of care for each management and not all types. We could not examine the time effect and the total number of care. The total number of care could be the result of intrinsic severity (severely ill children requiring more care and sometimes showing a fulminant evolution) or the result of previous suboptimal care (inadequate care could lead to worsened disease, which then requires more care). The time effect could have been considered in a marginal structural model (Figure S1), but such a model requires timely detailed information that cannot be obtained with a retrospective study. [26]

We did not include children with SBI who survived but were not hospitalized in a PICU. It could be argued that we over-evaluated the frequency of suboptimal care because children with SBI admitted to a PICU may have received more suboptimal care, which caused clinical worsening and then admission to a PICU as compared with children who received adequate care and would not have required admission to a PICU. Thus, this selection bias could have led to an under-evaluation of the association of suboptimal care and death because these children not hospitalized in a PICU and having received potentially more optimal care would most probably have survived.

The generalization of our results may be limited because the bacterial epidemiology may have changed since the study period. In France, conjugate vaccines against *Haemophilus influenzae, Neisseria meningitidis C and Streptococcus pneumoniae* with 7 and 13 valences were routinely recommended for all children by health authorities in 1992, 2009, 2002 and 2009, respectively. Invasive infection due to *H. influenzae* had almost disappeared during the study period. Reported cases of invasive pneumococcal infection decreased after vaccination introduction for only children younger than 2 years old. Incidences were 29 per 100 000 in 2001, 25 per 100 000 in 2004 and 18 per 100 000 in 2012 (meningitis and bacteremia). No significant changes were observed for older children. [27] Vaccine against meningococcus C had a too low coverage in the pediatric population to evidence a decrease in invasive infection due to *N. meningitidis* C since study period. [28] Thus, since the study period, the pattern of SBI may have changed for invasive pneumococcal infection in children less than 2 years old.

We did not observe a significant decrease in suboptimality of care across the years even though French recommendations concerning immediate administration of antibiotic therapy with purpura fuminans were largely diffused in 2000 and the Surviving Sepsis campaign began in 2003. [29,30] This finding highlights that simple diffusion of written recommendations are not enough to quickly modify practices of a large healthcare professional public. [31]

The analysis of suboptimal care determinants allowed us to identify potential targets for corrective actions. Young age (<1 year) was independently associated with increased risk of suboptimal care, whereas being under the care of a paediatric emergency specialist or a mobile medical unit physician was associated with reduced risk. Similar conclusions were reached by Dhamar *et al.* in a retrospective review of the quality of care received by 304 children with serious illnesses receiving treatment in 5 emergency departments in California between 2000 and 2003: after adjustment for confounding factors with a hierarchical model, younger children were at increased risk of receiving suboptimal care, and quality of care was better when provided by pediatric emergency physicians as compared with a GP. [32] Young age of children also appeared to be a barrier to optimal management of critical illness in community hospitals according to a qualitative study. [33] Corrective actions should then target the GP, in training and established, and focus on clinical evaluation of the youngest children.

Seeking medical care was considered delayed in 20% of our cases and accounted for 22% of the suboptimal care. We could not study the determinants of this delay, but French parents were previously found to poorly recognise purpuric rash. [34] Nevertheless, methods to recognize purpuric rash are warranted for not missing severe bacterial infections. [35] Parents worrying about their child's health has also been identified as a good marker of severe infection, although this sign is often missing, even with severe infection. [36] The better understanding of why parents are worried or not could be helpful to optimize early detection of sepsis.

Conclusions

Thanks to an adequate strategy for data analysis, we showed a significant association of suboptimal care for children with SBI and death. We identified determinants that could be acted on to optimize early management of SBI in children and then hopefully reduce the incidence of death. Physicians who are in charge of febrile children should pay particular attention to children younger than 1 year and systematically evaluate vital signs (pulse, respiratory rate, consciousness, capillary refill) that allow for early recognition of severe sepsis. Physicians and parents could be warned via widely distributed flyers or even television, as has been efficient in United Kindom by the meningitis research foundation. [37] Physicians who rarely experience vital emergency situations could also benefit from a simulated training program. [38]

Supporting Information

Figure S1 Theoretical causal diagrams between optimality of care and death reflecting time-dependance of exposure and confounding factors. a: summarized diagram with C representing confounding factors; E, exposition (optimality of care); F, risk factors for exposition (determinants of optimality); and Y, outcome (survival status). b: more complete diagram with H representing host factors (age, genetic and non-genetic susceptibility to infection); B, bacterial factors (type of infection, bacterial specie/serotype, virulence, inoculum); O, optimality of care; S, clinical severity; P, physician characteristics (qualification, clinical experience etc.); Pa, parent characteristics (educational/socioeconomic status, facility of access to health care systems etc.). Indices represent different time points (from 0 to k) (Inspired by Robins et al, Epidemiology, September 2000, Vol. 11 No. 5).

Figure S2 "Realistic" causal diagram between optimality of care before admission to a pediatric intensive care unit (PICU) and death. This diagram was established with DAGitty considering available variables. [16] The green circle with triangle inside represents exposure; blue circle with stick inside, outcome; green circles, exposure ancestors; pink circles, confounding factors; pink vectors, biasing pathway; green vectors, causal pathways; grey vectors, ancestor pathway. Clinical phenotype was represented by final diagnosis, severity signs at the first medical contact and first medical contact by a medical mobile unit.

Figure S3 Study flowchart.

Acknowledgments

This article is dedicated to the memory of Ms Albertine Aouba, MD, CépiDc-Inserm, Centre d'épidémiologie sur les causes médicales de décès, Le Vésinet, France.

Author Contributions

Conceived and designed the experiments: EL CGL CDT JCR MC. Performed the experiments: AM RA. Analyzed the data: EL CGL EM TB MC. Contributed reagents/materials/analysis tools: EL CGL MC. Contributed to the writing of the manuscript: EL MC. Critical revision of the manuscript for important intellectual concept: CGL AM RA CDT JCR.

References

1. Hartman ME, Linde-Zwirble WT, Angus DC, Watson RS (2013) Trends in the epidemiology of pediatric severe sepsis. Pediatr Crit Care Med 14: 686–693.
2. Harndern A, Mayon-White R, Mant D, Kelly D, Pearson G (2009) Child deaths: confidential enquiry into the role and quality of UK primary care. Br J Gen Pract 59: 819–824.
3. Launay E, Gras-Le Guen C, Martinot A, Assathiany R, Blanchais T, et al. (2010) Suboptimal care in the initial management of children who died from severe bacterial infection: a population-based confidential inquiry. Pediatr Crit Care Med 11: 469–474.
4. Han YY, Carcillo JA, Dragotta MA, Bills DM, Watson RS, et al. (2003) Early reversal of pediatric-neonatal septic shock by community physicians is associated with improved outcome. Pediatrics 112: 793–799.
5. McIntyre PB, Macintyre CR, Gilmour R, Wang H (2005) A population based study of the impact of corticosteroid therapy and delayed diagnosis on the outcome of childhood pneumococcal meningitis. Arch Dis Child 90: 391–396.
6. Nadel S, Britto J, Booy R, Maconochie I, Habibi P, et al. (1998) Avoidable deficiencies in the delivery of health care to children with meningococcal disease. J Accid Emerg Med 15: 298–303.
7. Ninis N, Phillips C, Bailey L, Pollock JI, Nadel S, et al. (2005) The role of healthcare delivery in the outcome of meningococcal disease in children: case-control study of fatal and non-fatal cases. BMJ 330: 1475.
8. Hernan MA, Cole SR (2009) Invited Commentary: Causal diagrams and measurement bias. Am J Epidemiol 170: 959–962; discussion 963–954.
9. Ahrens KA, Schisterman EF (2013) A time and place for causal inference methods in perinatal and paediatric epidemiology. Paediatr Perinat Epidemiol 27: 258–262.
10. von Elm E, Altman DG, Egger M, Pocock SJ, Gotzsche PC, et al. (2008) The Strengthening the Reporting of Observational Studies in Epidemiology (STROBE) statement: guidelines for reporting observational studies. J Clin Epidemiol 61: 344–349.
11. Conseil supérieur d'hygiène publique Opinion from the French High Committee on Public Health, Mars 10, 2000. Available: http://www.sante.gouv.fr/htm/dossiers/cshpf/a_mt_100300_meningite_01.htm. Accessed 2007 Dec 22.
12. Health Protection Agency (2006) Guidance for public health management of meningococcal disease in the UK. Health Protection Agency Meningococcus Forum.
13. Société de Réanimation de Langue Française Use of catecholamines during septic shock (adults and children). XV consensus conference of the French Society of Intensive cares 1996. Available: http://www.sfar.org/article/33/utilisation-des-catecholamines-au-cours-du-choc-septique-adultes-enfants-cc-1996. Accessed 2014 Jan 8.
14. Goldstein B, Giroir B, Randolph A (2005) International pediatric sepsis consensus conference: definitions for sepsis and organ dysfunction in pediatrics. Pediatr Crit Care Med 6: 2–8.
15. Landis JR, Koch GG (1977) The measurement of observer agreement for categorical data. Biometrics 33: 159–174.
16. Textor J, Hardt J, Knuppel S (2011) DAGitty: a graphical tool for analyzing causal diagrams. Epidemiology 22: 745.
17. Angus DC, van der Poll T (2013) Severe sepsis and Septic Shock. N Engl J Med 369: 840–851.
18. Launay E, Morfouace M, Deneux-Tharaux C, Gras le-Guen C, Ravaud P, et al. (2013) Quality of reporting of studies evaluating time to diagnosis: a systematic review in paediatrics. Arch Dis Child doi:101136.
19. Altman DG, Royston P (2006) The cost of dichotomising continuous variable. BMJ 332: 1080.
20. Ambler G, Royston P (2001) Fractional polynomial model selection procedures: investigation of type i error rate. J Statist Comput Simul 69: 89–108.
21. Snijders T, Bosker R (1999) Multilevel analysis: An introduction to basic and advanced multilevel modeling: London: Sage Publications Ltd.
22. Bouvier-Colle MH (2002) Confidential enquiries and medical expert committees: a method for evaluating healthcare. The case of Obstetrics. Rev Epidemiol Sante Publique 50: 203–217.
23. Casanova JL, Abel L (2007) Human genetics of infectious diseases: a unified theory. EMBO J 26: 915–922.
24. Thompson M (1996) Bacterial Pathogenesis. In: Baron S, editor. Medical Microbiology 4th edition. 2011/03/18 ed.
25. Thompson M, Mayon-White R, Harnden A, Perera R, McLeod D, et al. (2008) Using vital signs to assess children with acute infections: a survey of current practice. Br J Gen Pract 58: 236–241.
26. Robins JM, Hernan MA, Brumback B (2000) Marginal Structural Models and Causal Inference in Epidemiology. Epidemiology 11: 550–560.
27. Varon E, Janoir C, Gutmann L (2012) Centre national de référence du pneumocoque. Rapport d'activités 2013. Available: http://www.cnr-pneumo.fr/docs/rapports/CNRP2013.pdf. Accessed 2014 July 22.
28. Stahl J, Cohen R, Denis F, Gaudelus J, Lery T, et al. (2013) Vaccination against meningococcus C. Vaccinal coverage in the French target population. Med Mal Infect 43: 75–80.
29. Ministère des affaires sociales et de la santé Aide mémoire sur les infections invasives à méningocoque. Available: http://www.sante.gouv.fr/IMG/pdf/Annexe_-_Fiche_aide_memoire_sur_les_infections_invasives_a_meningocoques.pdf. Accessed 2014 Jan 8.
30. Slade E, Tamber PS, Vincent JL (2003) The Surviving Sepsis Campaign: raising awareness to reduce mortality. Crit Care 7: 1–2.
31. Giguere A, Legare F, Grimshaw J, Turcotte S, Fiander M, et al. (2012) Printed educational materials: effects on professional practice and healthcare outcomes. Cochrane Database Syst Rev 10: CD004398.
32. Dharmar M, Marcin JP, Romano PS, Andrada ER, Overly F, et al. (2008) Quality of care of children in the emergency department: association with hospital setting and physician training. J Pediatr 153: 783–789.
33. Gilleland J, McGugan J, Brooks S, Dobbins M, Ploeg J (2013) Caring for critically ill children in the community: a needs assessment. BMJ Qual Saf.
34. Aurel M, Dubos F, Motte B, Pruvost I, Leclerc F, et al. (2011) Recognising haemorrhagic rash in children with fever: a survey of parents' knowledge. Arch Dis Child 96: 697–698.
35. Mant D, Van den Bruel A (2011) Should we promote the tumbler test? Arch Dis Child 96: 613–614.
36. Van den Bruel A, Haj-Hassan T, Thompson M, Buntinx F, Mant D (2010) Diagnostic value of clinical features at presentation to identify serious infection in children in developed countries: a systematic review. Lancet 375: 834–845.
37. Meningitis Research Fondation Meningitis research fondation's website. Available: http://www.meningitis.org. Accessed 2014 July 22.
38. Katznelson J, Mills W, Forsythe C, Shaikh S, Tolleson-Rinehart S (2014) Project CAPE: a high-fidelity, in situ simulation program to increase critical access hospital emergency department provider comfort with seriously ill pediatric patients. Pediatr Emerg Care 30: 397–402.

12

Peri-Operative Morbidity Associated with Radical Cystectomy in a Multicenter Database of Community and Academic Hospitals

Luke T. Lavallée[1,2], David Schramm[2,3], Kelsey Witiuk[2], Ranjeeta Mallick[2], Dean Fergusson[2], Christopher Morash[1], Ilias Cagiannos[1], Rodney H. Breau[1,2]*

1 Division of Urology, Department of Surgery, The Ottawa Hospital, University of Ottawa, Ottawa, Ontario, Canada, 2 Clinical Epidemiology Program, Ottawa Hospital Research Institute, Ottawa, Ontario, Canada, 3 Department of Otolaryngology, The Ottawa Hospital, University of Ottawa, Ottawa, Ontario, Canada

Abstract

Objective: To characterize the frequency and timing of complications following radical cystectomy in a cohort of patients treated at community and academic hospitals.

Patients and Methods: Radical cystectomy patients captured from NSQIP hospitals from January 1 2006 to December 31 2012 were included. Baseline information and complications were abstracted by study surgical clinical reviewers through a validated process of medical record review and direct patient contact. We determined the incidence and timing of each complication and calculated their associations with patient and operative characteristics.

Results: 2303 radical cystectomy patients met inclusion criteria. 1115 (48%) patients were over 70 years old and 1819 (79%) were male. Median hospital stay was 8 days (IQR 7–13 days). 1273 (55.3%) patients experienced at least 1 post-operative complication of which 191 (15.6%) occurred after hospital discharge. The most common complication was blood transfusion (n = 875; 38.0%), followed by infectious complications with 218 (9.5%) urinary tract infections, 193 (8.4%) surgical site infections, and 223 (9.7%) sepsis events. 73 (3.2%) patients had fascial dehiscence, 82 (4.0%) developed a deep vein thrombosis, and 67 (2.9%) died. Factors independently associated with the occurrence of any post-operative complication included: age, female gender, ASA class, pre-operative sepsis, COPD, low serum albumin concentration, pre-operative radiotherapy, pre-operative transfusion >4 units, and operative time >6 hours (all p<0.05).

Conclusion: Complications remain common following radical cystectomy and a considerable proportion occur after discharge from hospital. This study identifies risk factors for complications and quality improvement needs.

Editor: Peter C. Black, University of British Columbia, Canada

Funding: The authors received no specific funding for this work.

Competing Interests: The authors have declared that no competing interests exist.

* Email: rbreau@toh.on.ca

Introduction

Bladder cancer is the ninth most common cancer worldwide and represents a significant disease burden with an estimated 72,570 new cases and 15,210 attributed deaths in the United States alone in 2013 [1,2]. Management of patients with muscle invasive bladder cancer remains challenging since the standard treatment involves removal of the bladder, reproductive organs, pelvic lymph nodes, and creation of a urinary diversion (radical cystectomy) [3]. This extensive resection and reconstruction is associated with considerable peri-operative morbidity to the patient. Common complications of radical cystectomy include significant blood loss, infections, wound complications, venous thrombosis, and metabolic disturbances [4–6].

Historical complication rates may not reflect the contemporary patient experience for several reasons. First, new technology and

surgical tools are available to reduce blood loss and surgical times [7–10]. Second, health care system changes such as pre-operative checklists and hospital care maps have been widely implemented and may improve quality of care and peri-operative outcomes. Finally, surgeon and hospital case volume have been shown to impact radical cystectomy outcomes and a trend toward centralization of radical cystectomy to tertiary care centers has been observed in some regions [11,12]. For these reasons we felt it was important to evaluate contemporary complication rates to verify if progress has been made.

The American College of Surgeons' National Surgical Quality Improvement Program (NSQIP) was initiated to supply feedback to participating hospitals by providing accurate information on patient outcomes within 30 days of surgery [13]. NSQIP provides risk-adjusted surgical outcome measures allowing hospitals to identify targets requiring quality improvement [13]. A previous

Table 1. Baseline patient and surgical characteristics of radical cystectomy cases in NSQIP from 2006–2012.

Variable	n (%)
Age (years)	Mean 67.9 (SD 11.2)
<65	800 (34.7)
65–70	388 (16.9)
70–75	400 (17.4)
>75	715 (31.1)
Race	
White	1911 (84.8)
Other	115 (5.1)
Missing	227 (11.2)
Gender	
Female	482 (20.9)
Male	1819 (79.0)
BMI	Mean 28.4 (SD 5.9)
<25	671 (29.4)
25–<30	836 (36.6)
30–<35	511 (22.4)
≥35	265 (11.6)
ASA class	
1–2	611 (26.5)
3–5	1690 (73.4)
Bleeding disorder	94 (4.1)
Pre-operative weight loss (>10% over 6 months)	77 (3.3)
Pre-operative sepsis	14 (0.6)
Steroid use (chronic)	71 (3.1)
Diabetes	446 (19.4)
Dialysis	16 (0.7)
Disseminated cancer	114 (5.0)
Chemotherapy (≤30 days before surgery)	
Yes	137 (6.0)
Missing	1024 (44.5)
Radiotherapy (≤90 days pre-operatively)	
Yes	11 (0.5)
Missing	1024 (44.5)
Dyspnea	241 (10.5)
Alcohol use (>2 drinks/day)	
Yes	56 (2.4)
Missing	1019 (44.3)
Current smoke	571 (24.8)
Smoking history	
≤50 pack years	852 (37)
>50 pack years	150 (6.5)
Missing	1301 (56.5)
Functional status	
Independent	2230 (96.8)
Dependent	70 (3.0)
Chronic obstructive pulmonary disease (severe)	191 (8.3)
Congestive heart failure (≤30 days pre-operatively)	19 (0.8)
Pre-operative albumin concentration (g/dl)	Mean 3.9 (SD 0.6)
>4.1	488 (21.2)
3.8–4.1	341 (14.8)

Table 1. Cont.

Variable	n (%)
3.5–3.7	261 (11.3)
<3.5	308 (13.4)
Missing	905 (39.3)
Pre-operative creatinine level (mg/dl)	Mean 1.17 (0.7)
≤1.3	1689 (73.3)
>1.3–<2	426 (185)
≥2	113 (4.9)
Missing	75 (3.3)
Emergency cystectomy	9 (0.4)
>4 units RBC transfusion (≤72 hours pre-operatively)	57 (2.48)
Surgical characteristics	
Operative time	
≤6 hours	1364 (59.5)
>6 hours	927 (40.5)
Continent urinary diversion	442 (19.2)

Missing data not shown for variables where <2% of patients had missing data.
BMI = body mass index.
ASA class = American Society of Anesthesiologists' classification.
NSQIP = National Surgical Quality Improvement Program.
RBC = red blood cells.

review of cystectomy patients treated from 1991–2001 at 123 NSQIP hospitals reported a 30% incidence of at least one peri-operative complication [5]. Since 2002, NSQIP has grown considerably and now includes over 500 hospitals.

The objective of this study is to characterize complications following radical cystectomy in a contemporary cohort and explore patient and surgical risk factors for adverse events. We hypothesize that despite advancements in peri-operative care, radical cystectomy continues to be associated with a high rate of peri-operative complications. Study results will inform healthcare professionals, facilitate pre-operative patient counseling, aid decision making by identifying vulnerable patients, and identify the most common complications that can be targeted for prophylactic intervention.

Patients and Methods

Institutional ethics review board approval was obtained from the Ottawa Health Science Network Research Ethics Board. Written informed consent was not obtained as patient information was anonymized and de-identified prior to analysis. De-identified and anonymized data was captured from *Participant Use Data Files* that include patients from hospitals enrolled in The American College of Surgeons' National Surgical Quality Improvement Program (NSQIP) from 2006 to 2012. NSQIP data is derived from academic and community hospitals, predominantly in North America, and provides highly accurate information including patient demographics, pre-operative comorbidities, and complications within 30 days of surgery. A combination of automated data collection and trained surgical clinical reviewers capture and extract data at each hospital site [13]. Information on outcome is strictly defined and confirmed through medical record reviews and, if necessary, direct patient contact. Frequent data audits are performed revealing an inter-rater reliability of approximately 98% [13]. Eligible procedures are sampled by

NSQIP from all participating centers by either capturing all cases at the center or by systematically including cases using a rotating 8-day cycle [13]. NSQIP hospitals are the source of data used in this analysis; however, NSQIP has not reviewed the methodology of this study and is not responsible for its content.

A consecutive cohort of radical cystectomy cases within NSQIP were included using Current Procedural Terminology codes. Patient demographics and medical comorbidities included: age, race, gender, body mass index, American Society of Anesthesiologists' classification (ASA class), bleeding disorder, pre-operative weight loss, pre-operative sepsis, chronic steroid use, diabetes, dialysis, disseminated cancer, pre-operative chemotherapy, pre-operative radiotherapy (in the last 90 days prior to surgery), dyspnea, alcohol use, smoking history, functional status, chronic obstructive pulmonary disease, congestive heart failure, pre-operative albumin concentration, pre-operative creatinine level, emergency status of cystectomy, >4 units of red blood cell transfusion prior to surgery, operative time, and urinary diversion type. In total 27 characteristics were available for baseline comparisons. Criteria for each characteristic are defined in the 2012 NSQIP User's Guide [13]. No information about treating institution, surgeon, or tumors (i.e. tumor stage or grade) was available.

The incidence of peri-operative complications within 30 days of surgery was reported. The NSQIP definition for each complication is available in the NSQIP User's Guide [13]. Complications examined in this analysis included: infectious complications (urinary tract infection, superficial and deep surgical site infection, sepsis), hematologic complications (bleeding [≥1 unit red blood cell transfusion intra-operatively or within 72 hours of surgery]), deep vein thrombosis/thrombophlebitis (DVT), and other complications (wound disruption/fascial dehiscence, acute renal failure, prolonged ventilation, unplanned intubation, cardiac arrest requiring cardiopulmonary resuscitation, myocardial infarction, and death). The severity of individual complications and management required for complications is not collected.

The primary study outcome was the occurrence of any peri-operative complication. Associations between individual patient and surgical factors with the occurrence of any complication was determined using log binomial regression to directly estimate relative risks with 95% confidence intervals. A multivariable log binomial regression analysis was then performed to adjust for confounding by incorporating variables that were statistically significant on univariable analysis and those that have been associated with cystectomy complications in previous studies.

Variables with >15% missing data (low serum albumin concentration, pre-operative radiotherapy, pre-operative chemo-therapy) were added to the baseline multivariable model to determine adjusted associations with post-operative complications in an exploratory analysis. For all analyses no adjustment was made for multiple testing and a p-value ≤0.05 was considered statistically significant. SAS software version 9.4 for Windows was used for analyses (Cary, NC, USA).

Results

From 2006 to 2012, 2303 radical cystectomy patients were captured by NSQIP. Patient and surgery characteristics are presented in Table 1. Of note, 1115 (48%) patients were 70 years old or older, 1911 (85%) were White, and 1819 (79%) were male. The median body mass index was 28 (IQR 24 to 32). Median hospital stay was 8 days (IQR 7 to 13 days).

Incidence and timing of complications

Overall, 1273 (55.3%) patients experienced at least 1 post-operative complication by the 30th post-operative day. The most common complication was blood transfusion within 72 hours of surgery (n = 875; 38.0%). If transfusion is not included as a complication, 659 (28.6%) experienced at least 1 post-operative complication by day 30. Infectious complications were common with 218 (9.5%) urinary tract infections, 193 (8.4%) surgical site infections, and 223 (9.7%) sepsis events. Seventy-three (3.2%) patients had fascial wound dehiscence. Eighty-two patients (4.0%) developed a DVT, 22 (1.0%) patients had cardiac arrest, and 67 (2.9%) patients died.

One hundred and ninety-one (15.6%) complications occurred after discharge from hospital including: 127 (58.8%) urinary tract infections, 37 (46.3%) DVTs, 28 (39.4%) wound dehiscences, and 25 (50.0%) deaths (Table 2 and Figure 1).

Associations between patient and surgical factors with the occurrence of at least one complication

On univariable analysis, several factors were significantly associated with an increased risk of at least one post-operative complication (primary outcome). This included female gender, high ASA classification (ASA 3–5), dependent functional status, chronic obstructive pulmonary disease, pre-operative weight loss, pre-operative dyspnea, pre-operative transfusion, and operative time >6 hours (Table 3). Many of these factors maintained clinical and statistical significance on multivariable analysis (Table 4).

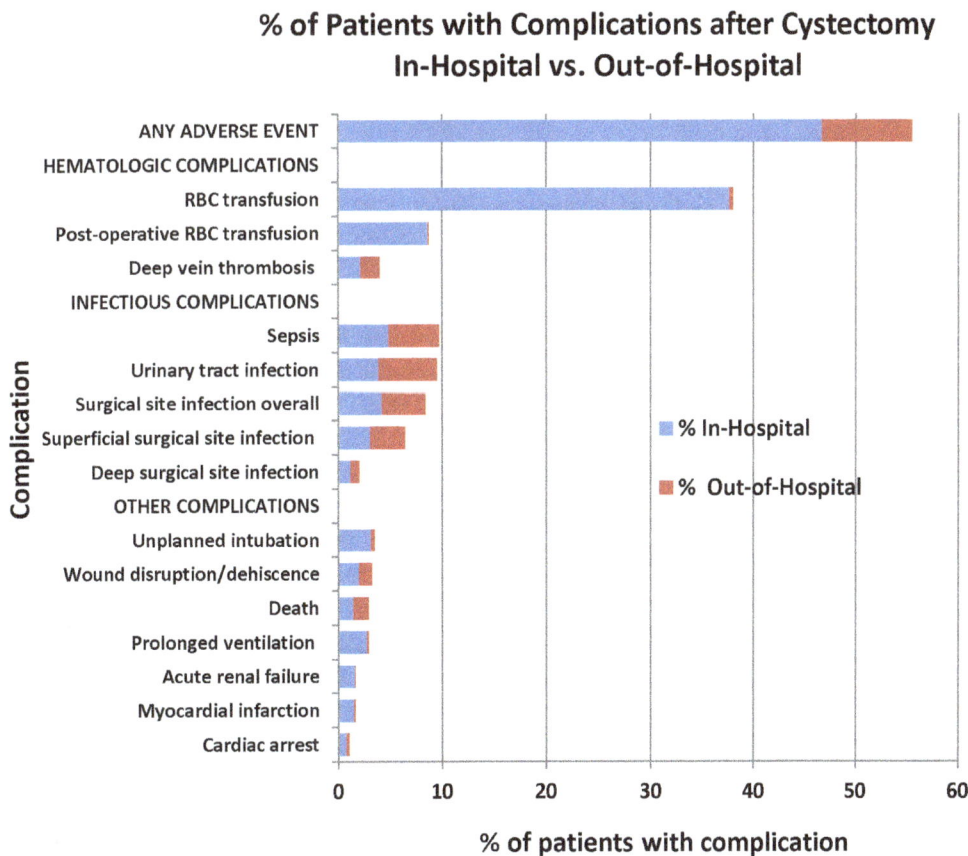

% of Patients with Complications after Cystectomy
In-Hospital vs. Out-of-Hospital

Figure 1. Percentage of patients who received radical cystectomy in NSQIP from 2006–2012 and experienced complications within 30 days of surgery. Complications are presented by type and by in-hospital versus out-of-hospital diagnosis. RBC = Red blood cell.

Table 2. Frequency of complications after radical cystectomy in NSQIP from 2006–2012.

Variable	n (%)	Days post cystectomy Median (IQR)	n (%) after discharge from hospital
Patients experiencing at least 1 complication	1273 (55.3%)	Mean 4.3 (SD 7.1)	191 (15.6)
Hematologic complications:			
Red blood cell transfusion (RBC)		Mean 0.6 (SD 2.3)	
Day of surgery (including intra-operative)	875 (38.0)		N/A
Within 72 hours post-operative	200 (8.7)		
Deep vein thrombosis	82 (4.0)	14 (8.5–20)	37 (46.3)
Infectious complications:			
Sepsis	223 (9.7)	12 (8–18)	111 (50.2)
Urinary tract infection	218 (9.5)	15 (9–21)	127 (58.8)
Surgical site infection overall	193 (8.4)		94 (50.3)
Superficial surgical site infection	147 (6.4)	13 (8–18)	75 (52.5)
Deep surgical site infection	46 (2.0)	12 (7–17)	19 (43.2)
Other complications:			
Death	67 (2.9)	14.5 (9–21)	25 (50.0)
Prolonged ventilation (>48 hours)	67 (2.9)	6 (3–11)	3 (4.6)
Unplanned intubation	80 (3.5)	6 (2–12)	9 (11.4)
Wound disruption/fascial dehiscence	73 (3.2)	11.5 (7.5–16)	28 (39.4)
Cardiac arrest requiring CPR	22 (1.0)	8 (5–15)	5 (25.0)
Myocardial infarction	37 (1.6)	3 (1.5–5.5)	2 (5.6)
Acute renal failure	36 (1.6)	8 (3.5–16.5)	6 (16.7)

Complications are presented by type. The absolute number, percentage, and occurrence of complications in-hospital versus out-of-hospital are shown.
CPR = cardiopulmonary resuscitation.
N/A = not available.

Variables with >15% missing data (low serum albumin concentration [39% missing], pre-operative radiotherapy [44% missing], pre-operative chemotherapy [44% missing]) were added to the baseline model to determine their adjusted associations with post-operative complications. Low serum albumin concentration (RR 1.16 95%CI 1.06–1.26, p = 0.0006) and pre-operative radiotherapy (RR 1.54 95%CI 1.13–2.09, p = 0.006) were independently associated with experiencing one or more complication.

Discussion

Accurate characterization of peri-operative morbidity facilitates patient counseling and identifies targets for quality improvement interventions. We studied a large historical cohort of patients treated from 2006 to 2012 at hospitals participating in The American College of Surgeons' National Surgical Quality Improvement Program (NSQIP) [13]. Two results of this study are particularly noteworthy: first, the incidence of complications after radical cystectomy remains high with 55.3% of patients experiencing at least one post-operative complication by 30 days. Second, a significant proportion (15.6%) of complications occurred after discharge from hospital, including 46.3% of DVTs.

Findings from this study are consistent with previous reports from multi-institutional cystectomy databases and large single center cohorts in which complication rates of 20–60% by 30 days were reported [3–6,14]. The most common complications in this study were: red blood cell transfusion (44.7%), urinary tract infections (9.5%), surgical site infections (8.4%), and sepsis (9.7%). The incidence of each of these complications is slightly higher than

reported in a previous review of the NSQIP hospitals from 1991–2002 and is in the higher range compared to other similar studies [5,15]. These differences may be due to differences in the study populations, as the earlier NSQIP cohorts were comprised of Veterans Affairs Medical Centers with only 1% of the sample being female, compared to 21% of our cohort. Consistent with previous studies, female gender is associated with complications (RR 1.18 95%CI 1.09–1.28), possibly due to vaginal entry and dissection [15,16]. A second reason that may explain a higher complication rate in this cohort is the rigor of complication assessment, which is a particular strength of NSQIP.

The timing of complications in this study has implications for physicians as a significant proportion (15.6%) occurred after discharge from hospital, most notably infectious complications, DVTs, and fascial dehiscence. A previous study of Surveillance, Epidemiology, and End Results (SEER)-Medicare data showed that as many as one quarter of patients require readmission after cystectomy with 33.8% of those having complications [17]. This high rate of out-of hospital complications should prompt physicians to examine ways to monitor these patients for complications using early follow-up visits/testing and to improve methods for preventing complications after discharge.

Despite ongoing efforts to improve radical cystectomy peri-operative care including refinement of surgical technique, technological advances, and thrombotic/infectious prophylaxis, complications remain high and improvement is needed. Improved outcomes begin with proper patient selection. This study and others have identified factors that are associated with poor outcomes such as: increased age, female gender, comorbid conditions, previous radio/chemotherapy, low albumin concen-

Table 3. Univariable analysis of patient and surgical factors with complications following radical cystectomy in NSQIP.

Variable	Relative Risk	95% Confidence Interval	p-value
Patient factors			
Age (Increase of 1 year)	1.00	1.00–1.01	0.01
Non Caucasian race	1.11	0.95–1.29	0.18
Female gender	1.19	1.10–1.29	<0.0001
Body mass index (≥35 vs <25)	1.08	0.96–1.21	0.19
ASA class 3–5	1.17	1.07–1.28	0.0006
Bleeding disorder	1.06	0.89–1.26	0.5
Pre-operative weight loss	1.21	1.02–1.42	0.02
Pre-operative sepsis	1.39	1.16–1.66	0.0004
Steroid use	1.10	0.91–1.33	0.33
Diabetes	1.01	0.92–1.11	0.79
Dialysis	1.13	0.77–1.66	0.52
Disseminated cancer	0.98	0.83–1.17	0.85
Pre-operative chemotherapy	1.09	0.93–1.28	0.28
Pre-operative radiotherapy	1.40	0.97–2.01	0.07
Dyspnea	1.15	1.04–1.28	0.009
Alcohol	0.89	0.67–1.18	0.41
Current smoker	1.00	0.92–1.08	0.93
Dependent functional status	1.12	0.92–1.35	0.26
COPD	1.15	1.03–1.30	0.02
History of TIA	0.92	0.60–1.40	0.70
Congestive heart failure	0.95	0.62–1.46	0.82
Decrease in pre-operative albumin	1.19	1.12–1.27	<0.0001
Increase in pre-operative creatinine	1.02	0.98–1.06	0.33
Pre-operative transfusion >4 units	1.34	1.15–1.58	0.0003
Emergency case	1.01	0.56–1.81	0.99
Operative factors			
Operative time greater than 6 hours	1.26	1.17–1.35	<0.0001
Continent urinary diversion	0.94	0.86–1.04	0.24

ASA class = American Society of Anesthesiologists' classification.
COPD = chronic obstructive pulmonary disease.
TIA = transient ischemic attack.

tration, and longer duration of surgery. Many risk factors cannot be modified, however knowledge of a high risk patient can aid the treating team to modify their approach and ensure proper patient counselling and monitoring. Some interventions have been shown to decrease surgical complications including: electrosurgical heat-sealing devices that reduce bleeding, pre-operative checklists, surgical care pathways, and adherence to antibiotic and deep vein thrombosis prophylaxis guidelines [7–9,15,18]. Physicians need to be aware of beneficial interventions at their disposal and ensure they are applied consistently in all cystectomy patients given their high risk of adverse outcomes.

This study has several strengths worth noting. First, compared to large single institution series, the results of this study are more generalizable because NSQIP currently includes data from 547 community and academic hospitals. Data from high volume centers of excellence are of value, however, they are not likely representative of outcomes for patient populations treated at a majority of hospitals [6,11,12]. Second, data used for analyses are likely valid. NSQIP collects data prospectively, using trained surgical clinical reviewers. They use pre-defined outcomes that

have been shown to be highly accurate [13]. Finally, the large number of procedures included in NSQIP each year makes it a powerful resource for measuring current practice outcomes compared to single institution series spanning several decades over which therapies and health care systems change [3].

NSQIP is a valuable resource; however, inherent restrictions of its data content limit this study's results and conclusions. Some pre-operative variables that are important to physicians treating bladder cancer are not available such as tumor stage and previous non-surgical treatments. Furthermore, data for some pre-operative variables, such as serum albumin concentration, and pre-operative chemotherapy or radiotherapy treatment have missing data, possibly limiting our ability to detect or characterize important risk factors for adverse events. Finally, we performed multiple tests of significance in our analysis to explore a range of independent variables; this may have allowed for some chance findings.

Table 4. Multivariable analysis of patient and surgical factors with complications following radical cystectomy in NSQIP.

Variable	Relative Risk	95% Confidence Interval	p-value
Age (Increase of 1 year)	1.01	1.00–1.01	0.004
Female gender	1.19	1.09–1.29	<0.0001
Current smoker	0.99	0.91–1.09	0.87
Body mass index (≥35 vs <25)	1.08	0.96–1.22	0.21
ASA class 3–5	1.13	1.03–1.25	0.01
Pre-operative weight loss	1.15	0.98–1.35	0.09
Pre-operative sepsis	1.23	1.01–1.49	0.04
Dependent functional status	1.02	0.83–1.25	0.87
COPD	1.14	1.02–1.29	0.02
Increase in pre-operative creatinine	1.02	0.96–1.09	0.50
Diabetes	0.98	0.89–1.08	0.65
Pre-operative transfusion >4 units	1.28	1.07–1.54	0.006
Operative factors			
Operative time greater than 6 hours	1.30	1.20–1.40	<0.0001
Continent urinary diversion	0.99	0.89–1.09	0.79

Multivariable analysis had a sample size of 2183.
ASA class = American Society of Anesthesiologists' classification.
COPD = chronic obstructive pulmonary diseaseReferences.

Conclusion

In summary, complications after radical cystectomy remain high with 55.3% of patients experiencing at least 1 complication within 30 days of surgery. Several randomized clinical trials are ongoing that attempt to reduce peri-operative complications in cystectomy patients with interventions such as: minimally invasive robotic surgery, intra-operative tranexamic acid to reduce blood loss, and pre-operative nutritional supplementation [19]. This study provides accurate information for pre-operative patient counseling and identifies targets for quality improvement interventions. Physicians performing radical cystectomy should be aware of risk factors, common complications, prevention strategies, and treatment of all complications to ensure optimal patient outcomes.

Acknowledgments

This research was made possible by the collaboration of the American College of Surgeons' National Surgical Quality Improvement Program (ACS NSQIP). The ACS NSQIP and the hospitals participating in the ACS NSQIP are the source of the data used herein; they have not verified and are not responsible for the statistical validity of the data analysis or the conclusions derived by the authors.

Author Contributions

Conceived and designed the experiments: LL DS DF CM IC RB. Performed the experiments: LL KW RM DS. Analyzed the data: LL KW RM. Contributed reagents/materials/analysis tools: LL RM RB DS. Contributed to the writing of the manuscript: LL DS KW RB.

References

1. Siegel R, Naishadham D, Jemal A (2013) Cancer statistics, 2013. CA Cancer J Clin 63: 11–30.
2. Ploeg M, Aben KK, Kiemeney LA (2009) The present and future burden of urinary bladder cancer in the world. World J Urol 27: 289–293.
3. Stein JP, Lieskovsky G, Cote R, Groshen S, Feng AC, et al. (2001) Radical cystectomy in the treatment of invasive bladder cancer: Long-term results in 1,054 patients. J Clin Oncol 19: 666–675.
4. Chang SS, Cookson MS, Baumgartner RG, Wells N, Smith JA Jr. (2002) Analysis of early complications after radical cystectomy: Results of a collaborative care pathway. J Urol 167: 2012–2016.
5. Hollenbeck BK, Miller DC, Taub D, Dunn RL, Khuri SF, et al. (2005) Identifying risk factors for potentially avoidable complications following radical cystectomy. J Urol 174: 1231–7; discussion 1237.
6. Shabsigh A, Korets R, Vora KC, Brooks CM, Cronin AM, et al. (2009) Defining early morbidity of radical cystectomy for patients with bladder cancer using a standardized reporting methodology. Eur Urol 55: 164–174.
7. Thompson IM, 3rd, Kappa SF, Morgan TM, Barocas DA, Bischoff CJ, et al. (2014) Blood loss associated with radical cystectomy: A prospective, randomized study comparing impact LigaSure vs. stapling device. Urol Oncol 32: 45.e11–45.e15.
8. Karl A, Buchner A, Becker A, Staehler M, Seitz M, et al. (2014) A new concept for early recovery after surgery for patients undergoing radical cystectomy for bladder cancer: Results of a prospective randomized study. J Urol 191: 335–340.
9. Cerantola Y, Valerio M, Persson B, Jichlinski P, Ljungqvist O, et al. (2013) Guidelines for perioperative care after radical cystectomy for bladder cancer:

Enhanced recovery after surgery (ERAS((R))) society recommendations. Clin Nutr 32: 879–887.
10. Haynes AB, Weiser TG, Berry WR, Lipsitz SR, Breizat AH, et al. (2009) A surgical safety checklist to reduce morbidity and mortality in a global population. N Engl J Med 360: 491–499.
11. Kulkarni GS, Urbach DR, Austin PC, Fleshner NE, Laupacis A (2013) Higher surgeon and hospital volume improves long-term survival after radical cystectomy. Cancer 119: 3546–3554.
12. Birkmeyer JD, Stukel TA, Siewers AE, Goodney PP, Wennberg DE, et al. (2003) Surgeon volume and operative mortality in the united states. N Engl J Med 349: 2117–2127.
13. National Surgical Quality Improvement Program (2005) American college of surgeons. Available: www.acsnsqip.org. Accessed 2014 January 27.
14. Yu HY, Hevelone ND, Lipsitz SR, Kowalczyk KJ, Nguyen PL, et al. (2012) Comparative analysis of outcomes and costs following open radical cystectomy versus robot-assisted laparoscopic radical cystectomy: Results from the US nationwide inpatient sample. Eur Urol 61: 1239–1244.
15. Lawrentschuk N, Colombo R, Hakenberg OW, Lerner SP, Mansson W, et al. (2010) Prevention and management of complications following radical cystectomy for bladder cancer. Eur Urol 57: 983–1001.
16. Lee KL, Freiha F, Presti JC, Jr, Gill HS. (2004) Gender differences in radical cystectomy: Complications and blood loss. Urology 63: 1095–1099.
17. Hu M, Jacobs BL, Montgomery JS, He C, Ye J, et al. (2014) Sharpening the focus on causes and timing of readmission after radical cystectomy for bladder cancer. Cancer.

18. Darouiche RO, Wall MJ, Jr, Itani KM, Otterson MF, Webb AL, et al. (2010) Chlorhexidine-alcohol versus povidone-iodine for surgical-site antisepsis. N Engl J Med 362: 18–26.

19. U.S.National Institutes of Health. Available: http://clinicaltrials.gov/. Accessed April 2014.

13

Cardiac Function in Patients with Early Cirrhosis during Maximal Beta-Adrenergic Drive: A Dobutamine Stress Study

Aleksander Krag[1,2]*, Flemming Bendtsen[2], Emilie Kristine Dahl[1], Andreas Kjær[3], Claus Leth Petersen[4], Søren Møller[4]

1 Department of Gastroenterology, Odense University Hospital, Odense, Denmark, 2 Gastro Unit, Medical Division, Hvidovre Hospital, University of Copenhagen, Copenhagen, Denmark, 3 Hvidovre Hospital, Department of Clinical Physiology Nuclear Medicine & PET, Rigshospitalet, Hvidovre Hospital, University of Copenhagen, Copenhagen, Denmark, 4 Centre of Functional Imaging and Research, Department of Clinical Physiology and Nuclear Medicine, Hvidovre Hospital, University of Copenhagen, Copenhagen, Denmark

Abstract

Background and aim: Cardiac dysfunction in patients with early cirrhosis is debated. We investigated potential cardiac dysfunction by assessing left ventricular systolic performance during a dobutamine stress test in patients with early cirrhosis.

Patients and methods: Nineteen patients with Child A and B cirrhosis (9 with non-alcoholic cirrhosis) and 7 matched controls were included. We used cardiac magnetic resonance imaging to assess left ventricular volumes and cardiac output (CO) at rest and during maximal heart rate induced by increasing dosages of dobutamine and atropine.

Results: Patients with cirrhosis and controls had an equal stress response, the heart rate and ejection fraction increased similarly and maximal heart rate was reached in all. At rest CO was higher in Child B patients than controls. During maximal stress, Child B patients had higher CO (10.6 ± 2.7 vs. 8.0 ± 1.8 L/min), left ventricle end diastolic volume (90 ± 25 vs. 67 ± 16 mL), left ventricular end diastolic volume (10 ± 4 vs. 6 ± 2 mL) and stroke volume (80 ± 23 vs. 61 ± 15 mL) than Child A patients. The systemic vascular resistance was lower in Child B than Child A patients (670 ± 279 vs. 911 ± 274 dyne*s*cm^{-5}). The left ventricle mass increased by 5.6 gram per model for end stage liver disease (MELD) point. MELD score correlated with the end diastolic and systolic volume, CO, and stroke volume at rest and at stress (all $p<0.05$).

Conclusion: In patients with early cirrhosis the chronotropoic and inotropic response to pharmacological stress induced by dobutamine is normal. With progression of the disease, the mass of the heart increases along with increase in cardiac volumes.

Editor: Xiongwen Chen, Temple University, United States of America

Funding: This study was supported by grants from the Lundbeck Foundation, Hvidovre Hospital Foundation for Liver Disease, and The Novo Nordic Foundation. Aleksander Krag received a grant from University of Copenhagen and The Capital Region of Denmark, Foundation for Health Research. Department of Radiology, Frederiksberg Hospital is thanked for the CMRI investigations. The author(s) received no specific funding for this work.

Competing Interests: The authors have declared that no competing interests exist.

* Email: Aleksander.Krag@rsyd.dk

Introduction

Several cardiac abnormalities have been described in cirrhosis. Diastolic and systolic dysfunction has been revealed in advanced cirrhosis and both seem to predict a poor outcome. Diastolic dysfunction is associated with reduced ascites clearance and increased mortality post transjungular intrahepatic portosystemic shunt (TIPS) operation [2]. Systolic dysfunction is associated with risk of developing hepatorenal syndrome [2–5]. Therefore a preserved systolic capacity with a high cardiac output at this stage of cirrhosis is related to better survival [5]. Furthermore, among patients who develop spontaneous bacterial peritonitis, a low cardiac output (CO) is associated with the development of hepatorenal syndrome and poor survival [6]. Several factors are found to differentiate patients with cirrhosis from healthy subjects. First, in advanced cirrhosis there are high levels of circulating noradrenaline and both beta-1 and -2 adrenoreceptors are down regulated. Beta-1 and -2 adrenoreceptors regulate the rate and the contractility of the heart [7,8]. Second, the adrenergic positive inotropic effect on the heart is reduced in experimental cirrhosis [9]. Third, impaired chronotropic response to stress is a predictor of low survival in healthy individuals and in sepsis [10]. A blunted chronotropic response is found in previous studies in cirrhosis both during exercise, tilting, paracentesis, and infections [6,11–13]. There is an increasing amount of data supporting a cardiac dysfunction in advanced cirrhosis with an impact on the risk of complications and survival [14]. However, cardiac systolic function in early cirrhosis has only been sparsely investigated. A cardiac dysfunction may be either subclinical, compensated at rest or in stable conditions and may only become clinically significant during circulatory stress [15]. Investigation of cardiac function by cardiac magnetic resonance imaging (CMRI) during maximal dobutamine stress is considered the gold standard for assessment of systolic abnormalities. We therefore aimed with CMRI to investigate left ventricular systolic performance at rest and during pharmacologically induced maximal beta-adrenergic drive in patients with mild cirrhosis.

Material and Methods

Nineteen patients with Child A and B cirrhosis and 7 matched controls participated. Nine out of 19 patients had non-alcoholic cirrhosis. Patients were included if they had mild cirrhosis Child A or B without known heart disease. Patients were excluded if they had experienced gastrointestinal bleeding within the month preceding the study, showed signs of insulin-dependent diabetes, acute or chronic intrinsic renal or cardiovascular disease, abnormal electrocardiogram (ECG) (apart from prolonged QT intervals), or any acute medical conditions, such as infections, acute heart or lung diseases. Furthermore, alcohol abstinence for two months was required. To make sure none of the patients had an undiscovered heart disease, all patients had a single photon emission computed tomography (SPECT) myocardial perfusion scan done the week before the study. A normal SPECT is associated with a good prognosis regarding cardiac events and excludes ischemic heart diseases with high accuracy [16]. A negative history of arterial hypertension, cardiac and pulmonary diseases together with a normal clinical examination, apart from signs of portal hypertension and cirrhosis, was required. Except from beta-blockers, none of the patients were receiving any drugs that could interfere with the cardiovascular or renal function, thus no patients had indications for cardiovascular medications. A normal serum creatinine, together with normal fasting blood glucose was also required. All patients were screened for diabetes before inclusion. Among patients 11 were smokers and 4 in the control group smoked. If the patient or control was a smoker, extra care during clinical examination was taken to be sure they did not have a chronic lung disease or signs of arteriosclerosis.

Treatment with diuretics or beta-blockers was temporarily discontinued for 7 days before the investigations to eliminate a pharmacological influence on cardiac work or volume status. In total, 5 patients were treated with furosemide 40–80 mg/day, 9 patients were treated with spironolactone 100–400 mg/day and 6 patients were treated with propranolol 80–160 mg/day. Nine patients did not receive any medication for their cirrhosis. Water overload may induce subtle cardiac dysfunction and therefore all were put on a sodium-restricted diet of 80 mmol/day in the last 7 days before the investigations. A dietician instructed them written and verbally about sodium restriction.

Stress testing

Dobutamine infusion started at 5 µg/Kg/min and was increased by 5 µg/Kg/min every third minute until a maximum of 40 µg/Kg/min or achievement of the pre-calculated age-adjusted maximal heart rate. The aim was to reach 85% of maximal heart rate defined as (220 – age) * 85%. If target heart rate was not achieved during maximal dobutamine infusion (40 µg/Kg/min), then atropine was added in refract doses of 0.25 mg. After reaching target maximal heart rate, infusion of dobutamine and atropine was continued throughout the CMRI.

The total workload of the heart, as expressed by heart rate times blood pressure product, was calculated from the maximal systolic blood pressure achieved during maximal stress times maximal heart rate.

Cardiac magnetic resonance imaging (CMRI)

The recordings were performed at Frederiksberg Hospital, University of Copenhagen in accordance with a standard protocol for CMRI as described in detail previously [17]. Briefly, CMRI was achieved with a 1.5 Tesla whole body scanner (Intera; Philips Medical Systems, MN, USA) using a dedicated hased array cardiac coil (Synergy; Philips Medical Systems, MN, USA). Following localisation of the long axis of the heart, continuous true short-axis slices were acquired using breath-hold ECG-triggered cine MRI gated prospectively. We applied 10 to 15 slices with 10 mm apart to measure the dimensions of the heart. The endocardial contours were drawn at the end-diastolic and end-systolic frame in all slices using standard software (Philips View Forum, release 3.2). End-diastolic volume (EDV) and end-systolic volume (ESV) were calculated by adding volume measurement in the end-diastole and end-systole, respectively from all slices. Based on EDV, ESV and heart rate LV stroke volume [1], ejection fraction (EF) and CO were calculated. For measurements of LV myocardial volume, epicardial contours were drawn at the end-diastolic frame in all slices. Myocardial mass was hereafter calculated by adding the differences between epi- and endocardial volumes with correction for the density of cardiac tissue (1.04 g/cm^3). Cardiac index (CI) was calculated as CO divided by the total body surface area [18]. Arterial compliance [19] was assessed as SV/puls-pressure (systolic minus diastolic blood pressure) and the systemic vascular resistance (SVR) as MAP*80/CO.

Hormones

A commercial available ELISA kit (Biomedica Gruppe, Vienna, Austria) was used to measure pro-atrial natriuretic peptide, ANP. Intra-assay and inter-assay coefficients of variation was 2% and 0.034 nmol/ml. An automated two-site sandwich immunoassay technique using chemilumin essence (ADVIA Centaur, Siemens, Germany) was used to measure BNP. The assay measures the physiologically active COOH-terminal peptide (77–108). The sensitivity of the assay was 2 pg/ml, intra-assay coefficient of variation was 1.2%, and inter-assay variation was 2.3%. Plasma renin concentration was determined by a commercially available two-site immunoradiometric assay (DGR International Inc., USA). Samples were collected in ice-chilled test tubes containing aprotinin-heparin and EDTA.

The Regional Ethics Committee for Copenhagen and Frederiksberg municipalities approved the study (journal number KF 01-270675) and it is registered on clinicaltrials.gov (NCT00250315). All patients gave their written informed consent to participate in accordance with the Helsinki II declaration.

Statistical analyses were performed by unpaired Student's t test or the Mann-Whitney test and paired Student's t test or the Wilcoxon test, as appropriate. All reported P-values are two-tailed with values less than 0.05 considered significant. Correlations were performed with Persons regression analyses. The SPSS 20 statistical package (SPSS Inc., Chicago) was applied throughout.

Results

Twenty patients were included in the study of which one was excluded due to hemochromatosis. The etiology of cirrhosis was alcohol in 10 patients, autoimmune in six patients, HCV in two patients and one had primary biliary cirrhosis. Demographic,

Table 1. Demographic, clinical, and biochemical characteristics of patients with cirrhosis and controls.

	Child A group (n = 12)	Child B group (n = 7)	Controls (n = 7)
Age (yr)	54±11	57±10	53±5
Gender (M/F)	4/8	5/2	2/5
Child-Pugh score	5.3±0.5	7.5±0.8	-
MELD score	6.3±4.0	10.3±2.8	-
BMI (kg/m²)	24±7	25±4	26±3
Aetiology (alcohol/no alcohol)	4/8	6/1	-
Diuretics (yes/no)	3/9	7/0	-
Beta-blocker treatment*	25%	43%	-
S-Sodium (135–145 mM)	142±4	139±5	-
S-Bilirubin (2–17 μmol/L)	13±9	15±5	-
S-Creatinine (49–121 μmol/L)	71±7	89±30	-
S-Albumin (37–48 g/L)	42±5	34±6	-
INR (0.9–1.2)	1.1±0.2	1.4±0.2	-
Pro-ANP nmol/L	2.9±1.4	3.6±1.2¤	2.1±0.3
BNP pg/mL	31.0±23	32.7±23.8	21.3±12.5
Renin ng/L	11 (6–19)	32 (18–98)¤	6 (4–9)

Mean ± SD, median and interquartile ranges. Reference interval in parentheses.
*The percentage of patients treated with beta-blockers before start of study. Compared with controls ¤ p<0.05.
Abbreviations:
Body Mass Index (BMI), International Normalized Ratio (INR), Model for End-stage Liver Disease (MELD).

clinical and biochemical characteristics of the participants are presented in table 1.

Baseline differences

At rest Child B patients had higher CO compared to Child A patients (6.9±1.4 vs. 5.0±1.3 L/min, p = 0.009); similarly CI differed (3.7±0.8 vs. 2.8±0.6 L/min/m², p = 0.02). The left ventricular mass correlated with MELD score (r = 0.58, p<0.01) and for each MELD point the left ventricle mass increased by 5.6 gram (Figure 1). At rest, the following volumes correlated positively with the MELD score and increased in volume for every MELD point: EDV (r = 0.70, p<0.01) ESV (r = 0.46, p< 0.05), CO (r = 0.66, p<0.01) and SV (r = 0.69, p<0.01).

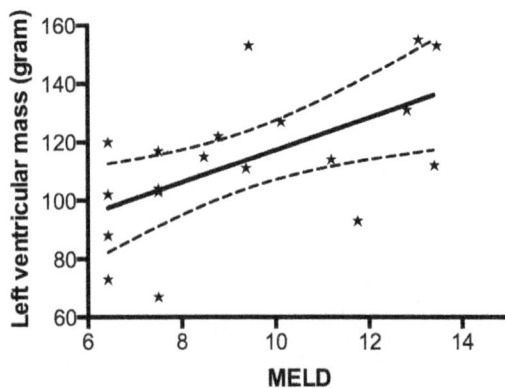

Figure 1. MELD score and left ventricular mass. The figure shows the correlation between Model for End-stage Liver Disease (MELD) score and the left ventricle mass at rest. For each MELD point the left ventricle mass increases with 5.6 gram, p<0.01. The two outer lines indicate a 95% confidence interval.

Stress testing

The pre-calculated maximal heart rate was reached in all patients and the heart rate increased by 80% (62±16 beats/min) and 92% (66±15 beats/min) in cirrhosis and controls, NS (Figure 2a, Table 2). The cardiac work, as reflected by the heart rate blood pressure product, increased by 84% (8854± 3915 mmHg/min) in Child A, 87% (9232±2418 mmHg/min) in Child B and 100% (9979±4857 mmHg/min) in controls, NS (Table 2). The dose of atropine (0.25 mg per dose) did not differ between cirrhosis and controls, p = 0.94 (0.26±0.7 vs. 0.29±0.5 dose of atropine). There was no difference in the increase in heart rate and heart rate blood pressure product between alcoholic and non-alcoholic cirrhosis. In all three groups, there were a significant increase from rest to stress in CO (mean difference 2.9±1.4, 3.7±1.8 and 4.2±1.9 L/min, all p<0.001) (Figure 2b), CI (mean difference 1.7±0.8, 1.9±0.9 and 2.2±1.0 L/min/m², all p< 0.001) and EF (mean difference 13±6, 11±5 and 13±5%, all p< 0.01) (Figure 2c) in Child A, Child B and controls, respectively. Likewise, there was a significant decrease in EDV (mean difference 21.3±16.5 mL p = 0.001, 17.1±12.8 mL p = 0.012 and 20.4±11.2 mL p = 0.003), ESV (mean difference 14.8±11.7 mL p = 0.001, 13.3±7.4 mL p = 0.003 and 16.4±7.1 mL p = 0.001) and SVR (mean difference 822±645 dyne*s*cm⁻⁵ p = 0.001, 438±150 dyne*s*cm⁻⁵ p<0.001 and 664±251 p<0.001 dyne*s*cm⁻⁵) during maximal stress, in Child A, Child B and controls, respectively (Table 2). SV decreased significantly in Child A patients from rest to stress (by 6.5±10.1 mL, p = 0.047) but not in Child B patients (3.9±13.3 mL, p = 0.47) or controls (4.0±9.8 mL, p = 0.32). AC decreased in Child A (by 0.4±0.4 mL/mmHg, p = 0.006) and Child B (by 0.7±0.7 mL/ mmHg, p = 0.035) but not in controls (by 0.5±0.8 mL/mmHg, p = 0.15). There was no difference in mean arterial pressure (MAP) from rest to stress in any of the three groups.

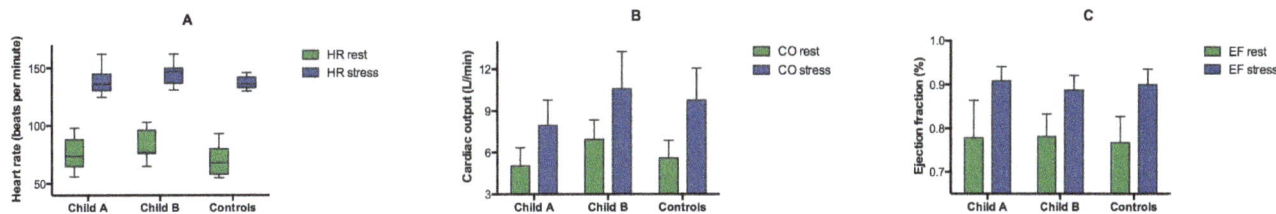

Figure 2. Response to dobutamine stress test. The figures show the response regarding heart rate (A), cardiac output (B) and ejection fraction (C) from rest to stress during maximal dobutamine infusion in Child A patients, Child B patients and controls. The bars show 95% confidence interval. Figure 2a: all groups show a similar significant increase in heart rate. Figure 2b: all groups show a similar significant increase in cardiac output. Cardiac output was significantly higher at rest in Child B patients compared to Child A patients, p<0.01. Figure 2c: all groups show a similar significant increase in ejection fraction.

Stress differences

At stress CO, SV, EDV, ESV and AC was significantly higher in Child B patients compared to Child A patients (all p<0.05), but EF and SVR did not differ. There were no differences in any volumes when comparing Child A and controls or Child B and controls.

As seen at baseline, EDV, ESV, SV, and CO correlated significant positively with the MELD score during maximal stress (EDV (r = 0.69, p<0.01), ESV (r = 0.56, p<0.01), SV (r = 0.68, p<0.01) and CO (r = 0.59, p<0.01)) (Figure 3). There was no difference in the response to stress between alcoholic and non-alcoholic cirrhotic patients.

Hormones

At rest, pro-ANP was higher in Child B patients compared to controls (3.6±1.2 vs. 2.1±0.3 nmol/L, p<0.01), Table 1. Both Child A and Child B patients had higher pro-ANP levels during maximal stress than controls (p<0.05 and p<0.01) but only in Child B patients pro-ANP significantly increased from rest to stress by 21% (0.77±0.38 nmol/L, p<0.05). BNP remained unchanged in both groups during stress. At rest, renin was slightly higher in

cirrhosis compared to controls, most pronounced in Child B patients (p<0.05). During dobutamine induced circulatory stress, renin increased similar in all groups (Child A (p<0.01, by 22.5 ng/L (11–75)), Child B (p<0.02, by 29 ng/L (6–200)), controls (p<0.02, by 11 ng/L (5–45)).

Discussion

The definition and consequences of cirrhotic cardiomyopathy is still debated [14,20]. Despite a considerable amount of research in this area many questions still remain unanswered. Most studies investigating cirrhotic cardiomyopathy have mainly been performed with various stress tests or echocardiography. The present study is the first to assess systolic cardiac function by dobutamine stress CMRI in early cirrhosis. Our main findings are: 1) A sufficient increase in heart rate suggesting intact beta-adrenergic response in early cirrhosis. 2) The increase in the blood pressure-heart rate product in Child A and Child B patients during dobutamine infusion was similar to controls. Thus, the chronotropic and inotropic response to dobutamine during stable conditions seems

Table 2. Cardiovascular function in 19 patients with cirrhosis and 7 controls at rest and after pharmacological stress with dobutamine +/− atropine.

	Child A group (n = 12)		Child B group (n = 7)		Controls (n = 7)	
	Rest	Stress	Rest	Stress	Rest	Stress
HR min^{-1}	76±13	138±10*	83±13	145±10*	71±14	137±5*
MAP mmHg	100±17	91±15	93±11	93±14	98±22	96±11
CO L/min	5.0±1.3	8.0±1.8*	6.9±1.4∞	10.6±2.7∞*	5.6±1.3	9.8±2.3*
CI L/min*m^2	2.9±0.6	4.5±0.9*	3.7±0.8∞	5.6±1.4*	2.9±0.9	5.2±1.5*
SV mL	68±16	61±15¤	84±22	80±23∞	80±13	76±17
EF %	78±9	91±3*	78±5	89±4*	77±6	90±4*
LV EDV ml	89±26	67±16*	107±27	90±25∞¤	105±16	86±17*
LV ESV ml	21±13	6±2*	23±8	10±4∞*	25±7	8±3∞*
LV mass g	108± 20		123±30		125±30	
AC mL/mmHg	1.2±0.5	0.9±0.2*	1.8±0.8	1.1±0.2∞¤	1.5±0.6	1.1±0.3
SVR dyne*s*cm^{-5}	1733±857	911±274*	1138±267	670±279*	1428±349	763±191*

Mean ± SD.
Comparison between rest and stress: ¤ p<0.05.
Comparison between rest and stress: * p<0.01.
Comparison with Child A patients: ∞ p<0.05.
Abbreviations:
Arterial Compliance (AC), Cardiac Index (CI), Cardiac Output (CO), Ejection Fraction (EF), Heart Rate (HR), Left Ventricle (LV), End-Diastolic Volume (EDV), End-Systolic Volume (ESV), Mean Arterial blood Pressunre (MAP), Stroke Volume (SV), Systemic Vascular Resistance (SVR).

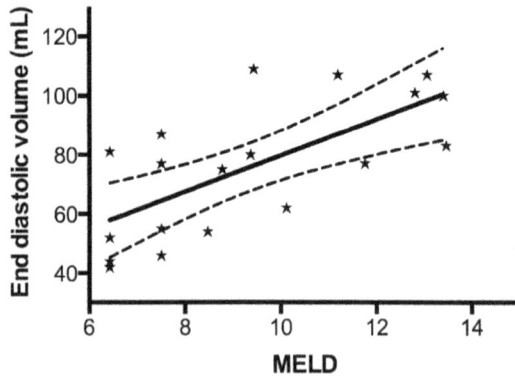

Figure 3. MELD score and end diastolic volume. The figure shows the correlation between model for end-stage liver disease (MELD) score and end diastolic volume during maximal stress, p = 0.001. The two outer lines indicate a 95% confidence interval.

intact in early cirrhosis. 3) With progression of the disease the mass of the heart increases along with an increase in cardiac volumes.

In an experimental study on cirrhotic rats a desensitization of myocardial beta-adrenoreceptors was found [7]. The rats where stimulated with isoprenaline and needed a significantly higher dose than controls before reaching target heart rate. Analyses showed a down-regulation of the density of beta-1-adrenoreceptors in the myocardial cells. We would therefore have expected a higher dose of dobutamine required to reach maximal heart rate in cirrhosis than controls. This difference is likely due to down regulation of beta-1-adrenoreceptors, which may not appear until advanced stages of cirrhosis where the sympathetic nervous system is highly activated [4–6,21]. However, it should be emphasized that heart rate is a surrogate readout of beta-adrenergic receptor responsiveness and does not provide mehanistic explanations such as downregulation or desensitization of receptors. However, it is easy to measure in a clinical setting and relate directly to cardiac output.

It has been proposed that stress could unmask cirrhotic cardiomyopathy. Two studies examined cirrhotic patients with bicycle ergometry and both found an inability to reach maximal heart rate with a lower total cardiac work [12,22,23]. Grose et al. found unaltered EF and an increase in EDV in patients with cirrhosis [12] and Wong et al. found a prolonged isovolumic relaxtion time, increased left ventricle wall thickening and less oxygen consumption in patients with cirrhosis [22]. Both studies suggest decreased diastolic and systolic functions as signs of cirrhotic cardiomyopathy. In accordance with this, Kim et al. found by stress echocardiography 25% of the patients to have blunted left ventricle response during maximal dobutamine infusion [24]. It has been questioned whether these bicycle or other exercise induced stress test indicate cirrhotic cardiomyopathy. Lemyze et al. suggest that the inability to reach maximal heart rate and thereby less produced work in bicycle ergometry tests may be explained by deconditioning, malnutrition-associated muscle weakness or anemia [25]. In support of this, studies have found that during exercise cirrhotic patients have decreased glucose uptake in the skeletal muscles, lower endogen glucose production together with a shift in oxidation from glucose towards lipids in energy production [26–28]. Furthermore, pulmonary dysfunction is common in cirrhosis [29] and may contribute to the insufficient amount of work produced during exercise tests [30].

In normal physiologic circumstances the systolic response at stress may be different from what is observed by dobutamine infusion. Sepsis, hypovolaemia, or physical work results in

differences in loading conditions. Thus the venous return and preload increase with physical work, whereas preload is low in advanced stages with central hypovolemia [31,32]. Our patients showed a normal response towards stress, but in the setting of a decreased afterload as reflected by the significant fall in SVR. Likewise, MAP remained unchanged during the whole study despite a steep increase in CO and heart rate. Dobutamine has a strong affinity for beta-1-adrenoreceptors and results in an increased heart rate, contractility and enhanced AV node conduction. But dobutamine also has affinity for beta-2-adreno-receptors and induces vasodilation [33]. This explains the observed decrease in SVR and afterload. In a previous study in patients with advanced cirrhosis we increased the afterload by terlipressin and observed a decrease in EF, CO and an increase in EDV. An increase in afterload requires an increase in total workforce, which was clearly impaired in these patients with advanced cirrhosis [34]. A number of factors related to the stage of cirrhosis may explain why systolic function as assessed in this study is adequate. Most patients with advanced cirrhosis have chronic elevation of proinflammatory cytokines, such as IL-6 and TNF-alfa and endotoxins, which represent a chronic low-grade inflammatory state [35]. The activation of cytokines, vasoactive hormones, and alteration in circulatory function in advanced cirrhosis and ascites without overt sepsis is similar to that seen in sepsis and septic shock without cirrhosis [35]. In septic shock it is estimated that approximately 40% of the patients develop myocardial dysfunction characterised by decreased systolic contractility and impaired diastolic relaxation [36,37]. In the cardiodepressant state, adrenal insufficiency (particularly with acute stresses), may result in critical illness related corticosteroid insufficiency [15,21]. In early stages of stable cirrhosis these factors are not in force. This study did not assess diastolic function. However, diastolic function has been investigated in a number of studies and seems related to clinical outcome and may be evident in all stages of disease including early stages. Two recent large studies assessed diastolic dysfunction in cirrhotic patients using echocardiography [24,38,39]. Nazar et al. found mild diastolic dysfunction frequent in cirrhotic patients and unrelated to circulatory dysfunction, ascites and HRS [38]. Ruiz-del-Arbol et al. did a one-year follow up study and found that the degree of left ventricular diastolic dysfunction correlated with survival rate and development of hepatorenal syndrome [39]. Furthermore, autonomic dysfunction may also play a role. In a previous study we found that after dobutamine stress the time to resume heart rate of 100 beats/min was longer in cirrhosis than in controls [40]. It is well known that patients with cirrhosis have altered hemodynamics leading to a hyperdynamic syndrome [14,41]. We found a significant higher CO in Child B patients compared to Child A patients. Furthermore, left ventricle mass correlated with the Child-Pugh score and increased with 2.8 gram per MELD score. Most likely, the observed increase in left ventricle mass is a physiology response to the increased work as reflected by increased CO. The increased CO also explains why Child B patients showed a significant higher stroke volume, end systolic volume and end diastolic volume than Child A patients during stress. These are likely the earliest changes towards the hyperdynamic syndrome seen in advanced cirrhosis with decreased SVR, increased CO, increased left ventricular mass together with subtle hormonal changes [42]. Physiological adaptions to protect the circulation and organ perfusion against the thread from progressive vasodilation [43]. Thus at this stage cardiac function and compensatory reserve in terms of ability to increase CO is intact and cardiac function is increased rather than depressed.

The slight increase in renin, mainly seen in Child B patients, support that the patients were in early stages of cirrhosis with a beginning of hemodynamic derangement and activation of vasoactive hormones [42]. This fit well with the fact that Child B patients had an increased CO compared to controls. The increase in renin after dobutamine infusion was similar in cirrhosis and controls and is likely a direct effect through stimulation of the beta$_1$ adrenergic receptors.

Conclusions

In stable early cirrhosis with normal loading conditions the cardiac systolic response to pharmacological stress is normal. With progression of the disease the mass of the heart increases along with an increase in cardiac volumes. Future follow-up studies should look for changes in patients with advanced cirrhosis and the long-term impact of cardiac dysfunction in the development of complications of cirrhosis.

Author Contributions

Conceived and designed the experiments: ALK FB SM ANK CLP. Performed the experiments: ALK. Analyzed the data: ALK ED ANK CLP. Wrote the paper: ALK ED FB SM.

References

1. De Minicis S, Rychlicki C, Agostinelli L, Saccomanno S, Candelaresi C, et al. (2014) Dysbiosis contributes to fibrogenesis in the course of chronic liver injury in mice. Hepatology 59: 1738–1749.
2. Cazzaniga M, Salerno F, Pagnozzi G, Dionigi E, Visentin S, et al. (2007) Diastolic dysfunction is associated with poor survival in patients with cirrhosis with transjugular intrahepatic portosystemic shunt 1. Gut 56: 869–875.
3. Rabie RN, Cazzaniga M, Salerno F, Wong F (2009) The use of E/A ratio as a predictor of outcome in cirrhotic patients treated with transjugular intrahepatic portosystemic shunt. Am J Gastroenterol 104: 2458–2466.
4. Ruiz-del-Arbol L, Monescillo A, Arocena C, Valer P, Gines P, et al. (2005) Circulatory function and hepatorenal syndrome in cirrhosis. Hepatology 42: 439–447.
5. Krag A, Bendtsen F, Henriksen JH, Moller S (2010) Low cardiac output predicts development of hepatorenal syndrome and survival in patients with cirrhosis and ascites. Gut 59: 105–110.
6. Ruiz-del-Arbol L, Urman J, Fernandez J, Gonzalez M, Navasa M, et al. (2003) Systemic, renal, and hepatic hemodynamic derangement in cirrhotic patients with spontaneous bacterial peritonitis. Hepatology 38: 1210–1218.
7. Lee SS, Marty J, Mantz J, Samain E, Braillon A, et al. (1990) Desensitization of myocardial beta-adrenergic receptors in cirrhotic rats. Hepatology 12: 481–485.
8. Ceolotto G, Papparella I, Sticca A, Bova S, Cavalli M, et al. (2008) An abnormal gene expression of the beta-adrenergic system contributes to the pathogenesis of cardiomyopathy in cirrhotic rats. Hepatology 48: 1913–1923.
9. Ma Z, Miyamoto A, Lee SS (1996) Role of altered beta-adrenoceptor signal transduction in the pathogenesis of cirrhotic cardiomyopathy in rats. Gastroenterology 110: 1191–1198.
10. Shujaat A, Bajwa AA (2012) Optimization of preload in severe sepsis and septic shock. Crit Care Res Pract 2012: 761051.
11. Laffi G, Lagi A, Cipriani M, Barletta G, Bernardi L, et al. (1996) Impaired cardiovascular autonomic response to passive tilting in cirrhosis with ascites. Hepatology 24: 1063–1067.
12. Grose RD, Nolan J, Dillon JF, Errington M, Hannan WJ, et al. (1995) Exercise-induced left ventricular dysfunction in alcoholic and non-alcoholic cirrhosis. J Hepatol 22: 326–332.
13. Ruiz-del-Arbol L, Monescillo A, Jimenez W, Garcia-Plaza A, Arroyo V, et al. (1997) Paracentesis-induced circulatory dysfunction: mechanism and effect on hepatic hemodynamics in cirrhosis. Gastroenterology 113: 579–586.
14. Moller S, Hove JD, Dixen U, Bendtsen F (2013) New insights into cirrhotic cardiomyopathy. Int J Cardiol 167: 1101–1108.
15. Krag A, Bendtsen F, Burroughs AK, Moller S (2012) The cardiorenal link in advanced cirrhosis. Med Hypotheses 79: 53–55.
16. Hachamovitch R, Berman DS, Shaw LJ, Kiat H, Cohen I, et al. (1998) Incremental prognostic value of myocardial perfusion single photon emission computed tomography for the prediction of cardiac death: differential stratification for risk of cardiac death and myocardial infarction. Circulation 97: 535–543.
17. Lenstrup M, Kjaergaard J, Petersen CL, Kjaer A, Hassager C (2006) Evaluation of left ventricular mass measured by 3D echocardiography using magnetic resonance imaging as gold standard. Scand J Clin Lab Invest 66: 647–657.
18. DuBois D, DuBois EF (1916) A formula to estimate the approximate surface area if height and weight be known. Archives of Internal Medicine 17: 863–871.
19. (1988) Prediction of the first variceal hemorrhage in patients with cirrhosis of the liver and esophageal varices. A prospective multicenter study. The North Italian Endoscopic Club for the Study and Treatment of Esophageal Varices. The New England Journal of Medicine 319: 983–989.
20. Timoh T, Protano MA, Wagman G, Bloom M, Vittorio TJ (2011) A perspective on cirrhotic cardiomyopathy. Transplant Proc 43: 1649–1653.
21. Theocharidou E, Krag A, Bendtsen F, Moller S, Burroughs AK (2012) Cardiac dysfunction in cirrhosis - does adrenal function play a role? A hypothesis. Liver Int 32: 1327–1332.
22. Wong F, Girgrah N, Graba J, Allidina Y, Liu P, et al. (2001) The cardiac response to exercise in cirrhosis. Gut 49: 268–275.
23. Bernardi M, Rubboli A, Trevisani F, Cancellieri C, Ligabue A, et al. (1991) Reduced cardiovascular responsiveness to exercise-induced sympathoadrenergic stimulation in patients with cirrhosis. J Hepatol 12: 207–216.
24. Kim MY, Baik SK, Won CS, Park HJ, Jeon HK, et al. (2010) Dobutamine stress echocardiography for evaluating cirrhotic cardiomyopathy in liver cirrhosis. The Korean journal of hepatology 16: 376–382.
25. Lemyze M, Dharancy S, Wallaert B (2013) Response to exercise in patients with liver cirrhosis: Implications for liver transplantation. Digestive and Liver Disease 45: 362–366.
26. Delissio M, Goodyear IJ, Fuller S, Krawitt EL, Devlin JT (1991) EFFECTS OF TREADMILL EXERCISE ON FUEL METABOLISM IN HEPATIC CIRRHOSIS. Journal of Applied Physiology 70: 210–215.
27. Selberg O, Burchert W, Vanderhoff J, Meyer GJ, Hundeshagen H, et al. (1993) INSULIN RESISTANCE IN LIVER-CIRRHOSIS - POSITRON-EMISSION TOMOGRAPHY SCAN ANALYSIS OF SKELETAL-MUSCLE GLUCOSE-METABOLISM. Journal of Clinical Investigation 91: 1897–1902.
28. Muller MJ, Lautz HU, Plogmann B, Burger M, Korber J, et al. (1992) ENERGY-EXPENDITURE AND SUBSTRATE OXIDATION IN PATIENTS WITH CIRRHOSIS - THE IMPACT OF CAUSE, CLINICAL STAGING AND NUTRITIONAL STATE. Hepatology 15: 782–794.
29. Moller S, Krag A, Henriksen JH, Bendtsen F (2007) Pathophysiological aspects of pulmonary complications of cirrhosis. Scand J Gastroenterol 42: 419–427.
30. Moller S, Krag A, Madsen JL, Henriksen JH, Bendtsen F (2009) Pulmonary dysfunction and hepatopulmonary syndrome in cirrhosis and portal hypertension. Liver International 29: 1528–1537.
31. Moller S, Bendtsen F, Henriksen JH (1995) Effect of volume expansion on systemic hemodynamics and central and arterial blood volume in cirrhosis. Gastroenterology 109: 1917–1925.
32. Moller S, Sondergaard L, Mogelvang J, Henriksen O, Henriksen JH (1995) Decreased right heart blood volume determined by magnetic resonance imaging: evidence of central underfilling in cirrhosis. Hepatology 22: 472–478.
33. Ruffolo RR Jr (1987) The pharmacology of dobutamine. Am J Med Sci 294: 244–248.
34. Krag A, Bendtsen F, Mortensen C, Henriksen JH, Moller S (2010) Effects of a single terlipressin administration on cardiac function and perfusion in cirrhosis. European Journal of Gastroenterology and Hepatology 22: 1085–1092.
35. Albillos A, de la HA, Gonzalez M, Moya JL, Calleja JL, et al. (2003) Increased lipopolysaccharide binding protein in cirrhotic patients with marked immune and hemodynamic derangement. Hepatology 37: 208–217.
36. Stahl W, Bracht H, Radermacher P, Thomas J (2010) Year in review 2009: Critical Care–shock. Crit Care 14: 239.
37. Hunter JD, Doddi M (2010) Sepsis and the heart. Br J Anaesth 104: 3–11.
38. Nazar A, Guevara M, Sitges M, Terra C, Sola E, et al. (2013) LEFT ventricular function assessed by echocardiography in cirrhosis: relationship to systemic hemodynamics and renal dysfunction. J Hepatol 58: 51–57.
39. Ruiz-Del-Arbol L, Achecar L, Serradilla R, Rodriguez-Gandia MA, Rivero M, et al. (2013) Diastolic dysfunction is a predictor of poor outcomes in patients with cirrhosis, portal hypertension, and a normal creatinine. Hepatology 58: 1732–1741.
40. Dahl EK, Moller S, Kjaer A, Petersen CL, Bendtsen F, et al. (2014) Diastolic and autonomic dysfunction in early cirrhosis: a dobutamine stress study. Scand J Gastroenterol 49: 362–372.
41. Schrier RW, Ecder T (2001) Gibbs memorial lecture. Unifying hypothesis of body fluid volume regulation: implications for cardiac failure and cirrhosis. Mt Sinai J Med 68: 350–361.
42. Moller S, Henriksen JH (2008) Cardiovascular complications of cirrhosis. Gut 57: 268–278.
43. Iwakiri Y, Groszmann RJ (2006) The hyperdynamic circulation of chronic liver diseases: from the patient to the molecule. Hepatology 43: S121–S131.

14

Adjuvant Potential of Selegiline in Attenuating Organ Dysfunction in Septic Rats with Peritonitis

Cheng-Ming Tsao[1,2], Jhih-Gang Jhang[3], Shiu-Jen Chen[4,5], Shuk-Man Ka[6], Tao-Cheng Wu[7,8], Wen-Jinn Liaw[2,9], Hsieh-Chou Huang[10*ⵑ], Chin-Chen Wu[3,11*ⵑ]

1 Department of Anesthesiology, Taipei Veterans General Hospital, and National Yang-Ming University, Taipei, Taiwan, R.O.C., 2 Department of Anesthesiology, Tri-Service General Hospital, National Defense Medical Center, Taipei, Taiwan, R.O.C., 3 Department of Pharmacology, National Defense Medical Center, Taipei, Taiwan, R.O.C., 4 Department of Nursing, Kang-Ning Junior College of Medical Care and Management, Taipei, Taiwan, R.O.C., 5 Department of Physiology, National Defense Medical Center, Taipei, Taiwan, R.O.C., 6 Graduate Institute of Aerospace and Undersea Medicine, National Defense Medical Center, Taipei, Taiwan, R.O.C., 7 Division of Cardiology, Department of Medicine, Taipei Veterans General Hospital, Taipei, Taiwan, R.O.C., 8 Cardiovascular Research Center, National Yang-Ming University, Taipei, Taiwan, R.O.C., 9 Department of Anesthesiology, Tungs' Taichung MetroHarbor Hospital, Taichung, Taiwan, R.O.C., 10 Department of Anesthesiology, Cheng-Hsin General Hospital, Taipei, Taiwan, R.O.C., 11 Department of Pharmacology, Taipei Medical University, Taipei, Taiwan, R.O.C.

Abstract

Selegiline, an anti-Parkinson drug, has antioxidant and anti-apoptotic effects. To explore the effect of selegiline on sepsis, we used a clinically relevant animal model of polymicrobial sepsis. Cecal ligation and puncture (CLP) or sham operation was performed in male rats under anesthesia. Three hours after surgery, animals were randomized to receive intravenously selegiline (3 mg/kg) or an equivalent volume of saline. The administration of CLP rats with selegiline (i) increased arterial blood pressure and vascular responsiveness to norepinephrine, (ii) reduced plasma liver and kidney dysfunction, (iii) attenuated metabolic acidosis, (iv) decreased neutrophil infiltration in liver and lung, and (v) improved survival rate (from 44% to 65%), compared to those in the CLP alone rats. The CLP-induced increases of plasma interleukin-6, organ superoxide levels, and liver inducible nitric oxide synthase and caspase-3 expressions were ameliorated by selegiline treatment. In addition, the histological changes in liver and lung were significantly attenuated in the selegiline -treated CLP group compared to those in the CLP group. The improvement of organ dysfunction and survival through reducing inflammation, oxidative stress and apoptosis in peritonitis-induced sepsis by selegiline has potential as an adjuvant agent for critical ill.

Editor: Cordula M. Stover, University of Leicester, United Kingdom

Funding: This work supported by grants from National Science Council, Taiwan, R.O.C. (NSC 97-2320-B-016-006-MY3, 98-2314-B-075-005-MY3 and 100-2320-B-016-008) and Cheng Hsin General Hospital, Taiwan, R.O.C. (CHGH 99-61). The funders had no role in study design, data collection and analysis, decision to publish, or preparation of the manuscript.

Competing Interests: The authors have declared that no competing interests exist.

* Email: hc1.huang@xuite.net (HCH); ccwu@office365.ndmctsgh.edu.tw (CCW)

ⵑ These authors contributed equally to this work.

Introduction

Despite advances in critical care medicine, sepsis continues to be a serious clinical entity with mortality rate still 30–50% for severe sepsis [1]. Numerous clinical trials of cytokine-specific therapies failed to improve survival in patients with sepsis, however recently, using pharmacological modulators to suppress apoptosis has been shown a striking efficacy in animal models of sepsis [2–5].

Selegiline (SEL, L-deprenyl), a monoamine oxidase-B (MAO-B) inhibitor, is a useful anti-Parkinson drug both in monotherapy and as an adjunct to levodopa therapy [6–8]. The MAO-B inhibitor could protect neuronal cells by its antioxidant and anti-apoptotic effects [9,10]. The neuroprotection effects of SEL in laboratory models may be associated with the decrease of oxidative stress, stabilization of mitochondria a)nd prevention of pro-apoptotic signaling process [11,12]. In addition to the treatment of neurodegenerative disorder, SEL reduces brain damage and enhances recovery after stroke in rats and humans [13–15]. Moreover, SEL increases free radical elimination and apoptosis

suppression in aged liver and collapsing heart [16,17]. SEL has been also shown to reduce vascular permeability and lung injury in a rodent hemorrhagic shock model, mostly due its anti-apoptotic action [18]. However, no studies have shown the impact of SEL at attenuating organ dysfunction and increasing survival in sepsis. In the current study, we have tested, using a rat model of cecal ligation and puncture (CLP)-induced sepsis, the hypothesis that SEL improved survival in an intra-abdominal sepsis via its antioxidant and anti-apoptotic effects.

Materials and Methods

Rat model of sepsis

Seventy-two male Wistar rats (280–350 g) were used in this study. All work was approved by the Committee on the Ethics of Animal Experiments of Cheng-Hsin General Hospital (Permit Number: CHGH 99-61), and the care and handling of the animals were in adherence to the National Institutes of Health Guidelines for ethical animal treatment. Rats were bred and maintained under a 12-h light/dark cycle at a controlled temperature $(21 \pm 2°C)$ with free access to food and tap water.

Surgical procedures

Catheter placements of left carotid artery and right jugular vein were performed for blood pressure measuring and drugs administering, respectively. The catheters were cannulated and exteriorized to the back of the neck under anesthesia of intraperitoneal sodium pentobarbital (40–50 mg/kg) and inhalational isoflurane (0.5%–1%) given via nosecone. After surgery, the cannulated animals were allowed to recover to the normal condition overnight with standardized pellet food and tap water *ad libitum*.

The intraperitoneal sepsis was induced by CLP using methods described previously [19]. Briefly, a midline laparotomy was performed under anesthesia of intravenous pentobarbital and inhalational isoflurane. The exposed cecum was ligated with a 3-0 silk ligature just distal to the ileocecal valve, punctured twice at opposite ends with an 18-gauge needle. The cecum was replaced into the abdominal cavity and the abdominal incision was closed. In addition, 0.2% lidocaine was used to infiltrate surgical wound in each rat after incision closure for post-operative analgesia. The rats in sham control were performed laparotomy and cecal exposure without any other manipulation. All animals immediately received normal saline solution (20 mL/kg subcutaneous) after operation.

Experimental design

Animals were divided into four groups: (1) sham operation (SOP) group: 0.9% saline (3 mL/kg intravenous for 10 min) at 3 h after sham operation, (2) SOP + SEL: SEL (3 mg/kg intravenous for 10 min) at 3 h after sham operation, (3) CLP group: same regimen of saline at 3 h after CLP surgery, and (4) CLP + SEL group: same regiment of SEL at 3 h after CLP surgery. The dose of SEL 3 mg/kg used in this study was based on our preliminary data showing that it was effective on reducing the superoxide level raised by CLP surgery in liver and lung, while 1 mg/kg of SEL did not improve the survival of CLP rats. SEL (Sigma-Aldrich, St. Louis, MO, USA) was dissolved in 0.9% saline at the concentration of 1 mg/mL.

All rats enrolled in the study were kept in the small in-house animal facility of our institute to enable optimal monitoring: the overall health status was checked every 2–3 h for signs of distress. As suggested by Nemzek et al. [20], we followed a more accurate, empirically established set of guidelines that offered, although a very narrow, yet a feasible window of opportunity for induction of death. Specifically, rats were euthanized only at the end of each experiment (at 18 h after CLP or sham surgery) or upon signs of imminent death (i.e. unresponsive to external stimuli, inability to maintain upright position/tremor and prolonged/deep hypothermia and/or agonal breathing) by using an overdose of pentobarbital (100 mg/kg, i.v.). Then, some tissue specimens of liver and lung were immediately exercised to analyze superoxide levels, Western blotting and histological changes. In addition, the survival rate at 18 h in each group was analyzed.

Measurement of hemodynamic parameters

At 0, 3, 6, 9 and 18 h after CLP or sham surgery, the carotid artery catheter was connected to a pressure transducer (P23ID, Statham, Oxnard, CA, USA) for the measurement of phasic blood pressure, mean arterial blood pressure (MAP) and heart rate, which were displayed on a polygraph recorder (MacLab/4e, AD Instruments Pty Ltd., Castle Hill, Australia). In addition, after

recording of hemodynamic parameters at 0 and 18 h, animals were intravenously given one dose of noradrenaline (NE, 1 μg/kg) to examine their pressor responses. The vasopressor reactivity was analyzed by integrating the area under the pressure waveform induced by NE bolus. In order to normalize results of pressor responses to NE in all groups, we calculated the values of pressor responses to NE at time 0 (baseline) of each group as 100%.

Quantification of organ function and injury

At 0, 9 and 18 h after CLP or sham surgery, the arterial blood samples were collected, and then immediately replaced by equal volumes of sterile saline. The total amount of blood removed was about 2.6 mL. Some blood (160 μL) was used to analyze the levels of pH, bicarbonate (HCO_3^-), arterial carbon dioxide tension ($PaCO_2$), base excess (BE) and potassium concentration by an arterial blood gas analyzer (AVL OPTI Critical Care Analyzer, AVL Scientific Corp., Roswell, GA, USA). In addition, 80 μL of plasma was used to analyze the biochemical parameters of liver (alanine aminotransferase (ALT) and aspartate aminotransferase (AST)) and renal (blood urea nitrogen (BUN) and creatinine) functions. In addition, plasma level of lactate dehydrogenase (LDH) was to evaluate the extent of tissue breakdown. All of these biochemical parameters were analyzed by Fuji DRI-CHEM 3030 (Fuji Photo Film Co., Ltd., Tokyo, Japan).

Measurement of plasma interleukin-6 concentrations

The plasma samples (150 μL) obtained at 0, 9 and 18 h were used. The plasma interleukin-6 (IL-6) was measured in duplicate with an enzyme-linked immunoadsorbent assay kit (R&D Systems, Inc., Minneapolis, MN, USA) according to the manufacturer's instructions.

Measurement of superoxide production in the plasma, liver and lung

At the end of experiment (i.e. 18 h after CLP), the plasma sample was obtained and liver and lung were freshly harvested and cleared of blood and cut into pieces. The 5×5 mm of lung and liver tissues and 100 μL of plasma were transferred to scintillation plates. These scintillation plates containing Krebs' buffer with 1.25 mM lucigenin (final volume of 250 μL) were then placed into a microplate luminometer (Hidex Microplate Luminometer, Turku, Finland) for analysis in duplicate. All tissues of liver and lung were then dried in a 95°C oven for 24 h. The results were expressed as counts per sec (in each mg of liver and lung or in each 100 μL of plasma).

Western blot analysis of tissues

Following protein isolation, equivalent amounts of protein were loaded onto a 10% (for inducible nitric oxide synthase (iNOS)) and 12% (for caspase-3) polyacrylamide gel for electrophoresis and blotting. After being blocked for 1 h at ambient temperature, the membrane was incubated overnight at 4°C with polyclonal anti-mouse iNOS antibody (BD Transduction Laboratories, Lexington, KY, USA) or polyclonal anti-rabbit cleaved caspase 3 antibody (Cell Signaling Technology, Danvers, CO, USA) at a 1: 1000 dilution. The blots were washed and incubated with horseradish-peroxidase-coupled secondary antibody (diluted 1:1500; BD Transduction Laboratories, Lexington, KY, USA) for 1 h at ambient temperature. The blots were then stripped and reprobed with β-actin antibody (1:3000; BD Transduction Laboratories, Lexington, KY, USA) as internal control. Immunoreactivity was visualized using an enhanced chemiluminescence reaction kit

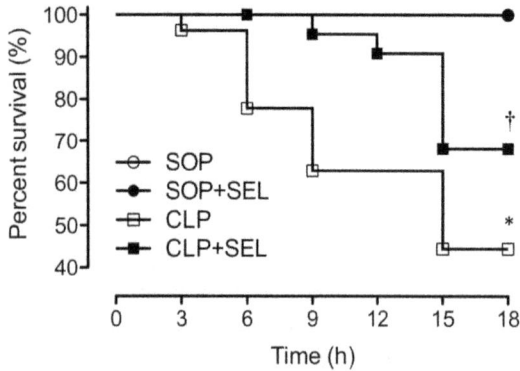

Figure 1. Administration of selegiline (SEL) improves survival after polymicrobial sepsis. A graph of the Kaplan-Meier survival of rats which received sham operation (SOP, n = 11), SOP and selegine administration (SOP + SEL, 3 mg/kg, i.v. at 3 h after SOP, n = 11), cecal ligation and puncture plus saline (CLP, n = 27) and CLP and SEL administration (CLP + SEL, 3 mg/kg, i.v. at 3 h after CLP, n = 23). The survival time was recorded for 18 hrs. *$P<0.05$, CLP vs. SOP; †$P<0.05$, with vs. without SEL in animals treated with CLP. Data are expressed as percentage of rats survived at the observed time point.

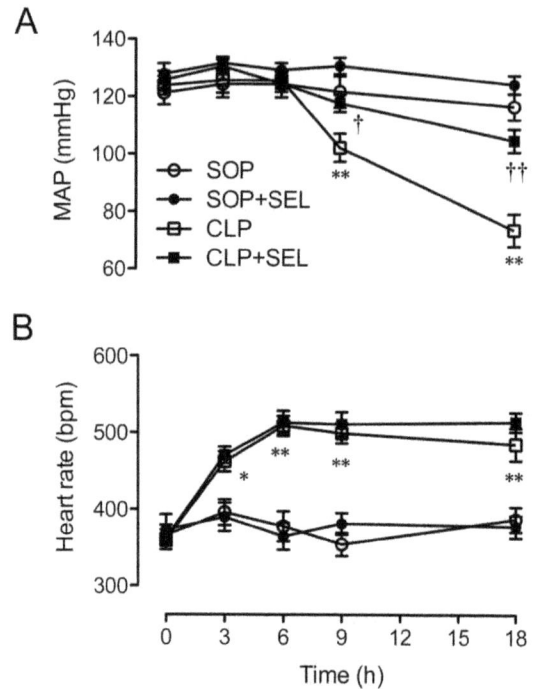

Figure 2. Effects of selegiline on hemodynamics. Alterations in (A) mean arterial pressure (MAP) and (B) heart rate during the experimental period. Rats underwent sham operation (SOP), SOP plus selegiline administration (3 mg/kg, i.v., SOP + SEL), cecal ligation and puncture (CLP), or CLP plus SEL administration (3 mg/kg, i.v., CLP + SEL). Data are expressed as mean ± SEM, n = 10 in each group for all time-points. *$p<0.05$ and **$p<0.01$, CLP vs. SOP; †$p<0.05$ and ††$p<0.01$, with vs. without SEL in animals treated with CLP.

(Amersham Pharmacia Biotech, Buckinghamshire, UK) and quantified by scanning densitometer.

Histological assessment

Specimens of liver and lung were harvested for histological analysis as previously described [19]. Briefly, the fixed tissues were dehydrated and embedded in paraffin. Each paraffin block was processed into 4-μm-thick slices that were stained with hematoxylin and eosin. This histological alteration was quantitatively analyzed as an index of the severity of neutrophil infiltration in 5 animals of each group. The index was determined by counting the numbers of neutrophil in 10 randomly selected high-power fields evaluated by a pathologist in a blinded fashion.

Cell cultures and cell viability assay

Human aortic endothelial cells (HAECs, Cascade Biologics) were grown in Medium 200 (Cascade Biologics) supplemented with low serum growth supplement (Cascade Biologics) in an atmosphere of 95% air and 5% CO_2 at 37°C in plastic flasks. The final concentrations of the components in Medium 200 contained 2% fetal bovine serum (Gibco–BRL), 1 μg/mL hydrocortisone, 10 ng/mL human epidermal growth factor, 3 ng/mL human fibroblast growth factor, 10 μg/mL heparin, and 1% antibiotic–antimycotic mixture (Gibco–BRL). At confluence, the cells were subcultured at a ratio 1:3 and used at passage numbers 3–8. Cell viability was always found to be greater than 95% by using the trypan blue exclusion method or a 3-(4,5-dimethylthiazol-2- yl)-2,5-diphenyl tetrazolium bromide assay (Sigma-Aldrich).

Measurement of reactive oxygen species production

We determined the effect of SEL on reactive oxygen species (ROS) production in HAECs by fluorometric assay using 2′,7′-dichlorofluorescein diacetate (DCFH-DA, Molecular Probes) as a probe for the presence of H_2O_2. HAECs were pre-treated with SEL in 24-well plates for 18 h, and subsequently combined with 25 ng/mL of lipopolysaccharide (LPS; *E. coli* serotype 0127:B8, L3127; Sigma-Aldrich) incubation for 3 or 24 h. Cells were subjected to incubation with DCFH-DA 20 μM for 45 min after the removal of SEL. Fluorescence intensity (relative fluorescence

units) was measured at 485-nm excitation and 530-nm emission using a fluorescence micro-plate reader (VICTPR2 Multilabel Readers, USA). Incubation of SEL (1–100 μg/mL) lasting 24 h had no effect on the cell viability of HAECs.

Western Blotting analysis of HAECs

Western blot analysis was conducted to determine the changes in expression of LPS-induced iNOS by SEL. Briefly, HAECs was lysed in a buffer containing 62.5 mM Tris-HCl, 2% SDS, 10% glycerol, 0.5 mM PMSF, 2 μg/mL aprotinin, 2 μg/mL pepstatin, and 2 μg/mL leupeptin. The whole-cell lysates were subjected to SDS-polyacrylamide (8%) gel electrophoresis, followed by electro-blotting. Membranes were incubated with monoclonal anti-mouse iNOS antibody (1:1000; BD Transduction Laboratories, Lexington, KY, USA), monoclonal anti-mouse β-actin antibody (1:10000; Chemicon, Temecula, CA, USA) for overnight, and then incubated for 2 h with a secondary antibody labeled with horseradish peroxidase. Bands were visualized by chemiluminescence detection reagents (NEN Life Science Products, Boston, MA, USA). Densitometic analysis was conducted with the Image Quant (Promega) software.

Statistical analysis

The data are presented as mean ± SEM of *n* determinations, where *n* represents the number of animals studied. The distribution of the variables was assessed with a normality test. Data with a normal distribution were analyzed by a one-way analysis of variance (ANOVA) or two-way ANOVA for repeated measures followed, where appropriate, by a Bonferroni correction

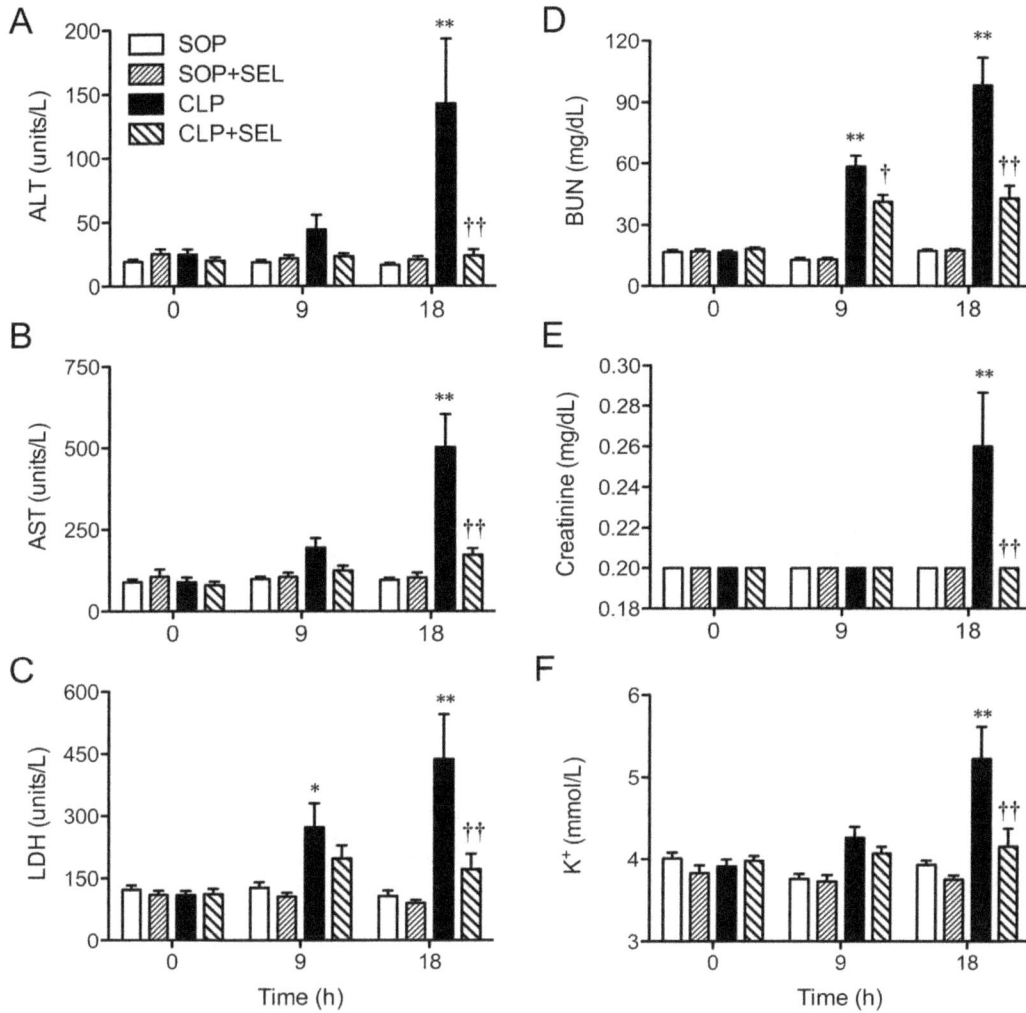

Figure 3. Effects of selegiline on organ function. Alterations in plasma levels of (A) alanine aminotransferase (ALT), (B) asparate aminotransferase (AST), (C) lactate dehydrogenase (LDH), (D) blood urea nitrogen (BUN), (E) creatinine, and (F) blood potassium concentration during the experimental period. Rats underwent sham operation (SOP), SOP plus selegiline administration (3 mg/kg, i.v., SOP + SEL), cecal ligation and puncture (CLP), or CLP plus SEL administration (3 mg/kg, i.v., CLP + SEL). Data are expressed as mean ± SEM, n = 10 in each group for all time-points. *$p < 0.05$ and **$p < 0.01$, CLP vs. SOP; †$p < 0.05$ and ††$p < 0.01$, with vs. without SEL in animals treated with CLP.

test. The score for tissue infiltration of neutrophils was compared by the Mann-Whitney U test. Kaplan-Meier estimates were constructed for overall survival, which was then analyzed by the log-rank test. A p value of less than 0.05 was considered to be statistically significant.

Materials

Unless otherwise stated all chemicals used were purchased from Sigma-Aldrich.

Results

Survival rate

No mortality was observed within 18 h in all SOP rats (n = 11 in each SOP group, figure 1). The survival rate was significantly decreased to 63% and 44% (i.e. 17/27 and 12/27 animals) at 9 and 18 h after CLP, respectively, whereas SEL (3 mg/kg) significantly increased the survival of CLP-treated rats to 96%

and 65% (i.e., 22/23 and 15/23 animals) at 9 and 18 h ($p < 0.05$, vs. CLP group). However, 1 mg/kg of SEL did not improve the survival of CLP rats in our preliminary data. Because of clot or kinking of arterial catheter, blood could not be withdrawn for above tests in some of rats, esp. in rats with CLP surgery.

Systemic hemodynamic parameters

As results shown in Fig. 2, the baseline values for MAP and heart rate among all groups were comparable. The CLP surgery led to a significantly substantial attenuation in MAP at 18 h ($p < 0.01$, vs. SOP group; Fig. 2A), whereas significant and sustained increases in heart rate was observed from 3 h after CLP ($p < 0.05$ or < 0.01, vs. SOP group; Fig. 2B). The treatment with SEL significantly prevented the severe hypotension at 18 h after CLP ($p < 0.01$, vs. CLP group). However, the CLP-induced tachycardia was not attenuated in rats treated with SEL. The SOP rats treated with saline or SEL exhibited stable hemodynamic conditions during the experimental period and there was no significant

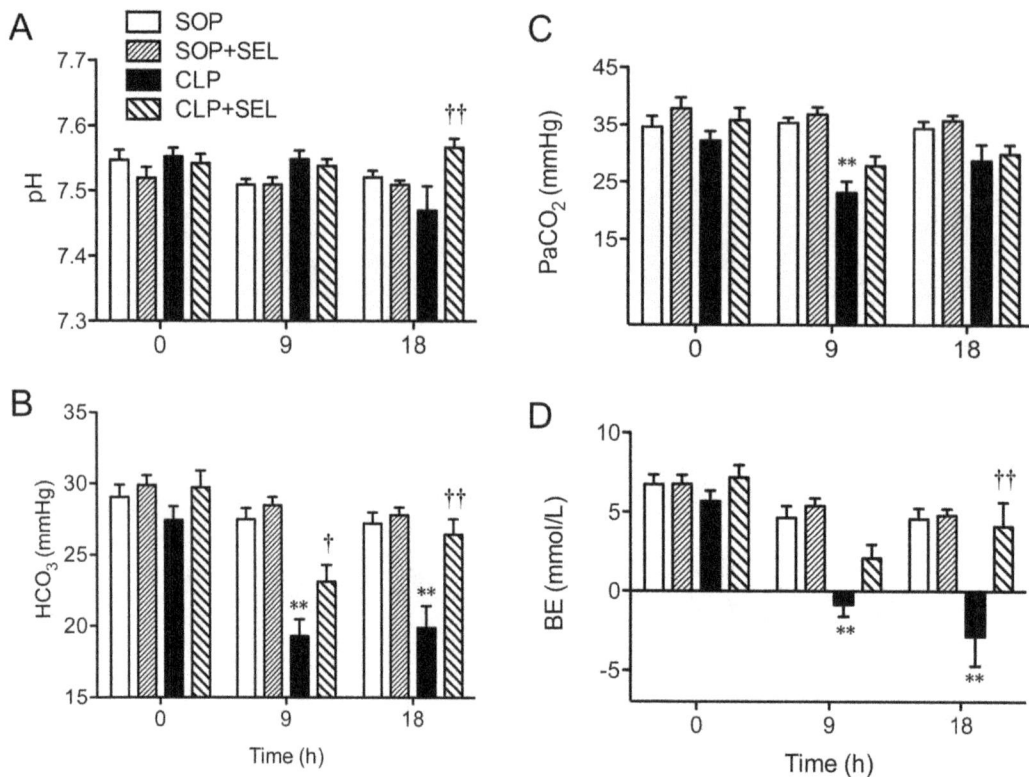

Figure 4. Effects of selegiline on blood potassium concentration and metabolic acidosis. Alterations in arterial blood levels of (A) pH, (B) bicarbonate (HCO_3^-), (C) carbon dioxide tension ($PaCO_2$), and (D) base excess (BE) during the experimental period. Rats underwent sham operation (SOP), SOP plus selegiline administration (3 mg/kg, i.v., SOP + SEL), cecal ligation and puncture (CLP), or CLP plus SEL administration (3 mg/kg, i.v., CLP + SEL). Data are expressed as mean ± SEM, n = 10 in each group for all time-points. **$p < 0.01$, CLP vs. SOP; †$p < 0.05$ and ††$p < 0.01$, with vs. without SEL in animals treated with CLP.

difference between both groups. In addition, the pressor response to NE at 18 h was significantly decreased to 19.5±2.3% of baseline in CLP rats ($p < 0.01$, vs. SOP group), which was attenuated by SEL (42.9±5% of baseline; $p < 0.01$, vs. CLP group). In SOP rats, the pressor response to NE at 18 h was 100.4±7.2% of baseline.

Biochemical and blood gas parameters

Baseline values of plasma biochemical and blood gas parameters were not significantly different among all groups. The administration of SEL in the SOP groups had little effect on the biochemical and gas parameters during the experimental period.

The CLP surgery caused time–dependent increases in plasma levels of ALT, AST, LDH, BUN, and creatinine ($p < 0.05$ or 0.01, vs. SOP group; Fig. 3). These increases were significantly attenuated by the treatment of CLP rats with SEL ($p < 0.01$, vs. CLP group), indicating that SEL ameliorates liver and kidney injuries induced by CLP. There was no difference in blood potassium concentration in all SOP rats. The rats treated with CLP caused hyperkalemia at 18 h ($p < 0.01$, vs. SOP group; Fig. 3F). However, this hyperkalemia induced by CLP were ameliorated by SEL ($p < 0.01$, vs. CLP group).

There was no difference in blood pH, HCO_3^-, $PaCO_2$ and BE in all SOP rats. The pH level in CLP rats was decreased at 18 h, although it was not significant. However, the rats treated with CLP for 18 h caused significant decreases of HCO_3^- and $PaCO_2$ and decreases of BE at 9 and 18 h ($p < 0.01$, vs. SOP group; Fig. 4).

This indicates that CLP-induced sepsis causes compensated metabolic acidosis. However, this decrease of HCO_3^- level induced by CLP was ameliorated by SEL at 9 h and 18 h ($p < 0.05$ and $p < 0.01$, respectively, vs. CLP group).

Plasma IL-6 and superoxide levels in the plasma, liver, and lung

In the SOP groups, no significant increase in plasma IL-6 level was observed during the experimental period, indicating that sham surgery and SEL treatment almost have no effect on plasma IL-6 level. The animals received CLP showed a significantly increase in the plasma level of IL-6 at 9 h ($p < 0.01$, vs. SOP group; Fig. 5A), and then declined to near baseline level. However, the treatment of CLP rats with SEL significantly attenuated the increases in plasma IL-6 level at 9 h ($p < 0.01$, vs. CLP group; Fig. 5A).

As results shown in Fig. 5B, animals received CLP had variable increases in the superoxide levels of plasma ($p < 0.01$), liver ($p < 0.05$) and lung ($p < 0.01$), whereas the treatment of CLP rats with SEL significantly attenuated the production of superoxide in these specimens. However, SEL alone had no effect on the changes of these superoxide levels in the SOP group.

iNOS and cleaved caspase-3 expression in tissues

The protein expression of iNOS was detectable in liver and lung homogenates obtained from the SOP groups, whereas a significant induction of iNOS protein was observed from the CLP rats ($p <$

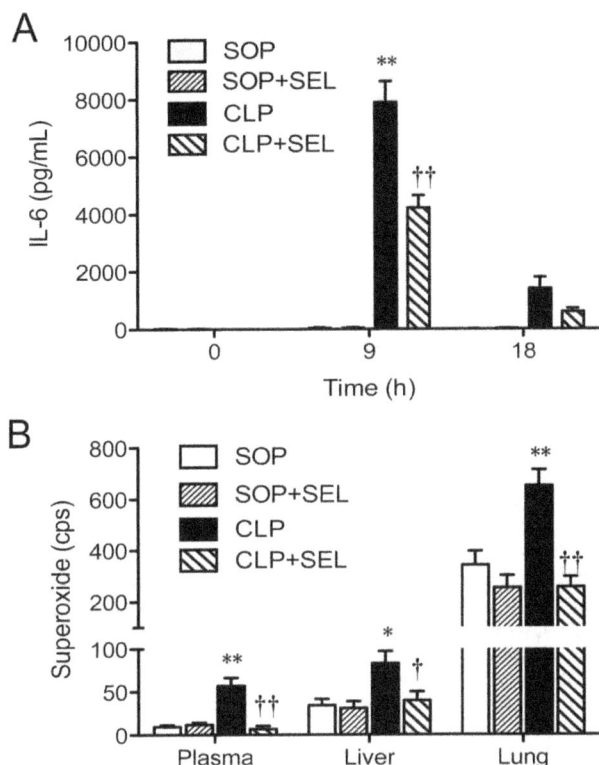

Figure 5. Effects of selegiline on interleukin-6 and superoxide levels. Alterations in (A) plasma interleukin-6 (IL-6) levels during the experimental period and (B) superoxide levels in plasma, liver and lung at 18 h after surgery. Rats underwent sham operation (SOP), SOP plus selegiline administration (3 mg/kg, i.v., SOP + SEL), cecal ligation and puncture (CLP), or CLP plus SEL administration (3 mg/kg, i.v., CLP + SEL). Data are expressed as mean ± SEM, n = 10 in each group for all time-points. *$p<0.05$ and **$p<0.01$, CLP vs. SOP; †$p<0.05$ and ††$p<0.01$, with vs. without SEL in animals treated with CLP.

0.01 in the liver and $p<0.05$ in the lung, vs. SOP group; Fig. 6A). The treatment of CLP rats with SEL significantly reduced the expression of iNOS ($p<0.05$, vs. CLP group) in liver and lung. The expression of caspase-3 was significantly higher in liver from the CLP group than from the SOP group ($p<0.01$; Fig. 6B), whereas the treatment of CLP rats with SEL significantly reduced this caspase-3 expression ($p<0.01$, vs. CLP group). However, the protein expression of caspase-3 in lung homogenates was not different among all groups (Fig. 6B).

Histopathological changes and neutrophil filtration

Stained specimens from CLP rats revealed (i) increased interstitial edema and marked necrosis in the liver (Fig. 7), and (ii) increased interstitial edema and decreased alveolar spaces in the lung compared to those from the SOP group (Fig. 8). However, the histopathological changes in these tissues were attenuated after SEL treatment. Light microscopy only showed a little infiltration or sequestration of neutrophil in liver and lung from the SOP group, whereas overt infiltrations of neutrophil in these tissues were observed in CLP rats (2.8±0.2 in liver and 3.2±0.2 in lung; $p<0.05$). However, in CLP rats treated with SEL, the neutrophil infiltrations were significantly reduced (1.6±0.4 in liver and 2±0.3 in lung; $p<0.05$).

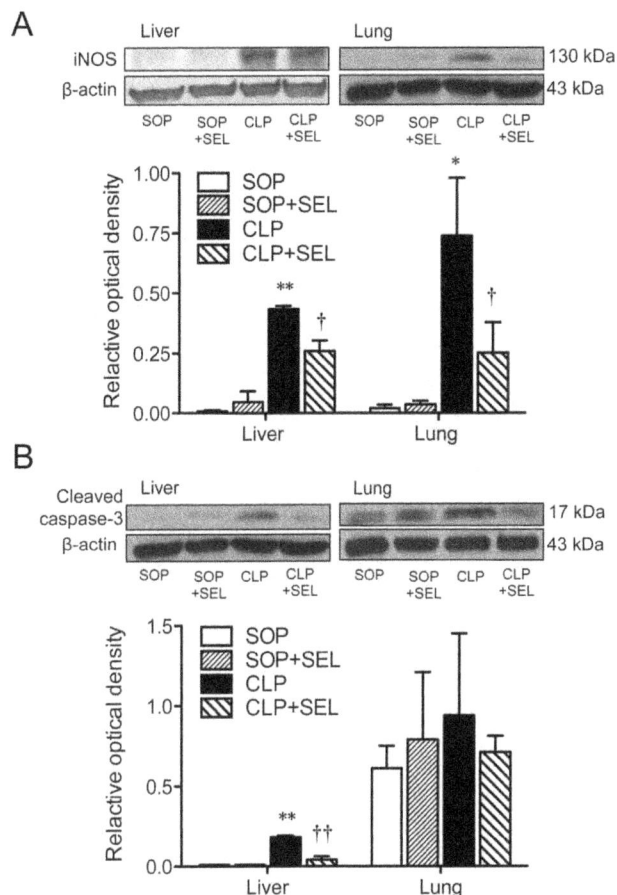

Figure 6. Immunoblot analysis of inducible nitric oxide synthase and cleaved caspase-3 expression in tissues. Rats underwent sham operation (SOP), SOP plus selegiline administration (3 mg/kg, i.v., SOP + SEL), cecal ligation and puncture (CLP), or CLP plus SEL administration (3 mg/kg, i.v., CLP + SEL). Liver and lung tissues were harvested at 18 h after surgery. The summary of quantification of densitometric measurement as ratio of (A) inducible nitric oxide synthase (iNOS) and (B) cleaved caspase-3 relative to β-actin is presented. Typical Western blots are shown on the upper panel of each figure. β-actin served as loading control. Data expressed as mean ± SEM, n = 3 in each group. *$p<0.05$ and **$p<0.01$, CLP vs. SOP; †$p<0.05$ and ††$p<0.01$, with vs. without SEL in animals treated with CLP.

ROS generation and iNOS expression in LPS-cultured HAECs

In the present study, intracellular ROS generation was increased by LPS and was unaffected by the pretreatment of SEL (0.1–10 µg/mL) (Figure 9). Western blot analysis also showed that pretreatment of HAECs with SEL (10 µg/mL) significantly increased endothelial iNOS expression (Fig. 10) in the conditioned medium.

Discussion

In this study, the administration of CLP-induced sepsis rats with SEL (3 mg/kg, i.v.) (i) increased arterial blood pressure and pressor response to NE, (ii) reduced plasma levels of biochemical parameters, (iii) attenuated metabolic acidosis and hyperkalemia, and (iv) ameliorated histopathological changes. This study provides novel evidence that the application of SEL seems to improve survival in the CLP-induced sepsis rats as a consequence

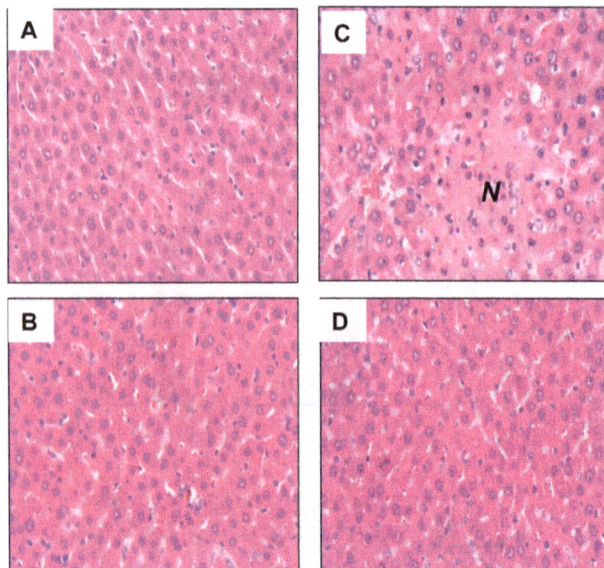

Figure 7. Histological analysis of liver. Liver tissue section stained with hematoxylin and eosin. Rats underwent (A) sham operation (SOP), (B) SOP plus SEL administration (3 mg/kg, i.v., SOP + SEL), (C) cecal ligation and puncture (CLP), or (D) CLP plus SEL administration (3 mg/kg, i.v., CLP + SEL). Tissues were harvested at 18 h after surgery. *N* indicates necrosis area. Shown are representative micrographs from 5 independent experiments in which the same results were obtained. Each, 400 X (original magnification).

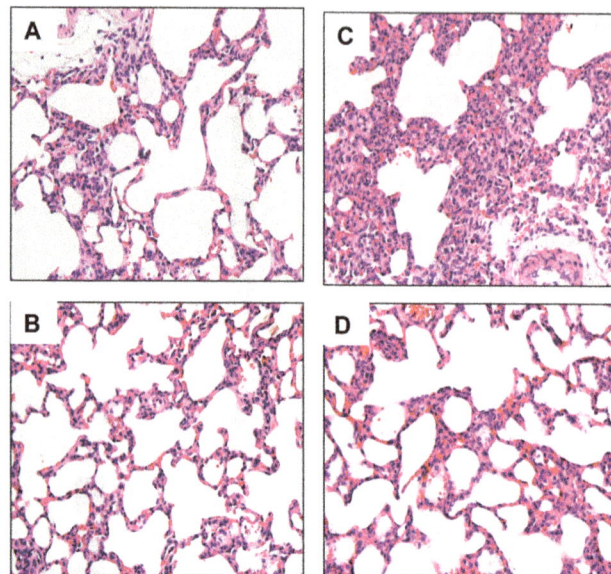

Figure 8. Histological analysis of lung. Lung tissue section stained with hematoxylin and eosin. Rats underwent (A) sham operation (SOP), (B) SOP plus SEL administration (3 mg/kg, i.v., SOP + SEL), (C) cecal ligation and puncture (CLP), or (D) CLP plus SEL administration (3 mg/kg, i.v., CLP + SEL). Shown are representative micrographs from 5 independent experiments in which the same results were obtained. Each, 400 X (original magnification).

of reduced dysfunction/injury of multiple organs. This could be due to attenuation of IL-6 production and superoxide formation and suppression of iNOS and caspase-3 expression by SEL in animals with CLP-induced sepsis.

This CLP-induced sepsis model, characterized by a biphasic process, mimics many of the pathophysiologic features of clinically relevant polymicrobial sepsis [21,22]. An early phase results from a surge of the unbridled reactive oxygen and nitrogen species and proinflammatory cytokines mediated primarily by neutrophils, macrophages and monocytes, whereas a late phase is marked by a sustained immunosuppressive response induced primarily by apoptosis of immune, epithelial and/or endothelial cells [23–26].

Although multiple reactive oxygen and nitrogen species produced by neutrophils and macrophages for killing invading bacteria in the body, these species can also damage host tissues when they are produced superfluously. Furthermore, together with increased amounts of nitric oxide (NO) that are produced by the iNOS, superoxide forms the highly reactive peroxynitrite that induces irreversible damage to proteins, causing mitochondrial dysfunction and organ failure [27]. Our present study demonstrated that superoxide production and iNOS expression were increased in CLP-induced septic rats, which were attenuated by SEL administration. These observations are consistent with previous studies showing that SEL prevents the increase of oxidative products in microvascular endothelial cells exposed to burn serum [28]. However, in our *in vitro* study, pretreatment of SEL (0.1–10 µg/mL) did not attenuate intracellular ROS generation and endothelial iNOS expression in HAECs treated with LPS. Similarly, Chakravarti *et al.* also revealed that 5 nM deprenyl (i.e. SEL) in cultures of RAW 264.7 cells did not affect iNOS expression [29]. Moreover, it has been shown that pro-inflammatory cytokines can also induce excessive productions of reactive oxygen and nitrogen species [30]. Our *in vivo* data

showed that CLP induced a significant increase of IL-6 in the early septic phase, which was suppressed by SEL. Thus, SEL decreased the inflammatory cytokine levels and the infiltration by neutrophils in organs (e.g. livers and lungs in this study) from sepsis animals. It has been shown that such neutrophil infiltration can lead to vascular dysfunction as well as parenchymal cell injury [31]. Based on these observations, we suggest that SEL prevents organ injury in sepsis most likely by its anti-inflammatory properties.

Indeed, we showed that SEL reduced the increased plasma levels of AST and ALT caused by CLP, which are intracellular

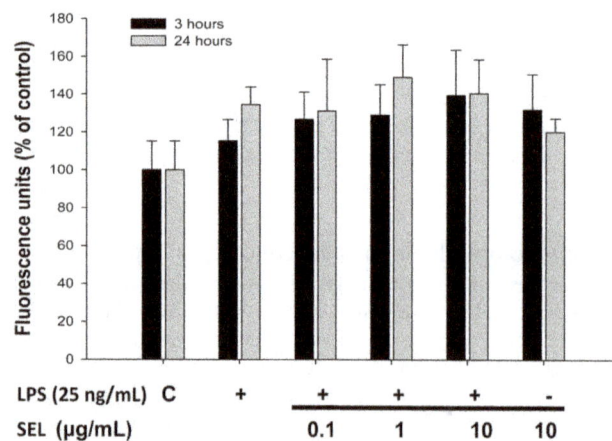

Figure 9. Effects of selegiline on reactive oxygen species in HAECs. Generation of reactive oxygen species induced by lipopolysaccharide (LPS) was unaffected by the treatment of selegiline (SEL) in HAECs. HAECs were pre-incubated with SEL for 18 h, followed by the incubation in 25 ng/mL of LPS for 3 or 24 h. Data are expressed as mean ± SEM of three independent experiments.

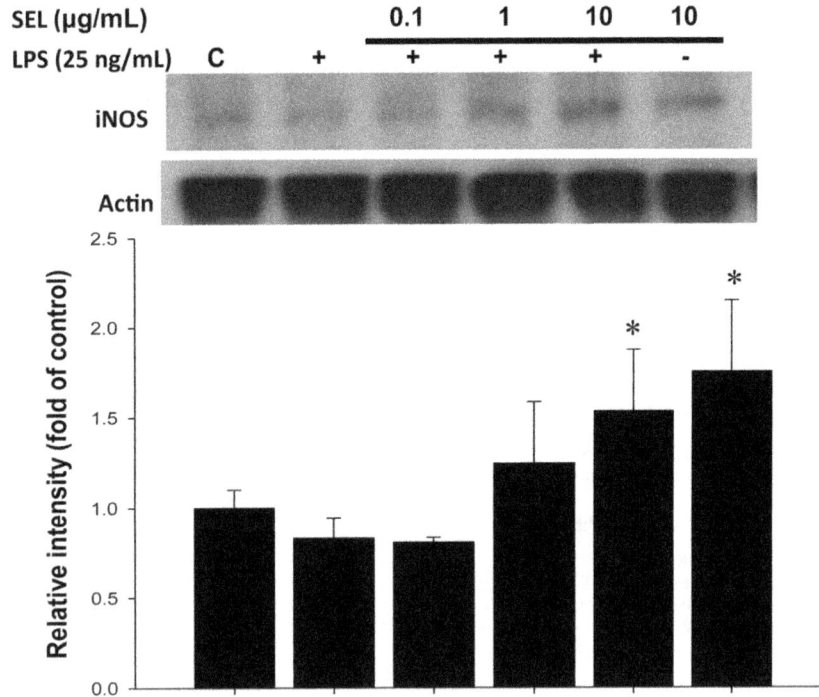

Figure 10. Immunoblot analysis of inducible nitric oxide synthase expression in HAECs. Selegiline (SEL) enhanced the iNOS expression in lipopolysaccharide (LPS)-cultured HAECs. HAECs were pre-treated with SEL for 18 h, and subsequently incubated in 25 ng/mL of LPS for 24 h. Data are expressed as mean ± SEM of three independent experiments. *$p < 0.05$ compared to LPS alone.

components of liver and released into serum during ongoing cell damage. This is consistent with the histological finding showing necrotic cells in the liver from CLP rats. There is increasing evidence that, in addition to cellular necrosis, the apoptotic mode of cell death also plays a pivotal role in the pathogenesis of sepsis syndrome [24,32]. Apoptotic cell death occurs primarily through extrinsic death-receptor pathway and/or intrinsic mitochondria pathway, which can be activated by diverse stimuli, including cytokines and free radicals [33]. The extrinsic or intrinsic pathway can activate caspase-3, leading to the degradation of cellular proteins and the destruction of cell integrity [34]. It has been shown that SEL reduces apoptosis by modulating Bcl-2 and BAX and inhibiting caspase-3 activity in a number of cell types [11,16,28]. Indeed, the decreased of the caspase-3 protein expression was also observed in the liver of the CLP + SEL group compared to that of the CLP group of animals in our present study. These results suggest that the beneficial effect of SEL on inflammation, tissue injury or apoptosis is further strengthened by the favorable survival outcome in the CLP group. The SEL-treated CLP animals had a 21% survival benefit over CLP controls.

In our study, SEL could attenuated caspase 3 expression in the liver of septic rats at 18 h after CLP, but not in the lung tissue. However, Tharaken et al. showed that SEL could prevent activation of caspase-3 in mesenteric vasculature in rats with hemorrhagic shock followed by 60 min of resuscitation [18]. Therefore, different experimental model, time point, and tissues may result in different effects of SEL on the caspase 3 expression.

It has been shown that amphetamine-like drugs, such as SEL and its major metabolites, L-methamphetamine and L-amphetamine, cause tachycardia [35,36], hypotension [37,38] or hypertension [39]. Allard et al. report that 3 mg/kg of SEL induces only a transient decrease in blood pressure, which returns to its baseline value after 4 min [40]. In addition, anorexia/nausea, musculoskeletal injuries, and cardiac arrhythmias occurred more often in patients receiving SEL compared with those receiving placebo [41]. Apart from these adverse effects, increased rates of elevated serum AST and ALT levels were noted [41]. However, 3 mg/kg of SEL used in this study neither affected MAP and heart rate, nor changed serum AST and ALT levels in sham control rats during the experimental period.

However, the current study has some limitations which need to be addressed. First, only one single intravenous dose of SEL was used, and consequently, we cannot exclude the possibility that multiple doses or continuous infusion could yield better outcome. Second, SEL was given at 3 h after CLP, nevertheless, the effect of SEL used in the late phase of sepsis is unknown. Third, this experimental sepsis model could not lead to profound hypoxemia at the end of study, indicating that the CLP is not a suitable experimental model of acute lung injury with significant blood gas exchange impairment, including a severe hypoxemic condition.

In conclusion, we used the most clinically relevant sepsis model to monitor sepsis-induced multiple organ dysfunction, and our findings support the hypothesis that SEL improved survival, minimized histological changes and prevented sepsis-induced multiple organ dysfunction by its anti-inflammatory and anti-apoptosis properties. This was based on the attenuation of IL-6 and superoxide production as well as the reduction of iNOS and caspase-3 expression in various tissues by SEL in animals with sepsis. Thus, we suggest that SEL could be a potential adjuvant for protecting tissues from oxidative stress and preventing organ dysfunction caused by CLP-induced sepsis.

Supporting Information

Checklist S1   The ARRIVE Guidelines Checklist.

References

1. Schlichting D, McCollam JS (2007) Recognizing and managing severe sepsis: a common and deadly threat. South Med J 100: 594–600.

2. Fisher CJ Jr, Agosti JM, Opal SM, Lowry SF, Balk RA, et al. (1996) Treatment of septic shock with the tumor necrosis factor receptor:Fc fusion protein. The Soluble TNF Receptor Sepsis Study Group. N Engl J Med 334: 1697–1702.

3. Hotchkiss RS, Swanson PE, Knudson CM, Chang KC, Cobb JP, et al. (1999) Overexpression of Bcl-2 in transgenic mice decreases apoptosis and improves survival in sepsis. J Immunol 162: 4148–4156.

4. Hotchkiss RS, Chang KC, Swanson PE, Tinsley KW, Hui JJ, et al. (2000) Caspase inhibitors improve survival in sepsis: a critical role of the lymphocyte. Nat Immunol 1: 496–501.

5. Bommhardt U, Chang KC, Swanson PE, Wagner TH, Tinsley KW, et al. (2004) Akt decreases lymphocyte apoptosis and improves survival in sepsis. J Immunol 172: 7583–7591.

6. Hauser RA (2009) New considerations in the medical management of early Parkinson's disease: impact of recent clinical trials on treatment strategy. Parkinsonism Relat Disord 15 Suppl 3: S17–21.

7. Chen JJ (2010) Parkinson's disease: health-related quality of life, economic cost, and implications of early treatment. Am J Manag Care 16 Suppl: S87–93.

8. Mizuno Y, Kondo T, Kuno S, Nomoto M, Yanagisawa N (2010) Early addition of selegiline to L-Dopa treatment is beneficial for patients with Parkinson disease. Clin Neuropharmacol 33: 1–4.

9. Nagatsu T, Sawada M (2006) Molecular mechanism of the relation of monoamine oxidase B and its inhibitors to Parkinson's disease: possible implications of glial cells. J Neural Transm Suppl 71: 53–65.

10. Naoi M, Maruyama W, Yi H, Inaba K, Akao Y (2009) Mitochondria in neurodegenerative disorders: regulation of the redox state and death signaling leading to neuronal death and survival. J Neural Transm 116: 1371–1381.

11. Tatton W, Chalmers-Redman R, Tatton N (2003) Neuroprotection by deprenyl and other propargylamines: glyceraldehyde-3-phosphate dehydrogenase rather than monoamine oxidase B. J Neural Transm 110: 509–515.

12. Magyar K, Szende B (2004) (-)-Deprenyl, a selective MAO-B inhibitor, with apoptotic and anti-apoptotic properties. Neurotoxicology 25: 233–242.

13. Knollema S, Aukema W, Hom H, Korf J, ter Horst GJ (1995) L-deprenyl reduces brain damage in rats exposed to transient hypoxia-ischemia. Stroke 26: 1883–1887.

14. Simon L, Szilagyi G, Bori Z, Orbay P, Nagy Z (2001) (-)-D-Deprenyl attenuates apoptosis in experimental brain ischaemia. Eur J Pharmacol 430: 235–241.

15. Sivenius J, Sarasoja T, Aaltonen H, Heinonen E, Kilkku O, et al. (2001) Selegiline treatment facilitates recovery after stroke. Neurorehabil. Neural Repair 15: 183–190.

16. Qin F, Shite J, Mao W, Liang CS (2003) Selegiline attenuates cardiac oxidative stress and apoptosis in heart failure: association with improvement of cardiac function. Eur J Pharmacol 461: 149–158.

17. Kiray M, Ergur BU, Bagriyanik A, Pekcetin C, Aksu I, et al. (2007) Suppression of apoptosis and oxidative stress by deprenyl and estradiol in aged rat liver. Acta Histochem 109: 480–485.

18. Tharakan B, Whaley JG, Hunter FA, Smythe WR, Childs EW (2010) (-)-Deprenyl inhibits vascular hyperpermeability after hemorrhagic shock. Shock. 33: 56–63.

19. Tsao CM, Chen SJ, Shih MC, Lue WM, Tsou MY, et al. (2010) Effects of terbutaline on circulatory failure and organ dysfunction induced by peritonitis in rats. Intensive Care Med 36: 1571–1578.

20. Nemzek JA, Xiao HY, Minard AE, Bolgos GL, Remick DG (2004) Humane endpoints in shock research. Shock 21: 17–25.

21. Oberholzer A, Oberholzer C, Moldawer LL (2001a) Sepsis syndromes: understanding the role of innate and acquired immunity. Shock 16: 83–96.

22. Yang S, Chung CS, Ayala A, Chaudry IH, Wang P (2002) Differential alterations in cardiovascular responses during the progression of polymicrobial sepsis in the mouse. Shock 17: 55–60.

23. Oberholzer A, Oberholzer C, Clare-Salzler M, Moldawer LL (2001b) Apoptosis in sepsis: a new target for therapeutic exploration. FASEB J 15: 879–892.

24. Hattori Y, Takano K, Teramae H, Yamamoto S, Yokoo H, et al. (2010) Insights into sepsis therapeutic design based on the apoptotic death pathway. J Pharmacol Sci 114: 354–365.

25. Olguner CG, Koca U, Altekin E, Ergür BU, Duru S, et al. (2013) Ischemic preconditioning attenuates lipid peroxidation and apoptosis in the cecal ligation and puncture model of sepsis. Exp Ther Med 5: 1581–1588.

26. Tsai KL, Liang HJ, Yang ZD, Lue SI, Yang SL, et al. (2014) Early inactivation of PKCε associates with late mitochondrial translocation of Bad and apoptosis in ventricle of septic rat. J Surg Res 186: 278–286.

27. Alvarez S, Evelson PA (2007) Nitric oxide and oxygen metabolism in inflammatory conditions: sepsis and exposition to polluted ambients. Front Biosci 12: 964–974.

28. Whaley JG, Tharakan B, Smith B, Hunter FA, Childs EW (2009) (-)-Deprenyl inhibits thermal injury-induced apoptotic signaling and hyperpermeability in microvascular endothelial cells. J Burn Care Res 30: 1018–1027.

29. Chakravarti R, Aulak KS, Fox PL, Stuehr DJ (2010) GAPDH regulates cellular heme insertion into inducible nitric oxide synthase. Proc Natl Acad Sci USA 107: 18004–18009.

30. Morgan MJ, Liu ZG (2011) Crosstalk of reactive oxygen species and NF-kappaB signaling. Cell Res 21: 103–115.

31. Jaeschke H, Hasegawa T (2006) Role of neutrophils in acute inflammatory liver injury. Liver Int 26: 912–919.

32. Hotchkiss RS, Nicholson DW (2006) Apoptosis and caspases regulate death and inflammation in sepsis. Nat Rev Immunol 6: 813–822.

33. Wesche-Soldato DE, Swan RZ, Chung CS, Ayala A (2007) The apoptotic pathway as a therapeutic target in sepsis. Curr Drug Targets 8: 493–500.

34. Boatright KM, Salvesen GS (2003) Mechanisms of caspase activation. Curr Opin Cell Biol 15: 725–731.

35. Reynolds GP, Elsworth JD, Blau K, Sandler M, Lees AJ, et al. (1978) Deprenyl is metabolised to methamphetamine and amphetamine in man. Br J Clin Pharmacol 6: 542–544.

36. Glezer S, Finberg JP (2003) Pharmacological comparison between the actions of methamphetamine and 1-aminoindan stereoisomers on sympathetic nervous function in rat vas deferens. Eur J Pharmacol 472: 173–177.

37. Abassi ZA, Binah O, Youdim MB (2004) Cardiovascular activity of rasagiline, a selective and potent inhibitor of mitochondrial monoamine oxidase B: comparison with selegiline. Br J Pharmacol 143: 371–378.

38. Finberg JP, Gross A, Bar-Am O, Friedman R, Loboda Y, et al. (2006) Cardiovascular responses to combined treatment with selective monoamine oxidase type B inhibitors and L-DOPA in the rat. Br J Pharmacol 149: 647–656.

39. Bexis S, Docherty JR (2006) Effects of MDMA, MDA and MDEA on blood pressure, heart rate, locomotor activity and body temperature in the rat involve alpha-adrenoceptors. Br J Pharmacol 147: 926–934.

40. Allard J, Bernabe J, Derdinger F, Alexandre L, McKenna K, et al. (2002) Selegiline enhances erectile activity induced by dopamine injection in the paraventricular nucleus of the hypothalamus in anesthetised rats. Int J Impot Res 14: 518–522.

41. Yamada M, Yasuhara H (2004) Clinical pharmacology of MAO inhibitors: safety and future. Neurotoxicology 25: 215–21.

Author Contributions

Conceived and designed the experiments: CMT HCH CCW. Performed the experiments: JGJ SJC. Analyzed the data: CMT SJC WJL HCH CCW. Contributed reagents/materials/analysis tools: SMK TCW. Wrote the paper: CMT CCW.

15

Tim-3 Negatively Mediates Natural Killer Cell Function in LPS-Induced Endotoxic Shock

Hongyan Hou, Weiyong Liu, Shiji Wu, Yanjun Lu, Jing Peng, Yaowu Zhu, Yanfang Lu, Feng Wang*, Ziyong Sun*

Department of Clinical Laboratory, Tongji Hospital, Tongji Medical College, Huazhong University of Science and Technology, Wuhan, China

Abstract

Sepsis is an exaggerated inflammatory condition response to different microorganisms with high mortality rates and extremely poor prognosis. Natural killer (NK) cells have been reported to be the major producers of IFN-γ and key players in promoting systematic inflammation in lipopolysaccharide (LPS)-induced endotoxic shock. T-cell immunoglobulin and mucin domain (Tim)-3 pathway has been demonstrated to play an important role in the process of sepsis, however, the effect of Tim-3 on NK cell function remains largely unknown. In this study, we observed a dynamic inverse correlation between Tim-3 expression and IFN-γ production in NK cells from LPS-induced septic mice. Blockade of the Tim-3 pathway could increase IFN-γ production and decrease apoptosis of NK cells in vitro, but had no effect on the expression of CD107a. Furthermore, NK cell cytotoxicity against K562 target cells was enhanced after blocking Tim-3 pathway. In conclusion, our results suggest that Tim-3 pathway plays an inhibitory role in NK cell function, which might be a potential target in modulating the excessive inflammatory response of LPS-induced endotoxic shock.

Editor: Laurel L. Lenz, University of Colorado School of Medicine, United States of America

Funding: This work was supported by the Infectious Diseases Control Project from Ministry of Health of China (2012zx10004-207). The funders had no role in study design, data collection and analysis, decision to publish, or preparation of the manuscript.

Competing Interests: The authors have declared that no competing interests exist.

* Email: Fengwang@tjh.tjmu.edu.cn (FW); tjszyong@163.com (ZS)

Introduction

Sepsis is characterized by an exaggerated systemic inflammatory response mainly caused by lipopolysaccharide (LPS) of Gram-negative bacterium, leading to serious effects such as multi-organ failure and even death [1]. The overwhelming release of proinflammatory cytokines, in particular TNF-α and IFN-γ, are involved in the development of sepsis [2]. Thus, strategies aimed at down-regulating the excessive inflammatory condition may be potentially useful for therapy of sepsis. Previous studies have indicated that macrophages, neutrophils and conventional T cells are activated and contribute to the sepsis-induced systemic inflammatory response [3]. Natural killer (NK) cells, which have been identified as the major producers of IFN-γ, also play a central role in the pathogenesis of sepsis. Depletion of NK cells provides protection against LPS or multi-bacteria-induced sepsis in mice [4–6].

T-cell immunoglobulin and mucin domain (Tim-3), a type I membrane glycoprotein, has been reported to be expressed on activated CD4[+] T cells, CD8[+] T cells, monocytes, dendritic cells (DCs) and NK cells [7–10]. Engagement of Tim-3 with its ligand galectin-9 [11] has been reported to play important roles in various immune responses such as infection, autoimmunity, and tumor immunity [12–14]. Moreover, the high expression of Tim-3 mRNA was observed in human NK cells when compared with other lymphocyte populations [15]. Previous studies have shown that Tim-3 acts as an activating coreceptor of human NK cells to enhance IFN-γ production among healthy individuals [16,17]. In

contrast, Tim-3 pathway might have different influence on NK cell function in patients with hepatitis B virus infection and atherogenesis, in which upregulation of Tim-3 on NK cells correlates with decreased IFN-γ production and cytotoxicity [10,18].

Tim-3 has also been proved to negatively regulate the toll-like receptor 4 (TLR-4)-mediated immune responses and plays important roles in maintaining the homeostasis of sepsis [19]. Our previous study also found that Tim-3 pathway could regulate LPS-induced endotoxic shock through CD4[+] T cells, CD8[+] T cells, and NK cells [20]. However, the precise mechanism by which the Tim-3 pathway regulates the phenotype and function of NK cells in sepsis still remains largely unknown. In this study, we dynamically detected the expression of Tim-3 on peritoneal NK cells during the development of LPS-induced endotoxic shock and further assessed its effect on NK cell activity. Our findings support the inhibitory role of Tim-3 on NK cells in LPS-induced endotoxic shock.

Materials and Methods

Mice

BALB/c mice (male, 6–8 weeks of age, weight 20–25 g) were purchased from Experimental Animal Center of Tongji Medical College, Huazhong University of Science and Technology, Wuhan, China. All mice were bred under specific pathogen-free conditions at Tongji Hospital animal facility. All experimental procedures on animals used in this study were carried out according to the protocol approved by the Institutional Animal Care and Use Committee at the Tongji Medical College. All surgery was performed under sodium pentobarbital anesthesia (50 mg/kg, i.p.), and all efforts were made to minimize animal discomfort.

Reagents and Abs

Abs to CD3 (11–0031), NKp46 (11–3351; 47–3351), Tim-3 (12–5871), CD69 (15–0691), IFN-γ (17–7311; 11–7311), CD107a (50–1071), granzyme B (50–8898), perforin (17–9392), CD4 (11–0042), CD8 (11–0081), CD11b (11–0112), CD11c (11–0114), F4/80 (11–4801), and Annexin V-PI Apoptosis Detection Kit (88–8007) were purchased from eBioScience (San Diego, CA). Anti-galectin-9 (136103) was purchased from Biolegend (San Diego, CA). Anti-Tim-3 blocking antibody (anti-Tim-3 Ab) (clone 8B.2C12; 16–5871) was purchased from eBioScience. Recombinant mouse Tim-3 Fc protein (1529-TM-050) was purchased from R&D Systems (Minneapolis, MN). Anti-CD3 microbead kit (130-094-973) and anti-NKp46 microbead kit (130-095-390) were purchased from Miltenyi Biotec (Miltenyi Biotec, GmbH). LPS (E. coli O55:B5) was obtained from Sigma-Aldrich, dissolved in PBS and stored at 4°C

Induction of experimental sepsis

Specific pathogen-free BALB/c mice were used to establish the LPS-induced sepsis model. Mice were injected i.p. with 15 mg/kg of LPS, as with previously described methods [20].

Cell preparation and culture

Mice were euthanized by cervical dislocation after sodium pentobarbital anesthesia (50 mg/kg, i.p.) at 24 h post-LPS injection. Spleen cells were separated through density gradient by mouse lymphocyte separation medium (DKW33-R0100). Spleen cells were plated at 1×10^5 cells/well in 96-well plates in RPMI 1640 supplemented with 10% fetal calf serum (FCS) and stimulated with LPS (1 µg/ml) in the presence of anti-Tim-3 Ab (1 µg/ml), Tim-3 Fc protein (5 µg/ml) or control IgG. Cell suspensions were cultured in 5% CO_2 incubator for 24 h, and then the cells were collected and analyzed by flow cytometry. For the analysis of intracellular IFN-γ production, monensin (1 µM, eBioScience) was added to cultures for the last 6 h of incubation.

Flow cytometry

Mice were euthanized by cervical dislocation after sodium pentobarbital (50 mg/kg, i.p.) anesthesia every 4 h in the initial 24 h after LPS injection. Peritoneal cells were harvested by peritoneal lavage using 10 ml PBS and the total numbers of cells were counted. Erythrocytes were removed by cell lysis in FACS lysing solution (BD Biosciences, Heidelberg, Germany). Peritoneal cells and spleen cells were pre-incubated for 10 min at room temperature in 10% FCS to block Fc receptors and non-specific binding. After washing three times, cells were stained with Abs specific for mouse CD3, NKp46, Tim-3, CD69, CD107a, CD4, CD8, CD11b, CD11c, F4/80, galectin-9 and incubated on ice for 30 min. For intracellular staining, the cells collected after surface staining were fixed and permeabilized with Fixation and Permeabilization Buffer (BD Pharmingen). After permeabilization, cells were stained with Abs to IFN-γ, granzyme B, perforin and analyzed using a FACScan flow cytometer (Becton Dickinson). NK cell apoptosis was assessed using an Annexin V-PI Apoptosis Detection Kit according to the manufacturer's instructions. Data analysis was performed using FlowJo version 7.6.1 software (TreeStar).

NK cell cytotoxicity analysis

NK cells were purified from the spleen cells of septic mice at 24 h after LPS injection by MACS according to the instructions of the manufacturer (Miltenyi Biotec). Briefly, $CD3^+$ cells were depleted from spleen cells with magnetic beads conjugated to anti-CD3, and from the negative cell fraction, $NKp46^+$ cells were isolated by positive selection with magnetic beads conjugated to anti-NKp46. The purity of NK cells ($CD3^-NKp46^+$) was more than 95% as assessed by flow cytometry. Purified NK cells were incubated with anti-Tim-3 Ab (1 µg/ml) or control IgG for 18 h. After incubation, the NK cells were collected as effector cells. Then carboxyfluorescein succinimidyl ester (CFSE) labeled K562 target cells were added to the cultures at effector: target (E: T) ratios of 0:1 (negative control) and 10:1 (test) and incubated at 37°C for additional 6 h. Immediately before acquisition, PI was added to each tube and the cells were analyzed by flow cytometry.

Statistical analysis

Data are expressed as the mean $\pm$ standard errors of measurement (SEM). Differences between groups were analyzed using two-tailed Student's t-test. GraphPad Prism (version 5.01, GraphPad) software was used for all statistical procedures. Values of $p < 0.05$ were considered as statistically significant.

Results

The dynamic expression of Tim-3 and intracellular IFN-γ in NK cells during the course of LPS-induced endotoxic shock

Tim-3 pathway has been described to play important roles in immune regulation of sepsis [19,20]. Our previous data have suggested that Tim-3 signaling pathway serves as a novel negative mediator in the development of sepsis and that the expression of Tim-3 is increased on NK cells [20]. In this study, we further determined the effect of Tim-3 on NK cell function during the development of sepsis. The expression of Tim-3 and intracellular IFN-γ was examined in peritoneal NK cells at different time points after LPS injection. Our results showed that the expression of Tim-3 on NK cells was significantly increased at 24 h after LPS injection (Fig. 1A). Furthermore, we observed that peritoneal NK cells exhibited low levels of Tim-3 and IFN-γ expression in the initial inflammatory response to LPS infection. Tim-3 expression on NK cells had a moderate increase at 4 h but declined to undetectable levels at 12 h after LPS injection. Meanwhile, the expression of IFN-γ in NK cells was steadily elevated and reached its peak at 12 h. In the following 12–24 h, the expression of Tim-3 on NK cells was increased gradually, while the expression of IFN-γ in NK cells was decreased (Fig. 1B). The percentages and absolute numbers of Tim-3^+ NK cells and IFN-γ^+ NK cells in the peritoneal cavity of septic mice at different time points are shown in Table 1. These data highlight a dynamic inverse correlation between Tim-3 expression and IFN-γ production of NK cells in LPS-induced endotoxic shock.

The relationship between Tim-3 expression and NK cell activity in LPS-induced endotoxic shock

To assess the effect of Tim-3 on NK cell function, we detected the activation and cytolytic effector molecules of NK cells from LPS-induced septic mice. Our data showed that Tim-3^- NK cells were the predominant subset that produced IFN-γ. We observed that Tim-3^- NK cells produced a higher percentage of IFN-γ compared with Tim-3^+ NK cells ($11.6 \pm 0.463\%$ versus $3.58 \pm 1.21\%$; $p < 0.01$) (Fig. 2A). CD69, as one of the early

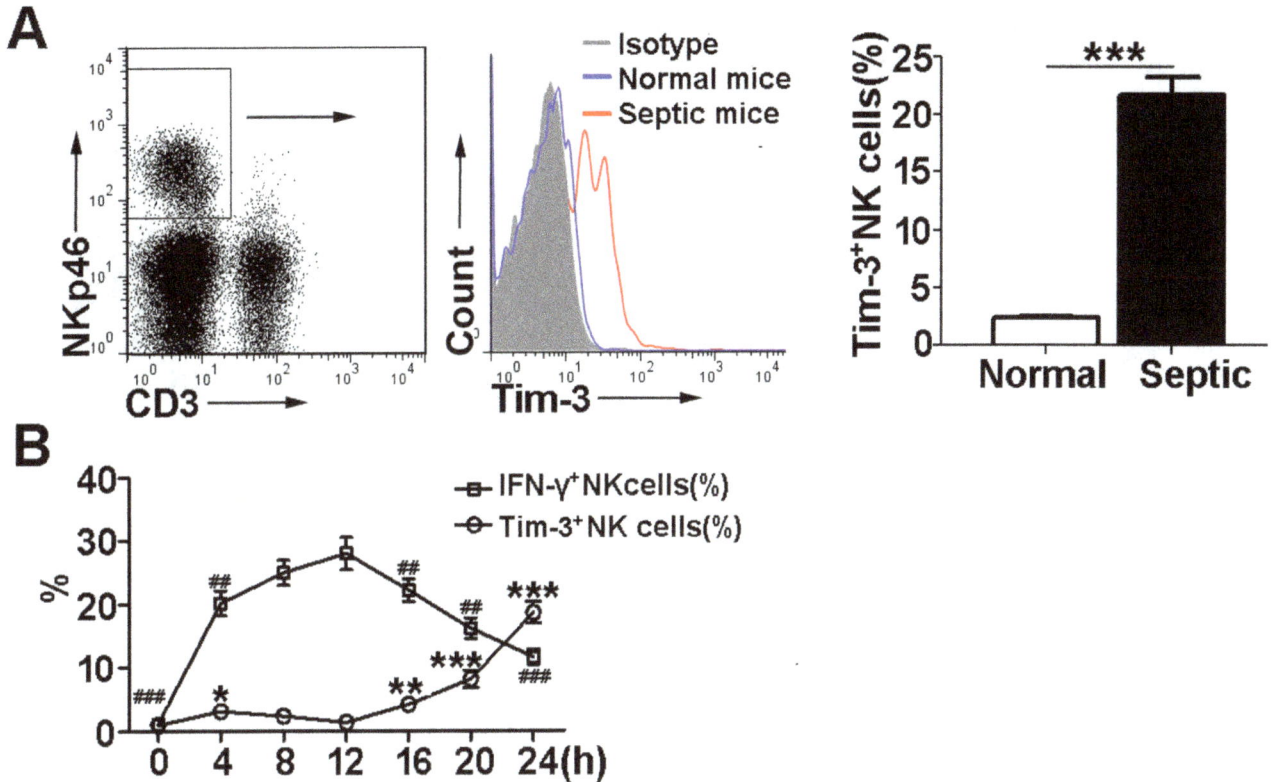

Figure 1. Expression of Tim-3 and IFN-γ in NK cells during the development of LPS-induced endotoxic shock. Peritoneal cavity cells were collected from normal and septic mice at different time points after LPS injection and were analyzed by flow cytometry. (A) NK cells were gated as the CD3⁻NKp46⁺ population. Representative flow cytometry histograms showed Tim-3 expression on NK cells from normal and septic mice at 24 h after LPS injection. The percentage of Tim-3⁺ NK cells was shown in the bar graphs. (B) The percentages of Tim-3⁺ NK cells and IFN-γ⁺ NK cells from septic mice at different time points after LPS injection were shown. Data are mean ± SEM of at least three independent experiments. $*p<0.05$, $**p<0.01$, $***p<0.001$ compared with septic mice at 0 h after LPS injection; $^{\#\#}p<0.01$, $^{\#\#\#}p<0.001$ compared with septic mice at 12 h after LPS injection.

activation markers, was expressed on peritoneal NK cells and continuously increased within 24 h after LPS injection (Fig. 2B). We observed that the mean fluorescence intensity (MFI) of CD69 expression on NK cells was significantly increased in septic mice when compared with normal mice (Fig. 2C). In addition, the percentage of CD69-expressing cells in Tim-3⁺ NK cell subset was significantly higher than that in Tim-3⁻ NK cell subset (Fig. 2D). Furthermore, to evaluate whether the expression of Tim-3 correlated with the cytotoxic potential of NK cells, we directly examined the cell surface degranulation marker CD107a and

intracellular cytotoxic effector molecules, including granzyme B and perforin. Our data showed that the expression of CD107a on NK cells was low at 0 h ($1.70\pm0.282\%$) and 4 h ($2.18\pm0.111\%$), but then increased at 12 h ($3.99\pm0.547\%$) and reached up to approximately 11% ($11.3\pm0.485\%$) at 24 h post-LPS injection (Fig. 3A). The percentage and MFI of CD107a expression on NK cells were significantly higher in septic mice than in normal mice (Fig. 3B). We also observed that Tim-3⁻ NK cells had higher expression of CD107a than Tim-3⁺ NK cells (Fig. 3C). In addition, we also detected the expression of cytotoxic effector

Table 1. The percentages and absolute numbers of Tim-3⁺ NK and IFN-γ⁺ NK cells.

	Tim-3⁺ NK %	(numbers ×10⁴ cells)	IFN-γ⁺ NK %	(numbers ×10⁴ cells)
0 h	0.880 ± 0.192	(2.16 ± 0.109)	$1.09\pm0.339^{\#\#\#}$	$(2.68\pm0.042^{\#\#\#})$
4 h	$3.05\pm0.202^{*}$	$(6.98\pm0.150^{***})$	$20.6\pm1.09^{\#\#}$	$(47.2\pm1.01^{\#\#})$
8 h	2.30 ± 0.178	$(5.13\pm0.017^{***})$	24.4 ± 1.51	(54.4 ± 2.39)
12 h	1.30 ± 0.435	$(2.83\pm0.041^{**})$	27.9 ± 0.897	(60.8 ± 2.63)
16 h	$4.13\pm0.278^{**}$	$(8.51\pm0.231^{***})$	$23.0\pm0.505^{\#\#}$	$(47.4\pm1.29^{\#\#})$
20 h	$8.15\pm0.362^{***}$	$(16.1\pm0.644^{***})$	$16.4\pm2.42^{\#\#}$	$(32.5\pm1.30^{\#\#\#})$
24 h	$17.5\pm2.64^{***}$	$(33.8\pm2.09^{***})$	$11.3\pm1.37^{\#\#\#}$	$(21.9\pm1.36^{\#\#\#})$

Data are mean ± SEM of at least three independent experiments. $*p<0.05$, $**p<0.01$, $***p<0.001$ compared with septic mice at 0 h after LPS injection; $^{\#\#}p<0.01$, $^{\#\#\#}p<0.001$ compared with septic mice at 12 h after LPS injection.

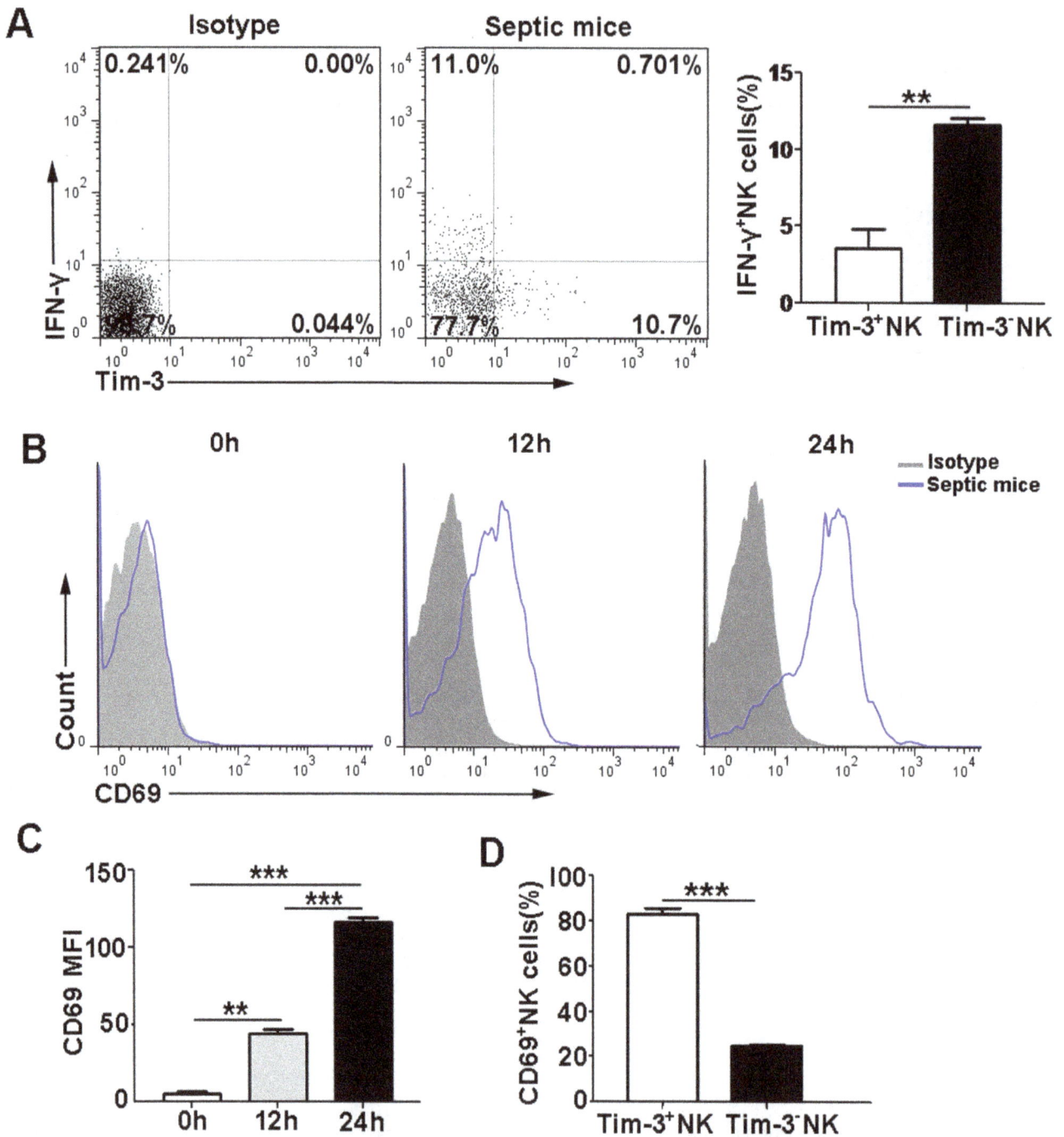

Figure 2. Tim-3 expression is inversely associated with NK cell activity. (A) The expression of Tim-3 and IFN-γ was analyzed in NK cells from septic mice at 24 h after LPS injection. The percentage of IFN-γ⁺ cells between Tim-3⁺ and Tim-3⁻ NK cell subsets was shown in the graphs. (B) Representative flow cytometry histograms of CD69 expression on NK cells from septic mice at 0, 12 and 24 h after LPS injection were shown. (C) The MFI of CD69 on NK cells was shown in the bar graphs. (D) The percentage of CD69⁺ NK cells between Tim-3⁺ and Tim-3⁻ NK cell subsets from septic mice at 24 h after LPS injection was shown. Data are mean ± SEM of at least three independent experiments. **$p < 0.01$, ***$p < 0.001$.

molecules in NK cells and found that the MFI of granzyme B and perforin expression in NK cells was increased in septic mice at 24 h after LPS injection (Fig. 3D, F). We then compared the expression of these two cytotoxic effector molecules between Tim-3⁺ and Tim-3⁻ NK cell subsets, but they had no statistical significance (Fig. 3E, G). The above data indicated that Tim-3

pathway was negatively correlated with NK cell activity in LPS-induced endotoxic shock.

Tim-3 blockade increases IFN-γ production and decreases apoptosis of NK cells

To further confirm the relationship between Tim-3 expression and NK cell function, we made use of an anti-Tim-3 Ab to block

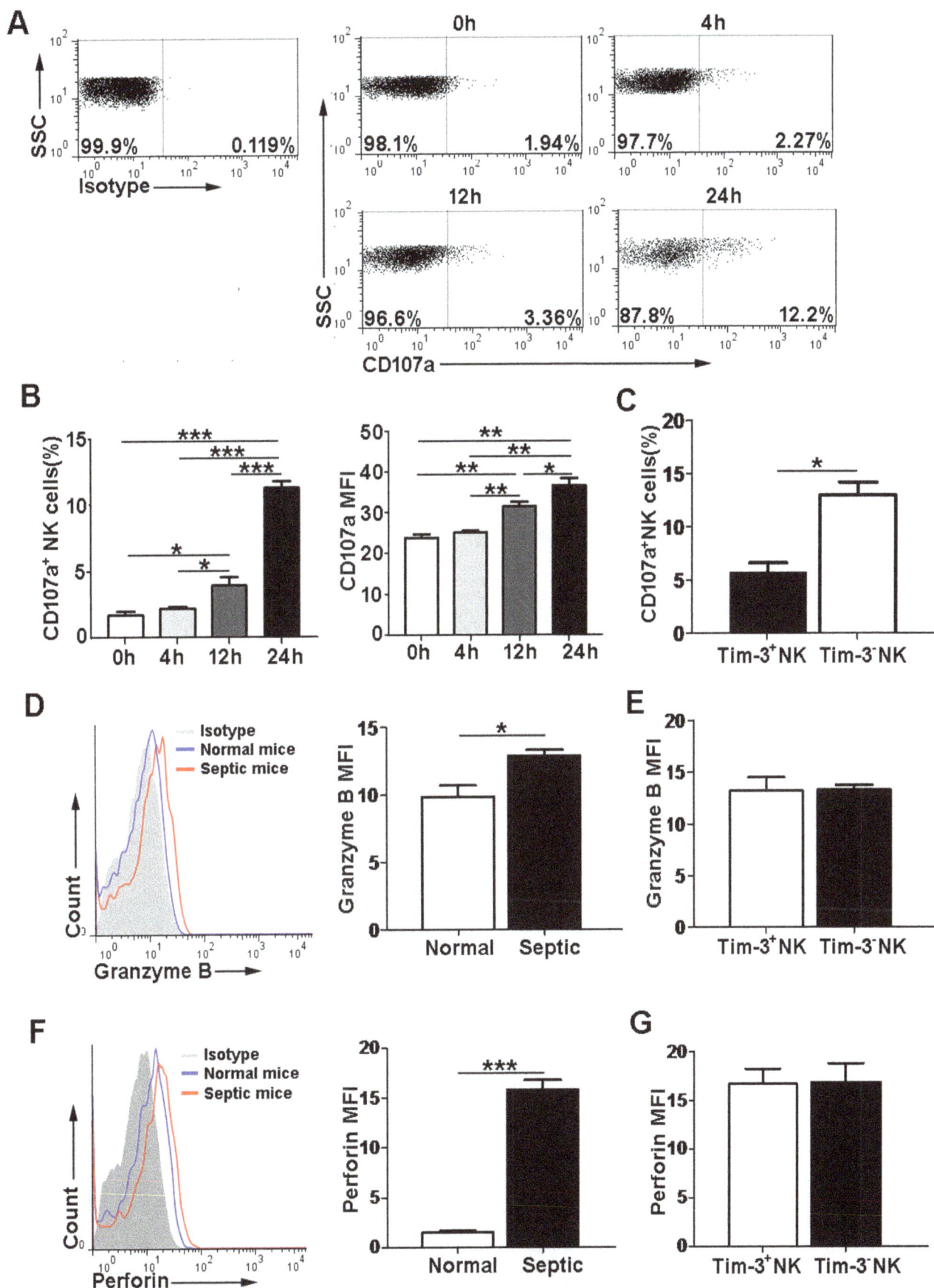

Figure 3. The relationship between Tim-3 expression and the cytotoxicity of NK cells. (A) Representative flow cytometric dot plots of CD107a expression on NK cells from septic mice at 0, 4, 12 and 24 h after LPS injection were shown. (B) The bar graphs showed the percentage and MFI of CD107a expression on NK cells at different time points. (C) The bar graphs showed the percentage of CD107a+ cells between Tim-3+ and Tim-3− NK cell subsets from septic mice at 24 h after LPS injection. (D, F) Representative flow cytometry histograms showed granzyme B and perforin expression in NK cells from normal and septic mice at 24 h after LPS injection. The MFI of granzyme B and perforin expression in NK cells was shown. (E, G) The MFI of granzyme B and perforin expression in NK cells was compared between Tim-3+ and Tim-3− NK cell subsets. Data are mean ± SEM of at least three independent experiments. *$p<0.05$, **$p<0.01$, ***$p<0.001$.

Tim-3 signaling pathway in vitro. Our results showed that the percentage of IFN-γ^+ NK cells had a near 2-fold increase after blocking Tim-3 pathway (Fig. 4A). On the other hand, we also used a recombinant Tim-3 Fc protein for interfering with Tim-3/Tim-3 ligand interaction. We observed that Tim-3 Fc protein had a similar effect with anti-Tim-3 Ab and could also significantly increase the production of IFN-γ by NK cells (Fig. 4A). However, no difference was observed in the expression of CD107a on NK cells after blockade of this pathway by using the anti-Tim-3 Ab (Fig. 4B). In addition, Annexin V/PI staining showed that blockade of Tim-3 pathway resulted in a significant decrease of NK cell apoptosis (Fig. 4C). These results suggested that blocking Tim-3 pathway could increase IFN-γ production and prevent the apoptosis of NK cells from LPS-induced septic mice.

Galectin-9, a ligand of Tim-3, has been reported to play important roles in regulating various inflammatory responses [12–14]. Thus, we also examined the surface galectin-9 expression on peritoneal lavage cells in this study. We observed that galectin-9 was expressed on both normal and septic mouse peritoneal macrophages and neutrophils, while it was not emerged on DCs, CD4+ T cells, CD8+ T cells and NK cells (Fig. 4D). The MFI of galectin-9 expression on macrophages was significantly increased in septic mice compared with that in normal mice. However, the expression of galectin-9 on neutrophils had no significant difference between the two groups (Fig. 4E). Our results demonstrated that Tim-3 ligand was present during sepsis, which suggested that Tim-3 signaling pathway might involve in the modulation of immune response of LPS-induced endotoxic shock.

The cytotoxicity of NK cells is enhanced after blocking Tim-3 pathway

We further determined the cytotoxic activity of NK cells after blockade of Tim-3 pathway. The cytotoxic activity of NK cells was tested for their ability to lyse the MHC class I-deficient K562 target cells. NK cells were isolated from spleen cells of septic mice and the purity of NK cells was more than 95% (Fig. 5A). Purified NK cells treated with anti-Tim-3 Ab or IgG control were used to lyse CFSE-labeled K562 cells. We observed that anti-Tim-3 Ab could significantly increase the cytotoxic activity of NK cells compared with IgG control ($12.0\pm0.423\%$ versus $7.77\pm0.327\%$; $p<0.01$) (Fig. 5B, C). These results indicated that Tim-3 might play an inhibitory role in NK cell-mediated cytotoxicity in LPS-induced endotoxic shock.

Discussion

NK cells are major effector cells of the innate immunity and participate in the defense against microbial infections, involving IFN-γ secretion, target cell elimination and shaping the adaptive immune response [21,22]. However, the function of NK cells are controversial in the process of sepsis [23]. It has been reported that depletion of NK cells can lead to significantly reduced inflammatory cytokine levels and improved survival of septic mice [4,23]. Moreover, the increased number of NK cells in the peripheral blood of patients with severe sepsis was associated with an increased risk of mortality [24]. On the contrary, other researchers

observed that high levels of NK cells were beneficial for the survival of septic patients [25,26]. The discrepancies concerning the number and function of NK cells in septic patients are probably due to the heterogeneity of patients in terms of either severity or involvement of pathogens [25]. Thus, the mechanism of how NK cells regulate the immune response of sepsis still needs further investigation.

Sepsis is a life-threatening condition and a major cause of death in intensive care units, which is characterized by an overzealous release of proinflammatory cytokines and inflammatory mediators [27]. It suggests that appropriate immune status would be beneficial to counter the severe infectious processes. Previous studies have shown that the Tim-3 pathway plays important roles in regulating the inflammatory responses, such as autoimmune diseases [13,28], transplant tolerance [29,30], antitumor immunity [31,32] and virus infection [12,33,34]. Tim-3 pathway has also been demonstrated to negatively regulate TLR-4 responses, resulting in down-regulation of the excessive inflammatory response and promoting the homeostasis of sepsis [19]. Our previous study have found that blockade of Tim-3 pathway can accelerate the death of septic mice [20], which suggests that Tim-3 serves as an important negative mediator in the development of LPS-induced endotoxic shock. Although our previous study mentioned the relationship between the upregulation of Tim-3 expression and the impairment of IFN-γ production in NK cells, the mechanism of Tim-3-mediated regulation of NK cell immunity during LPS-induced endotoxic shock still remains largely unknown. In the present study, we detected the dynamic expression of Tim-3 on NK cells and further determined the role of Tim-3 pathway in the regulation of NK cell function in LPS-induced endotoxic shock.

NK cells are the major producers of IFN-γ which can play an important role in regulating the process of experimental septic shock [4,6]. Developmental studies show that mice deficient in IFN-γ are resistant to LPS-induced toxicity [35], and blockade of IFN-γ can improve the survival of septic mice [36]. In this study, we dynamically observed that the expression of Tim-3 on NK cells was inversely associated with IFN-γ production during the initial 24 h of LPS-induced endotoxic shock, which suggested that Tim-3 might act as an exhausted marker of NK cells in the process of the inflammatory response. In addition, both the use of anti-Tim-3 Ab and Tim-3 Fc protein could increase the secretion of IFN-γ by NK cells in vitro. To further determine the effect of Tim-3 pathway on sepsis, we also examined the expression of galectin-9, a known ligand for Tim-3 [11], and we observed that galectin-9 was indeed expressed on the surface of mouse peritoneal macrophages and neutrophiles. These data suggest that Tim-3 signaling pathway is involved in the down-regulation of NK cell immune response in LPS-induced endotoxic shock.

Previous studies regarding the function of NK cells in the pathogenesis of sepsis have focused on the production of cytokines rather than the cytotoxic capability. NK cells possess large amounts of cytolytic granules containing perforin and various granzymes and have the ability to kill the target cells directly. It has been reported that septic patients with increased levels of granzyme A and/or B have a higher mortality rate and more

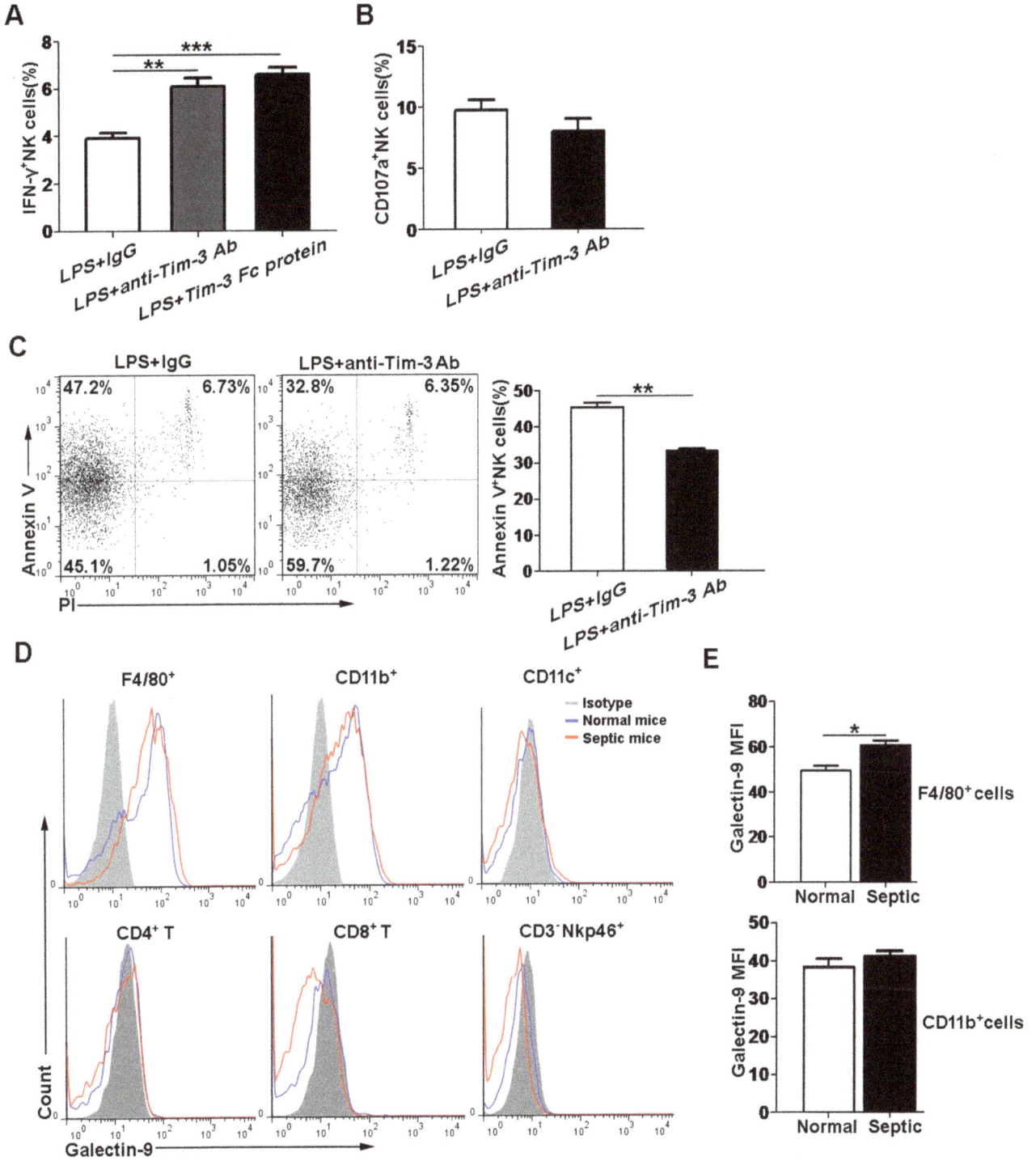

Figure 4. Blockade of Tim-3 pathway increased IFN-γ production and decreased apoptosis of NK cells in vitro. Spleen cells harvested from septic mice at 24 h after LPS injection were stimulated with LPS (1 μg/ml) in the presence of anti-Tim-3 Ab (1 μg/ml), Tim-3 Fc protein (5 μg/ml) or control IgG for 24 h. The bar graphs showed the percentages of (A) IFN-γ$^+$ NK cells and (B) CD107a$^+$ NK cells between the groups. (C) The apoptosis of NK cells (gated on CD3$^-$NKp46$^+$ cells) was analyzed by Annexin V/PI double staining. The percentage of Annexin V$^+$PI$^-$ cells (representative of apoptosis cells) was compared between the groups. (D) The expression of surface galectin-9 on peritoneal macrophages (F4/80$^+$ cells), neutrophils (CD11b$^+$ cells), DCs (CD11c$^+$ cells), CD4$^+$ T cells, CD8$^+$ T cells and NK cells from normal and septic mice at 24 h after LPS injection were analyzed. (E) The MFI of galectin-9 on F4/80$^+$ and CD11b$^+$ cell populations was shown in the bar graphs. Data are mean ± SEM of at least three independent experiments. *$p<0.05$, **$p<0.01$, ***$p<0.001$.

severe organ dysfunction [37]. Other researchers also observed that the elevated expression of granzyme B and perforin in the

cytotoxic cells of septic patients correlated with disease severity [38]. As the data obtained regarding the evaluation of NK cell

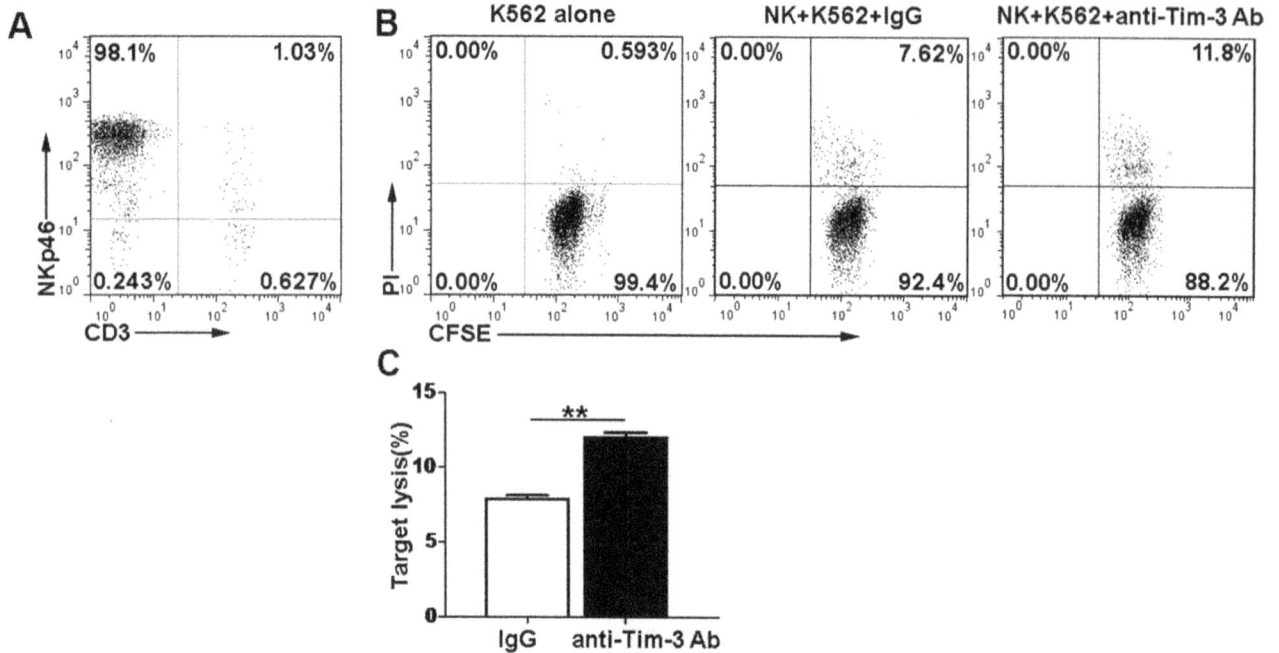

Figure 5. Blocking Tim-3 pathway enhances the cytotoxic activity of NK cells. NK cells were purified from the spleen cells of septic mice. Purified NK cells treated with anti-Tim-3 Ab (1 μg/ml) or control IgG for 18 h were used as effector cells. The effeteor cells were cocultured with CFSE-labeled K562 target cells at the E: T of 0:1 and 10:1 for 6 h. The death of target cells was detected by flow cytometry using PI staining. (A) The purity of NK cells was assessed by flow cytometric analysis of cells stained with anti-CD3 and anti-NKp46. (B) Representative flow cytometric dot plots showing the percentages of dead target cells in different experimental groups. (C) The percentage of target cell lysis was shown in the bar graphs. Data are expressed as the mean ± SEM of at least three independent experiments. **$p < 0.01$.

function are limited, we further assessed the cytotoxic activity of NK cells in LPS-induced endotoxic shock. CD107a, which is identified as a sensitive marker for degranulation of NK cells and activated CD8$^+$ T cells, is significantly correlated with the cytotoxic activity of NK cells [39]. We observed that the expression of CD107a on NK cells was elevated in septic mice and that Tim-3$^-$ NK cells had higher CD107a expression compared with Tim-3$^+$ NK cells. These data suggested that Tim-3 was an exhausted marker of NK cells in LPS-induced endotoxic shock, which was also consistent with previous findings [40]. Furthermore, the MFI of granzyme B and perforin expression in NK cells was elevated in septic mice. This trend was consistent with the change of CD107a expression. However, there was no difference regarding the MFI of these two cytotoxic effector molecules between Tim-3$^+$ and Tim-3$^-$ NK cell subsets. The expression of CD107a on NK cells also had no statistical significance after blocking Tim-3 pathway. These data indicated that blockade of Tim-3 pathway could enhance IFN-γ production in NK cells but have little effect on NK cell degranulation in LPS-induced endotoxic shock. Nevertheless, the cytotoxic activity of NK cells against K562 cells was enhanced after blocking Tim-3 pathway. However, the precise mechanism by which Tim-3 blockade increased NK cell cytotoxicity needs to be further investigated.

In addition, extensive lymphocyte apoptosis has been reported in patients with sepsis [41], but the consequence of cell apoptosis in sepsis still remains ambiguous. Previous study has shown that lymphocyte apoptosis leads to immunosuppression and is associated with the mortality of septic patients [35]. On the other hand,

other researchers have found that the reduced cell apoptosis of NK cells results in a further release of inflammatory cytokines and is harmful for the survival of septic shock patients [6]. Our previous results have shown that Tim-3$^+$ T cells are more prone to apoptosis than Tim-3$^-$ T cells in septic mice [20]. However, the effect of Tim-3 on the apoptosis of NK cells is still unknown. As expected, we observed that blockade of Tim-3 pathway could also reduce the apoptosis of NK cells from septic mice. These findings suggested that the increased expression of Tim-3 on NK cells might be associated with the down-regulation of inflammatory response, which could also be used to explain the mechanism of NK cell apoptosis in LPS-induced endotoxic shock.

Whereas Tim-3 expressed on normal human NK cells is proved to enhance IFN-γ production [16,17], other studies suggest that Tim-3 expressed on NK cells may serve an opposite role in patients with HBV infection and atherosclerosis [10,18]. Consistent with the latter observation, this study indicates that Tim-3 pathway plays an inhibitory role in NK cell function in LPS-induced endotoxic shock. This negative regulatory pathway represents a protective mechanism that can be used as a potential target in modulating the excessive inflammatory response of sepsis.

Author Contributions

Conceived and designed the experiments: HH FW ZS. Performed the experiments: HH FW WL Yanjun Lu JP. Analyzed the data: SW JP YZ. Contributed reagents/materials/analysis tools: YZ Yanfang Lu. Contributed to the writing of the manuscript: HH ZS.

References

1. Stearns-Kurosawa DJ, Osuchowski MF, Valentine C, Kurosawa S, Remick DG (2011) The pathogenesis of sepsis. Annu Rev Pathol 6: 19–48.

2. Hack CE, Aarden LA, Thijs LG (1997) Role of cytokines in sepsis. Adv Immunol 66: 101–195.

3. Hotchkiss RS, Karl IE (2003) The pathophysiology and treatment of sepsis. N Engl J Med 348: 138–150.

4. Emoto M, Miyamoto M, Yoshizawa I, Emoto Y, Schaible UE, et al. (2002) Critical role of NK cells rather than V alpha 14(+)NKT cells in lipopolysaccharide-induced lethal shock in mice. J Immunol 169: 1426–1432.

5. Barkhausen T, Frerker C, Putz C, Pape HC, Krettek C, et al. (2008) Depletion of NK cells in a murine polytrauma model is associated with improved outcome and a modulation of the inflammatory response. Shock 30: 401–410.

6. Etogo AO, Nunez J, Lin CY, Toliver-Kinsky TE, Sherwood ER (2008) NK but not CD1-restricted NKT cells facilitate systemic inflammation during polymicrobial intra-abdominal sepsis. J Immunol 180: 6334–6345.

7. Rodriguez-Manzanet R, DeKruyff R, Kuchroo VK, Umetsu DT (2009) The costimulatory role of TIM molecules. Immunol Rev 229: 259–270.

8. Anderson AC, Anderson DE, Bregoli L, Hastings WD, Kassam N, et al. (2007) Promotion of tissue inflammation by the immune receptor Tim-3 expressed on innate immune cells. Science 318: 1141–1143.

9. Ndhlovu LC, Leal FE, Hasenkrug AM, Jha AR, Carvalho KI, et al. (2011) HTLV-1 tax specific CD8+ T cells express low levels of Tim-3 in HTLV-1 infection: implications for progression to neurological complications. PLoS Negl Trop Dis 5: e1030.

10. Ju Y, Hou N, Meng J, Wang X, Zhang X, et al. (2010) T cell immunoglobulin- and mucin-domain-containing molecule-3 (Tim-3) mediates natural killer cell suppression in chronic hepatitis B. J Hepatol 52: 322–329.

11. Zhu C, Anderson AC, Schubart A, Xiong H, Imitola J, et al. (2005) The Tim-3 ligand galectin-9 negatively regulates T helper type 1 immunity. Nat Immunol 6: 1245–1252.

12. Jones RB, Ndhlovu LC, Barbour JD, Sheth PM, Jha AR, et al. (2008) Tim-3 expression defines a novel population of dysfunctional T cells with highly elevated frequencies in progressive HIV-1 infection. J Exp Med 205: 2763–2779.

13. Seki M, Oomizu S, Sakata KM, Sakata A, Arikawa T, et al. (2008) Galectin-9 suppresses the generation of Th17, promotes the induction of regulatory T cells, and regulates experimental autoimmune arthritis. Clin Immunol 127: 78–88.

14. Nobumoto A, Oomizu S, Arikawa T, Katoh S, Nagahara K, et al. (2009) Galectin-9 expands unique macrophages exhibiting plasmacytoid dendritic cell-like phenotypes that activate NK cells in tumor-bearing mice. Clin Immunol 130: 322–330.

15. Khademi M, Illes Z, Gielen AW, Marta M, Takazawa N, et al. (2004) T Cell Ig- and mucin-domain-containing molecule-3 (TIM-3) and TIM-1 molecules are differentially expressed on human Th1 and Th2 cells and in cerebrospinal fluid-derived mononuclear cells in multiple sclerosis. J Immunol 172: 7169–7176.

16. Ndhlovu LC, Lopez-Verges S, Barbour JD, Jones RB, Jha AR, et al. (2012) Tim-3 marks human natural killer cell maturation and suppresses cell-mediated cytotoxicity. Blood 119: 3734–3743.

17. Gleason MK, Lenvik TR, McCullar V, Felices M, O'Brien MS, et al. (2012) Tim-3 is an inducible human natural killer cell receptor that enhances interferon gamma production in response to galectin-9. Blood 119: 3064–3072.

18. Hou N, Zhao D, Liu Y, Gao L, Liang X, et al. (2012) Increased expression of T cell immunoglobulin- and mucin domain-containing molecule-3 on natural killer cells in atherogenesis. Atherosclerosis 222: 67–73.

19. Yang X, Jiang X, Chen G, Xiao Y, Geng S, et al. (2013) T cell Ig mucin-3 promotes homeostasis of sepsis by negatively regulating the TLR response. J Immunol 190: 2068–2079.

20. Wang F, Hou H, Xu L, Jane M, Peng J, et al. (2014) Tim-3 signaling pathway as a novel negative mediator in lipopolysaccharide-induced endotoxic shock. Hum Immunol 75: 470–478.

21. Vivier E, Tomasello E, Baratin M, Walzer T, Ugolini S (2008) Functions of natural killer cells. Nat Immunol 9: 503–510.

22. Vivier E, Raulet DH, Moretta A, Caligiuri MA, Zitvogel L, et al. (2011) Innate or adaptive immunity? The example of natural killer cells. Science 331: 44–49.

23. Chiche L, Forel JM, Thomas G, Farnarier C, Vely F, et al. (2011) The role of natural killer cells in sepsis. J Biomed Biotechnol 2011: 986491.

24. Andaluz-Ojeda D, Iglesias V, Bobillo F, Almansa R, Rico L, et al. (2011) Early natural killer cell counts in blood predict mortality in severe sepsis. Crit Care 15: R243.

25. Gogos C, Kotsaki A, Pelekanou A, Giannikopoulos G, Vaki I, et al. (2010) Early alterations of the innate and adaptive immune statuses in sepsis according to the type of underlying infection. Crit Care 14: R96.

26. Giamarellos-Bourboulis EJ, Tsaganos T, Spyridaki E, Mouktaroudi M, Plachouras D, et al. (2006) Early changes of CD4-positive lymphocytes and NK cells in patients with severe Gram-negative sepsis. Crit Care 10: R166.

27. Adib-Conquy M, Cavaillon JM (2009) Compensatory anti-inflammatory response syndrome. Thromb Haemost 101: 36–47.

28. Kanzaki M, Wada J, Sugiyama K, Nakatsuka A, Teshigawara S, et al. (2012) Galectin-9 and T cell immunoglobulin mucin-3 pathway is a therapeutic target for type 1 diabetes. Endocrinology 153: 612–620.

29. Wang F, He W, Yuan J, Wu K, Zhou H, et al. (2008) Activation of Tim-3-Galectin-9 pathway improves survival of fully allogeneic skin grafts. Transpl Immunol 19: 12–19.

30. Wang F, He W, Zhou H, Yuan J, Wu K, et al. (2007) The Tim-3 ligand galectin-9 negatively regulates CD8+ alloreactive T cell and prolongs survival of skin graft. Cell Immunol 250: 68–74.

31. Tang D, Lotze MT (2012) Tumor immunity times out: TIM-3 and HMGB1. Nat Immunol 13: 808–810.

32. Sakuishi K, Apetoh L, Sullivan JM, Blazar BR, Kuchroo VK, et al. (2010) Targeting Tim-3 and PD-1 pathways to reverse T cell exhaustion and restore anti-tumor immunity. J Exp Med 207: 2187–2194.

33. Wu W, Shi Y, Li S, Zhang Y, Liu Y, et al. (2012) Blockade of Tim-3 signaling restores the virus-specific CD8(+) T-cell response in patients with chronic hepatitis B. Eur J Immunol 42: 1180–1191.

34. Golden-Mason L, Palmer BE, Kassam N, Townshend-Bulson L, Livingston S, et al. (2009) Negative immune regulator Tim-3 is overexpressed on T cells in hepatitis C virus infection and its blockade rescues dysfunctional CD4+ and CD8+ T cells. J Virol 83: 9122–9130.

35. Heremans H, Dillen C, van Damme J, Billiau A (1994) Essential role for natural killer cells in the lethal lipopolysaccharide-induced Shwartzman-like reaction in mice. Eur J Immunol 24: 1155–1160.

36. Dinges MM, Schlievert PM (2001) Role of T cells and gamma interferon during induction of hypersensitivity to lipopolysaccharide by toxic shock syndrome toxin 1 in mice. Infect Immun 69: 1256–1264.

37. Zeerleder S, Hack CE, Caliezi C, van Mierlo G, Eerenberg-Belmer A, et al. (2005) Activated cytotoxic T cells and NK cells in severe sepsis and septic shock and their role in multiple organ dysfunction. Clin Immunol 116: 158–165.

38. Napoli AM, Fast LD, Gardiner F, Nevola M, Machan JT (2012) Increased granzyme levels in cytotoxic T lymphocytes are associated with disease severity in emergency department patients with severe sepsis. Shock 37: 257–262.

39. Aktas E, Kucuksezer UC, Bilgic S, Erten G, Deniz G (2009) Relationship between CD107a expression and cytotoxic activity. Cell Immunol 254: 149–154.

40. da Silva IP, Gallois A, Jimenez-Baranda S, Khan S, Anderson AC, et al. (2014) Reversal of NK-cell exhaustion in advanced melanoma by Tim-3 blockade. Cancer Immunol Res 2: 410–422.

41. Hotchkiss RS, Osmon SB, Chang KC, Wagner TH, Coopersmith CM, et al. (2005) Accelerated lymphocyte death in sepsis occurs by both the death receptor and mitochondrial pathways. J Immunol 174: 5110–5118.

16

Angiopoietin-1, Angiopoietin-2 and Bicarbonate as Diagnostic Biomarkers in Children with Severe Sepsis

Kun Wang[1,2], Vineet Bhandari[3], John S. Giuliano Jr[3], Corey S. O'Hern[2,4], Mark D. Shattuck[5], Michael Kirby[1]*

1 Department of Mathematics, Colorado State University, Fort Collins, Colorado, United States of America, 2 Department of Mechanical Engineering & Materials Science, Yale University, New Haven, Connecticut, United States of America, 3 Department of Pediatrics, Yale University School of Medicine, New Haven, Connecticut, United States of America, 4 Department of Applied Physics, Department of Physics, and Graduate Program in Computational Biology & Bioinformatics, Yale University, New Haven, Connecticut, United States of America, 5 Benjamin Levich Institute and Physics Department, The City College of New York, New York, New York, United States of America

Abstract

Severe pediatric sepsis continues to be associated with high mortality rates in children. Thus, an important area of biomedical research is to identify biomarkers that can classify sepsis severity and outcomes. The complex and heterogeneous nature of sepsis makes the prospect of the classification of sepsis severity using a single biomarker less likely. Instead, we employ machine learning techniques to validate the use of a multiple biomarkers scoring system to determine the severity of sepsis in critically ill children. The study was based on clinical data and plasma samples provided by a tertiary care center's Pediatric Intensive Care Unit (PICU) from a group of 45 patients with varying sepsis severity at the time of admission. Canonical Correlation Analysis with the Forward Selection and Random Forests methods identified a particular set of biomarkers that included Angiopoietin-1 (Ang-1), Angiopoietin-2 (Ang-2), and Bicarbonate (HCO_3) as having the strongest correlations with sepsis severity. The robustness and effectiveness of these biomarkers for classifying sepsis severity were validated by constructing a linear Support Vector Machine diagnostic classifier. We also show that the concentrations of Ang-1, Ang-2, and HCO_3 enable predictions of the time dependence of sepsis severity in children.

Editor: Jorge IF Salluh, D'or Institute of Research and Education, Brazil

Funding: This work was partially supported by DARPA (Space and Naval Warfare System Center Pacic) under award number N66001-11-1-4184 (http://www.darpa.mil/). Additional support for this work was provided by Infectious Disease Supercluster, Colorado State University, 2012 seed grant (http://infectiousdisease.colostate.edu/). The funders had no role in study design, data collection and analysis, decision to publish, or preparation of the manuscript.

Competing Interests: The authors have declared that no competing interests exist.

* Email: kirby@math.colostate.edu

Introduction

Pediatric sepsis continues to be a very significant cause of mortality in children [1,2]. Patients who develop organ dysfunction (i.e. severe sepsis or septic shock) have worse morbidity and mortality compared to those who do not [3,4]. Diagnosing and classifying the severity of sepsis is a significant challenge due to the highly variable and nonspecific nature of the signs and symptoms of sepsis. Biomarkers that play critical roles in the disease process show great promise in indicating the severity of sepsis. There are many biomarkers that have been studied for potential use in the early diagnosis and classification of sepsis [5,6]. However the complex and heterogeneous nature of sepsis makes the prospect of single biomarker classification less likely.

No single biomarker has sufficient specificity or sensitivity to be routinely employed in clinical practice. A combination of several sepsis biomarkers may be more effective, as has been suggested by other investigators [7–9]. Multivariate methods have the advantage of selecting an optimal subset of variables from a large number of variables and taking into account the relationship among the selected variables based on a specific outcome.

In this manuscript, we employ a discovery-oriented approach to identify a panel of diagnostic biomarkers. We systematically evaluate many commonly obtained clinical parameters and laboratory values using the multivariate diagnostic capacity of a scoring system that incorporates 17 potential variables to classify patients admitted to a tertiary care center's Pediatric Intensive Care Unit (PICU) with or without sepsis (PICU/sepsis group) versus those with severe sepsis (PICU severe sepsis group).

Materials

Study population

This study was approved by the Pediatric Protocol Review Committee and the Human Investigation Committee at Yale University School of Medicine. Patient records were anonymized and de-identified prior to analysis. The biological specimens and clinical data sets were obtained from a prospective observational study of critically ill pediatric patients with varying degrees of sepsis severity conducted at a tertiary care center PICU during the time period 9/2009–12/2011 [10].

All patients admitted to the PICU were evaluated for eligibility. Forty-five patients met the eligibility criteria and consented to participate in the study. Using the 2005 pediatric sepsis and organ dysfunction definitions [11], patients were divided into one of five categories based on clinical exam findings in the first 24-hours of PICU admission. The categories included systemic inflammatory response syndrome (SIRS), non-SIRS, sepsis, severe sepsis and septic shock. Briefly, SIRS required the presence of at least two of the following four criteria with one being abnormal temperature or leukocyte cout: abnormal core temperature, mean respiratory rate, leukocyte count, or tachycardia. Non-SIRS patients were admitted to the PICU but did not meet SIRS criteria. Patients with sepsis fulfilled SIRS criteria with suspected or proven infection. Patients with severe sepsis met the criteria for sepsis with organ failure, and septic shock patients were a subset of the severe sepsis group with cardiovascular organ failure [11]. Blood samples were collected every 12 hours for the first 3 days and then once a day for the last 4 days. Data collection was discontinued when the patient was discharged from the PICU. A maximum of 10 samples for 7 days were obtained from each patient. As a result of PICU discharge and line removal, the total number of samples available for analysis decreased with time for all patient groups. The number of samples for each time point is shown in Figure S1. Commercial enzyme-linked immunosorbent assay (ELISA) kits were used to measure plasma levels of Ang-1 and Ang-2. Descriptive data consisting of demographics and clinical data for all patients included in the clinical studies are provided in Tables S1 and S2 in File S1. Additional details can be found in Text S1 in File S1 and Ref. [10].

Biomarkers

To create a robust model of a specific combination of biomarkers for predicting the severity of sepsis in children in an unbiased manner, we selected multiple clinical and laboratory variables from the database of our study [10]. These 17 variables are as follows: (1) Age, (2) Weight (Wgt), (3) admission Pediatric Index of Mortality 2 (PIM-2) [12], (4) White Blood Cell count (WBC), (5) Hemoglobin count (Hgb), (6) Hematocrit (Hct), (7) Platelet count (Plt), and the levels of (8) Sodium (Na), (9) Potassium (K), (10) Chloride (Cl), (11) HCO_3, (12) Blood Urea Nitrogen (BUN), (13) Creatinine (Cr), (14) Ang-1, (15) Ang-2, (16) Ang-2/Ang-1 ratio, and (17) Vascular Endothelial Growth Factor (VEGF). To validate the data analysis, we augmented this data set to include (18) Gaussian distributed noise (g-Noise) and (19) uniformly distributed noise (u-Noise). These 19 variables were then used to develop sepsis severity prediction models.

Statistical analysis

Patients were classified within the first 24 hours of PICU admission into the five categories listed above based on the 2005 pediatric sepsis and organ dysfunction definitions [11]. We further consolidated these into the following two categories: 1) the PICU/sepsis group ($n=28$) included those not meeting SIRS criteria but were admitted to the PICU (non-SIRS) ($n=9$), SIRS ($n=8$), and sepsis ($n=11$); and 2) the PICU severe sepsis group ($n=17$) included those with severe sepsis ($n=3$), and septic shock ($n=14$). For the original study listed in Ref. [10], a two-sided Mann-Whitney test estimated a sample size of 50 (10 patients per group) to detect 1.5–1.8 standard deviations in the level of Ang-2 between comparison groups, assuming a standard deviation of 1,500 pg/mL, power of 80%, and a significance level (alpha) of 0.05.

Methods

Data Preprocessing

Our dataset (input), a $n \times p$ real-valued matrix x, contains $n=45$ attributes and $p=19$ biomarkers. Since the range of values of the biomarkers varies widely, it should be normalized so that each biomarker contributes approximately proportionally. We normalized x to have zero mean and unit standard deviation for each biomarker [13]:

$$x_{norm} = \frac{x - \bar{x}}{\sigma(x)}, \tag{1}$$

where x_{norm} is a $n \times p$ matrix, $\bar{x}$ and $\sigma(x)$ are the mean value and standard deviation of x for each biomarker. We also assigned each attribute $i = 1, \ldots, n$, a sepsis severity score, y_i. $y_i = -1$ is given to each in the PICU/sepsis group and $y_i = +1$ for the PICU severe sepsis group.

Canonical correlation analysis

CCA finds linear combinations of variables between two sets of data, x and y in our study, which have maximum correlation with each other [14,15]. Here we selected the optimal subset of biomarkers x that has the maximum correlation with y for $k = 1, \ldots, p$, by calculating the correlations between all possible k-combinations of x and y. The results are displayed in Table 1.

Linear support vector machines

In machine learning, a linear support vector machine (SVM) is a learning model used for classfication and regression analysis [16]. A SVM model separates two categories by a hyper-plane that has maximum margin for a given training dataset. New attributes are predicted to belong to a category based on which side of the hyper-plane they fall on.

The hyper-plane can be described by the equation:

$$f(x_i) = w^T x_i - b, \tag{2}$$

where w is the normal vector to the hyper-plane, b is the offset of the hyper-plane from the origin, and x_i is a p-dimensional vector of normalized biomarker values for attribute i in our study. The search of this hyper-plane can be translated into the following optimization problem:

$$\text{Minimize} \quad \|w\|_1 + C_+ \sum_{i:y_i=+1} \xi_i + C_- \sum_{j:y_j=-1} \xi_j$$

$$\text{subject to}$$
$$w^T x_i + b + \xi_i \geq 1, \ y_i = +1,$$
$$w^T x_j + b - \xi_j \leq -1, \ y_j = -1, \text{ and} \tag{3}$$
$$\xi \geq 0,$$

where $\|w\|_1 = \sum_i |w_i|$ is the 1-norm of a vector, which induces the sparsity in the weight vector w [17]. The slack variable, ξ_i, measures the degree of misclassification of x_i. The parameters C_+ and C_-, which determine the penalty assigned to the total error from misclassified samples, are chosen so that C_+/C_- is given by the ratio of the number of negative and positive training evaluations with $C_- = 1.0$.

Ensemble method

Due to the limited size and noise of our data, we follow the training procedure in Ref. [18]. A random one-third of the data is

Table 1. Stepwise Biomarker Selection using Canonical Correlation Analysis, Forward Selection and Random Forests.

Dim	Corr	Entering	Leave	Forward Selection	Random Forests
1	0.3811	Ang-2		Ang-2	Ang-2/Ang-1
2	0.4772	Ang-1		Ang-1	HCO3
3	0.5501	HCO3		HCO3	Ang-2
4	0.5842	Plt		Plt	Ang-1
5	0.6079	Age		Age	Cl
6	0.6183	Cl		WBC	PIM-2
7	0.6221	BUN, Hct, WBC	Cl, HCO3	Hct	Age
8	0.6286	VEGF		BUN	K
9	0.6311	PIM-2		VEGF	Hgb
10	0.6359	Cl, HCO3	PIM-2	PIM-2	VEGF
11	0.6395	Cr, Wgt	Age	g-Noise	Wgt
12	0.6409	Hgb, Na, Age	Cl, Wgt	Cl	Na
13	0.6414	Ang-2/Ang-1		Cr	g-Noise
14	0.6419	Wgt		u-Noise	Plt
15	0.6424	PIM-2		Ang-2/Ang-1	WBC
16	0.6427	Cl, u-Noise	Na	Hgb	u-Noise
17	0.6429	K		Wgt	Cr
18	0.6429	Na, g-Noise	K	K	BUN
19	0.6430	K		Na	Hct

We apply Canonical Correlation Analysis for all possible k-combinations ($k = 1, \ldots, 19$) to determine the subset of k biomarkers with the highest correlation with the sepsis severity score. The 'Enter' column indicates the biomarker that is added to achieve the highest correlation at each k. The 'Leave' column indicates the biomarker that is eliminated from the combination at each k. A biomarker will stay in the combination until it occurs in 'Leave' column. The 'Forward Selection' column gives the biomarker selected by the Forward Selection method when applied one biomarker at a time. The 'Random Forests' column gives the biomarker ranked by the mean decrease in accuracy measured by the Random Forests method.

selected as test set, T. The remaining data is used as training set, L. Bagging is used to construct the classifiers ensemble. Each new training set, L_i, is drawn, with replacement, from the original training set, L. Then a classifier, SVM or tree, is constructed on this new training set, L_i. In this study, we construct a classifiers ensemble 50 times, $i \in \{1, \ldots, 50\}$. The final classification is obtained by calculating the mean of the ensemble of 50 classifiers. This procedure is repeated 100 times and statistical measures on T are averaged.

Calculation of statistical measures

TPR, TNR, NPV, and PPV are statistical measures of the predictive performance of a binary classification test. TPR (or sensitivity) measures the proportion of actual positives that are correctly identified. TNR (or specificity) measures the proportion of actual negatives that are correctly identified. PPV (or precision) measures the proportion of positives that are true positive. NPV measures the proportion of negatives that are true negatives.

These statistical measures are calculated for each one of the 100 random divisions of test sets T by the classifier built on the bootstrap aggregation method. Their mean and standard error are calculated from the groups obtained from the 100 random divisions.

Results

Biomarkers selection

Feature selection is an important part of the data analysis given the fact that the data contains many redundant or irrelevant features. Redundant features provide no additional information

than the selected features, and irrelevant features provide no useful information. Feature selection is widely used in data sets with abundant features but comparatively few samples. In machine learning and statistics, the goal of a feature selection method is to select an optimal subset of relevant features for model construction.

In this study, there are 17 variables (features) augmented by 2 variables consisting of Gaussian and uniform noise to provide a baseline check for the data analysis. From the univariate correlation analysis, we found that this data set contained several possible redundant biomarkers and, not surprisingly, at least two irrelevant features (g-Noise and u-Noise). To extract an optimal subset of biomarkers, we analyzed the multivariate correlation between the outcome, sepsis severity score (0 for PICU/sepsis and 1 for PICU severe sepsis), and the input, which is a subset of variables.

A comparison of the univariate correlations for these two groups is shown in Fig. 1. The univariate analysis revealed that Na, K, Cl, HCO₃ form a group of highly correlated biomarkers (with correlations that range from 0.937 to 0.998) for the PICU/sepsis group. However, these variables are not strongly correlated for the PICU severe sepsis group (with correlations that range from 0.001 to 0.608). This notable difference between the PICU/sepsis and PICU severe sepsis groups indicates that these biomarkers may not independently provide information about the sepsis severity diagnosis. We also note that Ang-1 and Ang-2 are highly correlated with each other in the PICU severe sepsis group (0.76), but this correlation is significantly reduced for the PICU/sepsis group (0.21). Meanwhile, Ang-2/Ang-1 does not correlate very strongly with either Ang-1 (0.21 in PICU/sepsis, 0.24 in

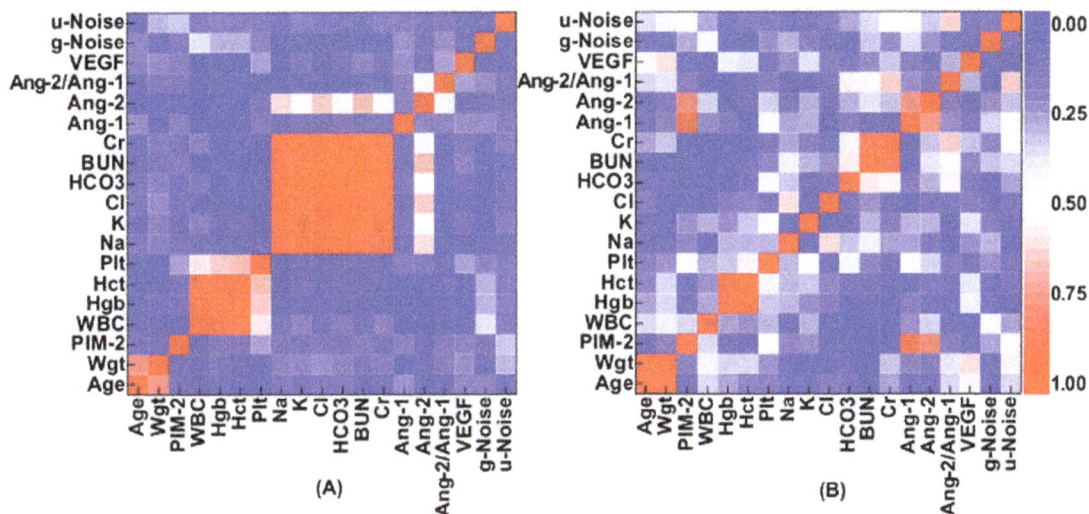

Figure 1. Heatmaps of pairwise correlations. Heatmaps of all pairwise correlations between the 17 variables (plus two noise samples) for patients in the (A) PICU/sepsis and (B) PICU severe sepsis groups. The color scale from blue to red indicates increasing correlations between the pair of biomarkers at the corresponding locations on the horizontal and vertical axes.

PICU severe sepsis) or Ang-2 (0.48 in PICU/sepsis, 0.17 in PICU severe sepsis). Based on these observations, we seek to identify an optimal set of non-redundant variables and biomarkers to predict the severity of sepsis.

In our recent study [19], we found that canonical correlation analysis (CCA) [14,15,20] can be applied effectively to identify an optimal subset of biomarkers with the maximum correlation with the outcome. As shown in Table 1, we found that the subset of Ang-2, Ang-1, and HCO_3 maximizes the correlation with the sepsis severity score. As expected, the two forms of random noise are selected near the end of the process when the correlation saturates for large subsets. We also applied the forward selection (FS) method to identify the optimal subset of biomarkers. FS is a greedy algorithm that adds the best feature at each step [21,22]. We found that the performance of the subset of biomarkers selected by FS was similar to that selected by CCA on this data set.

The optimal subset

In this study, we built a diagnostic classifier by selecting the subset of k biomarkers with the best diagnostic performance for each value of k. For each k, we applied the ensemble method [18,23] to construct a linear support vector machine (SVM) classifier [24] for the CCA-selected subset of biomarkers. SVM [17] finds a decision function that separates the high-dimensional data with the maximum margin. To quantify the classifier performance, we calculated the true positive rate (TPR), true negative rate (TNR), positive predictive value (PPV), and negative predictive value (NPV). See the Methods section for details.

In Figure 2, we find that all statistical measures reach a peak or saturate near $k=3$ using the CCA-selected biomarkers, Ang-2, Ang-1, and HCO_3, which suggests that these three biomarkers are the optimal subset for our data set (TPR $=0.69$, TNR $=0.87$, PPV $=0.79$, and NPV $=0.83$ at $k=3$). By adding HCO_3 to the optimal subset from $k=2$ to $k=3$, the combination has higher TPR (0.60 at $k=2$ versus 0.69 at $k=3$) and PPV (0.69 at $k=2$ versus 0.79 at $k=3$) when compared to the combination of Ang-2 and Ang-1. TNR (0.84 at $k=6$ versus 0.80 at $k=7$) and PPV (0.75 at $k=6$ versus 0.69 at $k=7$) begin to decrease from their plateau values when HCO_3 leaves the subset at $k=7$. The

improvement at $k=3$ and decrease at $k=7$ indicate the diagnostic importance of HCO_3.

Redundant biomarkers

Recent studies [10,25–27] suggest that plasma levels of Ang-2 and Ang-1 can serve as clinically informative biomarkers of sepsis severity. Further, the Ang-2/Ang1 ratio is considered to be a more relevant sepsis severity biomarker than isolated levels of each biomarker because of their antagonistic roles in regulating the tyrosine kinase receptor, Tie-2 [27]. However, both of our biomarker selection methods, CCA and FS, select Ang-2/Ang-1 to the optimal subset relatively late, *i.e.*, at large k ($k=13$ and $k=15$) as shown in Table 1. This suggests that a combination of Ang-2, Ang-1, and HCO_3, is potentially more effective than using the ratio of Ang-1 and Ang-2 with other biomarkers.

It is also interesting to consider the univariate and bivariate performance of these biomarkers. This analysis provides additional insight into the relative performance of different subsets of biomarkers and how they work together to provide inferences.

In Fig. 3(A), the relative performance of the univariate biomarkers performance is shown: 1) Ang-1 has consistent performance for all statistical measures compared to other biomarkers (see Table 2), 2) Ang-2 has a high TNR (0.85) and PPV (0.63) but relatively low TPR (0.38), and 3) HCO_3 has the highest TPR (0.87) and NPV (0.86) but relatively low TNR (0.42) and PPV (0.48). These observations indicate that the performances of these biomarkers did not correlate with each other. This supports the observation that the best subset of biomarkers includes both Ang-1 and Ang-2 since they provide distinct information. We also show that the combination of Ang-2, Ang-1 and HCO_3 improves the predictive capability by reducing overfitting in Fig. 2. The performance for the CCA-selected subsets decreases when $k>3$.

These results suggest, when examining groups of three, Ang-2/Ang-1 may be a redundant biomarker, *i.e.*, no additional information is gained when Ang-1 and Ang-2 data is known. We explore here how this ratio performs in isolation, *i.e.*, as a derived univariate statistic. We applied the same procedure as above to construct a SVM classifier for each single biomarker and

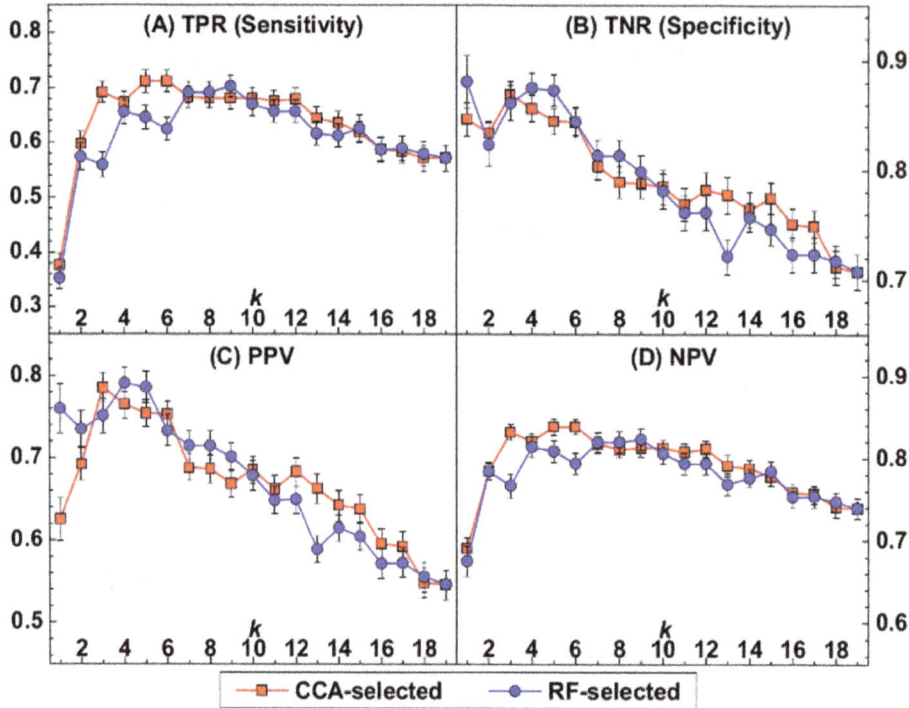

Figure 2. Prediction measures obtained from the Support Vector Machine (SVM) using the k-combinations selected by the Canonical Correlation Analysis (CCA) and Random Forests (RF) methods. The prediction measures (A) true positive rate (TPR), (B) true negative rate (TNR), (C) positive predictive value (PPV), and (D) negative predictive value (NPV) are shown for each step k. For each k, a SVM ensemble with bagging is constructed based on the CCA- and RF-selected subset of biomarkers.

show the statistical measures in Fig. 3(A). Overall, we find that Ang-2 and Ang-2/Ang-1 have comparable prediction performance (Fig. 3(A)). However, Ang-2/Ang-1 outperforms Ang-2 for PPV (0.76 for Ang-2/Ang-1, 0.63 for Ang-2), which suggests that

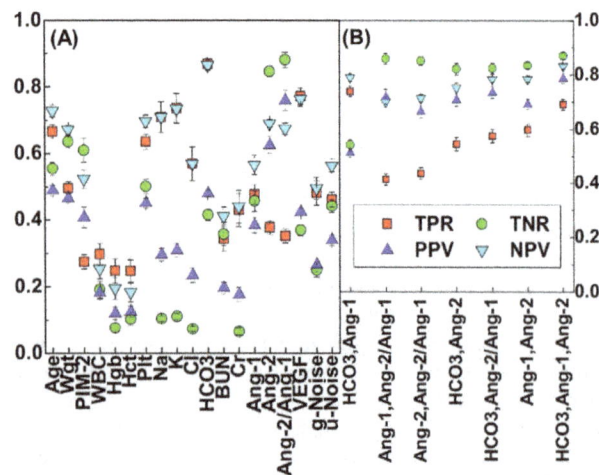

Figure 3. Prediction measures for single and pairs of biomarkers from the Support Vector Machine (SVM). True positive rate (TPR), true negative rate (TNR), positive predictive value (PPV), and negative predictive value (NPV) are shown for (A) each single biomarker and (B) all pairwise combinations of Ang-1, Ang-2, HCO_3 and Ang-2/Ang-1. The prediction measures for the CCA-selected optimal subset of biomarkers at $k=3$ (Ang-2, Ang-1, and HCO_3) are also shown in (B) for comparison.

Ang-2/Ang-1 alone may be a predictive biomarker. The similar performance of Ang-2 and Ang-2/Ang-1 suggest that these two biomarkers capture very similar information.

Of course it is not necessarily a fair assessment to compare true univariate biomarkers such as Ang-1 and Ang-2 to their ratio since this contains information from two measurements. Thus, we also compared the performance of combinations of Ang-1, Ang-2, HCO_3, and Ang-2/Ang-1 in Fig. 3(B). The combination of Ang-2 and Ang-2/Ang-1 does not notably improve each predictive measure compared to these biomarkers alone, which also indicates that these two biomarkers are redundant. In contrast, the combination of Ang-1 and Ang-2 has notably higher NPV (0.78) and TPR (0.60) and comparable values for the other prediction measures compared to each single biomarker (NPV $=0.69$ and TPR $=0.38$ for Ang-2, NPV $=0.57$ and TPR $=0.48$ for Ang-1) and Ang-2/Ang-1 (NPV $=0.67$ and TPR $=0.35$). This suggests that the ratio Ang-2/Ang-1 is less effective than using Ang-1 and Ang-2 separately.

For completeness, we also show the performance for the CCA-selected optimal subset of three biomarkers HCO_3, Ang-1 and Ang-2 on the far right of Fig. 3(B). This optimal subset notably improves the predictive capability as indicated by the small spread of values in the predictive measures.

The diagnostic classifier

We applied the linear SVM ensemble method [23,24] to construct a decision function using the CCA-selected optimal subset of biomarkers at $k=3$: Ang-2, Ang-1, and HCO_3. The optimal decision function is

Table 2. Prediction measures for single biomarker from Support Vector Machine.

Variable	TPR	TNR	PPV	NPV
Age	0.666	0.555	0.490	0.728
Wgt	0.496	0.636	0.466	0.671
PIM-2	0.276	0.611	0.407	0.524
WBC	0.298	0.192	0.183	0.255
Hgb	0.249	0.076	0.121	0.195
Hct	0.248	0.104	0.126	0.184
Plt	0.636	0.501	0.451	0.697
Na	0.710	0.105	0.297	0.710
K	0.737	0.112	0.309	0.735
Cl	0.570	0.073	0.236	0.570
HCO$_3$	0.868	0.415	0.480	0.865
BUN	0.343	0.358	0.197	0.411
Cr	0.430	0.065	0.177	0.440
Ang-1	0.477	0.457	0.384	0.566
Ang-2	0.378	0.846	0.625	0.690
Ang-2/Ang-1	0.353	0.881	0.760	0.675
VEGF	0.773	0.370	0.424	0.764
g-Noise	0.481	0.251	0.266	0.496
u-Noise	0.461	0.442	0.340	0.564

True positive rate (TPR), true negative rate (TNR), positive predictive value (PPV), and negative predictive value (NPV) are shown for each single variable.

$$\text{Score} = w_1 \, \text{Ang-2} + w_2 \, \text{Ang-1} + w_3 \, \text{HCO}_3 - b. \qquad (4)$$

Table 3 provides the weights w_i, errors e_i, means $\overline{x_i}$ and standard deviations σ_i of the biomarkers. Since the range of values of the biomarkers varies widely, all values of the biomarkers are normalized by subtracting the mean and then dividing by the standard deviation in Eq. 4. See the Methods section for details. With this decision function, if the sepsis severity score (Score) is greater than or equal to zero, the severity diagnosis is 1, otherwise it is 0. The magnitudes of weights w_i indicate the importance of the corresponding biomarker [28]. We find that Ang-2 has a larger weight than Ang-1 and HCO$_3$, which is consistent with the results for the single biomarker classification in Fig. 3(A), where the TNR, and PPV are larger for Ang-2 than Ang-1 and HCO$_3$. However, the TPR and NPV are larger for HCO$_3$ compared to that for Ang-2. The sign of each weight w_i indicates the sign of the correlation of the biomarker with the sepsis severity score. Thus, the sepsis severity score for a patient with a relatively high Ang-2 level and low Ang-1 and HCO$_3$ levels is most likely positive. This relation between biomarkers and sepsis severity score has been observed in clinical studies [25,29,30].

Longitudinal measurements of the predictor

A linear SVM finds the hyper-plane that separates data with maximum margin by categories. In our study, the sign of the sepsis severity score (Score) in Eq. 4 can predict the category for a patient. The magnitude of the Score represents the distance from the decision boundary and indicates the severity of sepsis. A large positive Score indicates critical severity.

Based on the fact that patients were hospitalized during the study, the longitudinal measurements should show a decrease in the number of patients in the PICU severe sepsis group. Fig. 4 shows that Scores in the PICU severe sepsis group are notably separated from the PICU/sepsis group for the first two days after admission. After two days, the Scores in the PICU severe sepsis group decrease and collapse with those from the PICU/sepsis group indicating the effectiveness of the treatment. Additionally, the sepsis severity score (Eq. 4) measured on the first 2 days after admission may allow for the early identification of patients with severe sepsis, which is important for the initiation of early goal-directed therapies.

Comparison with the random forests learning method

Random forests (RF) [31] is an ensemble method [18,23], which grows multiple classification and regression trees (CART) [32] for prediction. Every tree in the forests is constructed by a random selected bootstrap training set with replacement [18]. The splitting criteria for every decision node in a tree are also chosen from a random subset of the features without replacement. With the replacement from the original data, about two-thirds of the samples are used to construct a tree [18]. The out-of-bag (OOB) data, which are not chosen in the construction, are then used to estimate the prediction accuracy and the importance of the features [31,33]. Unlike a linear SVM, which constructs a hyper-plane to classify the data, a tree is a hierarchical classification procedure, which recursively partitions the data to increase the purity of the nodes with respect to the outcome [32].

RF provides two measures, the mean decrease in accuracy (MDA) and mean decrease in the Gini index [31,33], to estimate the importance of the features. In our study, the MDA is chosen to estimate the feature importance since the decrease in the Gini index is not as reliable as MDA [33,34]. By randomly permuting the values of a given feature in the OOB data for each tree, RF measures the accuracy difference between untouched and

Table 3. Parameters for the decision function that includes the CCA-selected optimal subset of biomarkers at $k = 3$.

i	Biomarker	Mean $\overline{x}_i$	Standard Deviation σ_i	Weight w_i $(b=0.313)$	Standard Error of Weight e_i
1	Ang-2	8518.1	13264	1.994	0.065
2	Ang-1	2649.2	4008.9	−1.396	0.050
3	HCO$_3$	27.270	24.361	−1.340	0.072

The values of the weights w_i, errors e_i, means $\overline{x}_i$, and standard deviations σ_i for the biomarkers in Eq. (4).

permuted OOB data. The average of this accuracy difference over all trees in the forest is the MDA for the given feature. The MDA is the average increase in misclassification rate due to the permutations. The larger the MDA the more important the corresponding feature is with respect to the outcome.

Following Ref. [31], we construct a forest with 1,000 trees to estimate the MDA for the biomarkers. We generated two RF: one for which Ang-2/Ang-1 is excluded (Fig. 5(A)) or included (Fig. 5(B)). Because of the interaction of Ang-2, Ang-1, and Ang-2/Ang-1, the existence of Ang-2/Ang-1 suppresses the importance of Ang-2 and Ang-1. However, both CCA and FS methods tend to select the combination of Ang-2 and Ang-1 as the most predictive feature. We notice that HCO$_3$ is considered important for all three methods, which suggests HCO$_3$ is also an important biomarker. The RF ranked biomarkers based on the importance are also shown in Table 1.

We also constructed a SVM ensemble using the RF-selected subset for each step k in Fig. 2 for comparison. Similar to the CCA-selected subset in Fig. 2, all prediction measures saturate at $k = 4$ and decrease for $k > 4$. We find that the RF-selected optimal subset, Ang-2/Ang-1, HCO$_3$, Ang-2, Ang-1 at $k = 4$, have comparable prediction performance with the CCA-selected optimal subset at $k = 3$.

Discussion

In this study, we employed machine learning approaches to analyze the clinical data of children with severe sepsis using feature selection methods, such as CCA, SVM, FS and RF. Feature selection methods are helpful in identifying biomarkers with minimum redundancy that can be useful in clinical diagnosis. Our multivariate feature selection methods select the combination of Ang-1, Ang-2, and HCO$_3$ as the optimal biomarkers for our data set. We demonstrated that this optimal combination of biomarkers significantly outperformed each single biomarker and all other combinations with redundant or irrelevant biomarkers for all statistical measures.

Our work [10,27], and that of others, has shown the biological plausibility and clinical relevance of Ang-2 and Ang-1 levels in PICU patients with severe sepsis. It is interesting to note that combining Ang-2 and Ang-1 with a well-established (and routinely measured) indicator of an imbalance in the acid-base levels performs much better than other scoring systems that are more complex (for example, PIM-2 [12]).

Our data driven approach indicates that there is an optimal set of biomarkers for diagnosing severe sepsis. We have demonstrated that the use of additional biomarkers actually reduces the quality of the diagnostic scoring system. This is a potentially important observation in the sense that it suggests that more feature rich data may not be helpful, but actually harmful to patient care.

In addition, a sepsis severity score function (Eq. 4) using this optimal combination of biomarkers was constructed by the SVM

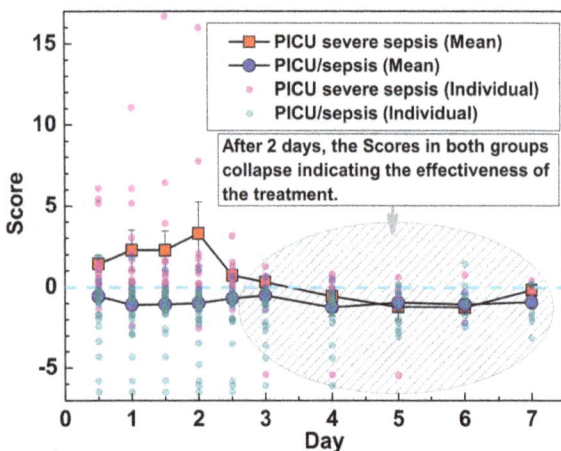

Figure 4. Longitudinal measurements of the sepsis severity score. The sepsis severity scores (Score) for patients from the PICU/sepsis group and the PICU severe sepsis during the 7 days of illness. Both the mean and individual severity scores are plotted.

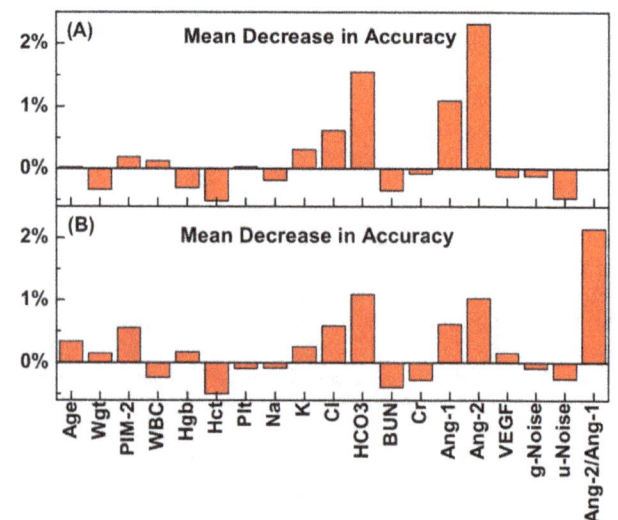

Figure 5. Measures of the biomarker importance obtained from the Random Forests method. Mean Decrease in Accuracy (MDA) are shown for biomarkers in (A) without Ang-2/Ang-1 and (B) with Ang-2/Ang-1 using the Random Forests method with 1,000 trees for each.

ensemble method. With this function, we can interpret the relation between these three biomarkers and the sepsis severity from the associate weights, w_i [28]. Even though these relations have been observed in clinical studies [10,25,26], we assert that our methodology is useful since it obtains similar results to those of the clinical studies using unbiased, rigorous statistical analyses. It also holds promise for the discovery of novel biomarkers.

The proposed sepsis severity score for each sample is also evaluated during the treatment. The patients in the PICU severe sepsis group have significantly high severity scores after admission. The sepsis severity scores measured on the first 2 days after admission may allow for the early identification of patients with severe sepsis. After two days treatment, the severity scores for each patient decline and collapse to match patients without severe sepsis. Based on the fact that all patients survived hospitalization, the change in the longitudinal measurements of this score function validates the robustness and effectiveness of this function as regards its potential utility at different stages of treatment.

It has been observed that single biomarkers, in isolation, have limited diagnostic capacity [5]. This study supports this conclusion. Our analysis strongly supports the conclusion that a combination of different biomarkers is more effective, i.e., using multiple biomarkers for diagnosis is superior to drawing conclusions from single biomarkers. The rationale for this observation may be that the biomarkers are not independent of each other but, as we have shown with our canonical correlation analysis, are correlated in groups. The identification of an optimal combination of biomarkers allows clinicians to focus on a small subset of indicators, which simplifies the diagnosis of sepsis in children with a spectrum of severities.

Despite the success in the classification of sepsis severity for this patient group, our study has several limitations. First, the data set was obtained from a single institution making generalizability difficult. Second, the biomarkers used to construct our models were based on clinical availability for most patients. It is possible that additional biomarkers, such as cytokines, would have improved the statistical measures for our models. Finally, since we have shown that measures of acid-base status are predictive biomarkers, it is likely that other acid-base determinants from blood gas analyses will also be predictive biomarkers. However, blood gas results were only available for the severe sepsis group

(not other groups), and thus including blood gas measurements would have biased our findings. We advocate new clinical studies that include additional clinical variables, such as blood gas panels, to address the question of finding the most predictive set of biomarkers for severe sepsis.

In conclusion, we have shown that a linear additive combination of 3 biomarkers, namely Ang-2, Ang-1 and HCO_3 provides a robust prediction of sepsis severity in patients admitted to the PICU. Additional independent studies are needed to confirm or refute the clinical utility of our biomarker combination for sepsis severity prediction. The collection of data sets with larger sample sizes would also be very useful for validating our statistical study.

Supporting Information

Figure S1 Sample size by study day. Samples were obtained twice per day for the first 3 days and then once per day for the last 4 days, for a maximum of 7 days and 10 samples. Sample collection was discontinued when the patient was discharged from the PICU, after the 7-day study completion, or when the clinical team deemed it unnecessary to draw further labs for patient care.

File S1 Contains Table S1, Infectious organisms: Causative organisms isolated in patients. N gives the number of patients with a given proven infection. Table S2, Baseline patient characteristics: Statistical analysis of the baseline patient characteristics based on the evaluation distributions of the PICU/sepsis group and PICU severe sepsis group. Categorical variables, presented as count (percentage), were analyzed using Fisher exact test. Continuous variables, presented as mean (standard deviation), were analyzed using the two-tailed t test. P values are comparisons between two groups. Any significance level of P less than 0.05 is associated with the diagnosis. Text S1, Supplementary Text.

Author Contributions

Conceived and designed the experiments: KW MK CSO VB MDS. Performed the experiments: JSG. Analyzed the data: KW. Contributed reagents/materials/analysis tools: KW MK. Wrote the paper: KW MK CSO VB JSG.

References

1. Watson RS, Carcillo JA (2005) Scope and epidemiology of pediatric sepsis. Pediatric Critical Care Medicine 6: S3–S5.
2. Kochanek KD, Kirmeyer SE, Martin JA, Strobino DM, Guyer B (2012) Annual summary of vital statistics: 2009. Pediatrics: peds–2011.
3. Proulx F, Joyal JS, Mariscalco MM, Leteurtre S, Leclerc F, et al. (2009) The pediatric multiple organ dysfunction syndrome. Pediatric Critical Care Medicine 10: 12–22.
4. Watson RS, Carcillo JA, Linde-Zwirble WT, Clermont G, Lidicker J, et al. (2003) The epidemiology of severe sepsis in children in the united states. American journal of respiratory and critical care medicine 167: 695–701.
5. Pierrakos C, Vincent JL, et al. (2010) Sepsis biomarkers: a review. Crit Care 14: R15.
6. Samraj RS, Zingarelli B, Wong HR (2013) Role of biomarkers in sepsis care. Shock 40: 358–365.
7. Wong HR, Salisbury S, Xiao Q, Cvijanovich NZ, Hall M, et al. (2012) The pediatric sepsis biomarker risk model. Crit Care 16: R174.
8. Wong HR, Weiss SL, Giuliano Jr JS, Wainwright MS, Cvijanovich NZ, et al. (2014) Testing the prognostic accuracy of the updated pediatric sepsis biomarker risk model. PLOS ONE 9: e86242.
9. Wong HR, Weiss SL, Giuliano Jr JS, Wainwright MS, Cvijanovich NZ, et al. (2014) The temporal version of the pediatric sepsis biomarker risk model. PloS one 9: e92121.
10. Giuliano Jr JS, Tran K, Li FY, Shabanova V, Tala JA, et al. (2014) The temporal kinetics of circulating angiopoietin levels in children with sepsis. Pediatric Critical Care Medicine 15: e1–e8.
11. Goldstein B, Giroir B, Randolph A, et al. (2005) International pediatric sepsis consensus conference: Definitions for sepsis and organ dysfunction in pediatrics. Pediatric critical care medicine 6: 2–8.
12. Slater A, Shann F, Pearson G (2003) Pim2: a revised version of the paediatric index of mortality. Intensive care medicine 29: 278–285.
13. Morik K, Brockhausen P, Joachims T (1999) Combining statistical learning with a knowledge-based approach-a case study in intensive care monitoring. In: Machine Learning-International Workshop Then Conference. Morgan Kaufmann Publishers, Inc., pp. 268–277.
14. Mardia KV, Kent JT, Bibby JM (1980) Multivariate analysis.
15. Tofallis C (1999) Model building with multiple dependent variables and constraints. Journal of the Royal Statistical Society: Series D (The Statistician) 48: 371–378.
16. Vapnik V (2000) The nature of statistical learning theory. springer.
17. Mangasarian OL (1999) Arbitrary-norm separating plane. Operations Research Letters 24: 15–23.
18. Breiman L (1996) Bagging predictors. Machine learning 24: 123–140.
19. Wang K, Bhandari V, Chepustanova S, Huber G, Stephen O, et al. (2013) Which biomarkers reveal neonatal sepsis? PloS one 8: e82700.
20. Björck A, Golub GH (1973) Numerical methods for computing angles between linear subspaces. Mathematics of computation 27: 579–594.
21. Efroymson M (1960) Multiple regression analysis. Mathematical methods for digital computers 1: 191–203.
22. Sjöstrand K, Clemmensen LH, Larsen R, Ersbøll B (2012) Spasm: A matlab toolbox for sparse statistical modeling. Journal of Statistical Software Accepted for publication.

23. Dietterich TG (2000) Ensemble methods in machine learning. In: Multiple classifier systems, Springer. pp. 1–15.

24. Kim HC, Pang S, Je HM, Kim D, Yang Bang S (2003) Constructing support vector machine ensemble. Pattern recognition 36: 2757–2767.

25. Ricciuto DR, dos Santos CC, Hawkes M, Toltl IJ, Conroy AL, et al. (2011) Angiopoietin-1 and angiopoietin-2 as clinically informative prognostic biomarkers of morbidity and mortality in severe sepsis. Critical care medicine 39: 702–710.

26. Fiusa M, Costa-Lima C, de Souza GR, Vigorito AC, Aranha F, et al. (2013) A high angiopoietin-2/angiopoietin-1 ratio is associated with a high risk of septic shock in patients with febrile neutropenia. Crit Care 17: R169.

27. Giuliano Jr JS, Lahni PM, Harmon K, Wong HR, Doughty LA, et al. (2007) Admission angiopoietin levels in children with septic shock. Shock (Augusta, Ga) 28: 650.

28. Mladenić D, Brank J, Grobelnik M, Milic-Frayling N (2004) Feature selection using linear classifier weights: interaction with classification models. In:

29. van der Heijden M, Pickkers P, van Nieuw Amerongen GP, van Hinsbergh VW, Bouw MP, et al. (2009) Circulating angiopoietin levels in the course of septic shock: relation with fluid balance, pulmonary dysfunction and mortality. Intensive care medicine 35: 1567–1574.

30. David S, Mukherjee A, Ghosh CC, Yano M, Khankin EV, et al. (2012) Angiopoietin-2 may contribute to multi-organ dysfunction and death in sepsis. Critical care medicine 40: 3034.

31. Breiman L (2001) Random forests. Machine learning 45: 5–32.

32. Breiman L, Friedman J, Stone CJ, Olshen RA (1984) Classification and regression trees. CRC press.

33. Pang H, Lin A, Holford M, Enerson BE, Lu B, et al. (2006) Pathway analysis using random forests classification and regression. Bioinformatics 22: 2028–2036.

34. Breiman L (2002) Manual on setting up, using, and understanding random forests v3. 1. Retrieved October 23: 2010.

Proceedings of the 27th annual international ACM SIGIR conference on Research and development in information retrieval. ACM, pp. 234–241.

17

Mortality Predictors in Renal Transplant Recipients with Severe Sepsis and Septic Shock

Mônica Andrade de Carvalho[1]*, **Flávio Geraldo Rezende Freitas**[1,2], **Hélio Tedesco Silva Junior**[1], **Antônio Toneti Bafi**[1,2], **Flávia Ribeiro Machado**[2], **José Osmar Medina Pestana**[1]

1 Unidade de Transplante, Disciplina de Nefrologia, Universidade Federal de São Paulo, São Paulo, SP, Brazil, 2 Disciplina de Anestesiologia, Dor e Terapia Intensiva. Universidade Federal de São Paulo, São Paulo, SP, Brazil

Abstract

Introduction: The growing number of renal transplant recipients in a sustained immunosuppressive state is a factor that can contribute to increased incidence of sepsis. However, relatively little is known about sepsis in this population. The aim of this single-center study was to evaluate the factors associated with hospital mortality in renal transplant patients admitted to the intensive care unit (ICU) with severe sepsis and septic shock.

Methods: Patient demographics and transplant-related and ICU stay data were retrospectively collected. Multiple logistic regression was conducted to identify the independent risk factors associated with hospital mortality.

Results: A total of 190 patients were enrolled, 64.2% of whom received kidneys from deceased donors. The mean patient age was 51±13 years (males, 115 [60.5%]), and the median APACHE II was 20 (16–23). The majority of patients developed sepsis late after the renal transplantation (2.1 [0.6–2.3] years). The lung was the most common infection site (59.5%). Upon ICU admission, 16.4% of the patients had ≤1 systemic inflammatory response syndrome criteria. Among the patients, 61.5% presented with ≥2 organ failures at admission, and 27.9% experienced septic shock within the first 24 hours of ICU admission. The overall hospital mortality rate was 38.4%. In the multivariate analysis, the independent determinants of hospital mortality were male gender (OR = 5.9; 95% CI, 1.7–19.6; p = 0.004), delta SOFA 24 h (OR = 1.7; 95% CI, 1.2–2.3; p = 0.001), mechanical ventilation (OR = 30; 95% CI, 8.8–102.2; p<0.0001), hematologic dysfunction (OR = 6.8; 95% CI, 2.0–22.6; p = 0.002), admission from the ward (OR = 3.4; 95% CI, 1.2–9.7; p = 0.02) and acute kidney injury stage 3 (OR = 5.7; 95% CI,1.9–16.6; p = 0.002).

Conclusions: Hospital mortality in renal transplant patients with severe sepsis and septic shock was associated with male gender, admission from the wards, worse SOFA scores on the first day and the presence of hematologic dysfunction, mechanical ventilation or advanced graft dysfunction.

Editor: Antonio De Maio, University of California, San Diego, United States of America

Funding: The project was supported by funding from the Coordenação de Aperfeiçoamento de Pessoal de Nível Superior (CAPES) programme and Hospital do Rim. The funders had no role in study design, data collection and analysis, decision to publish, or preparation of the manuscript.

Competing Interests: The authors have declared that no competing interests exist.

* Email: mactulha@hotmail.com

Introduction

Sepsis is the leading cause of death in non-cardiac intensive care units, although there is some evidence of a decline in mortality rates, at least in developed countries [1–4]. The scenario in emerging and limited-resources countries seems to be different with higher reported rates [5,6], although low mortality rates has also been reported [7]. The incidence of sepsis is increasing over the past years and the growing number of patients living with solid organ transplants is a factor that contributes to this finding [2–4,8].

The most common solid organ transplant procedure worldwide is the renal transplantation. It is the treatment of choice for end-stage renal disease. Compared with chronic dialysis, renal transplantation is cost-effective, offers improved quality of life and confers a progressive survival benefit [9,10]. The overall survival rate of kidney grafts has improved consistently during the past decades [11]. Moreover, the number of adult candidates on the waiting lists with kidney failure continues to increase [12]. Therefore, more renal transplant recipients with functioning grafts will be exposed to pathogens while in a sustained immunosuppressive state.

Because of immunosuppression, infection frequently occurs after kidney transplantation and greatly impacts patient morbidity and mortality. This explains why infection is the second leading cause of death in renal transplant recipients, following cardiovascular diseases [13]. The importance of infection as cause of death is higher in underdeveloped countries [14,15]. Surprisingly,

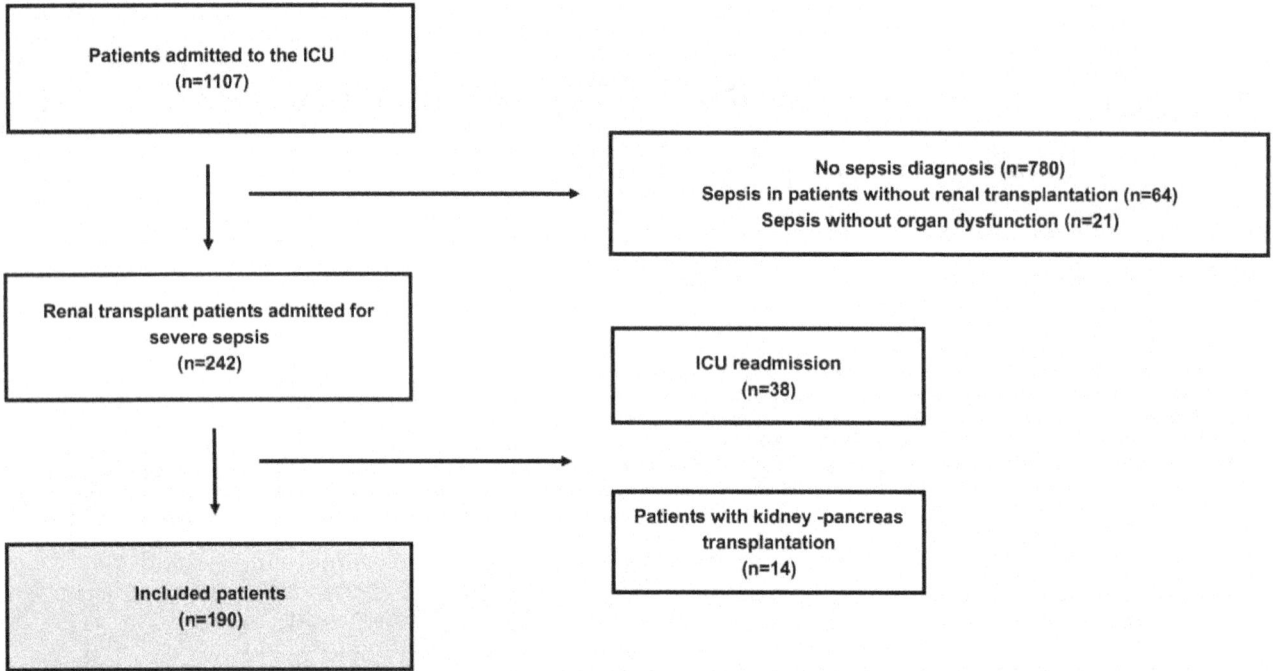

Figure 1. Study flowchart. ICU: intensive care unit.

relatively little is known about severe sepsis in this growing population. The aim of this study was to describe the characteristics of severe sepsis and septic shock in renal transplant patients who are admitted to the intensive care unit (ICU) and to evaluate the factors associated with hospital mortality.

Materials and Methods

This single center, retrospective, observational study was performed at a kidney transplant center in Brazil [16]. The institutional ethics committee approved the study and waived the informed consent requirement (Comité de Ética em Pesquisa – Universidade Federal de São Paulo, reference number: 1736–10). All consecutive adult renal transplant recipients (older than 18 years) diagnosed with severe sepsis or septic shock who were admitted to our 12-bed ICU from June 1, 2010 to December 31, 2011 were included. We excluded pregnant patients, patients who underwent kidney-pancreas transplantation, and patients with "do not resuscitate" orders. All patients were included only in their first episode of sepsis.

Data were retrospectively collected through medical records by a single author (MAC). We recorded the following data: patient demographics, comorbid chronic illnesses, severe sepsis characteristics and the severity scores Sequential Organ Failure Assessment (SOFA) and Acute Physiology and Chronic Health Evaluation II (APACHE II). We also collected data on the initial treatment, life support and fluid balance as well as pre-transplant, peritransplant and post-transplant variables. We assessed adequacy of treatment according to the compliance to the 6-hours Surviving Sepsis Campaign bundle available during the study period [17], which are similar to the recent published 3-hour and 6-hour bundles of the 2012 revised guidelines [18]. All transplant patients in our hospital are under continuous surveillance. Thus, the hospital database has all information about outpatient's visits,

hospital readmissions or death in other institutions. Thus, we collected not only the hospital mortality during the septic episode but also the one-year survival. The database was reviewed by two authors (FGRF and FRM). In cases of inconsistency, the sources documents were verified, and the data were corrected. Data were anonymized and de-identified prior to data analysis.

Severe sepsis was defined as a documented or presumed infection plus at least one organ failure secondary to infection. We did not use the systemic inflammatory response syndrome (SIRS) criteria, as depressed febrile response and diminished leukocytosis are frequently seen in solid-organ recipients [19]. Septic shock was defined as volume-refractory hypotension with the need for vasopressor. Organ dysfunction was diagnosed when one of the following factors was present: hypotension with systolic blood pressure <90 mmHg or mean arterial blood pressure <65 mmHg (cardiovascular); arterial oxygen partial pressure/oxygen inspiratory fraction (PaO_2/FiO_2) ratio ≤ 300 (respiratory); a bilirubin level $>$ twice the reference value (hepatic); a lactate level ≥ 1.5 times the reference value and a base deficit >5 (metabolic); an international normalized ratio (INR) >1.5 or a platelet count $<$ 100,000/mL (hematologic) and altered level of consciousness (neurologic). To define renal dysfunction, we used increased serum creatinine $>$ twice the baseline value. This cutoff was arbitrary chosen because of the lack of agreement on the definition of acute kidney injury (AKI) in this population. In parallel, we also used the definition recommended by Kidney Disease: Improving Global Outcomes (KDIGO) [20] to stage AKI during the ICU stay, without considering urine output.

The time to the sepsis diagnosis was defined as the number of hours elapsed between the onset of the first organ dysfunction and the recognition and management of sepsis by the healthcare provider, as described elsewhere [21]. The severe sepsis and septic shock treatment was analyzed based on compliance with the initial care bundle (within the first 6 hrs of presentation) [22].

Table 1. Patient characteristics and transplant variables.

	All Patients (n = 190)	Survivors (n = 117)	Non survivors (n = 73)	p value
Age (years)	51±13	50±13	52±13	0.300
Male gender	115 (60.5)	61 (52.1)	54 (73.9)	**0.002**
Body mass index (kg/m^2)	24±5	25±5	23±4	**0.003**
Comorbidities				
Hypertension	152 (80.0)	99 (84.6)	53 (72.6)	**0.040**
Diabetes mellitus	61 (32.1)	39 (33.3)	22 (30.1)	0.600
CAD	35 (18.4)	24 (20.5)	11 (15.0)	0.300
Stroke	8 (4.2)	6 (5.1)	2 (2.7)	0.700
CHF	5 (2.6)	3 (2.5)	2 (2.7)	1.000
Hepatitis C	13 (6.8)	7 (5.9)	6 (8.2)	0.500
Hepatitis B	6 (3.1)	3 (2.5)	3 (4.1)	0.600
COPD	6 (3.1)	1 (0.8)	5 (6.8)	**0.030**
ESRD etiology				0.220
Undetermined	67 (35.2)	41 (35.0)	26 (35.6)	
Glomerulonephritis	50 (26.3)	33 (28.2)	17 (23.2)	
Diabetes mellitus	36 (18.9)	18 (15.3)	18 (24.6)	
Hypertension	28 (14.7)	21 (17.9)	7 (9.5)	
Urologic disease	9 (4.7)	4 (3.4)	5 (6.8)	
Dialysis modality before transplant				0.480
Preemptive	8 (4.2)	7 (5.9)	1 (1.3)	
Hemodialysis	153 (80.5)	91 (77.7)	62 (84.9)	
Peritoneal	21 (11.0)	14 (11.9)	7 (9.5)	
Hemodialysis/peritoneal	8 (4.2)	5 (4.2)	3 (4.1)	
Time of dialysis (months)	34 (18–60)	32 (18–60)	36 (24–68)	0.170
Donor type				0.190
Deceased	122 (64.2)	71 (60.6)	51 (69.8)	
Living	68 (35.8)	46 (39.4)	22 (30.2)	
Donor gender [a]				0.330
Female	71 (42.0)	43 (40.6)	28 (44.5)	
Male	98 (58.0)	63 (59.4)	35 (55.5)	
Deceased donor [b]				
Cause of death [c]				0.930
Traumatic brain injury	33 (28.0)	21 (30.0)	12 (25.0)	
Subarachnoid hemorrhage	20 (16.9)	12 (17.1)	8 (16.6)	
Stroke	56 (47.5)	32 (45.7)	24 (50.0)	
Others	9 (7.6)	5 (7.2)	4 (8.4)	
Panel reactive antibodies [d]				0.660
0–50%	93 (84.5)	55 (83.3)	38 (86.3)	
>51%	17 (15.5)	11 (16.7)	6 (13.6)	
Final creatinine [e]				0.210
<1.5 mg/dL	31 (32.6)	21 (35.5)	10 (27.7)	
≥1.5 mg/dL	64 (67.4)	38 (64.5)	26 (72.3)	
Cold ischemia time (hours) [f]	23 (20–27)	23 (20–28)	22 (20–27)	0.630
Expanded criteria donor	31 (26.3)	13 (18.6)	18 (37.5)	**0.020**
Delayed graft function	82 (43.3)	44 (37.6)	38 (52.7)	**0.040**
Thymoglobulin use [g]	54 (28.5)	34 (29.0)	20 (27.7)	0.870
CMV disease treated	68 (35.9)	41 (35.0)	27 (37.5)	0.750
Current immunosuppression [h]				0.460
TAC+PRED+AZA	31 (16.3)	16 (13.6)	15 (20.5)	
TAC+PRED+MF	70 (36.8)	48 (41.0)	22 (30.1)	

Table 1. Cont.

	All Patients (n = 190)	Survivors (n = 117)	Non survivors (n = 73)	p value
CSA+PRED+AZA	17 (8.9)	12 (10.2)	5 (6.8)	
CSA+PRED+MF	7 (3.6)	4 (3.4)	3 (4.1)	
TAC/CSA+PRED+EVR/SRL	4 (2.1)	3 (2.5)	1 (1.7)	
SRL/EVR+PRED+MF	9 (4.7)	4 (3.4)	5 (6.8)	
Others	51 (26.8)	30 (25.6)	21 (28.7)	
Time between transplant and sepsis (years)	2.1 (0.6–7.2)	2.3 (0.6–7.8)	1.6 (0.6–7.0)	0.600
Acute rejection	55 (28.9)	34 (29.0)	21 (28.7)	0.960
Time rejection-sepsis (days) [i]	312 (130–776)	331 (115–817)	282 (152–849)	0.900

CAD coronary artery disease, CHF: congestive heart failure, COPD: chronic obstructive pulmonary disease, ESRD: end-stage renal disease, CMV: *cytomegalovirus*, TAC: tacrolimus, PRED: prednisone, AZA: azathioprine, MF: mycophenolate, CSA: cyclosporine, EVR: everolimus, SRL sirolimus.
a) 21 missing data,
b) 122 deceased donors,
c) 4 missing data,
d) 12 missing data,
e) final creatinine refers to the donors' last serum creatinine level, 27 missing data,
f) 3 missing data,
g) patients who used thymoglobulin for treating rejection and/or induction in transplantation,
h) 1 missing data and i) time between the occurrence of rejection and sepsis (total of patients with rejection, 55 patients, 3 patients among the survivors and 6 among the non-survivors were excluded for missing data). The results are expressed as number (%) or median (IQR, 25%–75%) or mean ± standard deviation. Chi-squared test, Mann-Whitney U-test, and Student's t-test (univariate analysis).

Statistical methods

The categorical variables are described as percentages, and the continuous variables are described as measures of central tendency and dispersion, according to distribution, as assessed by the Kolmogorov-Smirnov test. We compare hospital survivors and non-survivor using the two-tailed t-test, Mann-Whitney U-test, chi-squared test, and Fisher's exact test, as appropriate. Multiple logistic regression was conducted to identify the independent risk factors associated with hospital mortality, including all variables with a p value <0.10 in the univariate analysis (using a stepwise forward regression model). The time until the sepsis diagnosis was categorized using the best cutoff value in the receiver operating characteristic (ROC) curve for mortality (≥170 vs. <170 min). The number of organ dysfunctions (≥2 vs. <2) and the KDIGO classification (stage 3 vs. stage <3) of acute kidney injury during ICU stay were also categorized. All variables were checked for confounding and collinearity. The model calibration was assessed using the Hosmer-Lemeshow test, which was considered to be appropriate if p>0.10. We did not include the variables with missing data >10%, as the lack of data would result in serious inconsistencies. The patients were followed for one year, and a mortality curve was generated using the Kaplan-Meier methodology. A p value <0.05 was considered to be significant. Data were analyzed using SPSS 19.0 for Windows (SPSS, Chicago, IL, USA).

Results

During the study period, 1107 patients were admitted to the ICU, 242 (21.9%) of whom were renal transplant patients who were admitted for severe sepsis. Of these patients, 190 were enrolled, as shown in Figure 1.

The patients' characteristics and transplant variables are summarized in Table 1. The leading causes of end-stage renal disease were glomerulonephritis (26.3%), diabetes mellitus (18.9%) and hypertension (14.7%), although most patients (35.2%) did not have an identifiable cause. The majority of kidneys transplanted were from deceased donors (64.2%). All patients had immunosuppression suspended at ICU admission and used hydrocortisone

(50 mg every six hours). The majority of the patients developed sepsis late after the renal transplantation (2.1 years; range, 0.6–2.3 years). Fifty-five patients (28.9%) had histories of acute rejection that occurred at a median of 312 days (range, 130–776 days) before the ICU admission. The univariate analysis showed delayed graft function, and expanded criteria donor kidneys were associated with hospital mortality. No other clinical characteristic related to the transplant was significantly different between the survivors and non-survivors.

The lung was the most common site of infection (59.5%), followed by the urinary tract (16.8%) and abdomen (9.5%) (Table 2). We isolated the etiologic agents in the majority of the patients (57%). Most of these agents were bacteria (Gram-negative, 45.4%; Gram-positive: 20.4%). The other relevant agents were *Mycobacterium tuberculosis* (3.7%), Cytomegalovirus (3.7%) and fungi (24%), including *Pneumocystis jirovecii* (8.3%) (Table 3).

Upon ICU admission, 16.4% of the patients had ≤1 SIRS criterion (Figure 2). The most common SIRS criteria were tachypnea (74.7%) and tachycardia (67.9%). Two or more organ failures were present at admission in 61.5% of patients. Respiratory and hematological dysfunctions occurred more frequently in the non-survivors. Fifty-three patients (27.9%) experienced septic shock within the first 24 hours of ICU admission; however, 96 (50.5%) patients experienced septic shock during their ICU stays. The time for severe sepsis diagnosis was longer in the non-survivors. The patients who developed sepsis in the ward had worse outcomes than those patients in the emergency room (Table 2). The compliance rate with each component of the 6-hour bundle is shown in Table 2. The compliance rate for fluid administration (20 ml/kg crystalloid for hypotension or lactate ≥36 mg/dl) was higher among the survivors.

The clinical and biological variables at the ICU admission and during the ICU stay are shown in Table 3. In the univariate analysis, most of the variables were significantly different between the survivors and non-survivors. Note that more positive fluid

Table 2. Severe sepsis characteristics and treatment.

	All patients (n = 190)	Survivors (n = 117)	Non-survivors (n = 73)	p value
Site of infection				**0.006**
Respiratory	113 (59.5)	66 (56.4)	47 (64.3)	
Urinary	32 (16.8)	28 (23.9)	4 (5.4)	
Abdominal	18 (9.5	8 (6.8)	10 (13.7)	
Others	27 (14.2)	15 (12.8)	12 (16.4)	
SIRS criteria				
Tachypnea	142 (74.7)	84 (71.7)	58 (79.4)	0.230
Tachycardia	129 (67.9)	80 (68.3)	49 (67.1)	0.850
Leukocytosis	50 (26.3)	28 (23.9)	22 (30.1)	0.340
Leukopenia	31 (16.3)	16 (13.6)	15 (20.5)	0.210
Fever	46 (24.2)	32 (27.3)	14 (19.1)	0.200
Hypothermia	12 (6.3)	7 (5.9)	5 (6.8)	1.000
Organ failures				
Respiratory	84 (44.2)	43 (36.7)	41 (56.1)	**0.008**
Cardiovascular	78 (41.1)	49(41.8)	29 (39.7)	0.760
Renal	77 (40.5)	51 (43.5)	26 (35.6)	0.270
Hematologic	64 (33.9)	30 (25.6)	34 (46.6)	0.030
Neurologic	50 (26.3)	26 (22.2)	24 (32.8)	0.100
Metabolic	13 (7.9)	5 (4.8)	8 (12.9)	0.070
Hepatic	9 (4.7)	6 (5.1)	3 (4.1)	1.000
Admission				**<0.0001**
Emergency	110 (57.9)	83 (70.9)	27 (36.9)	
Ward	80 (42.1)	34 (29.0)	46 (63.0)	
Number of organs dysfunctions (≥2)	117 (61.5)	65 (55.5)	52 (71.2)	0.030
Glycemia (mg/dl)[a]	149 (121–194)	151 (121–195)	141 (119–193)	0.360
Time to sepsis diagnosis (hours)	2.5 (1.1–5.2)	2 (0.9–4.2)	3.5 (1.5–6.3)	**<0.001**
Time to antibiotics (minutes)	55 (30–120)	60 (30–120)	45 (20–80)	**<0.001**
Duration of ICU stay (days)	6 (3–13)	6 (3–11)	7 (3–16)	0.130
Duration of hospital stay (days)	20 (12–35)	21 (14–38)	15 (8–31)	0.010
Compliance to severe sepsis bundle				
Measure lactate	164 (86.3)	103 (88.0)	61 (83.5)	0.300
Broad-spectrum antibiotics	173 (91.0)	107 (91.5)	66 (90.4)	0.800
Blood cultures before antibiotics	151 (79.5)	93 (79.4)	58 (79.5)	0.990
Fluid resuscitation [b]	54 (62.3)	39 (75)	15 (44.1)	**0.004**
CVP >8 mm Hg [c]	6 (15.8)	2 (11.1)	4 (22.2)	0.370
ScvO2 >70% [c]	14 (36.8)	7 (38.9)	7 (38.9)	1.000
Initial care bundle	74 (39.0)	45 (38.5)	29 (39.7)	0.800

SIRS: systemic inflammatory response syndrome. ICU: intensive care unit. CVP: central venous pressure, $ScvO_2$: central venous oxygen saturation.
a) median glycemia during the first 24 h of sepsis,
b) indication to administer 20 ml/kg crystalloid for hypotension or lactate ≥36 mg/dl (n = 86),
c) indication to measure CVP or measure $ScvO_2$ (n = 38). The results are expressed as number (%) or median (IQR: 25%–75%). Chi-squared test and Mann-Whitney U-test (univariate analysis).

balance at 72 hours was also associated with hospital mortality; however this variable was not included in multiple logistic regression due to missing data.

The basal creatinine values (before severe sepsis) were 1.93 ± 1.44 mg/dL. Four patients were under dialysis before ICU admission because of acute Kidney dysfunction. Seventy seven (40.5%) had renal dysfunction (increased serum creatinine > twice the baseline value). Staging AKI according KDIGO, 48 (25.3%) patients reaching Stage 1, 27 (14.2%) a Stage 2, and 94 (49.5%) a Stage 3. There was a strong association between acute kidney injury stage 3 and hospital mortality (Table 4). During ICU stay, 77 (40.5%) patients underwent dialysis (conventional hemodialysis or sustained low-efficiency dialysis). The need for dialysis was higher among non-survivors (75.3% vs. 18.8%, p< 0.001). The need for dialysis was not included in our multivariate analysis because of its collinearity with AKI stage 3.

The overall hospital mortality rate was 38.4% (32.1% in severe sepsis patients and 54.7% in patients with septic shock in the first

Table 3. Frequencies of infectious agents identified.

	Frequency, n (%)
Gram-negative	49 (45.4)
Escherichia coli	16 (15.0)
Klebsiella pneumonia	13 (12.0)
Pseudomonas aeruginosa	8 (7.4)
Acinetobacter baumanii	6 (5.5)
Enterobacter sp	3 (2.7)
Proteus mirabilis	2 (1.8)
Citrobacter sp	1 (0.9)
Gram-positive	22 (20.4)
Staphylococcus aureus	10 (9.2)
Enterococcus sp	7 (6.5)
Staphylococcus epidermidis	3 (2.7)
Streptococcus pneumoniae	1 (0.9)
Streptococcus viridans	1 (0.9)
Fungi	26 (24.0)
Candida albicans	10 (9.2)
Pneumocystis jiroveci	9 (8.3)
Cryptococcus	2 (1.8)
Histoplasma capsulatum	3 (2.7)
Cândida sp	2 (1.8)
Others	11 (10.2)
Mycobacterium turbeculosis	4 (3.7)
Cytomegalovirus	4 (3.7)
Listeria monocytogenes	1 (0.9)
Neisseria meningitidis	1 (0.9)
Salmonella sp	1 (0.9)

24 hrs of ICU admission). In the multivariate analysis, the independent determinants of hospital mortality were male gender, delta SOFA score 24 h, mechanical ventilation, hematological dysfunction, admission from ward and AKI stage 3 (Table 5). We could assess the one-year mortality data in all patients and the rate was 42.6% (37.2% for severe sepsis and 56.6% for septic shock). Figure 3 shows the Kaplan-Meier curves for one-year survival after ICU admission.

Discussion

In our study, we were able to show that the independent risk factors for hospital mortality in renal transplant recipients with severe sepsis and septic shock admitted to ICU did not include the transplant characteristics. There was a lower incidence of SIRS criteria than previously described in other sepsis studies, and there was a higher frequency of opportunistic pathogens causing severe sepsis. We also demonstrated a low increment in the mortality rate one-year after discharge.

The hospital mortality rate for ICU renal transplant recipients varies greatly in the literature, and no study has specifically evaluated septic patients [23–29]. Old Brazilian sepsis data from private and public ICU have shown higher mortality rates than in the present study [21,30]. More recent data still shows a higher mortality rate in Brazil [5] than that reported in some studies conducted in developed countries [2–4]. There are some possible

explanations for this worst performance. In emerging countries, there are roughly enough resources but there is still limitation in access of care both in private and in public health systems. Sepsis awareness among lay people is restricted which contributes to a delay in searching for care. The gap between scientific evidence and bedside and staff's lack of knowledge, a frequent challenge even in the developed nations, is probably deeper in such settings. Our better findings might be partially explained by a shorter time to sepsis diagnosis [21], which was also associated with survival in our univariate analysis. In addition, the early management of these patients, as assessed by the compliance to Surviving Sepsis Campaign 6-hours bundle [17,18], was higher than those previously described [21,22]. The importance of high compliance with the resuscitation bundle to reduce mortality rate was demonstrated in Brazilian private hospitals [7]. In our study, there was a significant lower compliance to fluid administration in non-survivors. Interesting, non-survivors had higher fluid balance at 72 h. This finding suggests that fluids may be essential in the earliest phases of treatment, but late administration may be harmful.

Previous sepsis cohort studies have shown an increment in the mortality rate for sepsis patients (from 7% to 43%) 12 months after the initial assessment (hospital or 28-days mortality) [31]. In our study, no relevant increase in the 12-month mortality rate was observed compared to the in-hospital mortality rate (42.6% and 38.4%, respectively). This interesting and previously unreported

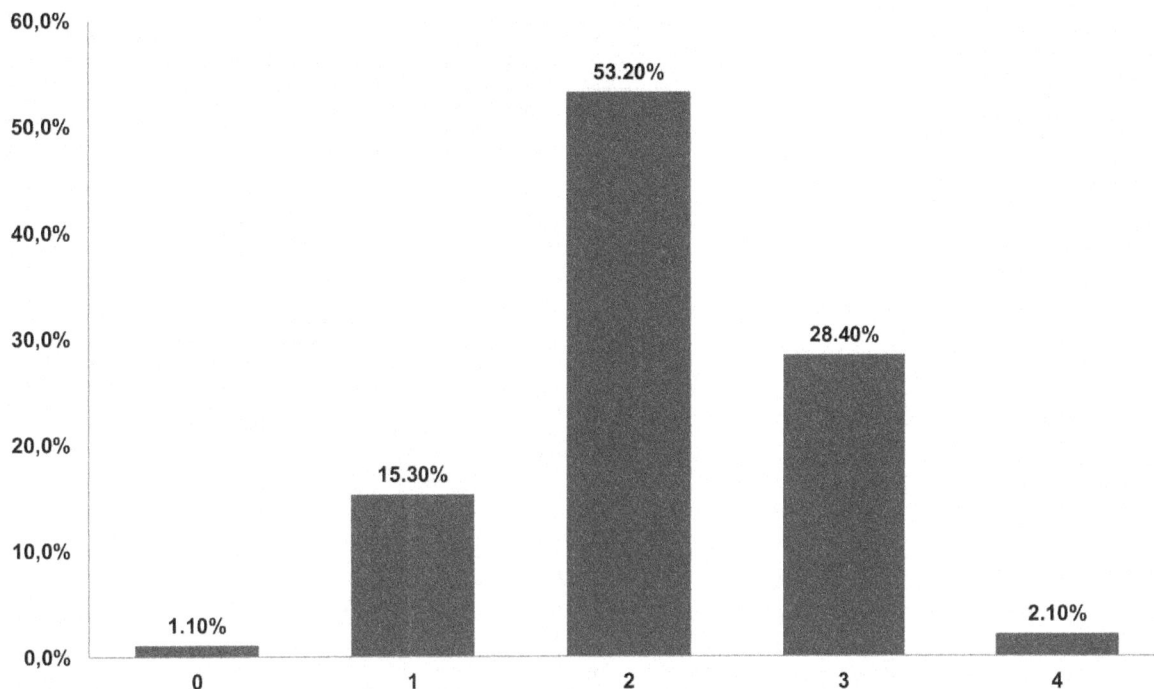

Figure 2. Frequency of systemic inflammatory response signs on intensive care unit admission.

finding might be explained, at least partially, by the fact that our patients were younger than those in other sepsis cohort studies [1,21]. Moreover, they were under continuous surveillance in a transplant center with adequate care during the entire follow-up period.

Considerable variations were present in our findings compared to other sepsis epidemiological studies. Our patients had fewer SIRS criteria. In a cohort, multicenter, observational study in European countries, Sprung et al. reported that approximately 90% of their septic patients had ≥3 SIRS criteria, while in our study only 30% of patients had ≥3 SIRS criteria [32]. Moreover, we found that 16.4% of the patients had ≤1 SIRS criteria. This profile of systemic inflammatory response has been previously suggested [19,33]. Sawyer et al. demonstrated that immunosuppressed solid organ transplant patients had significantly lower maximum temperatures and white blood cells counts compared to non-transplant patients [33]. These findings should be taken into account in sepsis studies involving transplant patients, as the need for meeting SIRS criteria to define sepsis could be flawed and may not adequately reflect the actual incidence of sepsis. In fact, the current SIRS criteria to define the presence of sepsis has been criticized even in immunocompetent patients [34].

In our study, the lung was the most common site of infection, which is in alignment with other sepsis cohort studies [22,35,36]. This finding was expected, as respiratory infection is the leading cause of ICU admission and acute respiratory failure in renal transplant recipients [23,26,29,37]. The second major source of sepsis was the urinary tract. Although this is the most common infectious complication after renal transplantation [38–40], urinary infection might not lead to severe sepsis as frequently as pneumonia even in these immunosuppressed patients. Interestingly, while the data may not be significant, urinary tract infection seems to be associated with lower mortality rates, as previously showed in immunocompetent patients [41]. We also found a higher frequency of microbiologically documented infection by opportunistic pathogens compared with non-transplant patients [1,8]. This finding was also expected, as infections caused by opportunistic pathogens in solid organ transplant recipient are frequent [42]. However, admissions for severe sepsis did not occur during periods of intensified immunosuppression (in the first months after transplantation or after treatment for acute rejection).

Our analysis showed that the classical factors usually associated with morbidity in this population, such as immunosuppressive regimens, previous rejection treatment and CMV disease, had no prognostic value. Although delayed graft function was associated with mortality, it did not remain in our final multivariate logistic regression model. The only other variable associated with mortality in the univariate analysis, expanded criteria donor, could not be included in the model as it was assessed only in the subgroup that received a deceased-donor kidney. This result aligns with other studies in critically ill renal transplant patients requiring ICU treatment [23,25,26,29].

Delta SOFA after 24 hours of ICU admission, the need of mechanical ventilation, the presence of hematologic dysfunction and admission from the ward and not from the emergency department were previously described as mortality risk factors in critically ill general septic patients [21,22,35,43–45]. The most controversial risk factor found in our study was male gender. Clinical sepsis studies evaluating gender-mortality relationships are inconsistent [46–49]. Recent studies have suggested that although the incidence of sepsis is greater in men, in-hospital mortality is significantly higher among women [48,49]. It is possible that gender influences outcomes differently in renal transplant patients. An example of these possible interactions is the reports that grafts from male donors show a trend towards better five-year survival compared to grafts from female donors [50]. Moreover, we did not have data about hormonal concentrations. The complexity of influencing factors did not allow us to evaluate the possible pathophysiological reasons for our finding.

Table 4. Severity scores at the ICU admission and the events during ICU stay.

	All patients (N = 190)	Survivors (N = 117)	Non survivors (N = 73)	p value
SOFA admission	5 (4–8)	5 (4–7)	6 (4–9)	**<0.0001**
SOFA at 24 h	5 (4–8)	4 (3–6)	7 (5–11)	**<0.0001**
SOFA at 72 h	5 (3–8)	4 (2–5)	8 (5–11)	**<0.0001**
Delta SOFA 24 h	0 (−1–1)	0 (−1–0)	1(0–3)	**<0.001**
Delta SOFA 72 h	−0.5 (−2–1)	−1 (−2–0)	2(−0.7–4)	**<0.001**
Lactate at admission (mg/dl)	10 (7–16)	10 (6–16)	10 (7–18)	0.670
Lactate at 6–12 h (mg/dl)	10 (7–16)	9 (6–13)	12 (8–25)	0.001
Lactate at 24 h (mg/dl)	8 (6–14)	8 (6–10)	13 (7–31)	**<0.0001**
Delta lactate 6–12 h (mg/dl)	1 (−3–4)	0 (−5–2)	4 (0–8)	**<0.001**
Delta lactate 24 h (mg/dl)	0 (−4–3)	−2 (−6–1)	3 (0–13)	**<0.001**
APACHE II score	20 (16–23)	18 (15–22)	21 (18–24)	**0.004**
Septic shock	53 (27.9)	24 (20.5)	29 (39.7)	**0.004**
Shock after 24 h	96 (50.5)	29 (24.7)	67 (91.7)	**0.004**
Mechanical ventilation	90 (47.4)	25 (21.3)	65 (89.0)	**<0.0001**
Hemodialysis	77 (40.5)	22 (18.8)	55 (75.3)	**<0.001**
AKI classification				**<0.0001**
Stage <3	96 (50.5)	80 (68.4)	16 (21.9)	
Stage 3	94 (49.5)	37 (31.6)	57 (78.1)	
Reinfection in ICU	34 (17.9)	18 (15.3)	16 (21.9)	0.200
Cumulative fluid balance				
First 6 h after severe sepsis[a]	500 (0–1500)	610 (0–1500)	250 (0–1500)	0.080
First 12 h after severe sepsis[b]	1500 (510–2640)	1500 (565–2569)	1175 (385–2736)	0.350
First 72 h after severe sepsis[c]	4634 (3192–6959)	4301 (3163–6208)	6099 (3657–8391)	**0.007**
First 6 h after septic shock[d]	1500 (774–2069)	1500 (790–2000)	1608 (750–2678)	0.710
First 12 h after septic shock[e]	2190 (1609–3231)	2000 (1394–3036)	2428 (1820–3330)	0.350
First 72 h after septic shock[f]	6928 (4598–8926)	5460 (2096–7117)	8750 (6928–13162)	**0.001**

SOFA: Sequential Organ Failure Assessment score, APACHE II: Acute Physiological and Chronic Health Evaluation II score, AKI: acute kidney injury (from KDIGO), ICU: intensive care unit.
a) n = 189,
b) n = 188,
c) n = 153,
d) n = 50,
e) n = 46,
f) n = 34. Results are expressed as number (%) or median (IQR: 25%–75%). Chi-squared test and Mann Whitney U-test (univariate analysis).

The degree of renal allograft dysfunction during ICU stay was also associated with hospital mortality. As there is no validated classification for AKI in renal transplant recipients, we used a KDIGO definition during the ICU stays [20]. Our results demonstrated that changes in graft function are important and associated with significant changes in outcomes. This result aligns with studies using RIFLE/AKIN definitions in which a worse RIFLE or AKIN class is associated with higher mortality and

Table 5. Multivariate logistic regression analysis in septic transplant patients with hospital mortality as dependent factor.

	OR (95% CI)	p value
Male gender	5.9 (1.7–19.6)	0.004
Delta SOFA 24 h (per point increase)	1.7 (1.2–2.3)	0.001
Mechanical ventilation	30.0 (8.8–102.2)	<0.0001
Hematological dysfunction	6.8 (2.0–22.6)	0.002
Sepsis admitted from ward	3.4 (1.2–9.7)	0.020
AKI stage 3	5.7 (1.9–16.6)	0.002

OR: odds ratio, CI: confidence interval, SOFA: Sequential Organ Failure Assessment, AKI stage 3: acute kidney injury stage 3.

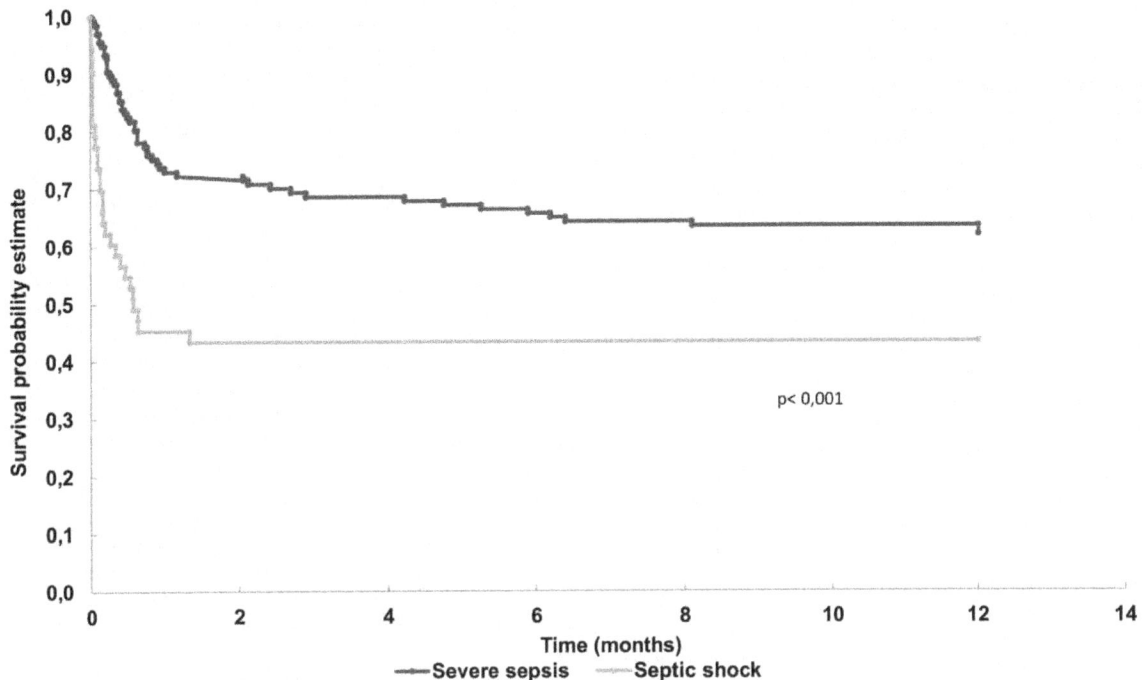

Figure 3. Kaplan-Meier curves (severe sepsis and septic shock) for one year survival after admission to the intensive care unit.

longer ICU or hospital stay [20]. This study is the first in renal transplant recipients to use a new approach of AKI classification to associate the degree of renal dysfunction with mortality. A previously reported by Nakamura *et al.*, higher acute kidney injury states correlate with lower graft survival rates. However, the authors did not present mortality as an outcome [51].

Our study had strengths and limitations. We included a homogeneous population of renal transplant recipients in a consecutive fashion. We assessed several transplant and sepsis characteristics, including treatment adequacy, which could interfere with patient outcomes. In addition, we used a new AKI classification approach. These contributions are relevant considering the paucity of data currently available in the literature. The study also has some limitations, the most important being the retrospective nature of our data collection. Second, our study has a single-center design, which limits the reproducibility of our findings. Third, we did not have a control group with septic non-transplanted patients and transplanted patients without sepsis. Fourth, we limited our analysis to ICU patients and did not include patients with severe sepsis in other hospital settings. The relevance of this limitation should have been minimized because in this institution, the vast majority of the septic patients are admitted to the ICU. Fifth, a better characterization of AKI is lacking. We do not have data regarding estimated glomerular filtration rate, time for dialysis onset or its duration, and long-term graft function. Moreover, we did not assess the role that acute rejection could have played in graft dysfunction. We also only consider creatinine and not diuresis in our AKI classification, which may have underestimated the number of patients with late stage diseases.

However, controversy exists regarding the impact of this assessment in the score ability to predict prognosis [52]. Sixth, we have no data regarding adrenal insufficiency in our study. Besides the possibility of corticosteroid insufficiency related to critical illness or sepsis, previous chronic use of prednisone in nearly all patients could suppress the hypothalamic-pituitary-adrenal axis (HPA). This was the main reason for hydrocortisone administration. Another reason was the need for immunosuppressant drugs to prevent rejection, since all other immunosuppressant agents were discontinued at ICU admission.

Conclusion

Hospital mortality in renal transplant patients with severe sepsis and septic shock was associated with male gender, admission from the wards, worse SOFA scores on the first day and the presence of hematologic dysfunction, mechanical ventilation or advanced graft dysfunction. Transplant-related variables had no prognostic value.

Acknowledgments

We thank Creusa Maria Roveri Dal Bó for support with the statistical analyses.

Author Contributions

Conceived and designed the experiments: MAC FGRF JOMP. Performed the experiments: MAC FGRF ATB. Analyzed the data: MAC FGRF HTSJ FRM. Contributed reagents/materials/analysis tools: MAC FGRF HTSJ FRM. Wrote the paper: MAC FGRF HTSJ FRM.

References

1. Angus DC, Linde-Zwirble WT, Lidicker J, Clermont G, Carcillo J, et al. (2001) Epidemiology of severe sepsis in the United States: analysis of incidence, outcome, and associated costs of care. Crit Care Med 29: 1303–1310.

2. Kaukonen KM, Bailey M, Suzuki S, Pilcher D, Bellomo R (2014) Mortality related to severe sepsis and septic shock among critically ill patients in Australia and New Zealand, 2000–2012. Jama 311: 1308–1316.

3. Walkey AJ, Wiener RS, Lindenauer PK (2013) Utilization patterns and outcomes associated with central venous catheter in septic shock: a population-based study. Crit Care Med 41: 1450–1457.

4. Lagu T, Rothberg MB, Shieh MS, Pekow PS, Steingrub JS, et al. (2012) Hospitalizations, costs, and outcomes of severe sepsis in the United States 2003 to 2007. Crit Care Med 40: 754–761.

5. Latin American Sepsis Institute (2014) Surviving Sepsis Campaign. Available: http://www.ilas.org.br/upfiles/fckeditor/file/Relat%C3%B3rio%20Nacional%20fev%202014.pdf

6. Phua J, Koh Y, Du B, Tang YQ, Divatia JV, et al. (2011) Management of severe sepsis in patients admitted to Asian intensive care units: prospective cohort study. Bmj 342: d3245.

7. Noritomi DT, Ranzani OT, Monteiro MB, Ferreira EM, Santos SR, et al. (2014) Implementation of a multifaceted sepsis education program in an emerging country setting: clinical outcomes and cost-effectiveness in a long-term follow-up study. Intensive Care Med 40: 182–191.

8. Angus DC, Pereira CA, Silva E (2006) Epidemiology of severe sepsis around the world. Endocr Metab Immune Disord Drug Targets 6: 207–212.

9. Gallon LG, Leventhal JR, Kaufman DB (2002) Pretransplant evaluation of renal transplant candidates. Semin Nephrol 22: 515–525.

10. Davis CL (2004) Evaluation of the living kidney donor: current perspectives. Am J Kidney Dis 43: 508–530.

11. Sam R, Leehey DJ (2000) Improved graft survival after renal transplantation in the United States, 1988 to 1996. N Engl J Med 342: 1837–1838.

12. Knoll G (2008) Trends in kidney transplantation over the past decade. Drugs 68 Suppl 1: 3–10.

13. Adams PL (2006) Long-term patient survival: strategies to improve overall health. Am J Kidney Dis 47: S65–85.

14. Reis MA, Costa RS, Ferraz AS (1995) Causes of death in renal transplant recipients: a study of 102 autopsies from 1968 to 1991. J R Soc Med 1995, 88(1): 24–7.

15. Ingsathit A, Avihingsanon Y, Rattanasiri S, Premasathian N, Pongskul C, et al. (2010) Different etiologies of graft loss and death in Asian kidney transplant recipients: a report from Thai Transplant Registry. Transplant Proc 42: 4014–4016.

16. Medina-Pestana JO (2010) More than 1,000 kidney transplants in a single year by the "Hospital do Rim" Group in Sao Paulo - Brazil. Clin Transpl: 107–126.

17. Dellinger RP, Levy MM, Carlet JM, Bion J, Parker MM, et al. (2008) Surviving Sepsis Campaign: international guidelines for management of severe sepsis and septic shock: 2008. Intensive Care Med 34: 17–60.

18. Dellinger RP, Levy MM, Rhodes A, Annane D, Gerlach H, et al. (2013) Surviving sepsis campaign: international guidelines for management of severe sepsis and septic shock: 2012. Crit Care Med 41: 580–637.

19. Pelletier SJ, Crabtree TD, Gleason TG, Raymond DP, Oh CK, et al. (2000) Characteristics of infectious complications associated with mortality after solid organ transplantation. Clin Transplant 14: 401–408.

20. KDIGO AKI Work Group (2012) KDIGO clinical practice guideline for acute kidney injury. Kidney inter 2: 1–138.

21. Conde KA, Silva E, Silva CO, Ferreira E, Freitas FG, et al. (2013) Differences in sepsis treatment and outcomes between public and private hospitals in Brazil: a multicenter observational study. PLoS One 8: e64790.

22. Levy MM, Dellinger RP, Townsend SR, Linde-Zwirble WT, Marshall JC, et al. (2010) The Surviving Sepsis Campaign: results of an international guideline-based performance improvement program targeting severe sepsis. Crit Care Med 38: 367–374.

23. Klouche K, Amigues L, Massanet P, Garrigue V, Delmas S, et al. (2009) Outcome of renal transplant recipients admitted to an intensive care unit: a 10-year cohort study. Transplantation 87: 889–895.

24. Mouloudi E, Massa E, Georgiadou E, Iosifidis E, Katsika E, et al. (2012) Infections related to renal transplantation requiring intensive care admission: a 20-year study. Transplant Proc 44: 2721–2723.

25. Mouloudi E, Massa E, Georgiadou E, Iosifidis E, Kydona C, et al. (2012) Course and outcome of renal transplant recipients admitted to the intensive care unit: a 20-year study. Transplant Proc 44: 2718–2720.

26. Arulkumaran N, West S, Chan K, Templeton M, Taube D, et al. (2012) Long-term renal function and survival of renal transplant recipients admitted to the intensive care unit. Clin Transplant 26: E24–31.

27. Aldawood A (2007) The course and outcome of renal transplant recipients admitted to the intensive care unit at a tertiary hospital in Saudi Arabia. Saudi J Kidney Dis Transpl 18: 536–540.

28. Candan S, Pirat A, Varol G, Torgay A, Zeyneloglu P, et al. (2006) Respiratory problems in renal transplant recipients admitted to intensive care during long-term follow-up. Transplant Proc 38: 1354–1356.

29. Canet E, Osman D, Lambert J, Guitton C, Heng AE, et al. (2011) Acute respiratory failure in kidney transplant recipients: a multicenter study. Crit Care 15: R91.

30. Beale R, Reinhart K, Brunkhorst FM, Dobb G, Levy M, et al. (2009) Promoting Global Research Excellence in Severe Sepsis (PROGRESS): lessons from an international sepsis registry. Infection 37: 222–232.

31. Winters BD, Eberlein M, Leung J, Needham DM, Pronovost PJ, et al. (2010) Long-term mortality and quality of life in sepsis: a systematic review. Crit Care Med 38: 1276–1283.

32. Sprung CL, Sakr Y, Vincent JL, Le Gall JR, Reinhart K, et al. (2006) An evaluation of systemic inflammatory response syndrome signs in the Sepsis Occurrence In Acutely Ill Patients (SOAP) study. Intensive Care Med 32: 421–427.

33. Sawyer RG, Crabtree TD, Gleason TG, Antevil JL, Pruett TL (1999) Impact of solid organ transplantation and immunosuppression on fever, leukocytosis, and physiologic response during bacterial and fungal infections. Clin Transplant 13: 260–265.

34. Vincent JL, Opal SM, Marshall JC, Tracey KJ (2013) Sepsis definitions: time for change. Lancet 381: 774–775.

35. Vincent JL, Sakr Y, Sprung CL, Ranieri VM, Reinhart K, et al. (2006) Sepsis in European intensive care units: results of the SOAP study. Crit Care Med 34: 344–353.

36. Alberti C, Brun-Buisson C, Burchardi H, Martin C, Goodman S, et al. (2002) Epidemiology of sepsis and infection in ICU patients from an international multicentre cohort study. Intensive Care Med 28: 108–121.

37. Veroux M, Giuffrida G, Corona D, Gagliano M, Scriffignano V, et al. (2008) Infective complications in renal allograft recipients: epidemiology and outcome. Transplant Proc 40: 1873–1876.

38. Alangaden GJ, Thyagarajan R, Gruber SA, Morawski K, Garnick J, et al. (2006) Infectious complications after kidney transplantation: current epidemiology and associated risk factors. Clin Transplant 20: 401–409.

39. Pourmand G, Pourmand M, Salem S, Mehrsai A, Taheri Mahmoudi M, et al. (2006) Posttransplant infectious complications: a prospective study on 142 kidney allograft recipients. Urol J 3: 23–31.

40. Ak O, Yildirim M, Kucuk HF, Gencer S, Demir T (2013) Infections in renal transplant patients: risk factors and infectious agents. Transplant Proc 45: 944–948.

41. Knaus WA, Sun X, Nystrom O, Wagner DP (1992) Evaluation of definitions for sepsis. Chest 101: 1656–1662.

42. Fishman JA (2007) Infection in solid-organ transplant recipients. N Engl J Med 357: 2601–2614.

43. Ferreira FL, Bota DP, Bross A, Melot C, Vincent JL (2001) Serial evaluation of the SOFA score to predict outcome in critically ill patients. Jama 286: 1754–1758.

44. Moreno R, Vincent JL, Matos R, Mendonça A, Cantraine F, et al. (1999) The use of maximum SOFA score to quantify organ dysfunction/failure in intensive care. Results of a prospective, multicentre study. Working Group on Sepsis related Problems of the ESICM. Intensive Care Med 25: 686–696.

45. Dhainaut JF, Yan SB, Joyce DE, Pettila V, Basson B, et al. (2004) Treatment effects of drotrecogin alfa (activated) in patients with severe sepsis with or without overt disseminated intravascular coagulation. J Thromb Haemost 2: 1924–1933.

46. Dombrovskiy VY, Martin AA, Sunderram J, Paz HL (2007) Rapid increase in hospitalization and mortality rates for severe sepsis in the United States: a trend analysis from 1993 to 2003. Crit Care Med 35: 1244–1250.

47. Adrie C, Azoulay E, Francais A, Clec'h C, Darques L, et al. (2007) Influence of gender on the outcome of severe sepsis: a reappraisal. Chest 132: 1786–1793.

48. Sakr Y, Elia C, Mascia L, Barberis B, Cardellino S, et al. (2013) The influence of gender on the epidemiology of and outcome from severe sepsis. Crit Care 17: R50.

49. Pietropaoli AP, Glance LG, Oakes D, Fisher SG (2010) Gender differences in mortality in patients with severe sepsis or septic shock. Gend Med 7: 422–437.

50. Glyda Glyda M, Czapiewski W, Karczewski M, Pieta R, Oko A (2011) Influence of donor and recipient gender as well as selected factors on the five-year survival of kidney graft. Pol Przegl Chir 83: 188–195.

51. Nakamura M, Seki G, Iwadoh K, Nakajima I, Fuchinoue S, et al. (2012) Acute kidney injury as defined by the RIFLE criteria is a risk factor for kidney transplant graft failure. Clin Transplant 26: 520–528.

52. Lopes JA, Jorge S (2013) Comparison of RIFLE with and without urine output criteria for acute kidney injury in critically ill patients: a task still not concluded! Crit Care 17: 408.

18

Acid Sphingomyelinase Serum Activity Predicts Mortality in Intensive Care Unit Patients after Systemic Inflammation: A Prospective Cohort Study

Matthias Kott[1]*[◊], Gunnar Elke[1◊], Maike Reinicke[1,2], Supandi Winoto-Morbach[2], Dirk Schädler[1], Günther Zick[1], Inéz Frerichs[1], Norbert Weiler[1], Stefan Schütze[2]

1 Department of Anesthesiology and Intensive Care Medicine, University Medical Center Schleswig-Holstein, Campus Kiel, Kiel, Germany, **2** Institute of Immunology, University Medical Center Schleswig-Holstein, Campus Kiel, Kiel, Germany

Abstract

Introduction: Acid sphingomyelinase is involved in lipid signalling pathways and regulation of apoptosis by the generation of ceramide and plays an important role during the host response to infectious stimuli. It thus has the potential to be used as a novel diagnostic marker in the management of critically ill patients. The objective of our study was to evaluate acid sphingomyelinase serum activity (ASM) as a diagnostic and prognostic marker in a mixed intensive care unit population before, during, and after systemic inflammation.

Methods: 40 patients admitted to the intensive care unit at risk for developing systemic inflammation (defined as systemic inflammatory response syndrome *plus* a significant procalcitonin [PCT] increase) were included. ASM was analysed on ICU admission, before (PCT_{before}), during (PCT_{peak}) and after (PCT_{low}) onset of SIRS. Patients undergoing elective surgery served as control (N = 8). Receiver-operating characteristics curves were computed.

Results: ASM significantly increased after surgery in the eight control patients. Patients from the intensive care unit had significantly higher ASM on admission than control patients after surgery. 19 out of 40 patients admitted to the intensive care unit developed systemic inflammation and 21 did not, with no differences in ASM between these two groups on admission. In patients with SIRS and PCT peak, ASM between admission and PCT_{before} was not different, but further increased at PCT_{peak} in non-survivors and was significantly higher at PCT_{low} compared to survivors. Survivors exhibited decreased ASM at PCT_{peak} and PCT_{low}. Receiver operating curve analysis on discrimination of ICU mortality showed an area under the curve of 0.79 for ASM at PCT_{low}.

Conclusions: In summary, ASM was generally higher in patients admitted to the intensive care unit compared to patients undergoing uncomplicated surgery. ASM did not indicate onset of systemic inflammation. In contrast to PCT however, it remained high in non-surviving ICU patients after systemic inflammation.

Editor: Lyle L. Moldawer, University of Florida College of Medicine, United States of America

Funding: This study was funded by a restricted grant of the Christian-Albrechts University Kiel, Germany and in part supported by a grant of the Deutsche Forschungsgemeinschaft (SCHU 733/9-2) given to S. Schütze. The funders had no role in study design, data collection and analysis, decision to publish, or preparation of the manuscript.

Competing Interests: The authors have declared that no competing interests exist.

* Email: matthias.kott@uksh.de

◊ These authors contributed equally to this work.

Introduction

Despite advances in critical care, systemic inflammatory response syndrome (SIRS) and sepsis syndrome with subsequent multi-organ failure still contribute to overall mortality in critically ill patients, equalling the number of deaths caused by acute myocardial infarction [1]. Besides specific treatment of the underlying cause of systemic inflammation, early diagnosis based on clinical findings and laboratory testing is of paramount importance to enable successful therapy [2]. The kinetics of biomarkers reflecting changes in the inflammatory condition can be helpful to identify patients at high risk for complications.

At present, procalcitonin (PCT) is regarded as the best available laboratory tool for the diagnosis of infection and systemic inflammation in combination with clinical symptoms [3,4] and has been introduced as a variable in the diagnostic criteria for sepsis in the recently updated Surviving Sepsis Campaign guidelines [5]. PCT has the advantage of an earlier peak level upon infection, a better specificity and correlation to disease severity and clinical outcome as compared to routine biomarkers such as white blood cell count or C-reactive protein (CRP) [6–9].

Activation of acid sphingomyelinase, a C-type phosphodiesterase leads to generation of ceramide from biological inert sphingomyelin derived from the cell membrane. Generation of ceramide at the outer leaflet of cell membranes induces changes in composition and spatial arrangement in terms of forming ceramide-enriched membrane lipid rafts, leading to receptor clustering and apoptosis signalling and modification of the cellular response to stress stimuli [10,11]. Clinical data concerning the potential role of acid sphingomyelinase serum activity (ASM) is infrequent. In a retrospective study of 12 patients with severe sepsis, Claus et al. showed that elevated ASM levels can be observed after the onset of sepsis, and that a further increase may be associated with worse outcome [12]. On the other hand, recent animal studies suggest a protective role of ASM secretion during the early host response as a first line of defence [13]. Due to its pathophysiological properties in the early host response, determination of ASM may also be used as an early diagnostic marker before the onset of systemic inflammation. The aim of our pilot study was to evaluate the role of ASM in a mixed intensive care unit (ICU) population at risk for the development of systemic inflammation. We hypothesized that ASM a) increases before the

onset of systemic inflammation, and b) may be used as a prognostic marker of outcome.

Materials and Methods

Study design and patients

This single-center prospective cohort study was conducted in two surgical intensive care units of a tertiary medical center (University Medical Center Schleswig-Holstein, Campus Kiel, Kiel, Germany) with the approval of the local ethics committee of the Christian-Albrechts University Kiel, Germany. Written informed consent was obtained from each patient or the legal representative, respectively.

We prospectively included patients (age≥18 years) who were admitted to the ICU and deemed to be at high risk for the development of systemic inflammation (ICU group). High risk criteria were defined as the following ICU admission diagnoses: extended surgery, polytrauma, respiratory insufficiency, and patients with an expected length of ICU stay >3 days. Patients were evaluated on a daily basis for new onset of systemic inflammatory response syndrome (SIRS) fulfilling two or more of the defined clinical criteria according to the ACCP/SCCM recommendations [14] *plus* an increase in PCT. This PCT peak was defined as a two-fold increase in PCT concentration compared to the value of the preceding day and exceeding a

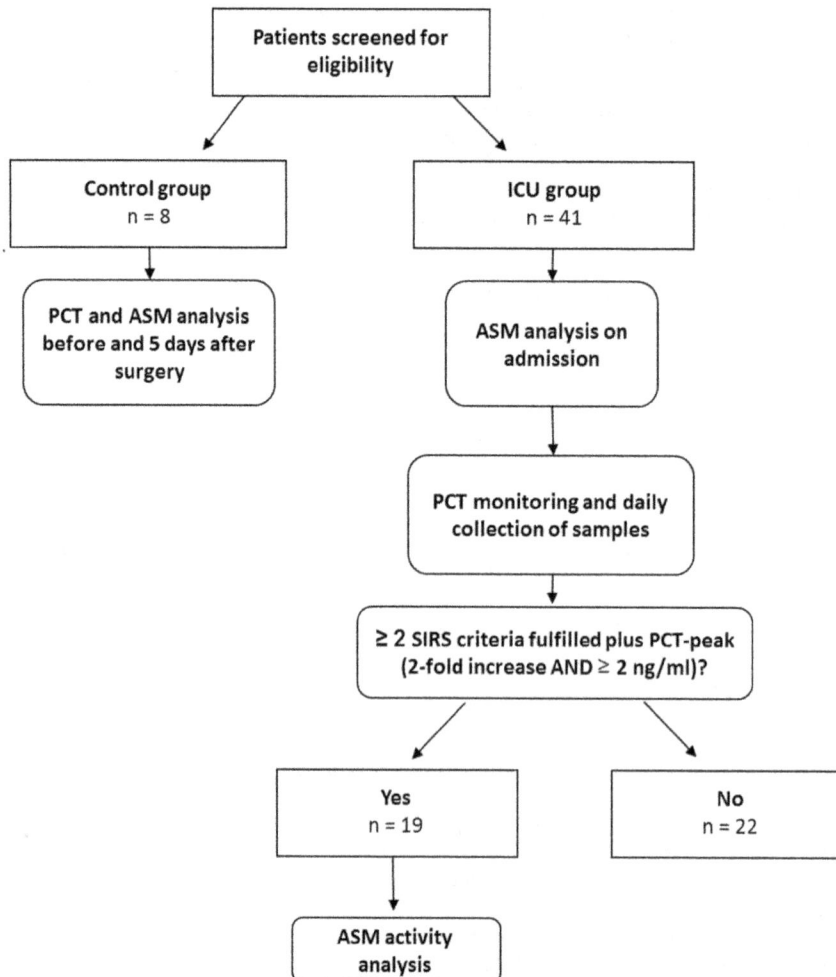

Figure 1. Study flow chart.

Table 1. Baseline patient characteristics and outcomes.

| | Total | ICU Group | | | Control |
		Total	SI	No SI	
Number	48	40	19	21	8
Age, median, years	69	69	69	69	65
Gender, male, n (%)	30 (62.5)	25 (63.4)	12 (63.2)	13 (66.6)	5 (62.5)
Mortality, n (%)	15 (31.2)	15 (36.6)	9 (47.4)	6 (27.3)	0
Main diagnosis, n (%)					
Abdominal surgery	22 (45.8)	14 (34.1)	8 (42.1)	6 (28.6)	8 (100)
Liver failure	1 (2.4)	1 (2.4)	1 (5.3)	-	-
Major bleeding	2 (4.9)	2 (4.9)	-	2 (9.5)	-
Major trauma	3 (7.3)	3 (7.3)	1 (5.3)	2 (9.5)	-
Mesenterial ischemia	2 (4.9)	2 (4.9)	-	2 (9.5)	-
Pancreatitis	2 (4.9)	2 (4.9)	2 (10.5)	-	-
Pneumonia	6 (14.6)	6 (14.6)	2 (10.5)	4 (19)	-
Soft tissue infection	3 (7.3)	3 (7.3)	-	3 (14.3)	-
Thoracic surgery	7 (17)	7 (17)	5 (26.3)	2 (9.5)	-

Systemic inflammation was defined as new onset of systemic inflammatory response syndrome plus a two-fold increase in PCT concentration compared to the value of the preceding day or exceeding a minimum of >2 ng/ml. PCT: procalcitonin, ICU: intensive care unit; SI: systemic inflammation.

minimum of >2 ng/ml. Exclusion criteria were diseases associated with hyperprocalcitoninaemia like small-cell lung cancer or C-cell carcinoma and administration of PCT inducing agents (Anti-Thymocyte globulin or OKT3 antibodies). Events with PCT elevations following re-operation during the ICU stay and patients receiving ASM inhibiting medications (amlodipin, sertralin, imipramin, desipramin, or steroids) were also excluded [15]. ASM was consecutively analysed at four time points: I), on ICU admission, II), the day before new onset of SIRS in combination with a PCT peak were detected (PCT_{before}), III), the first day of new onset of SIRS and a PCT peak (PCT_{peak}), and IV), on the first day when the PCT level was below 0.5 ng/ml or declined to a nadir with less than 30% of the PCT_{peak} concentration (PCT_{low}).

Patients undergoing uncomplicated elective major abdominal surgery were used as a control group to assess the peri-operative kinetics of ASM. In these patients, ASM was also determined before surgery to determine the influence of the surgical trauma on ASM. Serum samples for the analysis of ASM were collected

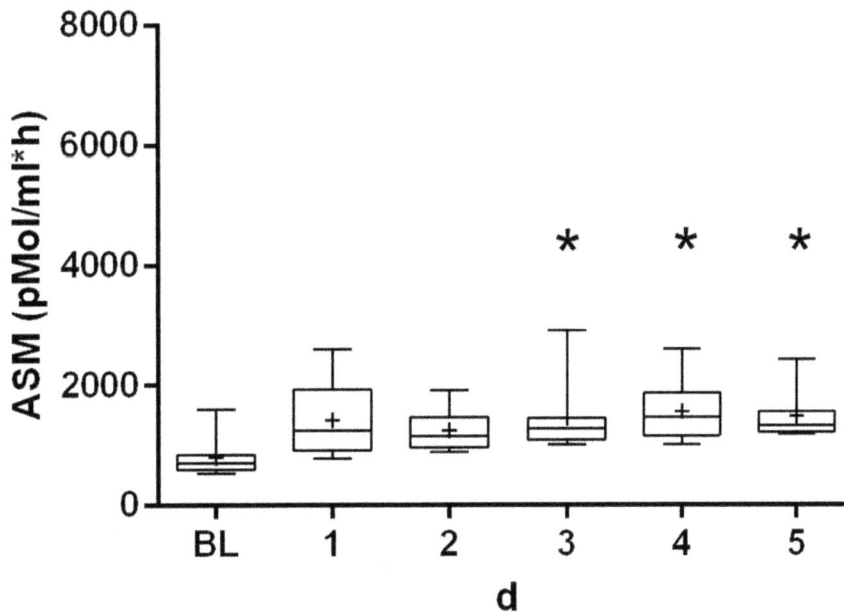

Figure 2. Kinetics of acid sphingomyelinase serum activity in the control group. The box plots display the minima/maxima (whiskers), 25%/75% percentile (box), median (−) and mean (+) values. Statistically significant differences (P<0.05) between baseline (BL) and post-operative values are marked with an asterisk (*). ASM: acid sphingomyelinase activity; BL: baseline (before surgery); d: days.

Table 2. Biomarker level and severity of illness measures of all study patients.

Variabe	ICU admission	ICU group		Control group
	(N = 40)	SI (N = 19)	No SI (N = 21)	(N = 8)
ASM (pMol/ml•h)	2593 (2021–4396)	2755 (1897–4396)	2529 (2041–4618)	709 (598–841)
PCT (ng/ml)	3.19 (1.03–8.15)	2.1 (0.75–4.88)	4.17 (1.57–10.38)	0.16 (0.12–0.23)
CRP (mg/l)	121 (35–274)	153 (12–235)	90 (35–304)	2.35 (0.97–25)
Lactate (mMol/l)	1.7 (0.9–2.5)	1.4 (0.8–2.6)	1.7 (1.1–2.5)	-
mSOFA score	7 (4–8)	7 (4–8)	6.5 (4–9)	-
SAPS II	46 (36–57)	46 (34–57)	48 (37–61)	-
TISS	19 (13–24)	14 (10–19)	22 (14–26)	-

In the ICU group, biomarker levels were measured in all patients at intensive care unit admission. For the control group, the pre-operative biomarker levels are displayed. Data are shown as median with interquartile ranges. Systemic inflammation was defined as new onset of systemic inflammatory response syndrome plus a two-fold increase in PCT concentration compared to the value of the preceding day or exceeding a minimum of >2 ng/ml. ASM: acid sphingomyelinase serum activity; CRP: C-reactive protein; mSOFA: modified Sequential Organ Failure Assessment score (excluding central nervous system); PCT: procalcitonin; SAPS II: Simplified Acute and Physiology Score II; SI: systemic inflammation; TISS: Therapeutic Intervention Scoring System.

prospectively on a daily basis and stored at $-20°$Celsius. ASM on the day of ICU admission was analysed in all included patients but due to financial restraints consecutive measurements of ASM (from PCT_{before} until patients' discharge or death) were performed only in those patients with a PCT peak.

Data collection

We collected baseline characteristics of the patients including demographic information, comorbidities and type of surgery. Severity of illness was determined by calculating the Simplified Acute and Physiology Score II (SAPS II) [16], Therapeutic Intervention Scoring System (TISS) [17] and a modified Sequential Organ Failure Assessment Score (mSOFA) [18]

(excluding central nervous system). Serum samples for the analysis of PCT and ASM (10 ml of either central venous or arterial blood) were prospectively collected on a daily basis in addition to routine laboratory including white blood cell count (WBC), lactate, C-reactive protein (CRP) serum levels. The patients' management was left at the discretion of the attending ICU physician. Patients were followed up until discharge from the ICU or death.

Measurements of ASM serum activity

Plasma was obtained and centrifuged at 3000 g for 5 minutes (Sorvall -Super TRI, Kendro Laboratory Products GmbH, Langenselbold, Germany) and stored at $-20°$C until assayed. Analytical determination of ASM depended on detection of radio-

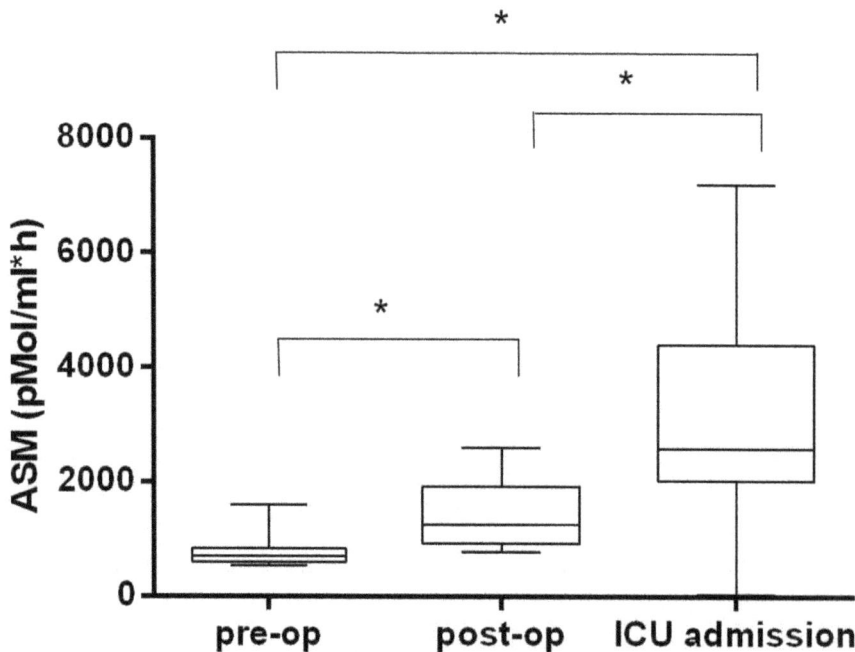

Figure 3. Acid sphingomyelinase serum activity in control and ICU patients. This figure indicates median pre- and post-operative acid sphingomyelinase serum activity of the control group and median acid sphingomyelinase serum activity of the ICU group on admission. Statistical significant differences between groups ($P<0.05$) are marked with an asterisk (*). The box plots display the minima/maxima (whiskers), 25%/75% percentile (box), and median (−) values. ASM: acid sphingomyelinase serum activity.

Table 3. Biomarker level and severity of illness measures in patients with systemic inflammation (N = 19) according to PCT time points.

Variable	Time point	All (N = 19)	Survivor (N = 9)	Non-survivor (N = 10)	P Value*
Procalcitonin	PCT_{before}	0.46 (0.29–2.08)	0.37 (0.19–1.38)	0.65 (0.42–2.78)	0.07
	PCT_{peak}	4.43 (2.54–11.74)	4.14 (2.42–21.43)	4.43 (2.81–10.65)	>0.99
	PCT_{low}	0.48 (0.43–1.09)	0.45 (0.41–0.72)	0.59 (0.44–1.12)	0.57
ASM	PCT_{before}	2782 (1991–3903)	2777 (1835–3244)	2874 (2278–4528)	0.40
	PCT_{peak}	3233 (1968–2907)	2501 (1953–3878)	3855 (1987–5122)	0.23
	PCT_{low}	2261 (2063–2907)	2205 (1596–2496)	2611 (2235–4402)	*0.03*
CRP	PCT_{before}	130 (87–220)	157 (74–210)	127 (80–233)	0.23
	PCT_{peak}	145 (95–256)	124 (77–237)	182 (111–295)	0.25
	PCT_{low}	98 (66–203)	70 (57–138)	141 (78–228)	*0.04*
Lactate	PCT_{before}	1.6 (1.1–3.8)	1.6 (0.9–3.05)	1.8 (1.3–4.5)	0.62
	PCT_{peak}	1.6 (1–3.2)	1.4 (1.1–3.2)	1.8 (1–3.9)	0.59
	PCT_{low}	1.1 (0.9–1.6)	1.1 (0.8–1.6)	1.1 (0.9–2.3)	0.54
mSOFA	PCT_{before}	7 (5–11)	7 (6–11)	7 (4–11)	0.67
	PCT_{peak}	8 (5–11)	8 (6–12)	6 (3–11)	0.39
	PCT_{low}	4 (2–6)	4 (3–7)	4 (1–6)	0.37
SAPS II	PCT_{before}	48 (37–50)	46 (37–49)	49 (29–55)	0.54
	PCT_{peak}	44 (37–51)	44 (40–46)	46 (30–58)	0.59
	PCT_{low}	41 (35–48)	39 (32–43)	43 (38–53)	0.17
TISS	PCT_{before}	21 (17–24)	22 (18–23)	20 (15–30)	0.88
	PCT_{peak}	18 (15–23)	18 (15–23)	20 (8–24)	0.73
	PCT_{low}	17 (6–23)	16 (9–19)	18 (0–26)	0.85

Time points were the day before the PCT peak (PCT_{before}), the day of the PCT peak (PCT_{peak}) and again lowered PCT (PCT_{low}).
*P value for comparison of survivors vs. non-survivors. Systemic inflammation was defined as new onset of systemic inflammatory response syndrome plus a two-fold increase in PCT concentration compared to the value of the preceding day or exceeding a minimum of >2 ng/ml. ASM: acid sphingomyelinase serum activity, CRP: C-reactive protein concentration, mSOFA: modified Sequential Organ Failure Assessment Score (excluding central nervous system); PCT: procalcitonin; SAPS II: Simplified Acute and Physiology Score II; TISS: Therapeutic Intervention Scoring System.

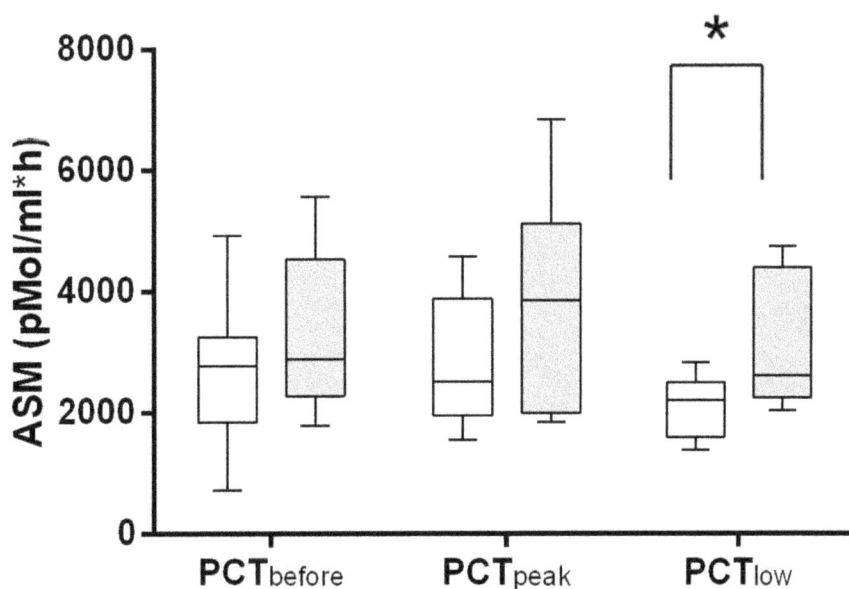

Figure 4. Acid sphingomyelinase serum activity in ICU patients with SIRS. Clear boxes represent survivors (n = 9) and grey boxes non-survivors (N = 10). Statistically significant difference (P<0.05) between survivors and non-survivors at PCT_{low} (*) for acid sphingomyelinase serum. The box plots show the minima/maxima (whiskers), 25%/75% percentile (box), and median (−) values. ASM: acid sphingomyelinase serum activity.

Table 4. Receiver operating characteristics curve analysis for patients with systemic inflammation at PCT_{low} (N = 19).

Variable	P Value	AUC	Optimal cut-off	Sensitivity (%)/Specifity (%)	LR
ASM (pMol/ml·h)	0.03	0.79	<2098	40/90	4
PCT	0.55	0.58	-	-	-
CRP	0.04	0.77	0.77	60/90	6
Lactate	0.52	0.58	-	-	-

At the two other time points, receiver operating characteristics curves were not significantly different from 0.5. Systemic inflammation was defined as new onset of systemic inflammatory response syndrome plus a two-fold increase in PCT concentration compared to the value of the preceding day or exceeding a minimum of > 2 ng/ml. ASM: acid sphingomyelinase serum activity; AUC: area under the curve; LR: likelihood ratio; CRP: C-reactive protein; PCT: procalcitonin.

labeled [14C]-Phosphorycholin that was generated by [14C]-sphingomyelin cleavage in aequimolar amounts to ceramide [19]. Protein quantity was determined by bicinchoninacid (BCA)-assays. 300 μg of purified protein were used in a total volume of 10 μl per assay. 100 μl ASM buffer and 40 μl of [14C]-substrate were added and incubated for at least 2 hours at 37°C. Reaction was stopped by adding 750 μl chloroforme/methanol (2:1) and 300 μl of destilled water. After 4 minutes of centrifugation by 14.000×g

revolutions per minute, 300 μl of the upper aqueous phase were pipetted and filled into a scintillation test tube. 4 ml of scintillation fluid were added (Aquasafe 300 plus, Zinsser Analytic, Frankfurt), and β-count of radio-labeled [14C]-Phosphorycholin was measured (LS 6000LL, Beckman Coulter GmbH, Krefeld, Germany). ASM was calculated as pmol/ml·h.

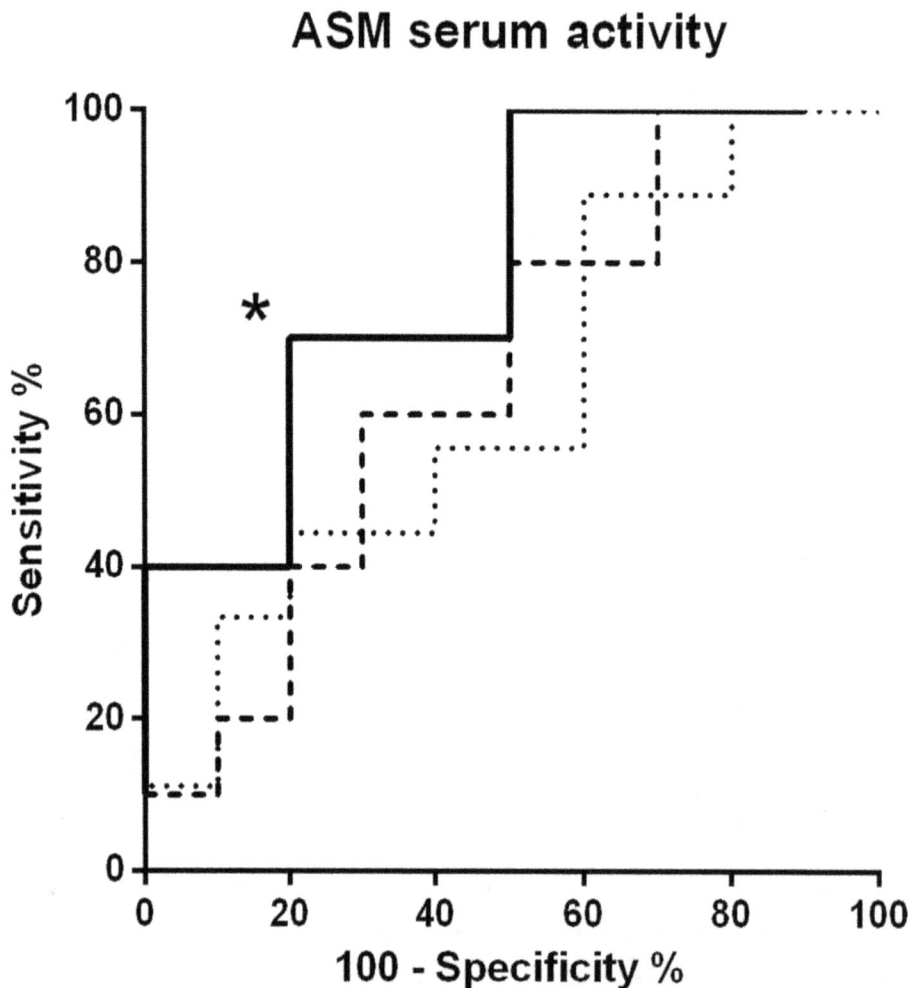

Figure 5. Receiver operating characteristics curve (ROC) analysis of acid sphingomyelinase serum activity. ROC analyses were performed at all three time points: PCT_{before} (fine dashed line), PCT_{peak} (dashed line), and PCT_{low} (solid line). ROC curves statistically significant different from 0.5 are marked with an asterisk (*). ASM: acid sphingomyelinase serum activity.

PCT measurements

PCT measurements were performed using a commercially available immunoluminometric assay (Elecsys BRAHMS PCT, BRAHMS-Diagnostica, Berlin, Germany) according to the manufacturer's instructions via the automated Kryptor platform (BRAHMS AG, Hennigsdorf, Germany). The direct measuring range of the assay is from 0.02–100 ng/ml, with automated dilution extending the upper range to 1.000 ng/ml. The functional assay sensitivity is 0.06 ng/ml, and the sample volume needed is 50 µl.

Statistical analysis

Means ± standard deviations (SD) or medians with interquartile ranges (IQR) are reported as appropriate. Differences in continuous variables between survivors and non-survivors were compared with the nonparametric Mann-Whitney test. Predictive values of serum ASM, PCT, CRP, WBC, body temperature and severity of illness measures regarding ICU mortality were evaluated. Discriminatory power (ability to distinguish between patients who die and those who survive) of laboratory tests and severity of illness scores were tested at all 3 time points to produce receiver operating characteristic (ROC) curves. The area under curve (AUC), with 95% confidence intervals (CI) and cut-offs for sensitivity and specificity were calculated in prediction of ICU mortality. A P value below 0.05 was considered statistically significant. Statistical analyses were performed with SPSS 17.0 (SPSS Inc., Chicago, IL, USA) and Prism 5 (GraphPad Software Inc., San Diego, CA, USA).

Results

Patient characteristics

A study flow chart is given in Figure 1. A total of 48 patients were included during the study period of whom 8 patients undergoing uncomplicated major abdominal surgery served as the control group. 40 patients fulfilled high-risk criteria and were included in the ICU group. Finally, 19 patients in the ICU group had new onset of SIRS *plus* a PCT peak (one patient with two episodes). Table 1 shows patients' baseline characteristics.

ASM, PCT and CRP levels in the control group

Figure 2 shows the pre- and post-operative kinetics of ASM in the control group. Median ASM measured before surgery was 709 pMol/ml•h (598–841 pMol/ml•h) and was significantly higher post-operatively (1320 pMol/ml•h; IQR: 1108–1565 pMol/ml•h). PCT and CRP both showed regular post-operative kinetics (data not shown).

ASM, PCT, CRP and lactate levels in the ICU group

ASM, PCT, CRP, lactate levels and severity of illness measures at ICU admission are shown in Table 2. Median ASM upon ICU admission in the ICU group was significantly higher than both baseline and post-operative values in the control group (Figure 3). In 21 patients of the ICU group, no newly developed SIRS plus a PCT peak were observed and median ASM upon ICU admission was not different when compared to the other 19 patients with PCT peak ($P = 0.8695$). Table 3 summarizes the course of biomarker level in the 19 patients with new onset of SIRS plus a PCT peak. Median PCT level at PCT_{before} was 0.46 ng/ml, increased markedly on PCT_{peak} to 4.43 ng/ml and subsequently returned to nearly baseline values at PCT_{low}. ASM showed no statistical significant differences between these three time points. Also, there was no difference in ASM in these patients between ICU admission and PCT_{before} ($P = 0.8995$). There were no

significant changes in CRP, lactate levels and severity of illness measures (table 3).

Survivors vs. non-survivors

Among the 19 patients with SIRS and a PCT peak, 9 patients (47.4%) died during their ICU stay as opposed to 6 of the 21 patients without PCT peak who died (27.3%). With PCT_{low} as the baseline of ASM (equalling 100%), ASM increased only in non-survivors (by 34%), whereas in survivors a decline (by 10%) of ASM was detected even at PCT_{peak}. ASM declined in all patients at PCT_{low} (91% vs. 79%), but remained significantly higher in non-survivors when compared to survivors ($P = 0.03$; Table 3 and Figure 4).

ROC analysis for ICU mortality in the ICU group

ROC analyses were performed at all four time points for all measured laboratory parameters. Only at PCT_{low}, the areas under receiver operating curves (AUC) for ASM in prediction of ICU mortality were significantly different from 0.5 (AUC: 0.79, $P = 0.03$) with a sensitivity of 40% and specificity of 90% at an optimal cut-off value of 2098 pMol/ml•h, (likelihood ratio: 4). For CRP, the sensitivity was 60% and specificity 90% at an optimal cut-off value of 77.1 mg/L (Table 4).

Discussion

This prospective pilot cohort study evaluated the role of ASM as a potential early diagnostic and prognostic marker in a mixed ICU population at high risk of developing systemic inflammation. We found that ASM was generally increased in a mixed ICU population as compared to patients who underwent uncomplicated surgery. ASM was not found to be an early marker before the clinical onset of systemic inflammation as defined by fulfilling clinical SIRS criteria plus a PCT increase. However, ASM remained elevated in the presence of a low PCT level in non-surviving patients after systemic inflammation.

To our best knowledge, only two clinical studies have yet evaluated the role of ASM in patients with systemic inflammation. In a retrospective study of 12 severely septic patients, Claus et al. were able to show that sphingolytic activity was significantly increased compared to 13 healthy volunteers and that a further increase during the clinical course was proportional to the severity of illness (as indicated by a higher SOFA score on the day of maximal ASM) and paralleled by fatal outcome [12]. Drobnik et al. accordingly reported that ASM as reflected by the ceramide/sphingomyelin ratio was higher in septic patients compared to healthy controls and associated with a poor clinical outcome [20]. While both studies included patients with established sepsis, we evaluated for the first time the kinetics of ASM in ICU patients before systemic inflammation became clinically evident as defined by SIRS criteria plus a PCT increase. We evaluated the potential of ASM to serve as an early marker of inflammation as compared to established biomarkers such as PCT and CRP during the course of disease, and used a pragmatic approach including patients at high risk for developing systemic inflammation. In the 19 ICU patients who developed systemic inflammation during their ICU stay, there were no significant increases in ASM on the day before patients developed new SIRS plus a PCT peak elevation (PCT_{before}). ASM levels were also not significantly different between patients with or without systemic inflammation upon ICU admission. Thus, ASM may not be a marker to indicate inflammation at an earlier stage than PCT.

In the control group, we observed a significant increase in median ASM after surgery parallel to a post-operative PCT and

CRP increase. This increase reflects a "post-trauma" effect that is most likely explained by a lysosomal release of ASM resulting from tissue damage during surgery. However, the pre-operative and median post-operative ASM levels in the control group were still significantly lower as compared to the ICU patients.

We were also able to show the potential of ASM as prognostic marker for mortality. Although we could not detect an association to severity of illness measures, ASM remained elevated in non-surviving patients while PCT and lactate levels were lowered or within the normal range again. ROC analysis revealed a discriminative power for ASM in predicting ICU mortality at PCT_{low} (see figure 5). It is not clear whether ASM is useful in guiding risk stratification of the critically ill patient, as an AUC of 0.79 indicates that sensitivity and specifity are not in a range where a clinically reliable discrimination between survivors and non-survivors can be derived. Other pro- and anti-inflammatory cytokines like Interleukin [IL]-10, IL-8, IL-6, IL-1β, or Tumor necrosis factor-α were shown to hold similar AUC [21]. Thus, it is most likely that the one particular biomarker for predicting outcome of patients with systemic inflammation may not exist due to the complexity of the immune response. One may speculate that ASM increases as a result of inflammation, as various inflammatory stimuli lead to activation of ASM mediated lipid signalling, including oxidative stress [22,23], induction by or of cytokines [24,25], platelet activating-factor (PAF)-mediated pulmonary oedema formation during acute lung injury [26] and ceramide accumulation in ischemia/reperfusion injury in mitochondria [27]. Due to the various pathophysiological properties of ASM in mediation of inflammation and apoptosis, we may also speculate that non-declining or continuously increased ASM in critically ill patients with systemic inflammation plays a putative causative role with respect to adverse outcome.

Our study has some limitations which have to be mentioned. The main limitation is the low number of patients included and that it was conducted as a single center study. Therefore, our results should be interpreted with caution as there is a high likelihood of a type II error. However, this study should be regarded in the context of a single center, pilot study aiming to gain more insight into the clinical usefulness of ASM kinetics in the course of systemic inflammation. A further limitation is that we did not perform consecutive ASM measurements in the ICU patients without systemic inflammation. This was due to financial restraints of this pilot study. Measurements of ASM are not yet comparable with established laboratory for PCT or CRP that are easier and cheaper to conduct. It is also likely that the time interval at which ASM was measured did not accurately capture an early change in ASM kinetics (24 hours range between measurement at PCT_{before} and PCT_{peak}). Future studies on ASM kinetics may address this potential limitation choosing an even closer measurement interval. Lastly, the potential of using ASM as a prognostic marker after systemic inflammation in clinical practice warrants further improvement of the assay to become more widely available.

Conclusions

Our study showed that patients who underwent uncomplicated surgery exhibited a significant post-operative increase in ASM. In a mixed ICU population, ASM was significantly higher compared to these patients. While ASM did not indicate the onset of systemic inflammation earlier than PCT in our group of patients, it was able to predict ICU mortality in patients after systemic inflammation in the presence of low PCT level. ASM may hold potential as a tool for risk stratification of these patients, but the clinical value has to be further evaluated in larger studies.

Supporting Information

File S1   Table S1, Procalcitonin (ng/ml) values of the included patients, sorted by survivors and non-survivors. Time points were the day before the PCT peak (PCT_{before}), the day of the PCT peak (PCT_{peak}) and again lowered PCT (PCT_{low}). **Table S2,** Acid sphingomyelinase (pMol/ml*h) values for the included patients, sorted by survivors and non-survivors. Time points were the day before the PCT peak (PCT_{before}), the day of the PCT peak (PCT_{peak}) and again lowered PCT (PCT_{low}). **Table S3,** C-reactive protein (mg/L) values of the included patients, sorted by survivors and non-survivors. Time points were the day before the PCT peak (PCT_{before}), the day of the PCT peak (PCT_{peak}) and again lowered PCT (PCT_{low}). **Table S4,** Lactate (mMol/L) values of the included patients, sorted by survivors and non-survivors. Time points were the day before the PCT peak (PCT_{before}), the day of the PCT peak (PCT_{peak}) and again lowered PCT (PCT_{low}). **Table S5,** Modified SOFA-Score (points) values of the included patients, sorted by survivors and non-survivors. Time points were the day before the PCT peak (PCT_{before}), the day of the PCT peak (PCT_{peak}) and again lowered PCT (PCT_{low}). **Table S6,** SAPS-Score (points) values of the included patients, sorted by survivors and non-survivors. Time points were the day before the PCT peak (PCT_{before}), the day of the PCT peak (PCT_{peak}) and again lowered PCT (PCT_{low}). **Table S7,** TISS-Score (points) values of the included patients, sorted by survivors and non-survivors. Time points were the day before the PCT peak (PCT_{before}), the day of the PCT peak (PCT_{peak}) and again lowered PCT (PCT_{low}). **Table S8,** Acid sphingomyelinase activity, Procalcitonin (PCT), C-reactive protein (CRP), Lactate, modified SOFA-Score (mSofa), SAPS II Score and TISS Score of the included patients on the day of intensive care unit (ICU) admission. **Table S9,** Patients' characteristics and outcomes of the included patients. **Table S10,** Patients' characteristics and outcomes of included patients with systemic inflammatory response syndrome (SIRS) plus Procalcitonin (PCT) peak. **Table S11,** Patients' characteristics and outcomes of included patients without systemic inflammatory response syndrome (SIRS) plus Procalcitonin (PCT) peak.

Author Contributions

Conceived and designed the experiments: MK GE NW SS. Performed the experiments: SWM MR. Analyzed the data: MK GE MR SWM DS GZ IF SS NW. Contributed to the writing of the manuscript: MK GE MR SWM DS GZ IF SS NW.

References

1. Angus DC, Linde-Zwirble WT, Lidicker J, Clermon G, Carcillo J, et al. (2001) Epidemiology of severe sepsis in the United States: analysis of incidence, outcome, and associated costs of care. Crit Care Med 7: 1303–1310.

2. Rivers E, Nguyen B, Havstad S, Ressler J, Muzzin A, et al. (2001) Early goal-directed therapy in the treatment of severe sepsis and septic shock. NEJM 19: 1368–1377.

3. Wacker C, Prkno A, Brunkhorst FM, Schlattmann P (2013) Procalcitonin as a diagnostic marker for sepsis: a systematic review and meta-analysis. Lancet Infect Dis 13: 426–35.

4. Prkno A, Wacker C, Brunkhorst FM, Schlattmann P (2013) Procalcitonin-guided therapy in intensive care unit patients with severe sepsis and septic shock - a systematic review and meta-analysis. Crit Care 17: R291.

5. Reinhart K, Brunkhorst FM, Bone HG, Bardutzky J, Dempfle CE, et al. (2010) Prevention, diagnosis, treatment, and follow-up care of sepsis. First revision of the S2k Guidelines of the German Sepsis Society (DSG) and the German Interdisciplinary Association for Intensive and Emergency Care Medicine (DIVI). Anaesthesist 59: 347–370.

6. Meisner M, Adina H, Schmidt J (2006) Correlation of procalcitonin and C-reactive protein to inflammation, complications, and outcome during the intensive care unit course of multiple-trauma patients. Crit Care 10: R1.

7. Castelli GP, Pognani C, Meisner M, Stuani A, Bellomi D, et al. (2004) Procalcitonin and C-reactive protein during systemic inflammatory response syndrome, sepsis and organ dysfunction. Crit Care 4: R234–242.

8. Herrmann W, Ecker D, Quast S, Klieden M, Rose S, et al. (2000) Comparison of procalcitonin, sCD14 and interleukin-6 values in septic patients. Clin Chem Lab Med 38: 41–46.

9. Uzzan B, Cohen R, Nicolas P, Cucherat M, Perret GY (2006) Procalcitonin as a diagnostic test for sepsis in critically ill adults and after surgery or trauma: a systematic review and meta-analysis. Crit Care Med 34: 1996–2003.

10. Jenkins RW, Canals D, Hannun YA (2009) Roles and regulation of secretory and lysosomal acid sphingomyelinase. Cell Signal 21: 836–46.

11. Grassmé H, Riethmüller J, Gulbins E (2007) Biological aspects of ceramide-enriched membrane domains. Prog Lipid Res 46: 161–70.

12. Claus RA, Bunck AC, Bockmeyer CL, Brunkhorst FM, Lösche W, et al. (2005) Role of increased sphingomyelinase activity in apoptosis and organ failure of patients with severe sepsis. FASEB J. 19: 1719–1721.

13. Jbeily N, Suckert I, Gonnert FA, Acht B, Bockmeyer CL, et al. (2013) Hyperresponsiveness of mice deficient in plasma-secreted sphingomyelinase reveals its pivotal role in early phase of host response. J Lipid Res 54: 410–424.

14. Levy MM, Fink MP, Marshall JC, Abrahams E, Angus D, et al. (2003) 2001 SCCM/ESICM/ACCP/ATS/SIS International Sepsis Definitions Conference. Crit Care Med 4: 1250–1256.

15. Kornhuber J, Tripal P, Reichel M, Muhle C, Rhein C, et al. (2010) Functional Inhibitors of Acid Sphingomyelinase (FIASMAs): a novel pharmacological group of drugs with broad clinical applications. Cell Physiol Biochem 26: 9–20.

16. Le Gall JR, Lemeshow S, Saulnier F (1993) A new simplified acute physiology score (SAPS II) based on a European/North American multicenter study. JAMA 270: 2957–2963.

17. Cullen DJ, Civetta JM, Briggs BA, Ferrara LC (1974) Therapeutic Intervention Scoring System: a method for quantitative comparison of patient care. Crit Care Med 2: 57–60.

18. Vincent JL, Moreno R, Takala J, Willatts S, De Mendonça A, et al. (1996) The SOFA (Sepsis-related Organ Failure Assessment) score to describe organ dysfunction/failure. On behalf of the Working Group on Sepsis-Related Problems of the European Society of Intensive Care Medicine. Intensive Care Med 22: 707–710.

19. Edelmann B, Bertsch U, Tchikov V, Winoto-Morbach S, Jakob M, et al. (2011) Caspase-8 and caspase-7 sequentially mediate proteolytic activation of acid sphingomyelinase in TNF-R1-receptosomes. EMBO-J 30: 379–394.

20. Drobnik W, Liebisch G, Audebert FX, Frohlich D, Gluck T, et al. (2003) Plasma ceramide and lysophosphatidylcholine inversely correlate with mortality in sepsis patients. J Lipid Res 44: 754–761.

21. Bozza FA, Salluh JI, Japiassu AM, Soares M, Assis EF, et al. (2007) Cytokine profiles as markers of disease severity in sepsis: a multiplex analysis. Crit Care 11: R49.

22. Castillo SS, Levy M, Wang C, Thaikoottathil JV, Khan E, et al. (2007) Nitric oxide-enhanced caspase-3 and acidic sphingomyelinase interaction: a novel mechanism by which airway epithelial cells escape ceramide-induced apoptosis. Exp Cell Res 313: 816–823.

23. Corda S, Laplace C, Vicaut E, Duranteau J (2001) Rapid reactive oxygen species production by mitochondria in endothelial cells exposed to tumor necrosis factor-alpha is mediated by ceramide. Am J Resp Cell Mol Biol 24: 762–768.

24. Garcia-Ruiz C, Colell A, Mari M, Morales A, Calvo M, et al. (2003) Defective TNF-alpha-mediated hepatocellular apoptosis and liver damage in acidic sphingomyelinase knockout mice. J Clin Invest 111: 197–208.

25. Tokuda H, Kozawa O, Harada A, Uematsu T (1999) Extracellular sphingomyelinase induces interleukin-6 synthesis in osteoblasts. J Bio Chem 172: 262–268.

26. Göggel R, Winoto-Morbach S, Vielhaber G, Imai Y, Lindner K, et al. (2004) PAF-mediated pulmonary edema: a new role for acid sphingomyelinase and ceramide. Nat Med 10: 155–160.

27. Gudz TI, Tserng KY, Hoppel CL (1997) Direct inhibition of mitochondrial respiratory chain complex III by cell-permeable ceramide. J Biol Chem 272: 24154–24158.

19

Identification of Novel Single Nucleotide Polymorphisms Associated with Acute Respiratory Distress Syndrome by Exome-Seq

Katherine Shortt[1,2], Suman Chaudhary[1], Dmitry Grigoryev[1,2], Daniel P. Heruth[1], Lakshmi Venkitachalam[2], Li Q. Zhang[1], Shui Q. Ye[1,2]*

1 Department of Pediatrics, Division of Experimental and Translational Genetics, Children's Mercy Hospital, University of Missouri - Kansas City School of Medicine, Kansas City, Missouri, United States of America, 2 Department of Biomedical and Health Informatics, University of Missouri - Kansas City School of Medicine, Kansas City, Missouri, United States of America

Abstract

Acute respiratory distress syndrome (ARDS) is a lung condition characterized by impaired gas exchange with systemic release of inflammatory mediators, causing pulmonary inflammation, vascular leak and hypoxemia. Existing biomarkers have limited effectiveness as diagnostic and therapeutic targets. To identify disease-associating variants in ARDS patients, whole-exome sequencing was performed on 96 ARDS patients, detecting 1,382,399 SNPs. By comparing these exome data to those of the 1000 Genomes Project, we identified a number of single nucleotide polymorphisms (SNP) which are potentially associated with ARDS. 50,190SNPs were found in all case subgroups and controls, of which89 SNPs were associated with susceptibility. We validated three SNPs (rs78142040, rs9605146 and rs3848719) in additional ARDS patients to substantiate their associations with susceptibility, severity and outcome of ARDS. rs78142040 (C>T) occurs within a histone mark (intron 6) of the Arylsulfatase D gene. rs9605146 (G>A) causes a deleterious coding change (proline to leucine) in the XK, Kell blood group complex subunit-related family, member 3 gene. rs3848719 (G>A) is a synonymous SNP in the Zinc-Finger/Leucine-Zipper Co-Transducer NIF1 gene. rs78142040, rs9605146, and rs3848719 are associated significantly with susceptibility to ARDS. rs3848719 is associated with APACHE II score quartile. rs78142040 is associated with 60-day mortality in the overall ARDS patient population. Exome-seq is a powerful tool to identify potential new biomarkers for ARDS. We selectively validated three SNPs which have not been previously associated with ARDS and represent potential new genetic biomarkers for ARDS. Additional validation in larger patient populations and further exploration of underlying molecular mechanisms are warranted.

Editor: You-Yang Zhao, University of Illinois College of Medicine, United States of America

Funding: Funding was in part provided by NHLBI/NIH Grant (HL080042 & HL080042-S1, Ye, SQ), start-up fund and endowments of Children's Mercy Hospitals and Clinics, UMKC (Ye, SQ), and a Sarah Morrison Student Research Award of UMKC (Shortt, K). The funders had no role in study design, data collection and analysis, decision to publish, or preparation of the manuscript.

Competing Interests: The authors have declared that no competing interests exist.

* Email: sqye@cmh.edu

Introduction

Acute respiratory distress syndrome (ARDS), a severe form of acute lung injury, is characterized by the inflammation and fluid build-up in the alveoli of the lungs, which reduces the ability of oxygen to cross over into the blood stream [1,2]. ARDS has an extremely high mortality rate where over a third of sufferers die, and many of the survivors experience complications such as brain damage due to prolonged oxygen deprivation [3,4]. The mortality rate is even higher in cases with common comorbidities such as sepsis with suspected pulmonary source (40.6%) and witnessed aspiration (43.6%) [3]. ARDS is estimated to have an age-adjusted incidence of 86.2 new cases per 100,000 person-years in adults age 15 and older. The total number of cases estimated to occur yearly in the US is about 190,000 [3]. Pneumonia and sepsis are most common causes of ARDS, and Sepsis is the leading cause of ARDS. There is a paucity of effective and specific therapy to

ARDS though low tidal volume ventilation has been demonstrated for some therapeutic utilities [5–8]. This is because the etiology and pathology of the disease are still not well understood and there remains a need for new specific and effective preventative measures and treatments.

The role of genetics in ARDS is increasingly recognized and it has recently been shown that complex diseases can be between 50 and 90% genetically determined [9]. Biomarkers that have been previously studied that are present in blood serum include surfactant-associated proteins (SP-A, B, and C), Mucin-associated antigens (KL-6 and MUC1), Cytokines (IL-1, 2, 6, 8, 10, and 15, TNFα), endothelium activation markers (E-selectin, L-selectin, I-CAM-1, V-CAM-1, and VWF), and neutrophil activation markers (MMP-9, LTB4, and Ferritin). Cytokine levels have been identified as a moderately effective measure of severity [10]. Additional biomarkers of ARDS severity have been obtained from breath analysis, including hydrogen peroxide levels and breath acidity [11]. Pre-B cell Colony Enhancing Factor (PBEF), also called nicotinamide phosphoribosyltransferase (NAMPT), was identified previously as a novel biomarker of ARDS by our group [12]. Analysis of two SNPs in the human PBEF promoter revealed an association with ARDS. The −1535T variant allele was associated with a decreased susceptibility to ALI/ARDS and a better outcome in septic patients in a Caucasian population when compared with patients without the variation. The −1001G variant allele was associated with increased susceptibility to acute lung injury and ARDS in African American and Caucasian populations. The −1001G variant was also associated with a higher ICU mortality rate in septic patients in a Caucasian

population [6,13–15]. Despite the previous identification of several available biomarkers, their available data are inconsistent and clinical relevance has not yet been established.

With the development of next-generation sequencing technologies and improvements in data analysis capabilities, it is now feasible to sequence and analyze whole genomes within a couple of days [16]. However, the cost of whole genome sequencing is still a prohibitive factor for sequencing more samples. Whole exome sequencing (WES) is faster and less expensive than whole-genome sequencing, making it ideal for the study of variants that cause changes to the protein-coding regions of genes [17]. WES has been used to identify genetic risk factors for both Mendelian and complex diseases alike [17–19]. The purpose of this study was to

Table 1. Participant demographics and comorbidities for the ARDS cases.

Whole-exome Sequencing Sample group	Participants*	Gender (%male)	Age± SD	APACHEII score ±SD	Ventilator-free days per 28 days ±SD	60-day mortality (% dead at 60 days post-onset)
ARDS total	96	46.9	50±14.6	97.2±30.4	12.6±10.2	29.4
Caucasian ARDS	70	44.3	50.7±13.8	94.5±30.2	13.6±10.0	23.9
African American ARDS	26	53.8	47.8±16.6	104.6±30.2	9.9±10.5	44
ARDS with Sepsis total	48	50	52.0±15.1	105.2±32.2	10.2±10.1	38.3
Caucasian ARDS with Sepsis	37	43.2	51.8±15.0	102.6±31.1	10.5±9.8	33.3
African American ARDS with Sepsis	11	72.7	52.9±16.1	113.6±35.8	9.3±11.7	54.5
ARDS with Pneumonia total	48	43.8	47.9±13.9	88.9±26.2	14.9±9.87	20
Caucasian ARDS with Pneumonia	33	45.5	49.5±12.4	85.0±26.6	17.0±9.2	12.9
African American ARDS with Pneumonia	15	40	44.1±16.6	97.6±24.0	10.3±10.0	35.7
TaqMan Genotyping Sample group	**Participants**	**Gender (%male)**	**Age± SD**	**APACHEII score ±SD**	**Ventilator-free days per 28 days ±SD**	**60-day mortality (% dead at 60 days post-onset)**
ARDS Total	117	46.2	50.8±16.6	105.1±32.7	12.0±10.5	31
Caucasian ARDs	75	40	52.1±15.4	104.3±31.4	11.8±10.5	29.2
African American ARDS	17	64.7	51.6±22.8	113.3±33.8	12.2±10.6	29.4
Other ancestry ARDS	25	52	46.4±15.3	101.8±36.2	12.6±10.7	37.5
ARDS with Sepsis total	59	52.5	51.5±17.3	112.9±31.5	11.3±11.0	37.9
Caucasian ARDS with Sepsis	34	50	51.1±15.6	113.6±29.7	10.9±11.1	33.3
African American ARDS with Sepsis	9	66.7	56.6±27.1	121.8±33.0	12.9±11.5	33.3
Other ancestry ARDS with Sepsis	16	50	49.6±14.8	106.4±34.7	11.4±11.0	50
ARDS with Pneumonia total	58	39.7	50.1±16.0	96.9±32.3	12.7±9.9	23.6
Caucasian ARDS with Pneumonia	41	31.7	52.9±15.3	96.4±31.0	12.6±10.0	25.6
African American ARDS with Pneumonia	8	62.5	46±16.9	103.8±34.3	11.4±10.2	25
Other ancestry ARDS with Pneumonia	9	55.6	46.8±15.2	92.4±39.7	14.9±10.3	12.5
Total ARDS	**Participants**	**Gender (%male)**	**Age± SD**	**APACHEII score ±SD**	**Ventilator-free days per 28 days ±SD**	**60-day mortality (% dead at 60 days post-onset)**
All ARDS patients	213	46.5	50.4±15.7	101.6±31.9	12.3±10.3	30.2

*, 8 samples, 4 exome sequenced and 4 TaqMan genotyped ARDS patients did not have these phenotypes available. An additional 2 exome sequenced ARDS patients did not have ventilator-free day's data. In addition to the 8 patients missing severity and mortality phenotype data, 2 patients were excluded from the regression because their phenotypes were thought to be missing until after the regressions were completed.

Table 2. Summary of the filtering applied to candidate SNPs.

Criteria for filtering	Number of remaining variants
SNPs detected in ARDS SNPs	1,382,399
matched in 1000 Genomes Project	169,376
common across 4 ARDS race and etiology groups*	50,190
χ^2 p-value <0.01 in top 5 ARDS groups**	99
χ^2 p-value <2.95×10^{-7} in at least 2/5 top 5 ARDS groups	76(in 65 genes)
coding variants	38(in 32 genes)
nonsynonymous	20
synonymous variants	18

*, African American with pneumonia, African American with sepsis, Caucasian with pneumonia, Caucasian with sepsis subgroups. Out of the 50,190 SNPs, 49,723 are bi-allelic. **, All ARDS, all pneumonia, all sepsis, all African American, all Caucasian groups.

discover new biomarkers for ARDS using WES. Exome sequencing of 96 ARDS patient DNA samples from the ARDSnet (www.ardsnet.org) and 48 race, gender and age matched normal healthy control subject DNAs from Coriell (www.coriell.org) was performed using Illumina's HiScanSQ system. By comparing SNP analysis of whole exome sequence data between the ARDS patient population (96 patients) and the normal healthy controls from Coriell (48 subjects) as well as the 1000 Genomes Project (440 total, 379 European Ancestry (EUR), 61 African Americans in the southwest (ASW), www.1000genomes.org) [20], we have identified a number of coding SNPs potentially associated with ARDS susceptibility. We also performed regression analyses within the

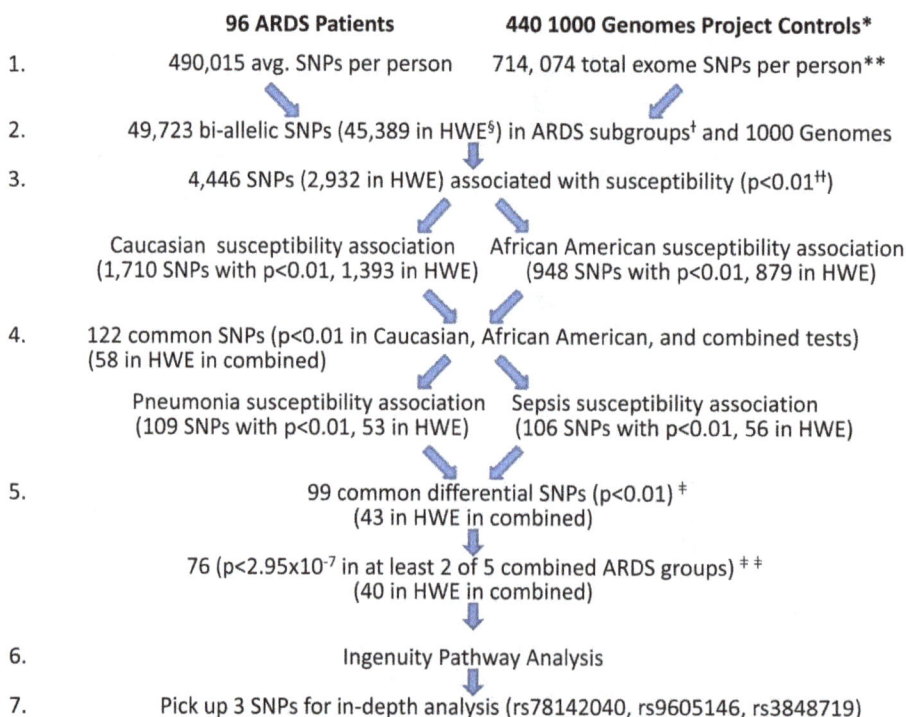

Figure 1. Pipeline of the exome-seq data analysis workflow. After processing the data using the GATK pipeline, this filtering workflow was derived to identify SNPs which were associated with measures of susceptibility across the racial and etiology groups of cases. SNPs were filtered based on strength of association, coding effect, and functional prediction prior to testing for association with other ARDS phenotypes. *, The sample contains African American and Caucasian patients, so the EUR and ASW healthy controls from 1000 Genomes were used for comparison; **, In the 1000 Genomes Project exome sequence, the same 714,074 SNPs are present for all 440 EUR and ASW; §, HWE = Hardy Weinberg Equilibrium, p> 0.0001; +, African American with pneumonia, African American with sepsis, Caucasian with pneumonia, Caucasian with sepsis; + +, χ^2 test of ARDS vs. respective 1000 Genomes Project control groups; ‡, SNPs with P-value <0.01 in the overall comparison, Caucasian ARDS comparison, and African American comparison with 1000 Genomes were filtered further by p<0.01 in the sepsis comparison and pneumonia comparison; ‡ ‡, All ARDS cases, all pneumonia cases, all sepsis cases, all African American cases, all Caucasian cases.

ARDS patient population to assess association of some newly identified SNPs with ARDS severity (APACHE II score) and outcome (60 day mortality). In addition, we validated three SNPs (rs78142040, rs9605146 and rs3848719) in an additional 117 ARDS patients for a total of 213 cases using TaqMan genotyping assays (Life Technologies) to substantiate their associations with the susceptibility, severity and outcome of ARDS.

Materials and Methods

ARDS patients and healthy control subjects

To perform this case-control study, we used 213 ARDS patient DNA samples from the ARDSnet (www.ardsnet.org) and 440 healthy control subjects (379 EUR and 61 ASW) from the 1000 Genomes Project (www.1000genomes.org). The African Ancestry 1000 Genomes Project panel used in our study is ASW (Americans of African Ancestry in Southwest USA). The European Ancestry 1000 Genomes Project panels used in our study include CEU (Utah residents with Northern and Western European ancestry), FIN (Finnish in Finland), GBR (British in England and Scotland), IBS (Iberian population in Spain), and TSI (Toscani in Italia). Clinical information for 213 ARDS cases was obtained from the NHLBI ARDS network 05: Fluid and Catheter Treatment Trial [21,22] as managed by the Biologic Specimen and Data Repository Information Coordinating Center (BioLINCC, http://biolincc.nhlbi.nih.gov.home). Limited demographic variables for normal control subjects were obtained from the 1000 Genomes Project (www.1000genomes.org).

Exome-seq and data analysis

Exome sequencing was performed on 96 ARDS cases using HiScanSQ (Illumina, CA, USA). Briefly, the libraries for exome sequencing were created using the TrueSeq Exome Enrichment Kit (http://www.illumina.com). Paired-end sequencing with 101 base pair read lengths was performed using Illumina's HiScanSQ, which provides a minimum average coverage depth of 50×. Consensus Assessment of Sequence And VAriations (CASAVA) software was used for the conversion of HiScanSQ reported.bcl files to.fastq format and for demultiplexing (http://www.illumina.com). The sequences were aligned to the hg19 human reference genome and variants alleles were called using the Genome Analysis Toolkit (GATK) (http://www.broadinstitute.org/gatk/). Sequencing data are submitted to the NCBI BioProject database (Accession ID: 262819, http://www.ncbi.nlm.nih.gov/bioproject/262819).

Both the lab-generated data for ARDS patient samples and the 1000 Genomes Project controls were processed using the GATK methodology [23]. GATK was also used to generate the list of SNPs from the sequence data. Sequencing data of the patient samples were considered to be high-confidence if the Phred-like quality was a minimum of 20 and there were at least 4× coverage depths. SNPs from the two data sources were merged by location from alpha ordered datasets and minor allele counts were determined from the merged data.

For the analysis of candidate SNPs associated with the ARDS susceptibility, the ARDS SNP data were compared with the 1000 Genomes Project SNP data. The total control sample size in the 1000 Genomes Project is 1092, and the data identifies about 15 million SNPs which underwent stringent quality control [20,24]. We studied the 440 ASW and EUR samples obtained from this dataset. In racially stratified analyses, the ASW population in the 1000 Genomes Project was used as a control population for the African American ARDS samples and the EUR population was used as a control for the Caucasian ARDS population (Table S1). SNPs in HWE in the cases with high data quality were selected for genotype validation. The detailed association analysis and Hardy-Weinberg equilibrium analysis are provided in Supporting Information S1 [25,26].

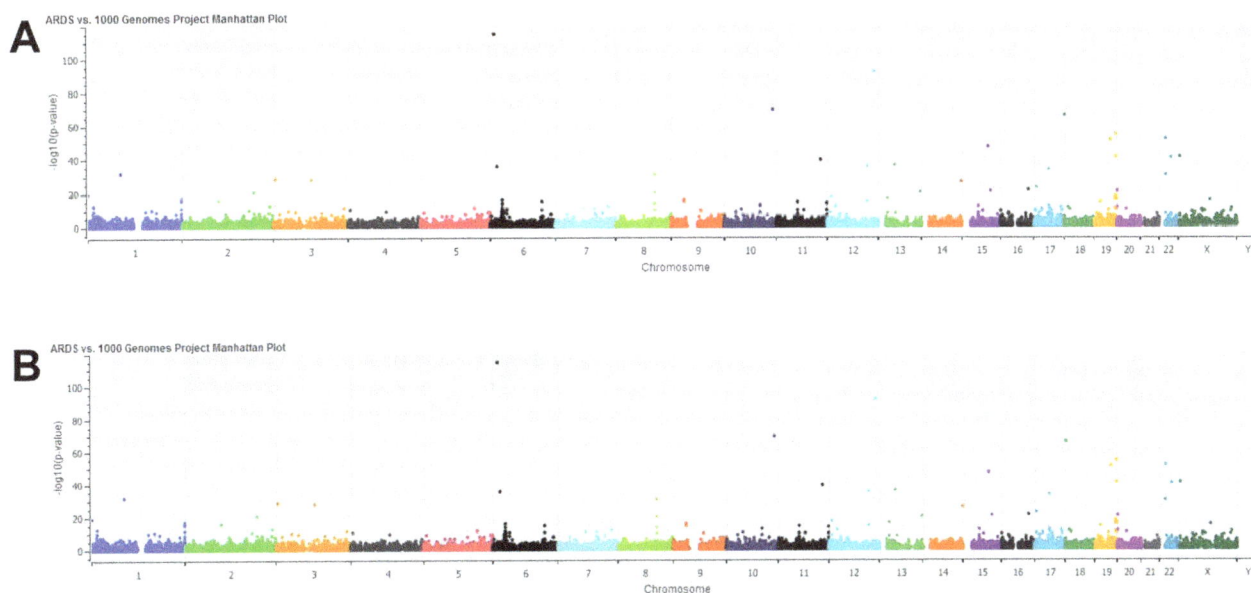

Figure 2. Manhattan plot of ARDS patients and 1000 genomes project controls. A number of strong associations with susceptibility to ARDS were observed using a χ^2 test. (**A**) A Manhattan plot of the whole exome sequence all ARDS cases vs. European Ancestry and ASW 1000 Genomes Project controls created using SVS v8.2.0. This is a graphic representation of the chromosome location (x axis) vs. the −log10 (χ^2 p-value) of the allele frequencies. SNPs whose chi-square tests yield a smaller p-value fall higher on the log scale are more significant [42]. (**B**) The same Manhattan plot with a zoomed Y-axis.

Table 3. Pathway analysis.

Top Canonical Pathways	p-value*	Ratio**	Molecules
Graft-versus-Host Disease Signaling	8.07×10^{-9}	6/48	KIR2DL1/KIR2DL3, HLA-DRB1, HLA-B, HLA-DQA1, HLA-DQB1, HLA-DRB5
Autoimmune Thyroid Disease Signaling	4.35×10^{-7}	5/49	HLA-DRB1, HLA-B, HLA-DQA1, HLA-DQB1, HLA-DRB5
Nur77 Signaling in T Lymphocytes	9.37×10^{-7}	5/57	HLA-DRB1, HLA-DQA1, HLA-DQB1, HLA-DRB5, SIN3A
Calcium-induced T Lymphocyte Apoptosis	1.68×10^{-6}	5/64	HLA-DRB1, HLA-DQA1, HLA-DQB1, ITPR1, HLA-DRB5
B Cell Development	3.75×10^{-6}	4/34	HLA-DRB1, HLA-DQA1, HLA-DQB1, HLA-DRB5

Top canonical pathways as predicted from the 65genes containing the76 SNPs that were identified using χ^2 tests. Pathway predictions were done using the Core Analysis function of Ingenuity Pathway Analysis. *, P-Value of <0.05 indicates a non-random association between the genes and pathway; **, Ratio of the number of genes in the dataset involved in the pathway to the total number of genes in the pathway.

For the analysis of candidate SNPs associated with the ARDS severity, the correlation between SNPs and the APACHEII score (a measure of the severity of a disease in adult patients) as well as the number of ventilator-free days per 28 days (an indication of a patient's ability to breathe on their own) was conducted.

For the identification of candidate SNPs associated with the ARDS outcome, the logistic regression analysis between SNPs and 60 day mortality was performed.

Following the results of the genetic association study the data were further analyzed through the use of the Variant Analysis component of SNP & Variation Suite v8.2.0 (SVS v8.2.0, Golden Helix, Inc., Bozeman, MT, www.goldenhelix.com). This software ranked the SNPs in order of likely importance based on location, as well as amino acid change predictions. This information was joined with predictions of protein functional effect changes made by Sift and Provean (http://provean.jcvi.org/index.php) as well as Polyphen2 (http://genetics.bwh.harvard.edu/pph2/index.shtml). Ingenuity Pathway Analysis Software (www.ingenuity.com/) from Ingenuity Systems was used to screen for SNPs which are likely to alter the function of relevant biologic pathways. To accomplish this a list of the genes that contain SNPs with χ^2 p-value of < 2.95×10^{-7} in at least 2 of the 5 main susceptibility comparisons and a χ^2 p-value of <0.01 in all of the 5 main comparisons of exome sequence data (All ARDS vs. 1000 Genomes, All Sepsis vs. 1000 Genomes, All Pneumonia vs. 1000 Genomes, African American ARDS vs. ASW1000 Genomes, and Caucasian ARDS vs. EUR 1000 Genomes) was submitted to IPA. Additional information on the statistical methods preformed in this study can be found in Supporting Information S1, which contains descriptions of the principal component analysis and genomic inflation factor calculations [27–31].

Genotyping of Selected Candidate SNPs

Three selected SNPs (rs78142040; rs9605146, and rs3848719) in the additional 117 ARDS patient DNA samples from the NHLBI Ardent were genotyped using TaqMan human SNP genotyping assays on the ViiA 7 Real Time PCR System (Life Technologies, Grand Island, NY) according to the supplier's instruction. Genotyping accuracy was validated using 10 previously exome-sequenced samples in-lab. Genotyping data from the additional samples was combined with the existing 96 patient sample to increase sample size for the 3 SNPs and association tests were repeated using the total 213 patient population.

Results

Identification of novel coding SNPs associated with the ARDS susceptibility

In order to identify novel coding SNPs associated with the ARDS susceptibility, we performed the exome-seq of 96 ARDS patient DNAs. These patients consisted of 70 Caucasian and 26 African Americans (Table 1). In Caucasian patients, 37 cases were due to the initiating etiology of sepsis and 33 were due to pneumonia. In African American patients, 11 cases were due to the initiating etiology of sepsis and 15 were due to pneumonia. We detected 1,382,399 SNPs in 96 ARDS patients by exome-seq (Table 2) and 490,015 SNPs per person on average (Figure 1). Among them, 169,376 SNPs matched records from 625 healthy control subjects in the 1000 human genome project. From 169,376 SNPs, there are 49,723 bi-allelic SNPs out of 50,190 total SNPs in all ARDS patient subgroups based on race and initiating etiologies: Caucasian sepsis, Caucasian pneumonia, African-American sepsis and African American pneumonia. Of our 1,382,399 ARDS SNPs, 608,723 were common between the sepsis and pneumonia cases while 369,639 and 404,037 are non-overlapping SNPs, respectively. There are 442,235 common SNPs between our African American cases and Caucasian cases while 337,738 and 602,426 are non-overlapping SNPs, respectively. 87.8% of the 1,382,399 ARDS SNPs (i.e., 1,213,023 ARDS SNPs) are not found in the 1000 Genomes Project Exome, but 85.4% of the 1,213,023 ARDS SNPs (i.e., 1,035,921 SNPs) were assigned RS numbers, suggesting our data collection and processing are reliable. By comparing the frequencies of the minor alleles in those newly detected SNPs in 96 ARDS patients with those in 440 Caucasian and African-Americans from the Southwest healthy control subjects of the 1000 human genome project, we found that there are 3,867 differential SNPs (p<0.01) (Figure 2). In Caucasians, between ARDS patients and healthy controls, there are 788 differential SNPs (p<0.01). In African-Americans, between ARDS patients and healthy controls, there are 948 differential SNPs (p<0.01). There are 122 common differential SNPs (p<0.01) between either Caucasian or African American patients or healthy controls. When we examined sepsis- or pneumonia-initiated ARDS separately, we found that 106 and 109 differential SNPs (p<0.01), respectively. Between them, there are 99 common differential SNPs (p<0.01). When the Bonferroni correction (p<2.95×10^{-7}) was applied, 76SNPs remains significantly different. These SNPs are potentially novel coding SNPs associated with the ARDS susceptibility.

Table 4. Profile of 3 SNPs.

	rs3848719	rs9605146	rs78142040
Location	20:44596545	22:17265194	X:2832771
Gene ID	ZNF335	XKR3	ARSD
Call Rate (Cases+Controls)	0.962	0.995	0.991
Call Rate (Cases)	0.883	0.986	0.972
HWE P-value (Cases)	2.86E-4	0.422	1.18E-3
HWE P-value (Controls)	0.887	3.72E-5	1
HWE P-value (Cases+Controls)	0.034	1.94E-12	0.471
Reference: Alternate Allele	G>A	G>A	C>T
Alt. Allele Freq. (Cases)	39.4%	38.6%	22.0%
Alt. Allele Freq. (Controls)	38.5%	4.0%	0%
Number AA (%) (Cases)	41 (21.8%)	34 (16.2%)	2 (1.0%)
Number AA (%) (Controls)	66(15.0%)	4(0.9%)	0(0%)
Number Ar (%) (Cases)	66 (35.1%)	94 (44.8%)	87 (42.0%)
Number Ar (%) (Controls)	207 (47.0%)	27 (6.1%)	0 (0%)
Number rr (%) (Cases)	81 (45.1%)	82 (39.1%)	118 (57.0%)
Number rr (%) (Controls)	339 (77.0%)	35 (8.0%)	0 (0%)
SNP classification	Coding	Coding	Intronic
Coding classification	Synonymous	Nonsynonymous	Intronic
Reference amino acid	S	P	NK
Alternate amino acid	S	L	NK
Provean prediction (cutoff = −25)[1]	Neutral	Deleterious	NK
Sift prediction (cutoff = 0.05)[1]	Tolerated	Tolerated	NK
Pph2 prediction[2]	NK	benign	NK

NK: Not known, HWE, Hardy-Weinberg equilibrium; AA, alternate genotype or homozygous minor genotype; Ar, heterozygous genotype; rr, reference genotype or homozygous major genotype; 1, http://provean.jcvi.org/genome_submit.php; 2, http://genetics.bwh.harvard.edu/pph2/.

Pathway Analysis

These 76 SNPs occur in 65 genes. To determine the functional consequences of these SNPs, Ingenuity Pathway Analysis was conducted on these 65 genes to identify biologic pathways in which these genes function. The top canonical pathway is *graft-versus-host disease signaling* and included 6 genes that contained associated SNPs, comprising 13% of the genes involved in the pathway ($p = 8.07 \times 10^{-9}$). The top 5 canonical pathways addi-

Table 5. Overall association summary.

	rs3848719	rs9605146	rs78142040
Susceptibility (cases vs. controls)			
Chi-squared p-value	0.780	1.68E-59	3.64E-47
Odds Ratio (95% CI)[1]	1.04(0.81–1.33)	15.16(10.25–22.41)	498.09 (30.83–8,047.51)
Severity (ventilator-free days/28 days)			
p-value	NS	NS	NS
Odds Ratio (95% CI)[2]	NS	NS	NS
Severity (APACHE II score)			
p-value	0.032	NS	0.061**
Odds Ratio (95% CI)[2]	0.55 (0.31–0.96)	NS	2.60(0.93–7.26)
Outcome (60-day mortality)			
p-value	NS*	NS	0.017
Odds Ratio (95% CI)[2]	NS	NS	2.04 (1.13–3.68)

NS, Not significant; *, significantly associated in genotyped Caucasian, pneumonia, and Caucasian pneumonia subgroups; **, for 117 genotyped samples only, not in total 213; 1, Odds ratio for alternate allele (allelic test); 2, additive genotypic model.

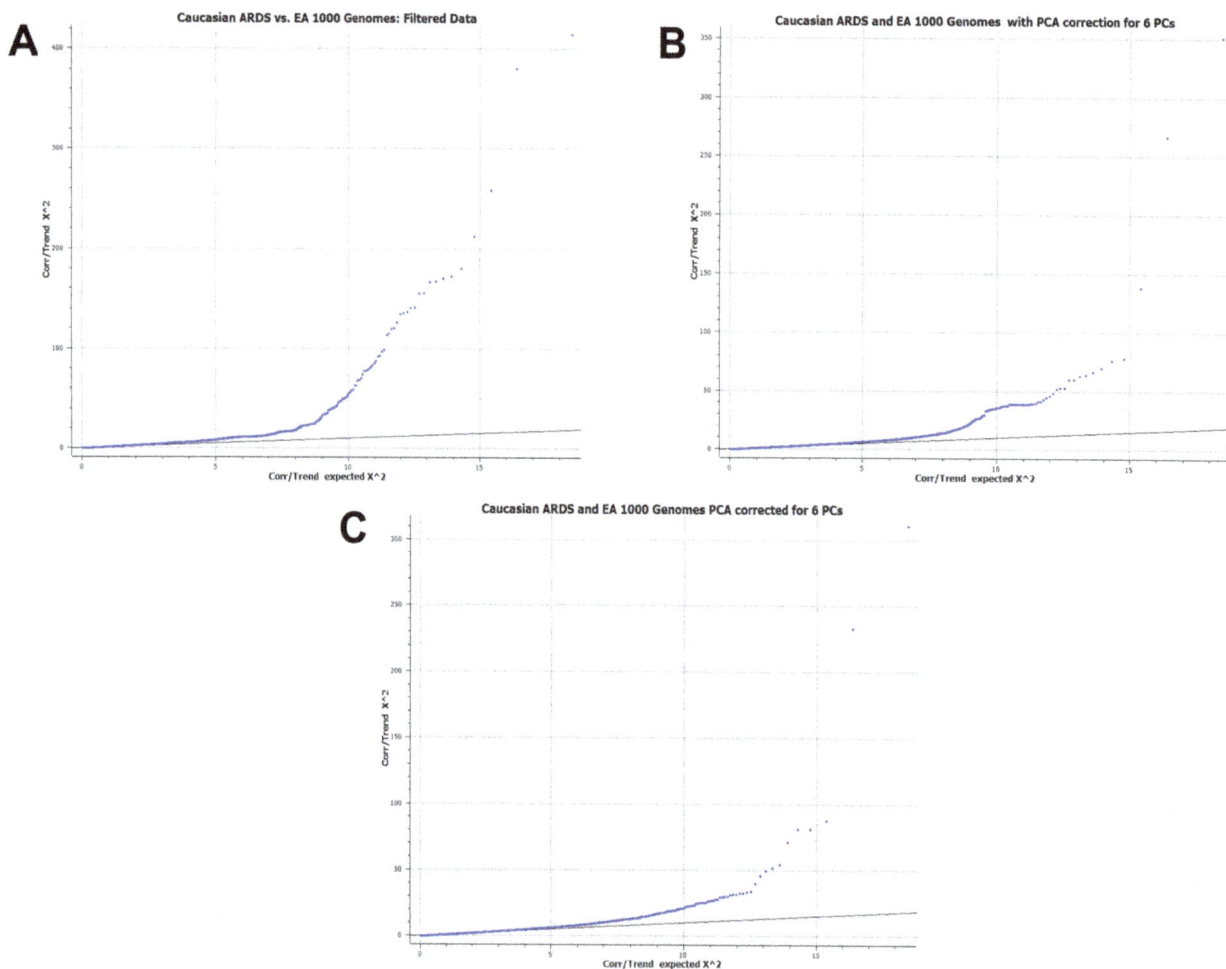

Figure 3. Quantile-quantile plots of Caucasian ARDS and EUR 1000 genomes. In the example of our Caucasian cases and EUR controls, we observe that correction for principal components improves the fit of our data with the expected distribution. (**A**) QQ plot of expected χ^2 values versus the actual χ^2 values for the genotypic trend test of case-control status. The data are filtered on HWE, LD, and SNP call rate but not PCA corrected. (**B**) QQ plot of expected χ^2 values versus the actual χ^2 values for the genotypic trend test of case-control status. The data have been filtered and corrected for 6 PCs. (**C**) QQ plot of expected χ^2 values versus the actual χ^2 values for the genotypic trend test of case-control status. The data have been filtered and corrected for 6 PCs and undergone sample outlier removal.

tionally include *autoimmune thyroid disease signaling, Nur77 signaling in T lymphocytes, calcium-induced T lymphocyte apoptosis*, and *B-cell development signaling* (Table 3). Among the 76 remaining significantly different SNPs after the Boneferroni correction (Figure 1), 38 SNPs are coding variants. Of these, 20 SNPs can cause nonsynonymous amino acid changes while 18 SNPs can cause synonymous amino acid changes (Table 2).

Selected validations of three SNPs (rs78142040, rs9605146 and rs3848719)in additional 117 ARDS patients

To validate the result of SNP identification by exome-seq, we selectively genotyped three SNPs (rs78142040, rs9605146 and rs3848719) in an additional 117 ARDS patients using the TaqMan genotype assay (Table 4). We then examined their association with the susceptibility, severity and outcome to ARDS in a combined 213 ARDS patients (96 by exome-seq +117 by TaqMan = 213) (Table 5, Table S2, Table S3, and Table S4).

rs78142040 has a major allele C and a minor allele T and is found on the X chromosome position X: 2832771 in the

Arylsulfatase D gene (ARSD). The SNP was determined to lie within a histone mark of intron 6 using the UCSC Genome Browser (http://genome.ucsc.edu/) and could potentially play a role in regulation of expression. The ARSD was associated with bone and cartilage development and was identified previously as having involvement in sphingolipid metabolism and as a potential biomarker for chronic lymphocytic leukemia [32]. The SNP is in Hardy-Weinberg Equilibrium (HWE p>1×10^{-4}) in the 1000 Genomes controls and the ARDS population and subgroups.

The SNP is associated significantly with susceptibility (p< $2.95\times10^{\wedge}-7$) in the total 213 patient population (MAF = 0.22) and the subgroups when compared with those from the 1000 Genomes Project (MAF = 0.00) (Table 5, Additional file 6: Table S5). rs78142040 approaches association with APACHEII score when the score quartiles are compared for the genotyped ARDS patients (p = 0.061, OR = 2.603, 95% CI = 0.933–7.260) (Table 5, Table S4). rs78142040 is associated with the 60-day mortality in the total ARDS population (p = 0.017, OR = 2.039, 95%CI 1.130–3.681) (Table S3).

rs9605146 (also known as rs114989947) has a major allele G and minor allele A. It is a nonsynonymous SNP found within exon 4 of chromosome 22 (22:17265194) in the "XK, Kell blood group complex subunit-related family, member 3" gene (XKR3) and causes a predicted amino acid change from proline to leucine. The protein encoded by XKR3 is a homolog of XK, which is a putative membrane transporter [33]. XKR3 has not been previously associated with human disease. This amino acid change has a deleterious effect predicted by a Provean score of -5.494, where a score of maximum -2.5 is considered to be deleterious. The SNP is in HWE ($p>1\times10^{-4}$) in the EUR 1000 Genomes Project samples as well as in the ARDS population and subgroups. rs9605146 is associated with disease susceptibility ($p<2.95\times10^{-7}$) in the total ARDS population (MAF = 0.39) and subgroups when compared with the 1000 Genomes controls (MAF = 0.04) with the exception of the African Americans when the sepsis and pneumonia etiologies are analyzed individually (Table 5, Table S6). The SNP also approaches significant association with 60-day mortality in the exome-sequenced patients with pneumonia ($p = 0.080$).

rs3848719 has a major allele of G and a minor allele A. It is a synonymous SNP in the 5th exon of the Zinc-Finger/Leucine-Zipper Co-Transducer NIF1 gene in chromosome 20 (ZNF335, location 20:44596545). The ZNF335 gene is expected to play a role in transcription regulation and is involved in neural progenitor cell proliferation and self-renewal. It is associated with the disease microcephaly [34,35]. The SNP is in Hardy-Weinberg Equilibrium (HWE $p>1\times10^{-4}$) in the 1000 Genomes controls and the ARDS population and subgroups.

The SNP was not associated with susceptibility in the total ARDS population (MAF = 0.39) when compared with the 1000 Genomes controls (MAF = 0.385) (Table 5, Table S7), however rs3848719 is associated with APACHEII score when the score quartiles are compared for total ARDS patients ($p = 0.032$, OR = 0.549, 95%CI = 0.313–0.96). The SNP is associated with 60-day mortality in the TaqMan genotyped Caucasian ARDS ($p = 0.012$, OR = 2.753, 95% CI = 1.196–6.336), TaqMan genotyped pneumonia ($p = 0.032$, OR = 2.511, 95% CI = 1.053–5.984), and TaqMan genotyped Caucasians with pneumonia ($p = 0.012$, OR = 4.045, 95% CI = 1.219–13.433).

Discussion

Overview of WES Findings

Whole-exome sequencing (WES) had been performed in 96 ARDS patients from the ARDSnet with the intent of identifying coding SNPs whose minor allele frequencies are significantly different in ARDS than those of healthy controls and of identifying those novel SNPs who may be predictors of ARDS severity and outcome. In the overall ARDS population 1,382,399 SNPs were detected by exome-seq (Table 2) and 490,015 SNPs per person on average (Figure 1) compared to 714,074 SNPs per person from 625 healthy control subjects in the 1000 Genome Project. Among them, only 169,376 SNPs overlapped between two populations. The majority of un-overlapped SNPs in ARDS patients may represent ARDS specific SNPs barring the individual variability, sequencing error and data analysis discrepancy. From 169,376 SNPs, there are 49,789 bi-allelic SNPs in all ARDS patient subgroups based on race and initiating etiologies: Caucasian sepsis, Caucasian pneumonia, African-American sepsis and African American pneumonia. These SNPs may represent sepsis or pneumonia etiology specific SNPs of ARDS. The reason why we initially focused on the identification of novel coding SNPs associated with ARDS in sepsis and pneumonia origins was that in

the original ARDS patient population, sepsis and pneumonia etiologies accounted for most cases [21,22]. We selectively genotyped and validated three SNPs (rs78142040, rs9605146 and rs3848719) in an additional 117 ARDS patients using the TaqMan genotype assay and performed in depth association analyses of these SNPs with the susceptibility, severity and outcome to ARDS in a combined 213 ARDS patients (96 by exome-seq +117 by TaqMan = 213). These validations lend a solid support to the validity and prowess of novel ARDS associated SNP identifications by exome-seq. This study provides a rich resource for further experimentation and replication to develop and establish new genetic biomarkers and therapeutic targets to ARDS.

Validation of selected three SNPs

Among three selectively validated SNPs (rs78142040, rs9605146 and rs3848719) in an additional 117 ARDS patients, rs78142040 in the ARSD gene is associated with increased ARDS susceptibility in the overall ARDS population (213 patients) as well as all racial and comorbidity subpopulations. It approaches significant association with an increase in APACHEII score ($p = 0.061$) when samples in the highest and lowest score quartiles are compared in ARDS patients. rs78142040 is associated significantly ($p<0.05$) with an increase in 60-day mortality in the total ARDS population ($p = 0.017$, OR = 2.039, 95%CI 1.130–3.681). The molecular mechanisms underlying these associations are presently unknown. The ARSD gene encodes a sulfatase that is associated with bone and cartilage development and has been identified previously as having involvement in sphingolipid metabolism (involved in signal transmission and cellular recognition) and as a potential biomarker for chronic lymphocytic leukemia [32]. ARSD protein isoforms have a highly conserved catalytic peptide domain when compared with other arylsulfatases [36,37]. ARSD is widely expressed and is suspected to play a role in housekeeping or multiple other processes, however specific substrates have not been identified [38]. It was reported that there were changes in activities of lung liposomal enzymes including sulfates during ARDS [39]. It may be interesting to explore whether rs78142040 causes the differential expression of the ARSD gene, thus sulfatase activity, which may link its role in the pathogenesis of ARDS.

rs9605146 in the XKR3 gene is associated with increased susceptibility in the ARDS population and all subgroups except the African American with sepsis etiology group and the African American with pneumonia etiology group when analyzed individually. XKR3 is a member of the XK/Kell complex in the Kell blood group system. XKR3 is a homolog of XK, which is a putative membrane transporter. XK is associated with McLeod syndrome (characterized by late-onset abnormalities in the central nervous system and neuromuscular system) and red cell acanthocytosis [33]. XKR3 has previously been indicated as a potential biomarker for blood transfusion compatibility [40]. While it is currently unknown what underlies the association of rs9605146 with susceptibility in ARDS, it causes a deleterious amino acid coding change from proline to leucine in the XKR3 gene as predicted by Provean (score = -5.494). These observations make rs9605146 a legitimate candidate for further study of its role in the pathogenesis of ARDS.

rs3848719 in the ZNF335 gene is not associated significantly with susceptibility, however the SNP is associated with a decreased APACHEII score when the highest and lowest score quartiles are compared in the total ARDS population ($p = 0.032$, OR = 0.55, 95%CI 1.27–2.05), and with an increased 60-day mortality in Caucasian and pneumonia groups ($p<0.05$). It is a synonymous

SNP in the 5th exon of the Zinc-Finger/Leucine-Zipper Co-Transducer NIF1 gene (ZNF335). ZNF335 gene is involved in neural progenitor cell proliferation and self-renewal as a component of the vertebrate-specific, trithorax H3K4-methylation complex. ZNF335 is associated with the disease microcephaly (a neurodevelopmental disorder), small somatic size and neonatal death. The gene is essential as homozygous knockout mouse models have a lethal effect [34,35]. The role of the gene in cellular differentiation and gene expression could implicate an effect on the fundamental physiology and neural signaling in the lungs, contributing to the pathogenesis of ARDS.

Limitations

Although we applied the Bonferroni correction ($p < 2.95 \times 10^{-7}$) and several SNP filtering steps during our data analysis as well as validations of three selected candidate SNPs to ARDS, our data come with potential limitations. First, we only performed exome-seq of 96 ARDS samples. Although we would argue that this is a very reasonable sample size considering the restriction of high exome-seq cost per sample, even though the exome-seq cost per sample is cheaper than whole genome-seq per sample, the sample size is not large. Our 76 SNPs which are associated strongly with susceptibility are all present in an age and race matched 48 sample control set, which will be used to validate our findings in further studies (117,35 out of the 169,376 SNPs which are in the ARDS cases and 1000 Genomes Project are found in this control set). Confirmation of our findings in larger patient populations is warranted. Second, during analysis of SNP associations with ARDS susceptibility, we used the healthy control subjects from the 1000 Genome Project. Both ARDS patients and healthy control subjects do not derive from the same population. Since population admixture is assumed in the African American cases, we have elected to compare these cases with the ASW subset of the 1000 Genomes Project African Ancestry panel. We feel this is the best fitting control group due to the observed reduction in genomic inflation factor (inflation factor = 1.18 when compared with ASW, after filtering for informative markers based on HWE, call rate, number of alleles, and LD) compared to the total African Ancestry controls (inflation factor = 1.70), YRI alone (inflation factor = 1.59), or LWK alone (inflation factor = 1.98) [41]. An ancestry-informative SNP panel with good coverage of our dataset was not available. Although we have applied HWE, PCA analysis and Q–Q plot determination as well as race specific comparison to filter the identified SNPs, it may not totally correct the population admixtures (Figure 3, Figure S1, Figure S2, Table S8). Two of the SNPs (rs9605146, control MAF 4.0% and rs78142040, control MAF 0% respectively) have extremely minor allele frequencies which causes inflation of the type-1 error of the Goodness-of-fit test for HWE [26]. In this study, we explicitly searched for SNPs in which the MAF differed between cases and controls, so we expect that we might see some deviation where the minor alleles are rare in healthy controls. The observed associations with other disease phenotypes within our case cohort support our conclusion that variations at these loci contribute to disease. Replication of our findings in larger and different populations may strengthen and develop the candidate SNPs identified here as` true genetic biomarkers of ARDS.

Conclusion

The primary focus of this study was to identify new and novel SNPs associated with ARDS susceptibility, severity and outcome using whole exome-sequencing. We have identified a number of potential ARDS associated SNPs, which has demonstrated that WES is a powerful tool to identify new biomarkers in ARDS. We

selectively validated 3 SNPs that are associated with the susceptibility (rs78142040 and rs9605146), severity (rs3848719) and outcome (rs78142040 and rs3848719) of ARDS. More validations in larger and different patient populations as well as further investigation of the underlying molecular mechanisms are warranted to establish them as true new diagnostic and therapeutic targets for ARDS.

Supporting Information

Figure S1   The scree plots of the eigenvalues generated by principal component analysis. The largest eigenvalues are used in corrections for population structure. (**A**) The All ARDS and ASW+EUR 1000 Genomes population eigenvalues. 535 principal components were measured and the largest eigenvalue is 7.32. (**B**) The Caucasian ARDS and EUR ARDS population eigenvalues. 449 principal components were measured and the largest eigenvalue is 1.52. (**C**) The African American ARDS and ASW 1000 Genomes population eigenvalues. 86 principal components were measured and the largest eigenvalue is 0.94.

Figure S2   The quantile-quantile plots of genotypic trend test χ^2 values for the African American ARDS and ASW 1000 Genomes population were derived using SVS v8.2.0. The straight line on each plot represents y = x. (**A**) QQ plot of expected χ^2 values versus the actual χ^2 values for the genotypic trend test of case-control status. The data are filtered on HWE, LD, and SNP call rate but not PCA corrected. (**B**) QQ plot of expected χ^2 values versus the actual χ^2 trend test of case-control status. The data are corrected for the 2 largest principal components. (**C**) QQ plot of expected χ^2 values versus the actual χ^2 for the genotypic trend test of case-control status. The data have been filtered and corrected for 2 PCs and undergone sample outlier removal.

Table S1   A summary of the comparison groups used for the genetic association analysis. Association of the exome-seq SNPs with susceptibility was explored by comparing 96 ARDS patients to 440 controls from the 1000 Genomes Project. Analysis was stratified by race and etiology.

Table S2   A summary of the susceptibility χ^2 tests for the 3 SNPs. The allelic chi-square test p-values for the exome sequenced ARDS patients ARDS patients and subgroups compared with the 1000 Genomes Project participants and subgroups, TaqMan genotyped ARDS patients and subgroups compared with the 1000 Genomes Project participants and subgroups, and the total ARDS patient population and subgroups compared with the 1000 Genomes Project participants and subgroups. P-values were considered to be significant if they were smaller than the Bonferroni corrected p-value of 2.95×10^{-7}.

Table S3   Logistic regression with 60-day mortality from the day of diagnosis was used to assess SNP association with outcome. Included in this table are the p-values of the logistic regression of 60-day mortality against genotype using an additive model in the ARDS exome samples, TaqMan genotyped samples, and total ARDS samples. Associations were considered significant if $p < 0.05$.

Table S4   Logistic regression with APACHE II score was used to assess SNP association with overall disease

severity. Included in this table are the p-values of the logistic regression of ARDS patient genotype and APACHEII score by quartile. The APACHEII scores are split into quartiles and the 1st and 4th quartiles are used in a logistic regression against genotype using an additive model in the ARDS exome samples, TaqMan genotyped samples, and total ARDS samples. Regressions were also run on the stratified sub-populations of the ARDS patients. Associations were considered to be significant if $P<0.05$.

Table S5 A summary of the descriptive statistics for SNP rs78142040 in the exome sequenced ARDS, TaqMan genotyped ARDS patients, and total ARDS patients, where the controls are 1000 Genomes Project participants. *, Chi-square tests were run on SNPs that were in both the controls and the cases; A, alternate allele; r, reference allele.

Table S6 A summary of the descriptive statistics for SNP rs9605146 in the exome sequenced ARDS, TaqMan genotyped ARDS patients, and total ARDS patients, where the controls are 1000 Genomes Project participants. *, Chi-square tests were run on SNPs that were in both the controls and the cases; A, alternate allele; r, reference allele.

Table S7 A summary of the descriptive statistics for SNP rs3848719 in the exome sequenced ARDS, TaqMan genotyped ARDS patients, and total ARDS patients, where the controls are 1000 Genomes Project partici-

pants. *, Chi-square tests were run on SNPs that were in both the controls and the cases; A, alternate allele; r, reference allele.

Table S8 A summary of the effect of the PCA adjustments on the genotypic trend test of the 3 SNPs. 2 of the 3 SNPs were present in the filtered Caucasian ARDS+EUR controls population. PCA, principal components analysis; PCs, principal components; AA, African American ARDS; ASW, African Americans in the southwest 1000 Genomes Project; EA, European Ancestry or Caucasian; corr/trend, trend association test.

Supporting Information S1 The Supporting Information contains a detailed description of statistical methods used in this study.

Acknowledgments

We would like to acknowledge the sponsorship of Roy G Brower, MD, Division of Pulmonary and Critical Care Medicine, Johns Hopkins University School of Medicine for our application to the ARDSnet to secure the ARDS patient DNA samples and the ARDSnet teams (www.ardsnet.org) for providing 213 ARDS patient DNA samples in this study.

Author Contributions

Conceived and designed the experiments: SQY LZ. Performed the experiments: KS SC. Analyzed the data: KS DG DPH. Contributed reagents/materials/analysis tools: SQY KS. Contributed to the writing of the manuscript: SQY LZ LV DPH DG KS.

References

1. Ashbaugh DG, Bigelow DB, Petty TL, Levine BE (1967) Acute respiratory distress in adults. Lancet 2: 319–323.
2. Bernard GR, Artigas A, Brigham KL, Carlet J, Falke K, et al. (1994) The American-European Consensus Conference on ARDS. Definitions, mechanisms, relevant outcomes, and clinical trial coordination. Am J Respir Crit Care Med 149: 818–824.
3. Rubenfeld GD, Caldwell E, Peabody E, Weaver J, Martin DP, et al. (2005) Incidence and outcomes of acute lung injury. N Engl J Med 353: 1685–1693.
4. Blank R, Napolitano LM (2011) Epidemiology of ARDS and ALI. Crit Care Clin 27: 439–458.
5. Flores C, Pino-Yanes MM, Casula M, Villar J (2010) Genetics of acute lung injury: past, present and future. Minerva Anestesiol 76: 860–864.
6. Garcia JG (2005) Searching for candidate genes in acute lung injury: SNPs, Chips and PBEF. Trans Am Clin Climatol Assoc 116: 205–219; discussion 220.
7. Gong MN (2006) Genetic epidemiology of acute respiratory distress syndrome: implications for future prevention and treatment. Clin Chest Med 27: 705–724; abstract x.
8. McGlothlin JR, Gao L, Lavoie T, Simon BA, Easley RB, et al. (2005) Molecular cloning and characterization of canine pre-B-cell colony-enhancing factor. Biochem Genet 43: 127–141.
9. Parks BW, Nam E, Org E, Kostem E, Norheim F, et al. (2013) Genetic control of obesity and gut microbiota composition in response to high-fat, high-sucrose diet in mice. Cell Metab 17: 141–152.
10. Tzouvelekis A, Pneumatikos I, Bouros D (2005) Serum biomarkers in acute respiratory distress syndrome an ailing prognosticator. Respir Res 6: 62.
11. Crader KM RJ, Repine JE (2012) Breath Biomarkers and the Acute Respiratory Distress Syndrome. J Pulmonar Respirat Med 2.
12. Ye SQ, Simon BA, Maloney JP, Zambelli-Weiner A, Gao L, et al. (2005) Pre-B-cell colony-enhancing factor as a potential novel biomarker in acute lung injury. Am J Respir Crit Care Med 171: 361–370.
13. Bajwa EK, Yu CL, Gong MN, Thompson BT, Christiani DC (2007) Pre-B-cell colony-enhancing factor gene polymorphisms and risk of acute respiratory distress syndrome. Crit Care Med 35: 1290–1295.
14. Lee KA, Gong MN (2011) Pre-B-cell colony-enhancing factor and its clinical correlates with acute lung injury and sepsis. Chest 140: 382–390.
15. Liu Y, Shao Y, Yu B, Sun L, Lv F (2012) Association of PBEF gene polymorphisms with acute lung injury, sepsis, and pneumonia in a northeastern Chinese population. Clin Chem Lab Med 50: 1917–1922.
16. Gullapalli RR, Desai KV, Santana-Santos L, Kant JA, Becich MJ (2012) Next generation sequencing in clinical medicine: Challenges and lessons for pathology and biomedical informatics. J Pathol Inform 3: 40.
17. Goh G, Choi M (2012) Application of whole exome sequencing to identify disease-causing variants in inherited human diseases. Genomics Inform 10: 214–219.
18. Takata A, Kato M, Nakamura M, Yoshikawa T, Kanba S, et al. (2011) Exome sequencing identifies a novel missense variant in RRM2B associated with autosomal recessive progressive external ophthalmoplegia. Genome Biol 12: R92.
19. Fang X, Bai C, Wang X (2012) Bioinformatics insights into acute lung injury/acute respiratory distress syndrome. Clin Transl Med 1: 9.
20. Abecasis GR, Altshuler D, Auton A, Brooks LD, Durbin RM, et al. (2010) A map of human genome variation from population-scale sequencing. Nature 467: 1061–1073.
21. Wheeler AP, Bernard GR, Thompson BT, Schoenfeld D, Wiedemann HP, et al. (2006) Pulmonary-artery versus central venous catheter to guide treatment of acute lung injury. N Engl J Med 354: 2213–2224.
22. Wiedemann HP, Wheeler AP, Bernard GR, Thompson BT, Hayden D, et al. (2006) Comparison of two fluid-management strategies in acute lung injury. N Engl J Med 354: 2564–2575.
23. McKenna A, Hanna M, Banks E, Sivachenko A, Cibulskis K, et al. (2010) The Genome Analysis Toolkit: a MapReduce framework for analyzing next-generation DNA sequencing data. Genome Res 20: 1297–1303.
24. Abecasis GR, Auton A, Brooks LD, DePristo MA, Durbin RM, et al. (2012) An integrated map of genetic variation from 1,092 human genomes. Nature 491: 56–65.
25. Melum E, Franke A, Schramm C, Weismuller TJ, Gotthardt DN, et al. (2011) Genome-wide association analysis in primary sclerosing cholangitis identifies two non-HLA susceptibility loci. Nat Genet 43: 17–19.
26. Lunetta KL (2008) Genetic association studies. Circulation 118: 96–101.
27. Pearson TA, Manolio TA (2008) How to interpret a genome-wide association study. Jama 299: 1335–1344.
28. Laurie CC, Doheny KF, Mirel DB, Pugh EW, Bierut LJ, et al. (2010) Quality control and quality assurance in genotypic data for genome-wide association studies. Genet Epidemiol 34: 591–602.
29. Price AL, Patterson NJ, Plenge RM, Weinblatt ME, Shadick NA, et al. (2006) Principal components analysis corrects for stratification in genome-wide association studies. Nat Genet 38: 904–909.
30. Hinrichs AL, Larkin EK, Suarez BK (2009) Population stratification and patterns of linkage disequilibrium. Genet Epidemiol 33 Suppl 1: S88–92.
31. Khrunin AV, Khokhrin DV, Filippova IN, Esko T, Nelis M, et al. (2013) A genome-wide analysis of populations from European Russia reveals a new pole of genetic diversity in northern Europe. PLoS One 8: e58552.

32. Trojani A, Di Camillo B, Tedeschi A, Lodola M, Montesano S, et al. (2011) Gene expression profiling identifies ARSD as a new marker of disease progression and the sphingolipid metabolism as a potential novel metabolism in chronic lymphocytic leukemia. Cancer Biomark 11: 15–28.

33. Calenda G, Peng J, Redman CM, Sha Q, Wu X, et al. (2006) Identification of two new members, XPLAC and XTES, of the XK family. Gene 370: 6–16.

34. Mahajan MA, Murray A, Samuels HH (2002) NRC-interacting factor 1 is a novel cotransducer that interacts with and regulates the activity of the nuclear hormone receptor coactivator NRC. Mol Cell Biol 22: 6883–6894.

35. Yang YJ, Baltus AE, Mathew RS, Murphy EA, Evrony GD, et al. (2012) Microcephaly gene links trithorax and REST/NRSF to control neural stem cell proliferation and differentiation. Cell 151: 1097–1112.

36. Franco B, Meroni G, Parenti G, Levilliers J, Bernard L, et al. (1995) A cluster of sulfatase genes on Xp22.3: mutations in chondrodysplasia punctata (CDPX) and implications for warfarin embryopathy. Cell 81: 15–25.

37. Urbitsch P, Salzer MJ, Hirschmann P, Vogt PH (2000) Arylsulfatase D gene in Xp22.3 encodes two protein isoforms. DNA Cell Biol 19: 765–773.

38. Dooley TP, Haldeman-Cahill R, Joiner J, Wilborn TW (2000) Expression profiling of human sulfotransferase and sulfatase gene superfamilies in epithelial tissues and cultured cells. Biochem Biophys Res Commun 277: 236–245.

39. Anasiewicz A, Maciejewski R, Juskiewicz W, Lakowska H, Madej B, et al. (1997) [Changes of lysosomal enzyme activity in the lungs during the course of acute pancreatitis]. Wiad Lek 50 Suppl 1 Pt 2: 96–100.

40. Le Goff GC, Bres JC, Rigal D, Blum LJ, Marquette CA (2010) Robust, high-throughput solution for blood group genotyping. Anal Chem 82: 6185–6192.

41. Devlin B, Roeder K (1999) Genomic control for association studies. Biometrics 55: 997–1004.

42. Robinson JT, Thorvaldsdottir H, Winckler W, Guttman M, Lander ES, et al. (2011) Integrative genomics viewer. Nat Biotechnol 29: 24–26.

20

Vancomycin Dosing in Neutropenic Patients

Michiel B. Haeseker[1,2]*, Sander Croes[3], Cees Neef[3], Cathrien A. Bruggeman[1,2], Leo M. L. Stolk[3], Annelies Verbon[1,4]

1 Department of Medical Microbiology, Maastricht University Medical Center, Maastricht, the Netherlands, 2 Care and Public Health Research Institute (CAPHRI), Maastricht, the Netherlands, 3 Department of Clinical Pharmacy and Toxicology, Maastricht University Medical Center, Maastricht, the Netherlands, 4 Department of Internal Medicine, Erasmus Medical Center, Rotterdam, the Netherlands

Abstract

Background: To compare vancomycin pharmacokinetic parameters in patients with and without neutropenia.

Methods: Patients ≥18 years admitted on general wards were included. Routinely vancomycin trough and peak plasma concentrations were measured with a fluorescence polarization immunoassay. Pharmacokinetic parameters of individual patients were determined with maximum a posterior Bayesian estimation (MW Pharm 3.60). Neutropenia was defined as neutrophils $<0.5\times10^9$ cells/L.

Principal Findings: A total of 171 patients were included. Patients with neutropenia (n = 56) had higher clearance of vancomycin (CLva), 67 (±26) mL/min, compared to patients without neutropenia (n = 115), CLva 50 (±22) mL/min (p< 0.001). No significant difference was found in serum creatinine and vancomycin volume of distribution. Neutropenia was positively associated with CLva, independently of relevant co-variables (B: 12.122, 95%CI: 1.095 to 23.149, p = 0.031). On average patients with neutropenia needed 33% higher doses of vancomycin to attain adequate exposure, i.e. AUC$_{24}$≥ 400 mg×h/L. Furthermore, 15 initially neutropenic patients in our study group received vancomycin for a second administration period. Ten patients received the second administration period during another neutropenic period and 5 patients during a non-neutropenic phase. All 5 patients with vancomycin during both neutropenic and non-neutropenic phase had higher CLva (91 (±26) mL/min) during the neutropenic period and lower CLva (45 (±10) mL/min) during the non-neutropenic phase (p = 0.009).

Conclusion: This study shows that most patients with neutropenia have augmented CLva. In a small group of patients that received vancomycin during two episodes, the augmented CLva seems to be reversible in the non-neutropenic period. Our data indicate that it is important to increase the daily dose with one third in patients with neutropenia (from 15 mg/kg twice daily to 13 mg/kg three times daily). Frequent performance of therapeutic drug monitoring in patients with neutropenia may prevent both therapy failure due to low AUCs and overcomes toxicity due to high vancomycin trough concentrations during recovery from neutropenia.

Editor: Jonghan Kim, Northeastern University, United States of America

Funding: The authors have no funding or support to report.

Competing Interests: The authors have declared that no competing interests exist.

* Email: m.haeseker@mumc.nl

Introduction

Mortality from infections after cytostatic conditioning regimens in hematologic neutropenic patients requiring hematopoietic cell transplantation is high [1]. Bacterial infections are common during neutropenic phases and antibiotics, such as vancomycin, are often required [2]. In a recent surveillance study, Gram positive organisms are the most common cause of bacteremia in hematology patients, i.e. coagulase negative staphylococci (36%), followed by, Streptococci (11%), *S. aureus* (8%) and Enterococci (4%) [3]. Antibiotics should be started within 1 hour in patients with severe sepsis. However, adequate dosing of vancomycin can be difficult. Augmented clearance has been increasingly described in critically ill patients at the Intensive Care Unit (ICU) [4–6]. Changes in volume of distribution (Vd), changes in renal function and severe hypoalbuminemia are often present, influencing

vancomycin plasma concentrations. Augmented clearance of vancomycin leads to lower vancomycin plasma concentrations, decreased 24-hour area under the curve (AUC$_{24}$) and leads to diminished clinical outcome [6]. Augmented clearance of vancomycin in patients with hematological malignancies has been reported, but the augmented clearance was not associated with population specific covariables [7]. In another study low teicoplanin trough concentrations in neutropenic patients were reported, suggesting augmented clearance of teicoplanin in neutropenic patients [8]. In addition, elevated clearance of piperacillin and ceftazidime has also been noticed in patients with febrile neutropenia [9,10]. The mechanism of augmented clearance of antibiotics is not completely understood and is poorly investigated in patients with hematologic malignancies or in patients with neutropenia. The aim of this study is to compare vancomycin pharmacokinetic parameters in patients with and without neutropenia at non-ICUs in a University Hospital.

Methods

Materials and Methods

Study group. In this observational study patients were prospectively followed. Patients older than 18 years treated with vancomycin intravenously (iv) and hospitalized at the Maastricht University Medical Center (MUMC), a 715 bed university hospital, were included from May 2011 until July 2013. Patients were excluded when admitted at the ICU or when insufficient data was collected. Vancomycin was started at the discretion of the attending physician, either empirically or as therapy for bacteria susceptible to vancomycin. Dose individualization was applied since an initial loading dose of 15 mg/kg was followed by dose adjustment based on therapeutic drug monitoring (TDM) and renal function. Demographic and clinical data, such as age, gender, weight, temperature, co-medication, length of hospital stay, time of administration of vancomycin and laboratory parameters, such as, serum creatinine (Jaffé method), and leucocytes were retrieved from the electronic patient file (SAP, the Netherlands). Neutropenia was defined as $<0.5 \times 10^9$ cells/L. Creatinine clearance (CLcr) was calculated with the Cockcroft and Gault formula [(140 - age in years) × weight in kg]/[serum creatinine in µmol × factor] using total bodyweight [11].

Ethics statement. This study was conducted according to the principles expressed in the Declaration of Helsinki. This study was registered at the Dutch Trial Register (NTR 1725). The Medical Ethical Committee of the Maastricht University Medical Center (MEC 08-4-063) approved this study and waived the necessity to obtain informed consent from participants because of the observational design. Electronic health records were anonymized prior to use.

Measurement of vancomycin. Vancomycin plasma concentrations were measured as standard clinical care with a fluorescence polarization immune assay using of Cobas Integra 800 system (Roche Diagnostics). The calibration curve ranged from 2.0 to 80 mg/L. The accuracy and coefficients of variation (CV) of the controls (6.9, 17.7 and 31.0 mg/L) were within 90%–110% and <3.3%, respectively. Patients with at least two plasma samples available, drawn in such a manner to ensure calculations of vancomycin clearance (CLva) were included. Blood samples were collected at least one hour after the end of infusion and trough levels were obtained just before the next dose.

PK-analysis. Pharmacokinetic parameters (CLva, Vd) of vancomycin in individual patients were calculated with maximum a posteriori (MAP) Bayesian estimation computer program (MW/Pharm 3.60, Mediware, the Netherlands). Bayesian priors from a two compartment open pharmacokinetic model based on previous studies, were applied: V1 0.21 ± 0.04 L/kg, k_{elm} 0.0143 ± 0.0029 h^{-1}, $k_{elr} = k_{slope} \times$ CLcr (mL/min), 0.00327 ± 0.00109 h^{-1}/mL/min, k_{12} 1.12 ± 0.28 h^{-1}, and k_{21} 0.48 ± 0.12 h^{-1} [12,13], where V1 is volume of distribution central compartment (L/kg); k_{elm}, metabolic elimination rate constant (h^{-1}); k_{slope}, renal elimination rate constant (h^{-1}/mL/min); k_{elr}, renal elimination rate constant (h^{-1}); k_{12} (h^{-1}), rate constant from the 1st to the 2nd compartment; and k_{21}(h^{-1}), vice versa. The elimination rate constant $k_{el} = k_{elm} + k_{elr} = k_{elm} + (k_{slope} \times$ CLcr$)$ [14]. With MAP Bayesian estimation all patient characteristics and measured vancomycin concentrations are fitted on an existing population model. With at least two concentrations per patient individual pharmacokinetic parameters can be adequately derived with MAP Bayesian estimation [15,16]. With these individual pharmacokinetic parameters, dosing simulations were made to adjust the dose individually; this MAP Bayesian

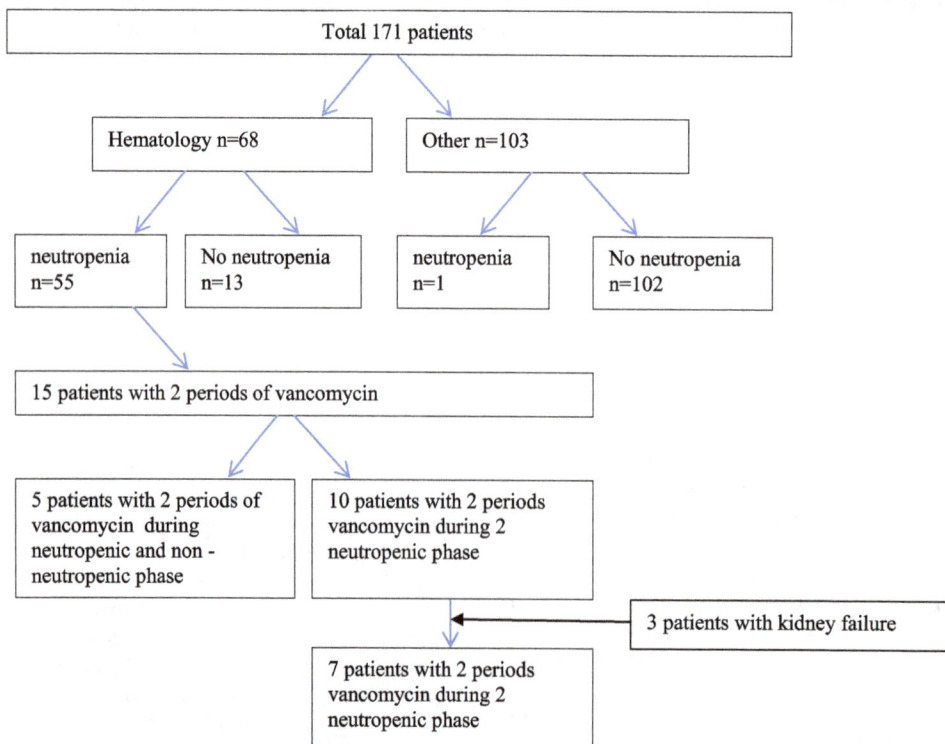

Figure 1. Flow of the 171 included patients with regard to hematology, neutropenia and two vancomycin administration periods.

Table 1. Mean (±SD) for Age, CLcr, CLva, Vd, Dose 24 h and AUC of patients with and without neutropenia in all patients (A) and in patients with haematological malignancy (B).

A) All patients (n=171)

Neutro-penia	N	Age year	CLcr mL/min	Creatinine μmol/L	CLva mL/min	Vd L	Dose 24 h mg	AUC mg*24 h/L
No	115	61(±14)	107 (±78)	95(±67)	50(±22)	56(±29)	1521(±727)	499(±102)
Yes	56	55(±13)	113 (±57)	80(±31)	67(±26)	62(±32)	2017(±719)	507(±87)
p		0.01	0.142	0.873	<0.001	0.304	<0.001	0.259

B) Patients with haematological malignancy (n=68)

Neutro-penia	N	Age Year	CLcr mL/min	Creatinine μmol/L	CLva mL/min	Vd L	Dose 24 h mg	AUC mg ×24 h/L
No	13	57(±11)	111(±58)	96(±59)	53(±16)	59(±18)	1604(±646)	502(±102)
Yes	55	55(±14)	114(±57)	79(±29)	68(±26)	62(±32)	2040(±705)	509(±87)
p		0.839	0.714	0.779	0.024	0.691	0.028	0.697

CLva: vancomycin clearance.
CLcr: creatinine clearance calculated from serum creatinine with Cockcroft and Gault [11].
Vd: volume of distribution.
AUC: 24 hour area under the curve.

estimation is a standard procedure in institutes which provide TDM service.

The AUC_{24} in steady-state was calculated with the formula: 24-hour dose/CLva.

Analysis of patients with and without neutropenia. Pharmacokinetic, clinical and demographic parameters were compared in patients with and without neutropenia in all patients and in patients with hematological malignancies. Furthermore, pharmacokinetic parameters of two vancomycin administration periods within the same patients were compared. Both patients with two vancomycin administrations during two different neutropenia periods and patients with two vancomycin administrations during one neutropenia period and one period without neutropenia were compared.

Statistical analysis. Normal distribution was evaluated for metric variables by means of the Shapiro-Wilk test and presented as mean (±SD). If not, median and ranges were given. Categorical variables are presented as frequencies and percentages. Metric and categorical variables were evaluated between patients with and without neutropenia using the Student t-test or non-parametric test (Kruskal Wallis), respectively.

First, the influence of co-variables on CLva was determined in univariable (Pearson) analysis. Subsequently, only the significant co-variables in the univariable analyses were included in the multivariable analysis, after checking the assumptions. The Enter method was used in the multivariable linear regression. CLcr is estimated with the C&G formula which includes serum creatinine, age, weight and gender [11]. To avoid multicollinearity, serum creatinine, age, weight and gender were left out of the multivariable model. Data analysis was done with IBM SPSS-pc version 20.0. A p-value of <0.05 was considered to be statistically significant.

Results

Study group

The mean age was 59 (±14) years and 61% were male. Patients were admitted on different general wards; hematology ward (40%, 68/171), surgery ward (19%, 32/171), internal ward (11%, 19/171), neurosurgery ward (11%, 18/171), orthopedic ward (10%, 17/171), cardiac (9%, 15/171) and eye ward (1%, 2/171). The majority of patients had sepsis (46%, 79/171), implant infection (16%, 27/171) or abdominal infection (15%, 25/171). A total of 171 patients with a mean (±SD) of 6 (±3) vancomycin plasma concentrations were included.

Pharmacokinetics analysis

The mean dose (±SD) of vancomycin per 24 hours was 1683 (±759) mg, with a mean Vd of 58 (±30) L and AUC_{24} of 502 (±97) mg×h/L. The mean (±SD) trough concentration in steady state (SS) was 13 (±4) mg/L, CmeanSS was 21 (±4) mg/L, peak concentration in SS was 49 (±14) mg/L, CLva was 56 (±25) mL/min and serum creatinine was 89 (±68) μmol/L.

Analysis of patients with and without neutropenia

Sixty eight patients had a hematological malignancy and 56 patients were neutropenic, Figure 1. Neutropenic patients (n = 56) had higher CLva, 67 (±26) mL/min, compared to non-neutropenic patients (n = 115), CLva 50 (±22) mL/min (p< 0.001). No significant difference in serum creatinine and Vd was found, Table 1 and Figure 2. Forty eight percent (27/56) of the neutropenic patients had CLva >70 mL/min, compared to 21% (24/115) without neutropenia. Of the 68 patients with a hematological malignancy, 55 patients were neutropenic and 13

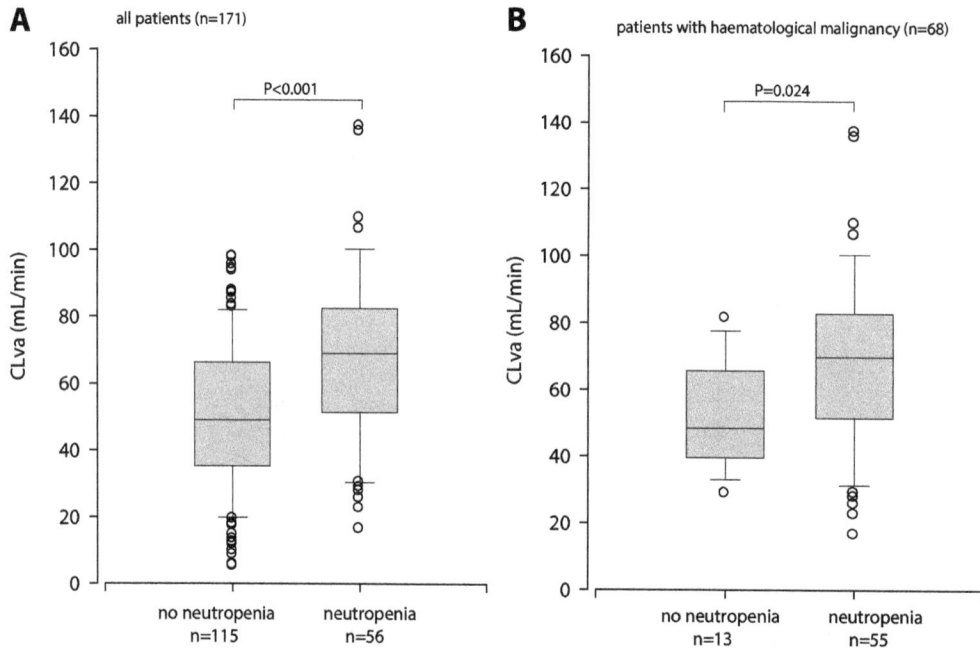

Figure 2. Boxplot for vancomycin clearance (CLva) in patients with and without neutropenia in all patients (A) and in patients with haematological malignancy (B). Lower and higher boundary of the box indicates 25th and 75th percentile, respectively, the line within the box marks the median, the whiskers above and below the box indicate the 90th and 10th percentiles and the open circles indicate outside the 90th and 10th percentiles.

were not neutropenic. Within the hematologic malignancy patients, neutropenic patients had higher CLva, than non-neutropenic patients, Table 1 and Figure 2. Physicians used TDM and adjusted vancomycin dosing as shown by the mean dose of vancomycin in patients with neutropenia of 2017 ($\pm$720) mg compared to 1521 ($\pm$727) mg in patients without neutropenia, p<0.001. On average, among patients with neutropenia the daily vancomycin dose was 33% (500 mg/day) higher to achieve the same AUC_{24} (Table 1). Patients with sepsis (n = 79) had higher CLva and were younger than patients without sepsis (n = 92). Vd and CLcr were not different, Table 2. Neutropenic patients with sepsis (n = 47) seemed to have slightly higher CLva of 69 ($\pm$27) mL/min than neutropenic patients without sepsis (n = 9) CLva 60 ($\pm$22) mL/min, p = 0.269. Both neutropenic patients with sepsis and without sepsis had higher CLva than non-neutropenic patients.

Of the 171 patients, 15 neutropenic patients received a second period of vancomycin, of which 5 patients received vancomycin during both an neutropenic and non neutropenic period. Ten patients received two vancomycin episodes during neutropenic periods. However, 3 patients developed kidney failure and were taken out. Leaving 7 patients with two vancomycin periods during neutropenia, Figure 1. Therefore, the data of 7 patients with two neutropenic periods and 5 patients with both a neutropenic and non-neutropenic period could be compared. The median (range) of time between the two vancomycin administrations was 30 (20–108) days for these 7 patients and 21 (14–136) days for the 5 patients with both a neutropenic and non neutropenic period. For the 7 patients with vancomycin administrations in two neutropenic periods, the CLva remained similar: 77 ($\pm$30) to 70 ($\pm$23) mL/min (p = 0.748), as did the serum creatinine 68 ($\pm$13) to 66 ($\pm$11) μmol/L (p = 0.701) and CLcr 120 ($\pm$41) to 117 ($\pm$35) mL/min (p = 0.848). The 5 patients with vancomycin administrations in both a neutropenic and non-neutropenic period had a statistically

significantly higher CLva, 91 ($\pm$26) mL/min, during the neutropenic phase compared to CLva, 45 ($\pm$10) mL/min during the non-neutropenic phase (p = 0.009). Serum creatinine, 65 ($\pm$10) and 69 ($\pm$11) μmol/L (p = 0.462) and CLcr, 141 ($\pm$70) and 113 ($\pm$48) mL/min during the neutropenic and non-neutropenic periods, respectively, were not significantly different (p = 0.402), Figure 3 and neither was the Vd was 74 ($\pm$24) L during neutropenic and 51 ($\pm$10) L during non-neutropenic phase (p = 0.175).

CLcr, neutropenia, hematologic malignancy and sepsis were correlated with CLva in the univariable analysis, Table 3. In the multivariable analysis, CLva was positively associated with CLcr (B: 0.205, 95%CI: 0.164–0.245, p<0.001) and neutropenia (B: 12.122, 95%CI: 1.095 to 23.149, p = 0.031), Table 3.

Discussion

Our study shows that higher doses of vancomycin are needed during neutropenic periods to achieve vancomycin target AUC_{24} and target trough concentrations. The augmented clearance of vancomycin in neutropenic patients seems reversible. Augmented clearance of vancomycin cannot be predicted with the estimated CLcr, as serum creatinine and estimated CLcr in our study are not significantly different in neutropenic and non-neutropenic patients. Moreover, the estimated CLcr is not reliable above 125 μmol/L and shows a poor agreement with measured CLcr in urine in critically ill patients displaying augmented clearance of creatinine [17,18]. Our Bayesian calculated CLva is in line with the population estimated CLva in patients with hematological malignancies in the simulations by Buelga *et al.* [7]. However, our routine patient care observations demonstrate that augmented clearance is associated with neutropenia rather than hematological malignancy and sepsis. In the multivariable analysis neutropenia (yes/no) was positively associated with CLva, independently of the

Table 2. Mean (±SD) for Age, CLcr, CLva, Vd, Creatinine for patients with sepsis and without sepsis.

	N	Age years	CLva mL/min	Vd L	CLcr mL/min	Creatinine μmol/L
Sepsis	79	56 (±13)	60 (±27)	57 (±26)	108 (±56)	84 (±38)
No sepsis	92	61 (±14)	52 (±23)	58 (±33)	110 (±83)	96 (±71)
p		0.017	0.048	0.639	0.535	0.894

CLva: vancomycin clearance.
CLcr: creatinine clearance calculated from serum creatinine with Cockcroft and Gault [11].
Vd: volume of distribution.

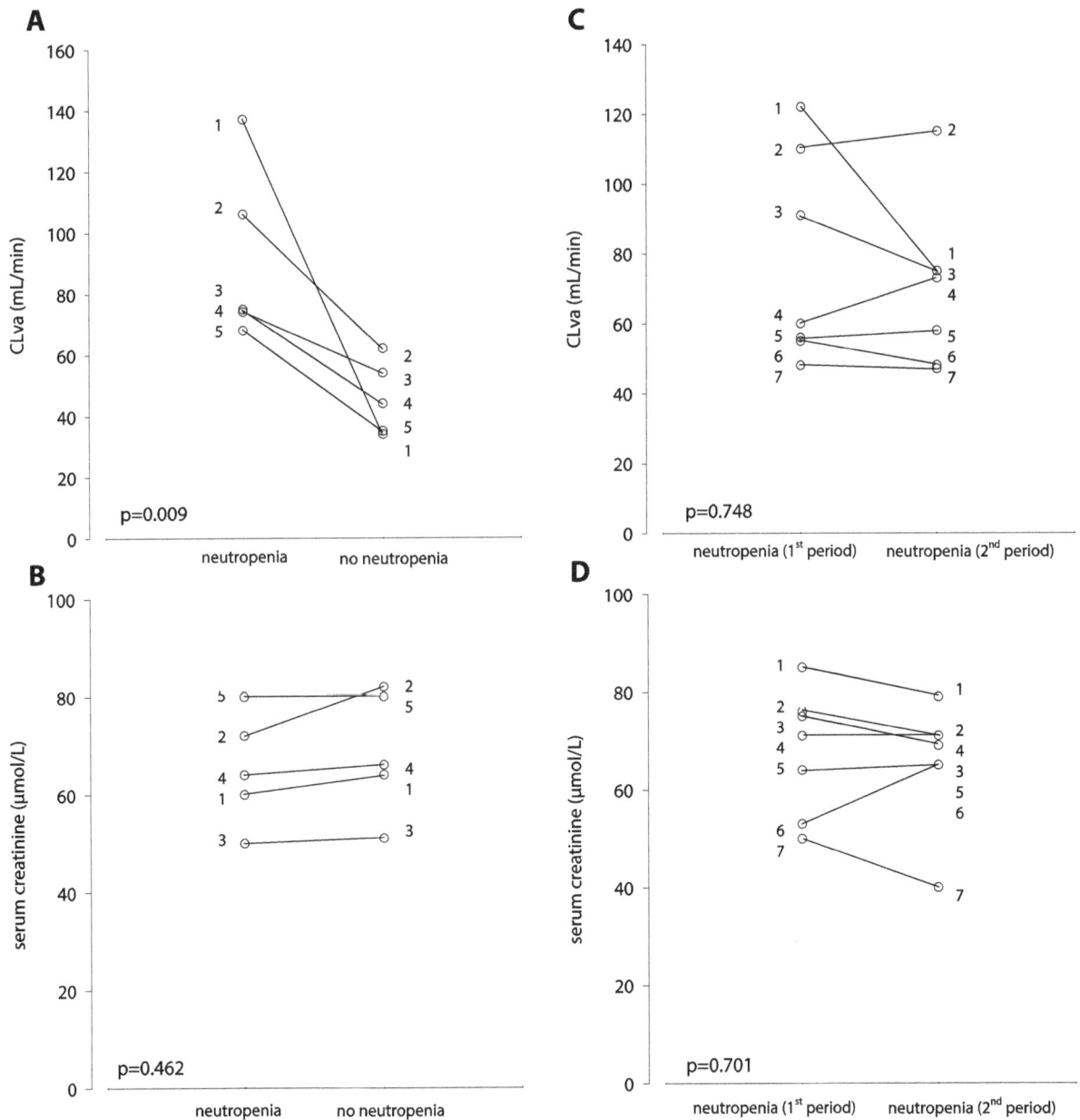

Figure 3. A. Vancomycin clearance (CLva) and B. serum creatinine of 5 patients (number 1–5) during both a neutropenic and a non-neutropenic phase and C. CLva and D. serum creatinine of 7 patients (number 1–7) during two neutropenic phases.

Table 3. Univariable and multivariable correlation coefficients between CLva and predictors used in this study.

| | Univariable[a] | | Multivariable[b] | | | |
| | R | P-value | B | 95% confidence interval for B | | p-value |
				Lower bound	Upper bound	
CLcr	0.599	<0.001	0.205	0.164	0.245	<0.001
Neutropenia	0.322	<0.001	12.122	1.095	23.149	0.031
Hematologic malignancy	0.300	<0.001	3.582	−8.404	15.569	0.556
Sepsis	0.170	0.027	0.427	−7.236	8.090	0.913
Vd	0.008	0.915	-	-	-	-

CLva: vancomycin clearance.
CLcr: creatinine clearance.
Vd: volume of distribution.
[a]Pearson correlation was performed as the univariable analysis.
[b]Only co-variates that were significantly correlated with CLva in the univariable analysis (P<0.05) were included in the multivariable analysis.

other co-variables. Although, our group of patients that received a second administration of vancomycin is small, the augmented clearance of vancomycin seems to be temporarily and reversible, as the CLva returned to normal during the non-neutropenic phase. The mechanism of augmented clearance is not completely clarified; most likely more than one factor is involved in developing augmented clearance. Young age, increased blood flow to the kidneys, genetic factors and other medication has been proposed to influence the CLva [5,6]. Neutropenia might be added to this list. Most likely augmented clearance also influences other renally cleared antibiotics [9,10]. Therefore, TDM of these antibiotics or/ and at least one 24-hour creatinine measurement in urine to determine the most accurate CLcr at the ICU is recommended [5,19,20]. Our data suggest that this recommendation may be extended to neutropenic patients.

Our study has a couple of limitations. Firstly, our study is a real-life observational study and we assumed the TDM protocol was strictly followed by clinicians, especially the timing of peak concentrations. Secondly, our group of patients with a second vancomycin administration was rather small to prove the demonstrated tendency of reversibility of elevated CLva, at the moment when patients are recovering from neutropenia. Further research is needed to fully understand the complex pharmacokinetics of vancomycin and other antibiotics in patients with

neutropenia. A prospective study may elucidate which other factors are involved in augmented CLva, but such a study would need a multicenter design and inclusion of many patients. Until, we fully understand augmented clearance, we suggest to increase the initial daily dose of vancomycin with 33% (13 mg/kg three times daily) in patients with neutropenia and to perform TDM after the first vancomycin dose in patients to prevent low plasma concentrations of vancomycin and consequently reduced efficacy. When patients are recovering from neutropenia, TDM is again necessary to adjust the vancomycin dose to prevent toxicity due to high vancomycin exposure.

Acknowledgments

The authors acknowledge the support provided by department of Pharmacy laboratory and the excellent statistical advice of Casper den Heijer.

Author Contributions

Conceived and designed the experiments: AV LMLS CAB CN. Performed the experiments: MBH SC LMLS. Analyzed the data: MBH SC LMLS AV. Contributed reagents/materials/analysis tools: MBH SC LMLS CN. Wrote the paper: MBH SC LMLS CN CAB AV.

References

1. Scott BL, Park JY, Deeg HJ, Marr KA, Boeckh M, et al. (2008) Pretransplant neutropenia is associated with poor-risk cytogenetic features and increased infection-related mortality in patients with myelodysplastic syndromes. Biol Blood Marrow Transplant 14: 799–806.

2. Sepkowitz KA (2002) Antibiotic prophylaxis in patients receiving hematopoietic stem cell transplant. Bone Marrow Transplant 29: 367–371.

3. Schelenz S, Nwaka D, Hunter PR (2013) Longitudinal surveillance of bacteraemia in haematology and oncology patients at a UK cancer centre and the impact of ciprofloxacin use on antimicrobial resistance. J Antimicrob Chemother 68: 1431–1438.

4. Revilla N, Martin-Suarez A, Perez MP, Gonzalez FM, Fernandez de Gatta Mdel M (2010) Vancomycin dosing assessment in intensive care unit patients based on a population pharmacokinetic/pharmacodynamic simulation. Br J Clin Pharmacol 70: 201–212.

5. Udy AA, Roberts JA, Boots RJ, Paterson DL, Lipman J (2010) Augmented renal clearance: implications for antibacterial dosing in the critically ill. Clin Pharmacokinet 49: 1–16.

6. Claus BO, Hoste EA, Colpaert K, Robays H, Decruyenaere J, et al. (2013) Augmented renal clearance is a common finding with worse clinical outcome in critically ill patients receiving antimicrobial therapy. J Crit Care 28: 695–700.

7. Buelga DS, del Mar Fernandez de Gatta M, Herrera EV, Dominguez-Gil A, Garcia MJ (2005) Population pharmacokinetic analysis of vancomycin in

patients with hematological malignancies. Antimicrob Agents Chemother 49: 4934–4941.

8. Pea F, Viale P, Candoni A, Pavan F, Pagani L, et al. (2004) Teicoplanin in patients with acute leukaemia and febrile neutropenia: a special population benefiting from higher dosages. Clin Pharmacokinet 43: 405–415.

9. Pea F, Viale P, Damiani D, Pavan F, Cristini F, et al. (2005) Ceftazidime in acute myeloid leukemia patients with febrile neutropenia: helpfulness of continuous intravenous infusion in maximizing pharmacodynamic exposure. Antimicrob Agents Chemother 49: 3550–3553.

10. Sime FB, Roberts MS, Warner MS, Hahn U, Robertson TA, et al. (2014) Altered pharmacokinetics of piperacillin in febrile neutropenic patients with haematological malignancy. Antimicrob Agents Chemother.

11. Cockcroft DW, Gault MH (1976) Prediction of creatinine clearance from serum creatinine. Nephron 16: 31–41.

12. Pryka RD, Rodvold KA, Garrison M, Rotschafer JC (1989) Individualizing vancomycin dosage regimens: one- versus two-compartment Bayesian models. Ther Drug Monit 11: 450–454.

13. Rodvold KA, Pryka RD, Garrison M, Rotschafer JC (1989) Evaluation of a two-compartment Bayesian forecasting program for predicting vancomycin concentrations. Ther Drug Monit 11: 269–275.

14. Manual MP. Available: http://www.mwpharm.nl/downloads/documentation/ UK-315-VOL3.PD.

15. van der Meer AF, Marcus MA, Touw DJ, Proost JH, Neef C (2011) Optimal sampling strategy development methodology using maximum a posteriori Bayesian estimation. Ther Drug Monit 33: 133–146.

16. Proost JH, Meijer DK (1992) MW/Pharm, an integrated software package for drug dosage regimen calculation and therapeutic drug monitoring. Comput Biol Med 22: 155–163.

17. Grootaert V, Willems L, Debaveye Y, Meyfroidt G, Spriet I (2012) Augmented renal clearance in the critically ill: how to assess kidney function. Ann Pharmacother 46: 952–959.

18. Hoste EA, Damen J, Vanholder RC, Lameire NH, Delanghe JR, et al. (2005) Assessment of renal function in recently admitted critically ill patients with normal serum creatinine. Nephrol Dial Transplant 20: 747–753.

19. Udy AA, Putt MT, Shanmugathasan S, Roberts JA, Lipman J (2010) Augmented renal clearance in the Intensive Care Unit: an illustrative case series. Int J Antimicrob Agents 35: 606–608.

20. Troger U, Drust A, Martens-Lobenhoffer J, Tanev I, Braun-Dullaeus RC, et al. (2012) Decreased meropenem levels in Intensive Care Unit patients with augmented renal clearance: benefit of therapeutic drug monitoring. Int J Antimicrob Agents 40: 370–372.

21

A Five-Year Experience of Carbapenem Resistance in Enterobacteriaceae Causing Neonatal Septicaemia: Predominance of NDM-1

Saswati Datta[1], **Subhasree Roy**[1], **Somdatta Chatterjee**[1], **Anindya Saha**[2], **Barsha Sen**[2], **Titir Pal**[3], **Tapas Som**[2], **Sulagna Basu**[1]*

1 Division of Bacteriology, National Institute of Cholera and Enteric Diseases, Kolkata, West Bengal, India, 2 Department of Neonatology, Institute of Postgraduate Medical Education & Research, SSKM Hospital, Kolkata, West Bengal, India, 3 AbsolutData Research and Analytics, Gurgaon, Haryana, India

Abstract

Treatment of neonatal sepsis has become a challenge with the emergence of carbapenemase-producing bacteria. This study documents the trend of carbapenem susceptibility in Enterobacteriaceae that caused septicaemia in neonates over a five year period (2007–2011) and the molecular characterisation of Enterobacteriaceae resistant to carbapenems and cephalosporins. Hundred and five Enterobacteriaceae including *Escherichia coli* (n = 27), *Klebsiella pneumoniae* (n = 68) and *Enterobacter spp.* (n = 10) were isolated from blood of septicaemic neonates followed by antibiotic susceptibility tests, determination of MIC values, phenotypic and genotypic detection of β-lactamases. Carbapenem was the most active antimicrobial tested after tigecycline. CTX-M type was the most prevalent ESBL throughout the period (82%). New Delhi Metallo-β-lactamase-1 (NDM-1), which is a recent addition to the carbapenemase list, was the only carbapenemase identified in our setting. Fourteen percent of the isolates possessed bla$_{NDM-1}$. Carbapenem non-susceptibility was first observed in 2007 and it was due to loss of Omp F/Ompk36 in combination with the presence of ESBLs/AmpCs. NDM-1 first emerged in *E. coli* during 2008; later in 2010, the resistance was detected in *K. pneumoniae* and *E. cloacae* isolates. NDM-1-producing isolates were resistant to other broad-spectrum antibiotics and possessed ESBLs, AmpCs, 16S-rRNA methylases, AAC(6')-Ib-cr, bleomycin resistant gene and class 1 integron. Pulsed field gel electrophoresis of the NDM-1-producing isolates indicated that the isolates were clonally diverse. The study also showed that there was a significantly higher incidence of sepsis caused by NDM-1-harbouring isolates in the male sex, in neonates with low birth weight and neonates born at an extramural centre. However, sepsis with NDM-1-harbouring isolates did not result in a higher mortality rate. The study is the first to review the carbapenem resistance patterns in neonatal sepsis over an extended period of time. The study highlights the persistence of ESBLs (CTX-Ms) and the emergence of NDM-1 in Enterobacteriaceae in the unit.

Editor: Jamunarani Vadivelu, University of Malaya, Malaysia

Funding: The study was partially supported by a fund from Department of Science and Technology (DST), West Bengal. Saswati Datta is now being supported by a fellowship from "Indian Council of Medical Research" but earlier she had been supported by a fellowship from Department of Science and Technology (DST), West Bengal. Somdatta Chatterjee has been supported by a fellowship from Department of Biotechnology, India. All other funds required for the study were provided by internal funding (Indian Council of Medical Research). The funders had no role in study design, data collection and analysis, decision to publish, or preparation of the manuscript. Co-author Titir Pal is employed by AbsolutData Research and Analytics. AbsolutData Research and Analytics provided support in the form of salary for author TP, but did not have any additional role in the study design, data collection and analysis, decision to publish, or preparation of the manuscript. The specific role of this author is articulated in the "author contributions" section.

Competing Interests: The authors have the following interests: co-author Titir Pal is employed by AbsolutData Research and Analytics. There are no patents, products in development or marketed products to declare. The authors also declare that none of the other authors have any potential conflicts of interests.

* Email: supabasu@yahoo.co.in

Introduction

Treatment of neonatal sepsis is a challenge. The treatment needs to be rapid, appropriate for the pathogen and safe for the neonate. The challenge seems to be increasing with each passing day due the escalating multidrug-resistant organisms [1]. In practice, ampicillin or amoxicillin along with an aminoglycoside (amikacin or gentamicin) is the common antibiotic regimen for neonatal sepsis. In case of severe infection due to multidrug-resistant members of the Enterobacteriaceae, including those with extended-spectrum β-lactamases (ESBLs) or AmpCs, carbapenems and quinolones are used as the last resort for treatment [2]. However, with the emergence of carbapenem-resistant isolates this treatment regimen is now under threat.

Carbapenem resistance may occur due to expression of ESBL/AmpC-type enzymes combined with the decreased cellular penetration of carbapenems caused by loss of outer membrane protein. Isolates with this mechanism of resistance often express variable susceptibility to the different carbapenem agents. However, isolates with carbapenemase-mediated resistance are of special clinical concern because multi-institutional outbreaks have been reported worldwide [3].

Carbapenemases are enzymes that not only hydrolyse carbapenems but almost all hydrolysable β-lactams, and most are resistant against inhibition by the β-lactamase inhibitors [4]. Carbapenemase-producing Enterobacteriaceae remained extremely rare for around 20 years after imipenem's introduction but recently, have begun to accumulate in the Enterobacteriaceae. In particular, *Klebsiella pnemoniae* carbapenemase (KPC, a class A carbapenemase), VIM (class B or metallo-carbapenemase) and OXA-48 (class D carbapenemase) [4] and recently the NDM-1 (metallo-carbapenemase) is widespread in Enterobacteriaceae throughout the world [5].

The New Delhi Metallo-β-lactamase-1 (NDM-1) is the most recent addition to the list of carbapenemases. It is a zinc–requiring metallo–β–lactamase (MBL) that can hydrolyse all penicillins, cephalosporins, carbapenems and spares only the monobactam aztreonam [6]. NDM-1 is often associated with other antibiotic resistance genes and plasmids carrying bla_{NDM-1}, can have up to 14 other antibiotic resistance determinants and can easily transfer this resistance to other bacteria [7].

This study was carried out in a neonatal intensive care unit (NICU) in which carbapenem resistance in Enterobacteriaceae was rare before 2008. Resistance to carbapenems was more a problem with lactose nonfermenting bacteria like *Acinetobacter baumannii* in the same unit [8], but not in Enterobacteriaceae. However, with the emergence of carbapenem resistance in Enterobacteriaceae it was necessary to evaluate the carbapenem susceptibility patterns in the NICU and the genetic determinants responsible for the resistance. This study focuses on (i) the trend of carbapenem susceptibility in Enterobacteriaceae causing septicaemia in neonates, over a five year period (includes period before and after the emergence of carbapenem resistance) and (ii) the molecular characterisation of carbapenem-resistant and cephalosporin-resistant genes in Enterobacteriaceae isolated during that period. The study is the first to evaluate the carbapenem resistance patterns in neonatal sepsis over an extended period of time.

Materials and Methods

Ethics Statement

The study protocol was carefully reviewed and approved by the Institutional Ethics Committee of the National Institute of Cholera and Enteric Diseases (Indian Council of Medical Research) (No. C-48/2010 T & E and NO. C-48/2011- T & E respectively). Individual informed consent was waived because this study used currently existing sample collected during the course of routine diagnosis of sepsis and did not pose any additional risks to the patients. The patient records/information was anonymized and de-identified prior to analysis.

Setting and patients

The study was conducted at a 20-bed level III unit of the IPGMER and SSKM Hospital, Kolkata, India between 2007 and 2011. The unit is the only Level III unit in the state. This unit has about 1000 admissions per year (departmental census 2010), including both intramural and extramural births.

Bacterial strains

During 2007–2011, a total of 1985 blood specimens had been drawn from the admitted neonates suspected for sepsis on the basis of criteria set earlier by authors [9], and blood culture procedures followed were as described previously [10]. Of the specimens cultured, 285 were positive (including gram-positive bacteria, gram-negative bacteria and fungal isolates). The clinical data were noted from the hospital registers.

Laboratory procedures

All Enterobacteriaceae isolated were identified by the ID 32 E kit (bioMerieux, Marcy l'E toile, France). Antibiotic susceptibility profiles and minimum inhibitory concentrations (MIC) were evaluated along with phenotypic tests for the detection of β-lactamases and carbapenemases. Detailed molecular characterization and outer membrane permeability were carried out for the ertapenem-non-susceptible isolates. Molecular typing was performed only for carbapenemase-producing (more specifically NDM-1-producing) isolates.

Antimicrobial susceptibility and MIC

Antimicrobial susceptibility testing was done by the Kirby-Bauer standard disk diffusion method [11] according to CLSI guidelines [12] for different antimicrobial agents like: ceftazidime (30 μg), cefotaxime (30 μg), cefpodoxime (10 μg), ceftriaxone (30 μg), cefepime (30 μg), aztreonam (30 μg), ampicillin (10 μg), piperacillin (100 μg), cefoxitin (30 μg), gentamicin (120 μg), amikacin (30 μg), ciprofloxacin (5 μg), tetracycline (30 μg), minocycline (30 μg), chloramphenicol (30 μg), trimethoprim/sulfamethoxazole (1.25 μg/23.75 μg), colistin (10 μg), ertapenem (10 μg) and meropenem (10 μg) (BD Diagnostics, Franklin Lakes, NJ, USA).

The MIC values (mg/L) of cefotaxime, ertapenem, meropenem, amikacin, gentamicin and tigecycline were determined using Etest method (AB Biodisk, Solna, Sweden) and were interpreted according to CLSI guidelines as modified in 2013. The clinical breakpoints for meropenem were as follows: susceptible (S) ≤ 1.0 mg/L, intermediate (I) 2.0–3.0 mg/L, and resistant (R) ≥ 4.0 mg/L. The same for ertapenem were as follows: S ≤0.5 mg/L, I: 1.0 mg/L, R ≥2 mg/L. MIC50 and MIC90 of meropenem were calculated as the MIC at which 50% and 90% of the isolates were inhibited.

Screening for ESBLs, AmpCs and Carbapenemases

For all Enterobacteriaceae, the MIC value for ertapenem ≥ 0.5 mg/L was set as the screening breakpoint to detect carbapenemases [13]. The presence of ESBL was determined according to CLSI guidelines. The AmpC screening breakpoint was set as zone diameter of ≤18 mm for cefoxitin (30 μg) disc [14].

Detection of β-lactamase and carbapenemase phenotypes

The production of ESBLs, AmpCs, KPC and MBLs were evaluated using cephalosporin/clavulanic acid (BD Diagnostics, Franklin Lakes, NJ, USA) combination disc, cefoxitin (30 μg)/boronic acid (300 μg) (Sigma-Aldrich, St Louis, MO, USA) combination disc [14], meropenem (10 μg)/boronic acid (300 μg) combination disc and imipenem (10 μg)/EDTA (750 μg) (Sigma-Aldrich, St Louis, MO, USA) combination disc test [15] respectively. Isolates exhibiting an increase of ≥5 mm in the inhibition zone of the combination disc were categorized as positive.

Molecular characterization of β-lactamases, carbapenemases, 16S rRNA methylases and integrons

On the basis of results of the phenotypic tests, PCR was carried out for presence of carbapenemase genes ($bla_{VIM,IMP,SPM-1,GIM-1,SIM-1,KPC,SME,SPM,NDM,GES}$) [16–19], β-lactamase genes ($bla_{SHV,TEM,OXA-1,CTX-M}$) [20,21], and AmpC genes ($bla_{MOX, CMY, DHA, ACC, MIR/ACT, FOX}$) [22]. For ertapenem-non-susceptible isolates, all amplified β-lactamase products were further sequenced on both DNA strands in an automated DNA sequencer (Applied Biosystems 3730, DNA Analyzer, Perkin Elmer, USA) and aligned with the gene sequences available from Genbank (http://www. ncbi.nlm.nih.gov/genbank).

For isolates resistant to either aminoglycoside, genotypic detection for 16S rRNA methylase-encoding genes (*rmtA, rmtB, rmtC, rmtD & armA*) were done [23]. Investigation of integron classes (*IntI1, IntI2* and *IntI3* genes) were carried out for all 105 isolates [24].

In case of NDM-1 producing isolates only, association of plasmid-mediated quinolone resistance gene, *aac(6')-Ib-cr* and bleomycin resistant gene, ble_{MBL} were also investigated in addition to other genes listed above [25]. Amplified ble_{MBL} gene was further sequenced on both DNA strands to confirm its position with respect to bla_{NDM-1}.

Outer membrane permeability

Whole-cell extracts of the ertapenem-non-susceptible Enterobacteriaceae isolates were separated on 11% SDS–polyacrylamide gels [16], and were transferred to Immobilon-P membrane (Millipore) following standard procedures. From our collection, an isolate of *E. coli* (S205) (resistant to all generations of cephalosporins, aminoglycosides, carbapenems, fluoroquinolones and only susceptible to minocycline and colistin) which retained both the porins (Omp C/F) has been used as a control for the western blots. Porins were detected using polyclonal anti-OmpC/F antibody as described earlier [10].

Pulsed field gel electrophoresis (PFGE) of NDM-1-producing Enterobacteriaceae

PFGE was carried out for all NDM-1-possessing isolates by following PulseNet standardized procedures (http://www.cdc. gov/pulsenet/protocols.htm) in a CHEF-DR III apparatus (Bio-Rad Laboratories, Hercules and CA). XbaI macrorestriction patterns were compared and interpreted according to the criteria of Tenover *et al.* [26]. The dendrogram was generated by FPQuest software, version 4.5 (BioRad Laboratories, Hercules, CA, USA).

Statistical analysis

Data generated for the above samples and tests were analyzed systematically using established statistical procedures. All data analysis and statistics was done using R version 3.1.1. Association of clinical factors with sepsis caused by NDM-1-harbouring bacteria was evaluated by a multivariate logistic regression. All available clinical factors were entered into the regression at the same time and a backward selection process was used to identify the clinical factors with a significant association with neonates having sepsis due to NDM-1-carrying Enterobacteriaceae. P-values <0.05 were considered statistically significant. The association of the presence of NDM-1-producing bacteria with mortality was tested using a Chi-square test.

Results and Discussion

Bacterial isolates

During 2007–2011, 37% of the 285 culture positive isolates yielded Enterobacteriaceae. The 105 non-duplicate clinical isolates of Enterobaceriaceae including *Escherichia coli* (n = 27, 26%), *Klebsiella pneumoniae* (n = 68, 65%), *Enterobacter cloacae* (n = 8, 7.6%) and one each of *Enterobacter amnigenus* and *Enterobacter sakazakii* (0.95%) were analyzed.

Distribution of MIC values of different groups of antibiotics with focus on carbapenems

Tigecycline was the most active antimicrobial tested against *E. coli*, with 100% susceptibility followed by carbapenems (74% for meropenem and 67% for ertapenem), over the five year period. All other broad-spectrum agents had susceptibility rates ranging between 22% and 74% (22% for cefotaxime, 41% for gentamicin and 74% for amikacin) (Table 1). The resistance to carbapenems in *E. coli* first emerged in 2008 (11% for meropenem, 22% for ertapenem) and the resistance was highest in 2011 (37.5% for meropenem and ertapenem both).

In case of *K. pneumoniae*, tigecycline was again the most active antimicrobial with 96% susceptibility, closely followed by carbapenems (91% for meropenem and 87% for ertapenem). All other broad-spectrum agents had susceptibility rates ranging between 9% and 56% (9% for cefotaxime, 19% for gentamicin and 56% for amikacin). (Table 1). The resistance to carbapenems in *K. pneumoniae* isolates did not appear until 2009 (30% for ertapenem) and the resistance to meropenem emerged in 2010. The resistance to carbapenems was highest in 2010 (33% for meropenem and ertapenem both). In contrast, in 2011, there was only 9% resistance towards carbapenems indicating decreasing resistance rates.

A comparison of the susceptibility profiles of the two organisms revealed that susceptibility rates for cefotaxime, gentamicin and amikacin among *K. pneumoniae* isolates are lower than *E. coli* isolates. But with respect to carbapenems, susceptibility rates for *K. pneumoniae* isolates are higher than *E. coli* isolates during the study period (Table 1). However, with very few *E. coli* isolates these differences should not be overemphasized.

For *E. cloacae* (n = 8), the highest resistance was observed with cefotaxime (100%) followed by amikacin and gentamicin (87.5%), ertapenem (50%) and meropenem (37.5%). Tigecycline was the only agent for which 100% susceptibility was found. The resistance to ertapenem in *E. cloacae* isolates emerged in 2008 (n = 1) but resistance to meropenem was observed in late 2010 (n = 1); and was highest during 2011 (n = 2). Due to small number of *Enterobacter* isolates, percentage calculation as well as MIC50, MIC90 determination was not carried out. *Enterobacter amnigenus* and *Enterobacter sakazakii* were susceptible to all antimicrobial agents tested in this study.

The MIC values inhibiting 50% (MIC50) and 90% (MIC90) of the organisms tested against cefotaxime, ertapenem, meropenem, amikacin, gentamicin and tigecycline are presented in Table 1. As this study focuses on carbapenem resistance, detailed distribution of meropenem MIC values of *E. coli* and *K. pneumoniae* isolates for each year has been depicted in Figure 1a and 1b, respectively.

The distribution of the MIC90 values indicated an upward shift of meropenem MICs among the *E. coli* isolates from 2007 to 2011. Since for *E. coli*, the sample number is small, particularly for the numbers in an individual year, the MIC50 and MIC90 obtained in this study should not be overstated as a few strains with high MICs may skew the result. For *K. pneumoniae* isolates, the range of MIC values and MIC90 values indicated an abrupt upward shift from 2009 to 2010, which did not persist in the following year (2011).

MIC50 values for both *E. coli* and *K. pneumoniae* isolates remained within the susceptible range based on the CLSI guidelines as modified in 2013. In addition, a comparison of the two organisms revealed that the number of *E. coli* isolates non-susceptible to meropenem increased constantly throughout the study period while among *K. pneumoniae*, non-susceptible isolates were first detected in 2010 but the number of such isolates declined in 2011.

As the MIC value for ertapenem ≥0.5 mg/L was selected as the screening breakpoint for carbapenemases, a comparison of the

Table 1. Antimicrobial activity of meropenem and 5 broad-spectrum comparator agents tested against Enterobacteriaceae during the study period (2007–2011).

Organism (no. tested)/antimicrobial agent	% susceptible[a]						MIC (mg/L)		
	5 years	2007	2008	2009	2010	2011	50%	90%	Range
Escherichia coli (27)		(4)	(9)	(2)	(4)	(8)			
Meropenem	74	100	88.89	50	75	62.5	0.094	32	0.016–≥32
Ertapenem	67	100	77.78	50	75	62.5	0.064	≥32	0.004–≥32
Cefotaxime	22	50	0	0	0	50	32	≥256	0.006–≥256
Amikacin	74	100	88.89	50	50	62.5	8	≥256	2–≥256
Gentamicin	41	50	44.45	50	0	50	32	≥1024	0.125–≥1024
Tigecycline	100	100	100	100	100	100	0.094	0.38	0.047–0.5
Klebsiella pneumoniae (68)		(20)	(12)	(10)	(15)	(11)			
Meropenem	91	100	100	100	66.7	91	0.094	2	0.047–32
Ertapenem	87	100	100	70	66.7	91	0.125	12	0.012–≥32
Cefotaxime	9	15	8.33	10	0	9	32	≥256	0.032–≥256
Amikacin	56	50	66.7	100	20	63.6	12	≥256	1.5–≥256
Gentamicin	19	25	0	30	26.7	9	96	≥1024	0.38–≥1024
Tigecycline	96	100	91.7	90	100	91	0.5	1.5	0.19–8

[a] the susceptibility was determined according to the CLSI-2013 MIC interpretative criteria.

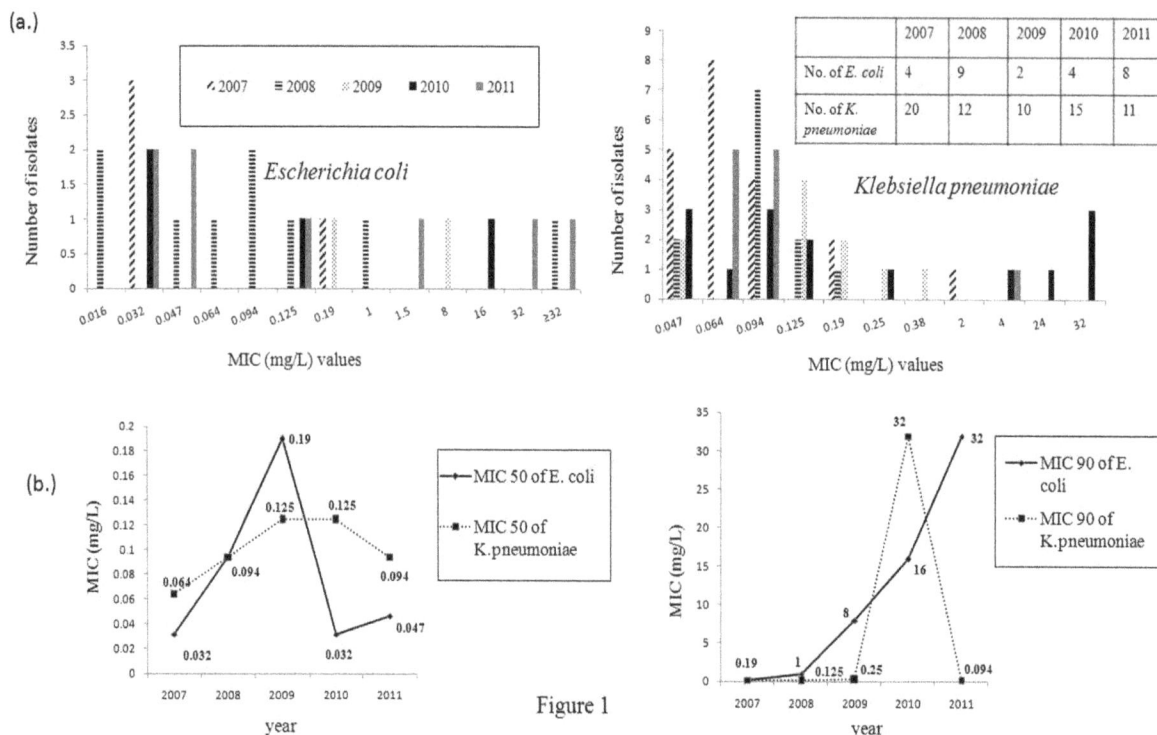

Figure 1. Meropenem MIC values : (a) Distribution of Meropenem MIC values among 27 *E. Coli* isolates and 68 *K. pneumoniae* isolates as determined by the Etest method during the study period (2007–2011); (b) Graphical representation of MIC50 and MIC90 values of the isolates throughout five year period.

susceptibilities to other antibiotics (cefotaxime, amikacin, genta-micin and tigecycline) among ertapenem-susceptible and ertape-nem-non-susceptible isolates (Table S1) was carried out. This showed that ertapenem non-susceptible isolates had decreased susceptibilities to other antibiotics. This result supports other earlier studies from different countries where carbapenem-non-susceptible isolates show reduced susceptibility to other classes of antibiotics [27,28].

Detection of β–lactamases based on phenotypic tests

Ten Enterobacteriaceae isolates (4 *E. coli*, 4 *K. pneumoniae*, each of *Enterobacter amnigenus* and *Enterobacter sakazakii*) were susceptible to all generations of cephalosporins, monobactam and carbapenems as tested by the disc diffusion test. The remaining Enterobacteriaceae (n = 95) were further analysed for production of β-lactamases by phenotypic tests (Figure S1). Seventy six percent (n = 80) and 8.5% (n = 9) were detected as ESBL- and AmpC-producers, respectively.

Twenty-six isolates with elevated ertapenem MICs (≥0.5 mg/L) were considered for KPC and MBL analysis. None were positive for KPC production but fifteen isolates (6 *E. coli*, 6 *K. pneumoniae* and 3 *E. cloacae*) produced MBLs. These fifteen isolates were also non-susceptible to meropenem (>1 mg/L). MBL-producing bacteria showed inconclusive phenotypic results for ESBLs and AmpCs. Therefore, the presence of ESBLs and AmpCs in these isolates was confirmed by PCR subsequently (Figure S1).

The phenotypic detection of ESBLs and AmpCs in presence of MBLs is challenging, indicating that further development of phenotypic tests for ESBL detection in MBL–producing isolates is of utmost importance. The failure to detect the ESBLs in the MBL–producing clinical isolates may lead to the hidden spread of such β- lactamases complicating the situation even further.

Genotypic distribution of β-lactamases among Enterobacteriaceae

Isolates categorized as positive by the different phenotypic tests were further analysed for the cephalosporin-resistant and carba-penem-resistant genes. Isolates harboured different combinations of any of the three ESBL types (CTX-M, SHV and TEM), two AmpC types (CMY and ACT) and only one carbapenemase type (NDM) (Table S2). The most common β-lactamase was CTX-M group 1, present in 82% of the isolates (n = 86), followed by TEM in 70% (n = 74) and SHV in 45% of the isolates (n = 47). The most common AmpC β-lactamase type was CMY (n = 5), followed by ACT (n = 2). The yearwise breakup of the ESBLs, AmpCs and carbapenemases are presented in Table 2. There were very few isolates that did not possess any of these genes.

Sequencing for all the genes on both strands have been carried out in the ertapenem-non-susceptible isolates. Table 3 and Table 4 demonstrates the distribution of β-lactamases in these isolates.

NDM-1 was present in 14% (n = 15) of the isolates and was the only carbapenemase type identified. No other carbapenemases were detected in this study. Class 1 integron was observed in 69 isolates (66%).

Figure S2 depicts the prevalence of ESBLs, AmpCs and NDM-1 over the period of five years. ESBLs have a consistently high prevalence throughout the period while AmpCs have a variable trend after their emergence in 2008. It is noteworthy that NDM-1 has an increasing trend after its emergence in 2008.

We had earlier reported the presence of NDM-1 in *K. pneumoniae* in 2 cases of neonatal septicaemia in 2010 [19]. However, this retrospective study showed that NDM-1 in *E. coli* had actually emerged in 2008 and much later (2010) in *K. pneumoniae*.

Table 2. Distribution of resistance determinants among Enterobacteriaceae isolates (2007–2011).

Isolate and resistance determinants	Total (%)	2007	2008	2009	2010	2011
		No. of strains				
Escherichia coli	27 (26)	4	9	2	4	8
bla_{SHV}	6 (26)	0	3	0	1	2
bla_{TEM}	16 (69)	0	7	1	3	5
bla_{OXA}	8 (35)	2	2	1	0	3
bla_{CTXM}	20 (87)	2	6	1	4	7
bla_{CMY}	5 (19)	0	2	1	0	2
bla_{NDM}	**6 (22)**	**0**	**1**	**1**	**1**	**3**
Negative for all determinants	4 (15)	2	2	0	0	0
Klebsiella pneumoniae	68 (65)	20	12	10	15	11
bla_{SHV}	40 (63)	14	2	10	10	4
bla_{TEM}	51 (80)	17	11	8	11	4
bla_{OXA}	30 (47)	11	6	3	5	5
bla_{CTXM}	58 (91)	17	9	8	14	10
bla_{NDM}	**6 (9)**	**0**	**0**	**0**	**5**	**1**
Negative for all determinants	4 (6)	2	1	0	0	1
Enterobacter cloacae	8 (7.6)	1	2	1	3	2
bla_{SHV}	1 (12)	0	0	0	1	0
bla_{TEM}	7 (87)	1	1	1	2	2
bla_{OXA}	6 (75)	1	1	1	2	1
bla_{CTXM}	8 (100)	1	1	1	3	2
bla_{ACT}	2 (25)	0	1	0	1	0
bla_{NDM}	**3 (37)**	**0**	**0**	**0**	**1**	**2**
Negative for all determinants	0 (0)	0	0	0	0	0

Molecular characterization of ertapenem-non-susceptible isolates which did not produce NDM-1

Eleven (7 *K. pneumoniae*, 2 *E. coli* and 2 *E. cloacae*) out of twenty-six ertapenem-non-susceptible isolates did not produce NDM-1 or any other carbapenemases. Microbiological and molecular characterization of these isolates has been documented in Table 3. All possessed different combinations of ESBLs, particularly CTX-M-15. Two isolates also produced AmpCs (CMY-4 and ACT-7). Evaluation of the porins showed that all of them lack a structural protein, OmpF (in *E. coli*)/OmpK36 (in *K. pneumoniae*). A loss of porin in combination with ESBLs/AmpCs is the reason for carbepenem-resistance in these isolates; these mechanisms of resistance have been documented earlier by other authors also [29].

Co-existence of multiple resistant-genes along with NDM-1

The molecular characterization of NDM-1-producing Enterobacteriacae (n = 15) is represented in Table 4. Most NDM-1-producing isolates possess multiple β-lactamases, aminoglycoside-resistant genes *armA* or *rmtB* and plasmid mediated quinolone resistant gene *aac(6′)-Ib-cr*. This result indicates that the NDM-1 possessing isolates are associated with unrelated broad-spectrum resistance genes, suggesting that they have been selected by wide range antibiotics. Two novel β-lactamases were also identified in two isolates harbouring NDM-1, a new SHV-type, SHV-167 (GenBank accession no. AB733453) and an AmpC gene, ACT-16 (GenBank accession no. AB737978). The presence of these novel β-lactamases has been reported [30]. Fourteen NDM-1 carrying isolates also possessed ble_{MBL} immediately downstream of the bla_{NDM-1} gene. This association has been quite systematically identified throughout the world [25].

The fact that class1 integrons were detected in nearly all isolates harbouring NDM-1 makes the situation even more worrisome. Class1 integrons are important players in driving the evolution of complex and laterally mobile multidrug-resistant units [31,32]. Class 1 integrons have been isolated earlier from NDM-1 harbouring isolates and other multidrug-resistant isolates [33,34].

The distribution of different classes of resistant determinants among NDM-1-harbouring isolates and isolates not harbouring NDM-1 is described in Table 5. This genetic distribution clearly indicated the association of multiple resistance genes along with NDM-1 gene as has also been reported by other authors [35]. With a wide battery of resistance determinants, NDM-1-possessing isolates remain only suscepltible to colistin and tigecycline. Aztreonam as an alternative also does not stand a chance, as a substantial proportion of the NDM-1 isolates are reported to co-produce CTX-Ms [5]. This study also shows that all NDM-1 isolates possessed CTX-M-15 which is probably widespread in this setting.

Outer membrane permeability of NDM-1-possessing isolates

The wide range of MIC values (1.5–≥32 mg/L) for meropenem among NDM-1 positive isolates prompted us to examine whether loss of porin was associated with such differences.

All 15 NDM-1-producing isolates retained normal levels of OmpA, a structural protein but OmpF/OmpK36 was not detected

Table 3. Microbiological and molecular characterization of non-NDM-harbouring Enterobacteriaceae isolates with ertapenem MIC ≥0.5 mg/L.

Isolate no.	Period of isolation	organism	MIC Values (mg/L)								Genetic determinants	Integrons	Porins
			CT	ETP	MP	AK	GM	CI	TGC	CL			
I1	Mar, 2007	Klebsiella pneumoniae	>256	0.5	0.094	8	96	3	ND$^{\#}$	ND	bla_{SHV-28}, bla_{TEM-1}, bla_{OXA-1}, $bla_{CTX-M-28}$		Ompk35, Omp A
I2	Aug, 2007	Klebsiella pneumoniae	>256	0.5	0.094	24	13	4	ND	ND	bla_{SHV-61}, bla_{TEM-1}, bla_{OXA-1}, $bla_{CTX-M-22}$	Intl1	Ompk35, Omp A
I3	Aug, 2007	Escherichia coli	>256	0.5	0.19	16	128	>32	ND	ND	bla_{OXA-1}, $bla_{CTX-M-28}$, rmt B		Omp C, Omp A
I4	Sep, 2007	Enterobacter cloacae	>256	0.5	0.19	≥256	≥1024	>32	ND	ND	bla_{TEM-1}, bla_{OXA-1}, $bla_{CTXM-15}$		Omp C, Omp A
I5	Jan, 2008	Enterobacter cloacae	>256	24	0.25	16	≥1024	>32	0.125	0.25	bla_{TEM-1}, bla_{OXA-1}, $bla_{CTXM-15}$, bla_{ACT-7}		Omp C, Omp A
I6	Sep, 2008	Klebsiella pneumoniae	>256	0.5	0.047	12	162	>32	0.5	0.16	bla_{TEM-1}, bla_{OXA-1}, $bla_{CTXM-15}$	Intl1	Ompk35, Omp A
I7	Dec, 2008	Escherichia coli	>256	>32	1	≥256	≥1024	>32	0.064	0.125	bla_{TEM-1}, bla_{OXA-1}, $bla_{CTXM-15}$, bla_{CMY-4}	Intl1	Omp C, Omp A
I8	Jan, 2009	Klebsiella pneumoniae	>256	2	0.19	8	48	>32	8	1	bla_{SHV-11}, bla_{TEM-1}, bla_{OXA-1}, $bla_{CTXM-15}$	Intl1	Ompk35, Omp A
I9	Jul, 2009	Klebsiella pneumoniae	>256	32	0.125	8	128	>32	1	0.38	bla_{SHV-1}, bla_{TEM-1}, bla_{OXA-1}, $bla_{CTXM-15}$	Intl1	Ompk35, Omp A
I10	Aug, 2009	Klebsiella pneumoniae	>256	1	0.125	2	>1024	>32	1	0.25	bla_{SHV-1}, bla_{TEM-1}, bla_{OXA-1}, $bla_{CTXM-15}$	Intl1	Ompk35, Omp A
I11	Dec, 2009	Klebsiella pneumoniae	>256	0.5	0.38	2	0.75	0.75	0.75	0.5	bla_{SHV-1}	Intl1	Ompk35, Omp A

CT: Cefotaxime, ETP: Ertapenem, MP: Meropenem, AK: Amikacin, GM: Gentamicin, CI: Ciprofloxacin, TGC: Tigecycline, CL: Colistin; Intl1: class 1 integron; Omp: Outer membrane protein. #ND: Not Determined.

in 6 *K. pneumoniae* (K1-K6), 3 *E. cloacae* (EC1-EC3) and 1 *E. coli* (E1) isolates (Table 4). OmpF/OmpK36 is generally lost or has reduced expression in most ESBL-producing strains. However, loss of porins could not be correlated to differences in MIC values of meropenem. Loss of porin was observed in isolates with MIC values of 4 mg/L, 6 mg/L as well as 24 mg/L, ≥32 mg/L in case of *K. pneumoniae*. All the porins were detected in 5 *E. coli* (E2-E6) isolates with MIC values 1.5 mg/L, 8 mg/L, 16 mg/L, 32 mg/L and ≥32 mg/L. Therefore, loss of porin seemed to be species specific and the differences in MIC values of the NDM-1 possessing isolates probably did not result due to absence of porins. Further work is in progress to understand the reason for such differences which can occur due to alterations in the expression of the enzymes or other changes in the outer membrane proteins.

However, it should be noted that all eleven ertapenem-non-susceptible isolates showed loss of porin which along with the ESBLs was the cause for carbapenem-nonsusceptibility.

Diversity of the NDM-1 possessing isolates

PFGE revealed that all NDM-1 carrying Enterobacteriaceae isolates were clonally diverse (Figure 2) and most cases did not cluster in time. No epidemic clone was found to exist during this period. This indirectly indicated the horizontal transmission of carbapenem resistance among these isolates and not cross-transmission among the neonates. However, the fact that most neonates with septicaemia due to NDM-1 possessing Enterobactericeae were referred from other hospitals (Table 4) could also be a reason for the diversity of the clones.

Clinical presentation of the neonates carrying NDM-1

An evaluation of the demographics and clinical data (Table 4) revealed that most neonates with septicaemia where the causative organism harboured NDM-1 were of low birth weight (n = 7) or very low birth weight (n = 5), preterm (n = 10), ventilated (n = 8), male (n = 12) and born at an extramural centre (outborn) (n = 9). Most of these neonates survived after treatment and were discharged (n = 11).

Cefotaxime along with amikacin or gentamicin was used in the NICU as a pre-emptive antimicrobial therapy for clinically suspected cases of sepsis during 2007-2008. This was changed to piperacillin/tazobactam and amikacin due to the high prevalence of CTX-M gene in the unit. For serious cases of infection, meropenem, ofloxacin and colistin in different combinations were used particularly after the emergence of carbapenem resistance.

Association of clinical factors and mortality of the neonates with the presence of NDM-1 harbouring-Enterobacteriaceae

The results of a comparison of neonates with presence of NDM-1-producing bacteria in their blood sample and those without NDM-1 are shown in Table 6. Multivariate logistic regression identified significantly higher incidence of sepsis with NDM-1-harbouring Enterobacteriaceae in male neonates as compared to females [Odds ratio (OR) 14.2; p-value 0.01521]. In addition, outborn neonates were also found to have a significantly higher incidence of sepsis due to NDM-1-carrying bacteria[OR 0.19; p-value 0.01877]. Finally, neonates with a low birth weight also had a significantly higher incidence of NDM-1-producing Enterobacteriaceae in their blood sample [OR 9.04; p-value 0.04989]. None of the other clinical factors tested had a significant association with the presence of NDM-1-possessing bacteria.

In order to get an indication of the association between the presence of NDM-1-carrying Enterobacteriaceae in blood with

Table 4. Antibiotic susceptibility and molecular characterization of NDM-1- harbouring Enterobacteriaceae along with clinical features of the neonates harbouring the same isolates in their blood specimens.

Patient no./ Organism (isolate no.)	Sex	Inborn Or Outborn	Birth weight	Gestational Age$	Mode Of delivery	ventilation	Prescribed antibiotics	Outcome	CT	ETP	MP	AK	GM	CI	TGC	CL	Genetic determinants	Integron	Porins
P1/$Escherichia\ coli$ (E1)	M	Inborn	LBW	preterm	LUCS	No	PipTaz/ Amika	discharge	>256	>32	>32	>256	>1024	>32	0.25	1	bla_{TEM-1}, $bla_{CTXM-15}$, bla_{CMY-6}, $rmt\ C$, $aac(6')-Ib$, ble_{MBL}	Int1	Omp C, Omp A
P2/$Escherichia\ coli$ (E2)	M	Inborn	VLBW	preterm	LUCS	Yes	PipTaz/ Amika	discharge	>256	>32	8	>256	>1024	>32	0.25	0.5	bla_{TEM-1}, bla_{OXA-1}, bla_{CMY-42}, $arm\ A$, $aac(6')-Ib-cr$, ble_{MBL}	Int1	Omp C, Omp F, Omp A
P3/$Klebsiella$ $pneumoniae$ (K1)	M	Outborn	NW	term	NVD	Yes	colistin	discharge	>256	>32	32	>256	>1024	>32	0.75	0.25	bla_{SHV-11}, $aac(6')-Ib$, ble_{MBL}	Int1	Ompk35, Omp A
P4/$Klebsiella$ $pneumoniae$ (K2)	M	Outborn	LBW	preterm	LUCS	No	ofloxacin	discharge	>256	>32	24	>256	>1024	3	1.5	0.38	$bla_{SHV-167}$, $bla_{CTXM-15}$, $arm\ A$, $aac(6')-Ib-cr$, ble_{MBL}	Int1	Ompk35, Omp A
P5/$Klebsiella$ $pneumoniae$ (K3)	M	Outborn	LBW	preterm	NVD	Yes	ofloxacin	discharge	>256	12	4	>256	>1024	>32	1	0.75	bla_{TEM-1}, bla_{OXA-1}, $bla_{CTXM-15}$, $aac(6')-Ib$, ble_{MBL}	Int1	Ompk35, Omp A
P6/$Klebsiella$ $pneumoniae$ (K4)	M	Outborn	LBW	term	LUCS	Yes	colistin	discharge	>256	>32	32	>256	>1024	>32	1	0.38	bla_{TEM-1}, bla_{OXA-1}, $bla_{CTXM-15}$, $aac(6')-Ib$, ble_{MBL}	Int1	Ompk35, Omp A
P7/$Escherichia\ coli$ (E3)	M	Inborn	LBW	preterm	NVD	No	meropenem	death	>256	>32	16	>256	>1024	>32	0.25	0.38	bla_{TEM-1}, $bla_{CTXM-15}$, $rmt\ B$, ble_{MBL}	Int1	Omp C, Omp F, Omp A
P8/$Klebsiella$ $pneumoniae$ (K5)	F	Outborn	VLBW	preterm	LUCS	Yes	meropenem	discharge	>256	>32	32	>256	>1024	>32	0.38	0.75	bla_{SHV-11}, bla_{OXA-1}, $bla_{CTXM-15}$, $aac(6')-Ib$, ble_{MBL}	Int1	Ompk35, Omp A
P9/$Enterobacter$ $cloacae$ (EC1)	M	Outborn	LBW	preterm	NVD	Yes	colistin/ ofloxacin	LAMA	>256	>32	>32	>256	>1024	4	0.25	1.5	bla_{OXA-1}, $bla_{CTXM-15}$, bla_{ACT-16}, $rmt\ C$, $aac(6')-Ib$, ble_{MBL}	Int1	Omp C, Omp A
P10/$Enterobacter$ $cloacae$ (EC2)*	M	Outborn	VLBW	preterm	NVD	Yes	colistin	discharge	>256	8	6	>256	>1024	2	0.5	0.5	bla_{TEM-1}, bla_{OXA-1}, $bla_{CTXM-15}$, $rmt\ B$, $aac(6')-Ib-cr$, ble_{MBL}	Int1	Omp C, Omp A
P10/$Escherichia\ coli$ (E4)*	M	Outborn	VLBW	preterm	NVD	Yes	colistin	discharge	>256	>32	>32	>256	>1024	>32	0.125	0.75	bla_{TEM-1}, $bla_{CTXM-15}$, bla_{CMY-42}, $rmt\ B$, ble_{MBL}	Int1	Omp C, Omp F, Omp A
P11/$Escherichia\ coli$ (E5)	M	Inborn	LBW	term	LUCS	No	ofloxacin	discharge	>256	>32	32	>256	>1024	>32	0.38	1.5	$bla_{CTXM-15}$, $rmt\ B$, $aac(6')-Ib-cr$, ble_{MBL}	Int1	Omp C, Omp F, Omp A

Table 4. Cont.

Patient no./ Organism (isolate no.)	Sex	Inborn Or Outborn	Birth weight	Gestational Age[S]	Mode Of delivery	ventilation	Prescribed antibiotics	Outcome	MIC Values (mg/L)							Genetic determinants	Integron	Porins
P12/*Klebsiella pneumoniae* (K6)**	No clinical data available								>256	12	4	>1024	8	0.75	1	bla_{TEM-1}, bla_{OXA-1}, $bla_{CTX-M-15}$, rmt B, aac(6')-Ib, bla_{MBL}	Int1	Ompk35, Omp A
P13/*Enterobacter cloacae* (EC3)	M	Outborn	VLBW	preterm	NVD	Yes	PipTaz/ Amika	death	>256	>32	32	>1024	8	1.5	1	bla_{TEM-1}, $bla_{CTX-M-15}$, aac(6')-Ib, bla_{MBL}	Int1	Omp C, Omp A
P14/*Escherichia coli* (E6)	M	Outborn	VLBW	preterm	NVD	No	ofloxacin	discharge	>256	1.5	>32	>1024	>32	0.094	0.75	bla_{TEM-1}, bla_{OXA-1}, $bla_{CTX-M-15}$, bla_{CMY-42}, rmt B, aac(6')-Ib	Int1	Omp C, Omp F, Omp A

M: male; F: female; LBW: low birth weight (<2500 gm); VLBW: very low birth weight (<1500 gm); NW: normal weight (>2500 gm); NVD: normal vaginal delivery; LUCS: low uterine caesarean delivery; Omp: Outer membrane protein; LAMA: left against medical advice.

CT: Cefotaxime; ETP: Ertapenem; MP: Meropenem; AK: Amikacin; GM: Gentamicin; CI: Ciprofloxacin; TGC: Tigecycline; CL: Colistin; PipTaz: Piperacillin/Tazobactam; Amika: Amikacin;

[S]Gestational age <37 weeks is considered as preterm.

*Two different Enterobacteriaceae isolates (1 *E. coli* and 1 *E. cloacae*) were isolated from blood of a single patient.

**No clinical data was available for this patient.

mortality, a simple association analysis between the two was conducted. The results showed that neonates with NDM-1-harbouring Enterobacteriaceae in their blood actually had a mortality rate of 13.33% (2 out of 15 neonates). In comparison, the neonates without NDM-1-possessing Enterobacteriaceae in their blood had a mortality rate of 22.22% (20 out of 90 neonates). The difference in the mortality between septicaemic neonates with and without the presence of NDM-1-producing Enterobacteriaceae was not statistically significant [P-value 0.6595].

As there are no previous studies that have analysed the association of clinical factors with sepsis due to NDM-1-carrying organisms in neonates, comparisons with earlier studies is not possible. Comparisons could only be made with studies where risk factors for neonatal sepsis have been investigated. One particular study has shown that male sex is associated with sepsis in neonates [36]. Low birth weight is a risk for sepsis as seen in other studies [37,38]. Neonates with low birth weight are more vulnerable to infections and thus the association with NDM-1 harbouring Enterobacteriace seems plausible. Neonates born at an extramural centre (outborn) were found to have a significantly higher incidence of sepsis with NDM-1-possessing Enterobacteriacae lending support to the diversity of the isolates as seen by PFGE in this study.

Sepsis caused by NDM-1-producing Enterobateriacae was not associated with mortality of the neonates in this study though one particular study in adults have shown that infections with carbapenem- resistant isolates had a higher mortality rate [39].

Conclusion

The emergence of carbapenem resistance particularly in Enterobacteriaceae is a considerable burden on the neonatal healthcare system in developing countries. This is the first analysis of the carbapenemases in a neonatal intensive care unit for an extended period of time. The study tries to capture the trend in resistance for a period before and after the emergence of NDM-1 in the unit. The study shows the persistence of the CTX-M-15 gene throughout the five year period. In fact, a prelude to carbapenem resistance, as observed in this study, has been the presence of ESBLs particularly CTX-Ms. Earlier studies from our laboratory and other studies from India have shown the extensive dissemination of this gene [40,41]. Before the emergence of NDM-1, CTX-M-15 along with porin-loss were the reason for carbapenem-non-susceptibility. However, the prevalence of the AmpC–β- lactamases or the aminoglycoside resistance has shown a rise with the emergence of NDM-1. The association of NDM-1 with other resistance genes has been frequently observed in Enterobacteriacae in other studies also [35].

Though present in the same setting, *K. pneumoniae* and *E. coli* displayed differences in susceptibility patterns. *K. pneumoniae* showed higher susceptibility to carbapenems but lower to cefotaxime, gentamicin and amikacin. Such differences in the species has also been noted in other studies [42]. However, with very few *E. coli* isolates, particularly in individual years, these differences should not be overstated.

Though a number of variants of the NDM gene have been reported till date, no variants of this gene were identified in this study. All isolates possessed NDM-1. In addition throughout the five-year period no other MBL was detected in these isolates. The diversity of the isolates indicates probable horizontal transfer of the NDM-1 gene either through plasmids or by the transposons related acquisition. The capability of NDM-1 to associate with other resistance genes raises serious concerns. The other cause for

Table 5. Comparison of the presence of resistance determinants and integrons between NDM-1- producing and non-producing Enterobacteriaceae isolates.

Resistance determinants	NDM-1 isolates (%) (n = 15)	Non-NDM-1 isolates (%) (n = 90)
ESBL- producer	15 (100)	80 (89)
bla_{CTX-M}	13 (87)	73 (81)
bla_{SHV}	3 (20)	44 (49)
bla_{TEM}	10 (67)	64 (71)
bla_{OXA-1}	8 (53)	36 (40)
AmpC- producer	5 (33)	2 (2)
bla_{CMY}	4 (27)	1 (1)
bla_{ACT}	1 (7)	1 (1)
16s r-RNA methylase producer	10 (67)	7 (7)
Integrons	14 (93)	64 (71)

ESBL: Extended Spectrum β Lactamase; NDM: New Delhi Metallo-β-lactamase.

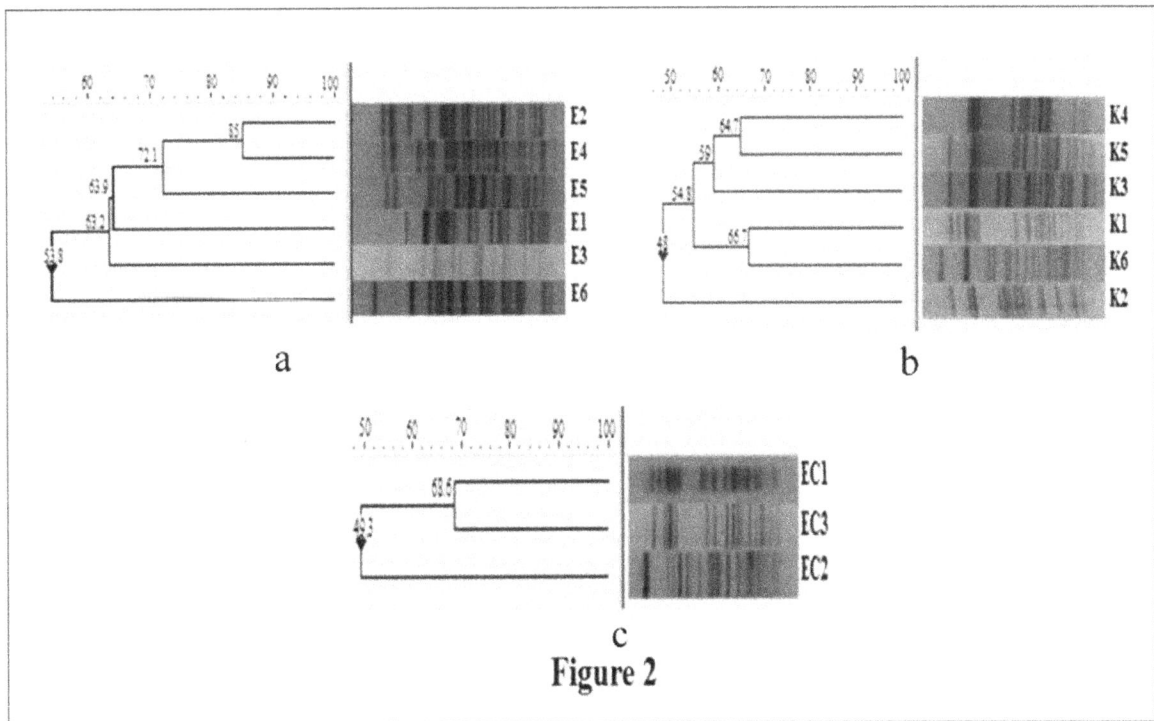

Figure 2. Analysis of the genetic relationship according to Dice's similarity coefficient and the unweighted pair group method with arithmetic mean (UPGMA) (the position tolerance and optimization were set at 1.0 and 1.0% respectively) of the XbaI patterns of *E. coli* (E1-E6) (a), *K. pneumoniae* (K1-K6) (b) and *E. cloacae* (EC1-EC3) (c). *Salmonella* serotype Braenderup H9812 has been used as reference standard.

Table 6. Association of clinical factors with sepsis caused by NDM-1 harbouring Enterobacteriaceae in neonates.

Clinical factors		Neonates with NDM-1 harbouring Enterobacteriaceae in Blood (n = 14)$^\$$		Neonates without NDM-1 harbouring Enterobacteriaceae in Blood (n = 87)$^\#$		P value
No. of Neonates		n	%	n	%	
Sex	Male	13	93	43	49.4	0.01521**
	Female	1	7	44	50.6	
Gestational Age	Pre-term	11	78.6	52	59.8	-
	Term	3	21.4	35	40.2	
Inborn/Outborn	Inborn	4	28.6	59	67.8	0.01877**
	Outborn	10	71.4	28	32.2	
Birth Weight	Low birth weight	13	93	60	69	0.04989**
	Normal birth weight	1	7	26	29.8	
Baby on Ventilation	Yes	9	64.3	36	41.4	-
	No	5	35.7	49	56.3	
Onset of Sepsis*	Early	4	28.6	34	39	-
	Late	9	64.3	52	59.8	
Mode of Delivery	Caesarean delivery	5	35.7	34	39	
	Normal vaginal delivery	8	57	53	61	

**Significant at 95% confidence.
$^\$$No clinical data was available for one patient.
$^\#$No clinical data was available for three patients.
*Early onset of sepsis (<72 hours of birth), Late onset sepsis (>72 hours of birth).
Description of other clinical factors has been described in the footnote of Table 4.

concern is the difficulty in detection of ESBLs in the presence of NDM-1 which hydrolyse carbapenems and also cephalosporins.

The high prevalence of ESBLs and the increasing presence of carbapenemases, both of which can be attributed to horizontal transfer, are indeed worrisome. Added to this is a vulnerable group of critical patients, the hectic environment of the ICU where lapses in infection control may happen and extremely capable pathogens. This is a fatal combination and necessary systemic steps need to be implemented soon.

Supporting Information

Figure S1   Schematic representation of the molecular analysis of Enterobacteriaceae isolates enrolled in this study.

Figure S2   Graphical representation of percentage of Enterobacteriaceae isolates producing ESBLs, AmpC and NDM during the study period.

Table S1   Susceptibility patterns of the ertapenem susceptible and non-susceptible Enterobacteriaceae isolates for 4 broad spectrum antibiotics.

Table S2   Microbiological and molecular characterization of 105 Enterobacteriaceae isolates included in this study.

Acknowledgments

We extend our thanks to Dr. Arun K. Singh and Dr. Rajlakshmi Viswanathan for their support during the study. We wish to thank George A. Jacoby, Anne Marie Queenan, Olivier Moquet & Kyungwon Lee for providing control strains for the PCRs and Heinz Schwarz & Helen I. Zgurskaya for the antibodies.

Author Contributions

Conceived and designed the experiments: SB. Performed the experiments: SD SR SC. Analyzed the data: SD SR SC TP. Contributed reagents/materials/analysis tools: AS BS TS TP SB. Contributed to the writing of the manuscript: SD SB TP. Coordinated collection of specimens, maintenance of clinical data: AS BS TS.

References

1. Viswanathan R, Singh AK, Basu S, Chatterjee S, Sardar S, et al. (2012) Multi-drug resistant gram negative bacilli causing early neonatal sepsis in India Arch Dis Child Fetal Neonatal Ed 97(3): F182–7.
2. Polin RA (1989) Neonatal Sepsis: progress in diagnosis and management In: St Geme III JW. New Ethicals; 25(6): 133–41(part 1) and 25(7): 109–31 (part 2).
3. Patel JB (2009) Carbapenemases in Enterobacteriaceae: Activity, Epidemiology, and Laboratory Detection. Clin Microbiol Newslett 31(8): 55–62.
4. Queenan AM, Bush K (2007) Carbapenemases: the Versatile β-Lactamases. Clin Microbiol Rev 20(3): 440–58.

5. Nordmann P, Poirel L, Walsh TR, Livermore DM (2011) The emerging NDM carbapenemases Trends in Microbiology 19(12): 588–595.
6. Yong D, Toleman MA, Giske CG, Cho HS, Sundman K, et al. (2009) Characterization of a new metallo-beta-lactamase gene, bla(NDM-1), and a novel erythromycin esterase gene carried on a unique genetic structure in *Klebsiella pneumoniae* sequence type 14 from India Antimicrob Agents Chemother 53: 5046–54.
7. Walsh TR, Weeks J, Livermore DM, Toleman MA (2011) Dissemination of NDM-1 positive bacteria in the New Delhi environment and its implications for

human health: an environmental point prevalence study. Lancet Infect Dis 11(5): 355–62.

8. Roy S, Viswanathan R, Singh A, Das P, Basu S (2010) Gut colonization by multidrug-resistant and carbapenem-resistant *Acinetobacter baumannii* in neonates. Eur J Clin Microbiol Infect Dis 29(12): 1495–500.

9. Das P, Singh AK, Pal T, Dasgupta S, Ramamurthy T, Basu S (2011) Colonization of the gut with Gram-negative bacilli, its association with neonatal sepsis and its clinical relevance in a developing country. J Med Microbiol 60(11): 1651–60.

10. Roy S, Datta S, Viswanathan R, Singh AK, Basu S (2013) Tigecycline susceptibility in *Klebsiella pneumoniae* and *Escherichia coli* causing neonatal septicaemia (2007–10) and role of an efflux pump in tigecycline non-susceptibility. J Antimicrob Chemother 68(5): 1036–42.

11. Bauer AW, Kirby WM, Sherris JC, Turck M (1966) Antibiotic susceptibility testing by a standardized single disk method. Am. J. Clin. Pathol 45: 493–496.

12. Clinical and Laboratory Standards Institute. Performance Standards for Antimicrobial Susceptibility Testing: Eighteenth Informational Supplement M100-S18 CLSI, Wayne, PA, USA, 2008.

13. Nordmann P, Poirel L, Carrër A, Toleman MA, Walsh TR (2011) How To Detect NDM-1 Producers, J Clin Microbiol 49(2): 718–21.

14. Coudron PE (2005) Inhibitor-Based Methods for Detection of Plasmid-Mediated AmpC β-Lactamases in *Klebsiella spp.*, *Escherichia coli*, and *Proteus mirabilis*. J. Clin. Microbiol 43: 4163–4167.

15. Cohen Stuart J, Leverstein-Van Hall MA (2010) Dutch Working Party on the Detection of Highly Resistant Microorganisms. Guideline for phenotypic screening and confirmation of carbapenemases in Enterobacteriaceae. Int J Antimicrob Agents 36(3): 205–10.

16. Woodford N, Tierno PM Jr, Young K, Tysall L, Palepou MF, et al. (2004) Outbreak of *Klebsiella pneumoniae* producing a new carbapenem-hydrolyzing class A β-lactamase, KPC-3, in a New York Medical Center. Antimicrob Agents Chemother 48: 4793–9.

17. Ellington MJ, Kistler J, Livermore DM, Woodford N (2007) Multiplex PCR for rapid detection of genes encoding acquired metallo-β-lactamases. J Antimicrob Chemother 59: 321–2.

18. Gröbner S, Linke D, Schütz W, Fladerer C, Madlung J, et al. (2009) Emergence of carbapenem-non-susceptible extended-spectrum β-lactamase-producing *Klebsiella pneumoniae* isolates at the university hospital of Tübingen, Germany. J Med Microbiol 58: 912–22.

19. Roy S, Viswanathan R, Singh AK, Das P, Basu S (2011) Sepsis in neonates due to imipenem resistant *Klebsiella pneumoniae* producing NDM-1 in India. J Antimicrob Chemother 66(6): 1411–3.

20. Colom K, Pérez J, Alonso R, Fernández-Aranguiz A, Lariño E, et al. (2003) Simple and reliable multiplex PCR assay for detection of blaTEM, bla(SHV) and blaOXA-1 genes in Enterobacteriaceae. FEMS Microbiol Lett 223(2): 147–51.

21. Saladin M, Cao VT, Lambert T, Donay JL, Herrmann JL, et al. (2002) Diversity of CTX-M β-lactamases and their promoter regions from Enterobacteriaceae isolated in three Parisian hospitals. FEMS Microbiol Lett 209(2): 161–8.

22. Perez-Perez FJ, Hanson ND (2002) Detection of plasmid-mediated AmpC beta-lactamase genes in clinical isolates by using multiplex PCR. J. Clin. Microbiol 40(6): 2153–2162.

23. Berçot B, Poirel L, Nordmann P (2011) Updated multiplex polymerase chain reaction for detection of 16S rRNA methylases: high prevalence among NDM-1 producers. Diagn Microbiol Infect Dis 71(4): 442–445.

24. Shibata N, Doi Y, Yamane K, Yagi T, Kurokawa H, et al. (2003) PCR typing of genetic determinants for metallo-β-lactamases and integrases carried by gram-negative bacteria isolated in Japan, with focus on the class 3 integron. J Clin Microbiol 41(12): 5407–13.

25. Poirel L, Dortet L, Bernabeu S, Nordmann P (2011) Genetic Features of bla NDM-1-Positive Enterobacteriaceae. Antimicrob Agents Chemother 55(11): 5403–5407.

26. Tenover FC, Arbeit RD, Goering RV, Mickelsen PA, Murray BE, et al. (1995) Interpreting chromosomal DNA restriction patterns produced by pulsed-field gel electrophoresis: criteria for bacterial strain typing. J Clin Microbiol 33: 2233–9.

27. Kumarasamy KK, Toleman MA, Walsh TR, Bagaria J, Butt F, et al. (2010) Emergence of a new antibiotic resistance mechanism in India, Pakistan, and the UK: a molecular, biological, and epidemiological study. Lancet Infect Dis 10(9): 597–602.

28. Williamson DA, Sidjabat HE, Freeman JT, Roberts SA, Silvey A, et al. (2012) Identification and molecular characterisation of New Delhi metallo-β-lactamase-1 (NDM-1) and NDM-6-producing Enterobacteriaceae from New Zealand hospitals. Int J Antimicrob Agents 39(6): 529–33.

29. Jacoby GA, Mills DM, Chow N (2004) Role of β-Lactamases and Porins in Resistance to Ertapenem and Other- β-Lactams in *Klebsiella pneumoniae*. Antimicrob Agents Chemother 48(8): 3203–3206.

30. Datta S, Mitra S, Viswanathan R, Saha A, Basu S (2014) Characterisation of novel plasmid-mediated β-lactamases (SHV-167 and ACT-16) associated with New Delhi Metallo-β-lactamase-1 harbouring isolates from neonates in India. J Med Microbiol 63: 480–82.

31. Bonnet R (2004) Growing group of extended-spectrum beta-lactamases: the CTX-M enzymes. Antimicrob Agents Chemother 48(1): 1–14.

32. Poirel L, Lartigue MF, Decousser JW, Nordmann P (2005) ISEcp1B-mediated transposition of blaCTX-M in Escherichia coli. Antimicrob Agents Chemother 49(1): 447–50.

33. Roy S, Singh AK, Viswanathan R, Nandy RK, Basu S (2011) Transmission of imipenem resistance determinants during the course of an outbreak of NDM-1 *Escherichia coli* in a sick newborn care unit. J Antimicrob Chemother 66(12): 2773–80.

34. Patel G, Bonomo RA (2013) "Stormy waters ahead": global emergence of carbapenemases. Front Microbiol 14(4): 48.

35. Johnson AP, Woodford N (2013) Global spread of antibiotic resistance: the example of New Delhi metallo-β-lactamase (NDM) - mediated carbapenem resistance. J Med Microbiol 62: 499–513.

36. Shakil S, Akram M, Ali SM, Khan AU (2010) Acquisition of extended-spectrumb-lactamase producing *Escherichia coli* strains in male and female infants admitted to a neonatal intensive care unit: molecular epidemiology and analysis of risk factors; J Med Microbiol 59: 948–954.

37. Tsai MH, Chu SM, Lee CW, Hsu JF, Huang HR, et al. (2014) Recurrent late-onset sepsis in the neonatal intensive care unit: incidence, clinical characteristics and risk factors Clin Microbiol Infect. doi: 10.1111/1469-0691.12661.

38. Viswanathan R, Singh AK, Basu S, Chatterjee S, Sardar S, et al. (2011) Multi-drug resistant gram negative bacilli causing early neonatal sepsis in India Arch Dis Child Fetal Neonatal Ed. 97:F182–F187.

39. Chang YY, Chuang YC, Siu LK, Wu TL, Lin JC, et al. (2014) Clinical features of patients with carbapenem nonsusceptible *Klebsiella pneumoniae* and *Escherichia coli* in intensive care units: a nationwide multicenter study in Taiwan J Microbiol Immunol Infect. doi: 10.1016/j.jmii.2014.05.010.

40. Roy S, Gaind R, Chellani H, Mohanty S, Datta S, et al. (2013) Neonatal septicaemia caused by diverse clones of *Klebsiella pneumoniae* & *Escherichia coli* harbouring blaCTX-M-15. Indian J Med Res 137(4): 791–9.

41. Mohamudha Parveen R, Manivannan S, Harish BN, Parija SC (2012) Study of CTX-M Type of Extended Spectrum β-Lactamase among Nosocomial Isolates of *Escherichia coli* and *Klebsiella pneumoniae* in South India. Indian J Microbiol 52(1): 35–40.

42. Romero L, López L, Rodríguez-Baño J, Ramón Hernández J, Martínez-Martínez L, et al. (2005) Long-term study of the frequency of *Escherichia coli* and *Klebsiella pneumoniae* isolates producing extended-spectrum beta-lacta mases. Clin Microbiol Infect 11(8): 625–31.

22

Presence of Neutrophil Extracellular Traps and Citrullinated Histone H3 in the Bloodstream of Critically Ill Patients

Tomoya Hirose[1]*[9¶], **Shigeto Hamaguchi**[2¶], **Naoya Matsumoto**[1], **Taro Irisawa**[1], **Masafumi Seki**[2], **Osamu Tasaki**[3], **Hideo Hosotsubo**[1], **Norihisa Yamamoto**[2], **Kouji Yamamoto**[4], **Yukihiro Akeda**[5], **Kazunori Oishi**[5], **Kazunori Tomono**[2], **Takeshi Shimazu**[1]

1 Department of Traumatology and Acute Critical Medicine, Osaka University Graduate School of Medicine, Osaka, Japan, 2 Division of Infection Control and Prevention, Osaka University Graduate School of Medicine, Osaka, Japan, 3 Department of Emergency Medicine, Unit of Clinical Medicine, Nagasaki University Graduate School of Biomedical Sciences, Nagasaki, Japan, 4 Department of Medical Innovation, Osaka University Hospital, Osaka, Japan, 5 International Research Center for Infectious Diseases, Research Institute for Microbial Diseases, Osaka University, Osaka, Japan

Abstract

Neutrophil extracellular traps (NETs), a newly identified immune mechanism, are induced by inflammatory stimuli. Modification by citrullination of histone H3 is thought to be involved in the in vitro formation of NETs. The purposes of this study were to evaluate whether NETs and citrullinated histone H3 (Cit-H3) are present in the bloodstream of critically ill patients and to identify correlations with clinical and biological parameters. Blood samples were collected from intubated patients at the time of ICU admission from April to June 2011. To identify NETs, DNA and histone H3 were visualized simultaneously by immunofluorescence in blood smears. Cit-H3 was detected using a specific antibody. We assessed relationships of the presence of NETs and Cit-H3 with the existence of bacteria in tracheal aspirate, SIRS, diagnosis, WBC count, and concentrations of IL-8, TNF-α, cf-DNA, lactate, and HMGB1. Forty-nine patients were included. The median of age was 66.0 (IQR: 52.5–76.0) years. The diagnoses included trauma (7, 14.3%), infection (14, 28.6%), resuscitation from cardiopulmonary arrest (8, 16.3%), acute poisoning (4, 8.1%), heart disease (4, 8.1%), brain stroke (8, 16.3%), heat stroke (2, 4.1%), and others (2, 4.1%). We identified NETs in 5 patients and Cit-H3 in 11 patients. NETs and/or Cit-H3 were observed more frequently in "the presence of bacteria in tracheal aspirate" group (11/22, 50.0%) than in "the absence of bacteria in tracheal aspirate" group (4/27, 14.8%) ($p<.01$). Multiple logistic regression analysis showed that only the presence of bacteria in tracheal aspirate was significantly associated with the presence of NETs and/or Cit-H3. The presence of bacteria in tracheal aspirate may be one important factor associated with NET formation. NETs may play a pivotal role in the biological defense against the dissemination of pathogens from the respiratory tract to the bloodstream in potentially infected patients.

Editor: Nades Palaniyar, The Hospital for Sick Children and The University of Toronto, Canada

Funding: This work was supported by a Grant-in-Aid for Scientific Research from the Ministry of Education, Culture, Sports, Science and Technology in Japan (no. 21390163, no. 25293366 and no. 25861718) and by ZENKYOREN (National Mutual Insurance Federation of Agricultural Cooperatives). The funders had no role in study design, data collection and analysis, decision to publish, or preparation of the manuscript.

Competing Interests: The authors have declared that no competing interests exist.

* Email: htomoya1979@hp-emerg.med.osaka-u.ac.jp

⑨ These authors contributed equally to this work.

¶ These authors are joint first authors on this work.

Introduction

Neutrophils play an important role as the first line of innate immune defense [1]. One function of neutrophils, called "neutrophil extracellular traps" (NETs), has been discovered recently. NETs are fibrous structures that are released extracellularly from activated neutrophils in response to infection and also the sterile inflammatory process [2–5]. This distinctive phenomenon was first reported by Brinkmann et al in 2004 [6]. The main components of NETs are deoxyribonucleic acid (DNA) and histones H1, H2A, H2B, H3, and H4; other components such as neutrophil elastase, myeloperoxidase, bactericidal/permeability-

increasing protein, cathepsin G, lactoferrin, matrix metalloproteinase-9, peptidoglycan recognition proteins, pentraxin, and LL-37 have also been reported [5–11]. The type of active cell death involving the release of NETs is called NETosis [12], which differs from apoptosis and necrosis. Because formation of NETs does not require caspases and is not accompanied by DNA fragmentation, it is believed that this process is independent of apoptosis [12]. Despite several in vitro and animal experiments that have clearly shown the biological importance of NETs, little is known about the function of NETs in the human body [13,14].

Before the discovery of NETs, several studies reported on an increase in the concentration of circulating free DNA (cf-DNA) in the blood in various diseases including sepsis, trauma, stroke, autoimmune disorders, and several cancers [15–20]. This cf-DNA is thought to be derived from necrotic and/or apoptotic cells [21]. Recent articles have suggested that NETs and cf-DNA are related [15,16]. In these reports, cf-DNA was quantified directly in plasma, and the cf-DNA in plasma was treated the same as NETs in blood. However, it remains unknown whether cf-DNA is derived from NETs.

Citrullination of histone H3 is considered to be involved in NET formation in vitro. Neutrophils show highly decondensed nuclear chromatin structures during NETosis, and hypercitrullination of histone H3 by peptidylarginine deiminase 4 (PAD4) plays an important role in chromatin decondensation [14,22,23]. Inhibition of PAD4 prevents citrullination of H3 and NET formation [23]. Thus, measuring the presence of citrullinated histone H3 (Cit-H3) in conjunction with the presence of NETs may help clarify the kinetics of the response of NETs to systemic stress.

In preliminary studies, we recently identified NETs immunocytochemically in sputum and blood smear samples from intensive care unit (ICU) patients [24,25], whereas NETs could not be detected in blood smears from healthy volunteers [25].

In the present study, we used immunofluorescence to prospectively explore the existence of NETs and Cit-H3 in the blood of critically ill patients hospitalized in an ICU.

The respiratory tract is considered one of the most vulnerable places for bacterial invasion of the body, and NETs might start to be produced in response to pathogens before infection is completely apparent. Therefore, in this study we evaluated the presence of bacteria by Gram staining in tracheal aspirate as the preclinical stage of manifested infection to highlight its relationship with the induction of NETs in blood. The purpose of this study was to evaluate the relationships between NET or Cit-H3 and various clinical and biological parameters.

Materials and Methods

Patients and Setting

This study was a prospective observational study and was approved by the Ethics Committee of Osaka University Graduate School of Medicine. The institutional review board waived the need for informed consent. From April to June 2011, we examined blood samples collected from all patients who required intubation at the time of admission into the ICU of the Trauma and Acute Critical Care Center at the Osaka University Hospital (Osaka, Japan).

Evaluation of Clinical Background and Severity of Illness

Age, sex, Acute Physiological And Chronic Health Evaluation (APACHE) II score, and Sequential Organ Failure Assessment (SOFA) score were recorded at the time of admission. Systemic inflammatory response syndrome (SIRS) was diagnosed at the time of admission on the basis of the criteria for SIRS defined by the American College of Chest Physicians/Society of Critical Care Medicine Consensus [26]. At admission, the blood samples were analyzed to obtain the following laboratory data: white blood cell (WBC) count and concentrations of lactate, IL-8, TNF-α, HMGB1, and cf-DNA. WBC count was measured by an automated hematology analyzer (KX-21N; Sysmex, Hyogo, Japan). Lactate concentration was measured by a blood gas analyzer (ABL 835 Flex; Radiometer, Brønshøj, Denmark). The serum levels of IL-8 (R&D Systems, Minneapolis, MN, USA), TNF-α (R&D Systems), and HMGB1 (Shino-Test Corporation, Tokyo, Japan) were measured by enzyme-linked immunosorbent assay (ELISA) kits, and cf-DNA concentration was quantified using the Quant-iT PicoGreen dsDNA Assay kit (Invitrogen, Carlsbad, CA, USA), according to the manufacturer's instructions.

Immunofluorescence Analysis to Identify the Presence of NETs and Cit-H3

For histological analysis, each blood sample collected at the time of admission to the ICU was immediately smeared in a thin layer on a glass slide. After drying, the specimens were stored at −80°C until immunostaining was performed. We confirmed that this sample preparation method did not induce additional generation of NETs or citrullination of histone H3 using neutrophils isolated from healthy donors on the smear (Fig. S1). To identify NETs, DNA and histone H3, the main components in NETs, were visualized simultaneously by immunofluorescence, and Cit-H3 was also detected using a specific antibody as follows. The sample on the glass slide was fixed with 4% paraformaldehyde for 30 min, washed with phosphate-buffered saline (PBS) (pH 7.4), and then blocked with a solution containing 20% Block-Ace (Dainippon-Sumitomo Seiyaku, Osaka, Japan) and 0.005% saponin in PBS for 10 min. The samples were then incubated for 60 min with the primary antibody as follows: anti-human histone H3 mouse monoclonal antibody (diluted 1:100) (MABI0001; MAB Institute, Inc., Hokkaido, Japan) and anti-human Cit-H3 rabbit polyclonal antibody (1:100) (ab5103; Abcam, Cambridge, UK). After washing in PBS, each primary antibody was visualized using secondary antibodies coupled to 1:500 Alexa Fluor 546 goat anti-mouse IgG (Invitrogen) and 1:500 Alexa Fluor 488 goat anti-rabbit IgG (Invitrogen). The primary and secondary antibodies were diluted with 5% Block-Ace and 0.005% saponin in PBS. After incubation for 60 min with the secondary antibodies, the specimens were washed with PBS, and the DNA was stained with 4′,6-diamidino-2-phenylindole (DAPI; Invitrogen) in PBS for 5 min. All procedures were performed at room temperature. The specimens were analyzed using a confocal laser-scanning microscope (BZ-9000; Keyence Corporation; Osaka, Japan).

The validity of immunostaining was ensured by the negative results of control experiments in which whole mouse or rabbit IgG (Abcam) was used instead of primary antibodies or primary antibodies were omitted in the procedure (Fig. S2). In addition, neutrophils stimulated with phorbol myristate acetate from healthy donors were used as a positive control for immunostaining (Fig. S3).

In the preliminary experiments, string-like structure extending from the cell body, which was positive for DNA and histone, was exclusively also positive for neutrophil elastase (Fig. S4). Hence, we considered the extracellular component that is double-positive for DNA and H3 to be a NET. The production of NETs and the specific expression of the citrullination of histone H3 in neutrophils were confirmed using anti-CD66b antibody (Fig. 1). Diff-Quik staining revealed the presence of a variety of blood cells in the smears (Fig. S5).

For the purpose of estimating the presence of NETs and the occurrence of citrullination of histone H3 concurrently, triple staining for DNA, H3, and citrullinated H3 was performed in this study. Samples were considered negative for the presence of NETs or Cit-H3 if cells harboring NETs or Cit-H3 were not identified in 300 neutrophils by immunostaining. If at least one of NETs and Cit-H3 was positive in the smear according to the definition mentioned above, the corresponding patient was classified into the "NET- and/or Cit-H3-positive" group.

Detection of the presence of bacteria in tracheal aspirate

Aspiration is defined as the inhalation of oropharyngeal or gastric contents into the larynx and lower respiratory tract, and

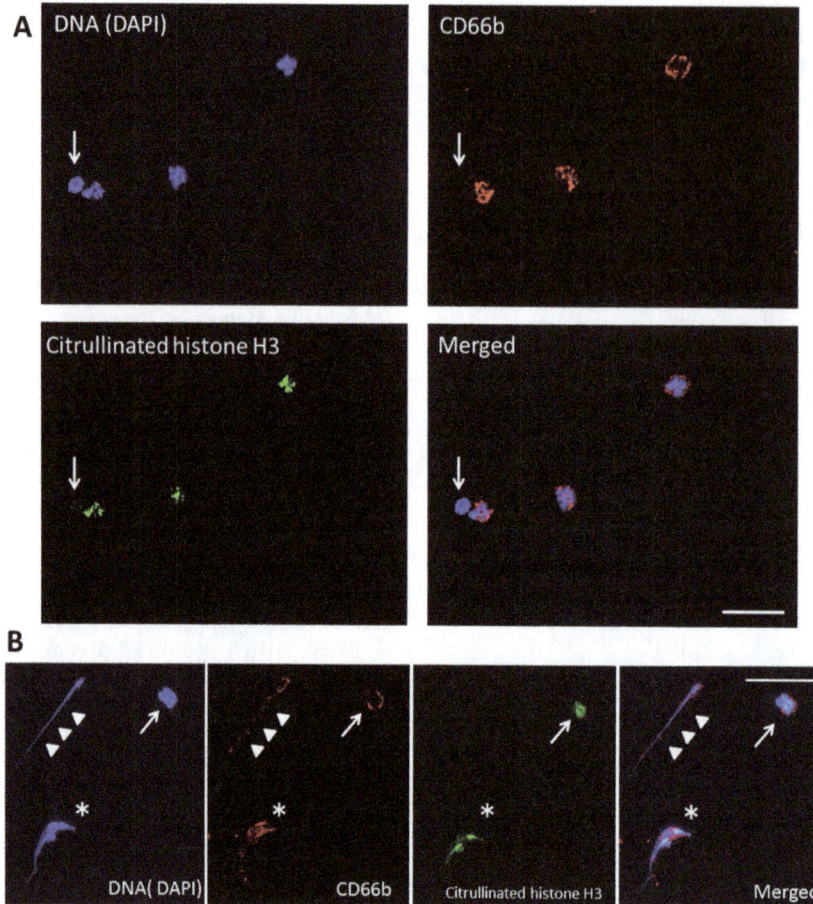

Figure 1. Representative images of immunostaining using anti-CD66b antibody in the blood smear sample from a critically ill patient. Triple staining by DAPI, anti-CD66b antibody, and anti-citrullinated histone H3 was performed using the blood smear sample obtained from a critically ill patient. A. The CD66b-positive cells were subjected to citrullination of histone H3 in their nuclei. Citrullination of histone H3 was not detected in the CD66b-negative cell (arrow). B. Arrow indicates the occurrence of citrullination of histone H3 in a neutrophil that had immunoreactivity against CD66b. Arrowheads indicate NETs stained with CD66b, whose appearance was of a string-like structure extending from the cell body. Asterisk indicates a neutrophil that was beginning to release NETs from its ruptured cell body. Interestingly, freshly produced NETs (asterisk) held immunoreactivity against citrullination of histone H3. In contrast, elongated NETs (arrowheads) were not stained with anti- citrullinated histone H3 antibody. Blue, DAPI; Red, CD66b; Green, citrullinated histone H3. (Magnification ×400). Scale bar; 50 μm.

aspiration pneumonia is an infectious process caused by the inhalation of oropharyngeal secretions that are colonized by pathogenic bacteria [27]. The presence of bacteria in tracheal aspirate by Gram staining is regarded as part of aspiration that favors the development of infection. In this study, we evaluated the presence of bacteria in tracheal aspirate as the preclinical stage of manifested infection. To screen for the presence of bacteria in tracheal aspirate, an aspirated sputum smear was also prepared independently from immunostaining at the time of each patient's admission to the ICU. For Gram staining, the smear was dried, stained with crystal violet (Merck KGaA, Darmstadt, Germany) followed by iodine (Merck KGaA), washed with 99.5% ethanol (Wako Pure Chemical Industries, Ltd., Osaka, Japan), and stained with Safranin (Merck KGaA). Images were captured on an optical microscope system (ECLIPSE 50i; Nikon Instruments Inc., Tokyo, Japan).

Statistical Analysis

Continuous variables are presented as the median and interquartile range (IQR). The Wilcoxon rank-sum test and Pearson's chi-square test were used to compare two patient groups.

Single and multiple logistic regression analyses were used to identify associations between the presence of NETs and/or Cit-H3 and the clinical and biological parameters studied. A p-value of < .05 was considered significant. All statistical analyses were performed using JMP 9.0.2 (SAS Institute Inc., Cary, NC, USA) and reviewed by a statistician.

Results

Patient Characteristics

During the study period, 263 patients were admitted to the ICU; 49 of these 263 patients were intubated patients and were included in this study. We excluded patients with cardiopulmonary arrest (CPA) who could not be resuscitated on admission. The patients' characteristics are shown in Table 1. The study group comprised 29 men and 20 women with a median age of 66.0 (IQR, 52.5–76.0) years. The median APACHE II score was 18.0 (IQR, 12.5–21.5), and the median SOFA score was 5.0 (IQR, 4.0–8.0). Thirty-eight patients (77.6%) were diagnosed as having SIRS, and 22 patients (44.9%) were judged as positive for "the presence of bacteria in tracheal aspirate". Thirty-six patients (73.5%)

survived and 13 patients died. The ICU mortality rate of intubated patients during this study period was 26.5%. The median WBC count was 10,900/μL (IQR, 8215–14,915/μL). The diagnoses included trauma (n = 7, 14.3%), infection (n = 14, 28.6%), resuscitation from CPA (n = 8, 16.3%), acute poisoning (n = 4, 8.1%), heart disease (n = 4, 8.1%), brain stroke (n = 8, 16.3%), heat stroke (n = 2, 4.1%), and others (n = 2, 4.1%) (Table 2).

Presence of NETs and Cit-H3 in the Bloodstream

NETs were identified as extracellular string-like structures that were simultaneously immunoreactive for DNA and histone H3 (Fig. 2). Cit-H3 was detected by a specific antibody, and its presence was confirmed to be located inside lobulated nuclei and histone H3 (Fig. 3). In the blood smears surveyed in this study, we identified NETs in 5 patients and Cit-H3 in 11 patients (Table 2). Both NETs and Cit-H3 were identified concurrently in one patient with infection. We detected the presence of circulating NETs and/or Cit-H3-positive cells in samples from patients with infection (4/14, 28.6%), resuscitation from CPA (5/8, 62.5%), acute poisoning (1/4, 25.0%), brain stroke (3/8, 37.5%), and heat stroke (1/2, 50.0%). We found no NETs or Cit-H3-positive cells in samples from patients with trauma (0/7) or heart disease (0/4).

Identification of Factors Related to the Presence of NETs and Cit-H3 in the Bloodstream

We tried to identify the factors that are related to the presence of NETs or Cit-H3 in the bloodstream. We first examined clinical parameters recorded at the time of admission including age, APACHE II and SOFA scores, number of patients who presented with SIRS or with the presence of bacteria in tracheal aspirate, and biological parameters such as the total WBC count and concentrations of lactate, IL-8, TNF-α, HMGB1, and cf-DNA. We also recorded the number of survivors. We compared these variables between the patients positive or negative for NETs and/or Cit-H3. The results are shown in Table 3. Among the factors evaluated in this research, only "the presence of bacteria in tracheal aspirate" differed significantly between the NET- and/or Cit-H3-positive and -negative groups ($p<.01$, Wilcoxon rank-sum test and Pearson's chi-square test). The other factors were not significantly related to the presence of NETs and/or Cit-H3. In patients classified into two groups based on the presence or absence of bacteria in tracheal aspirate, the occurrence rate of NETs and/or Cit-H3 was significantly higher in "the presence of bacteria in tracheal aspirate" (BTA (+)) group (11/22, 50.0%) than

in "the absence of bacteria in tracheal aspirate" (BTA (−)) group (4/27, 14.8%) ($p<.01$) (Table S1). In patients with SIRS on admission, there was a trend toward greater expression of NETs and/or Cit-H3 ($p = .079$) (Table S2).

Logistic regression analysis was performed to identify the factors related to the presence of NETs and Cit-H3 in the bloodstream. The results of single logistic regression analysis of factors associated with the presence of NETs and Cit-H3 are shown in Table 4. Only BTA (+) at the time of intubation was a significant factor associated with the presence of NETs and Cit-H3 ($p = .0112$). Although there were indications of a trend toward an association between the presence of circulating NETs and/or Cit-H3 and the comorbid conditions of SIRS or elevated cf-DNA concentration ($p = .1093$ and.3003, respectively), these were not statistically significant. Table 5 shows the results of multiple logistic regression analysis of factors associated with the presence of NETs and/or Cit-H3 and model selection. Two methods of multiple regression analysis, backward and forward regression, yielded similar models. Again, "the presence of bacteria in tracheal aspirate" was the only factor that was significantly related to the presence of NETs and/or Cit-H3 in the bloodstream; the odds ratio for aspiration was 5.750.

Discussion

A series of in vitro and animal experiments have uncovered a suppressive function of NETs against the dissemination of microorganisms in blood by mechanical trapping and by exploiting coagulant function to segregate these microorganisms within the circulation [28,29]. However, direct evidence remains scarce in living human systems. In this clinical study of blood smears, we attempted to identify morphologically the presence of NETs and Cit-H3 in the bloodstream of critically ill patients at the time of admission to the ICU and to characterize the factors associated with the presence of NETs and Cit-H3.

Among the 49 enrolled patients, immunofluorescence analysis revealed blood-borne NETs in five patients (10.2%), Cit-H3 in 11 patients (22.4%), and NETs and/or Cit-H3 in 15 patients (30.6%) (Table 2). These data replicate the results of our previous preliminary study in which NETs were present in patients in a critical condition [25] and show for the first time, to our knowledge, the presence of Cit-H3 in circulating blood cells. Cit-H3-positive cells possessed a multi-segmented nucleus, and most were immunoreactive for CD66b (Fig. 1), suggesting that citrullination of histone H3 occurred exclusively in neutrophils.

Table 1. Patient characteristics.

Variable	Value
No. of patients (M/F)	49 (29/20)
Age (years, median, IQR)	66.0 (52.5–76.0)
APACHE II score (median, IQR)	18.0 (12.5–21.5)
SOFA score (median, IQR)	5 (4–8)
No. of patients with SIRS	38 (77.6%)
The presence of bacteria in tracheal aspirate	22 (44.9%)
No. of survivors	36 (73.5%)
WBC (median, IQR)	10,900 (8215–14,915)

During the study period, 263 patients were admitted to the ICU of whom 49 were intubated and were included in this study. We excluded patients with cardiopulmonary arrest who could not be resuscitated on admission. IQR: interquartile range, APACHE: Acute Physiological And Chronic Health Evaluation, SOFA: Sequential Organ Failure Assessment, SIRS: systemic inflammatory response syndrome, WBC: white blood cell.

Table 2. Diagnoses and the number of patients exhibiting neutrophil extracellular traps and citrullinated histone H3 in each diagnostic group.

Diagnosis	NET positive (n)	Cit-H3 positive (n)	NET and/or Cit-H3 positive (%)
Trauma (n = 7)	0	0	0/7 (0)
Infection (n = 14)	3	2	4/14 (28.6)
Resuscitated from cardiopulmonary arrest (n = 8)	2	3	5/8 (62.5)
Acute poisoning (n = 4)	0	1	1/4 (25.0)
Heart disease (n = 4)	0	0	0/4 (0)
Brain stroke (n = 8)	0	3	3/8 (37.5)
Heat stroke (n = 2)	0	1	1/2 (50.0)
Others (n = 2)	0	1	1/2 (50.0)
Total (n = 49)	5	11	15/49 (30.6)

In the blood smears surveyed in this study, we identified NETs in 5 patients and Cit-H3 in 11 patients. Both NETs and Cit-H3 were identified concurrently in one patient with infection. We found no NETs or Cit-H3-positive cells in samples from patients with trauma (0/7) or heart disease (0/4). NETs: neutrophil extracellular trap, Cit-H3: citrullinated histone H3.

Citrullination of histone H3 is considered an important process in the release of NETs through decondensation of chromatin [14,22,23]. Interestingly, the occurrence ratio of Cit-H3 was twice that of NETs. In vitro experiments imply that a substantial period of time is necessary to expel NETs extracellularly after the initiation of cell death by a stress stimulus [12,30,31]. However, it is still not clear how much time is required in vivo for NETs to appear intravascularly. The number of patients who exhibited circulating NETs in this study was lower than anticipated. We collected blood samples on admission to the ICU, and the timing might have been too early to detect NETs after the onset of a critical illness. The 11 Cit-H3-positive patients could be considered to have been in an early stage of NET formation. The change in the appearance of NETs and Cit-H3 during the course of hospitalization should be studied. If it can be shown clinically that Cit-H3 expression is followed by NET formation, it might be important to evaluate Cit-H3 expression in the blood upon admission to an ICU.

Table 2 shows that NETs and Cit-H3 were detected in patients with infection, resuscitation from CPA, acute poisoning, brain stroke, or heat stroke; surprisingly, we could not detect NETs or Cit-H3 in patients with trauma or heart disease. NETs are formed

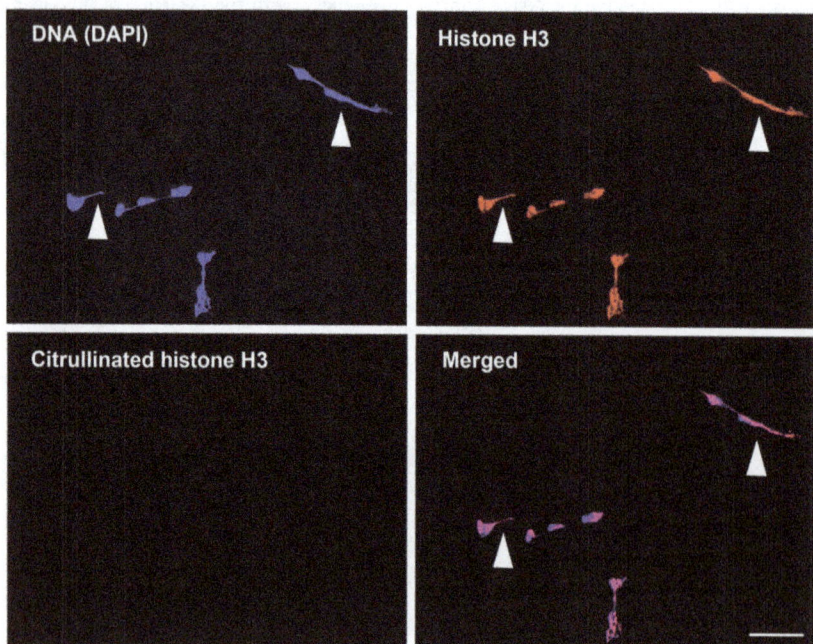

Figure 2. Representative images of immunofluorescence staining to detect neutrophil extracellular traps (NETs). NETs were visualized in the blood smear samples by immunocytochemistry and identified as extracellular string-like structures composed of chromatin (DNA and histone H3). NETs were present in the bloodstream of critically ill patients. Citrullination of histone H3 was not recognized in these images. In the blood smears surveyed in this study, we identified NETs in five patients (5/49, 10.2%). Blue, 4′,6-diamidino-2-phenylindole (DAPI); red, histone H3; green, citrullinated histone H3. Arrowheads indicate the double-stained areas containing NETs (Magnification ×400). Scale bar; 50 μm.

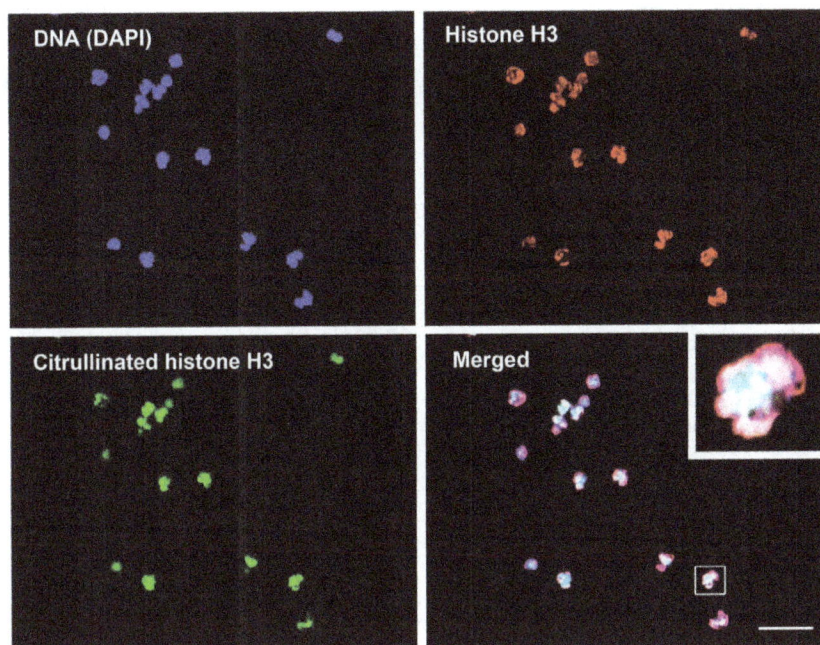

Figure 3. Representative images of immunofluorescence staining to detect citrullinated histone H3 (Cit-H3). Citrullination of histone H3, which is a critical enzymatic process to produce NETs through decondensation of chromatin, was visualized in the blood smear samples using anti-citrullinated histone H3 antibody by immunohistochemistry. Cit-H3 was present in the bloodstream of critically ill patients. The inset in the merged image is the magnified image of a representative cell (white rectangle) expressing citrullinated histone H3 in the nucleus. Neutrophil extracellular traps are not recognized here. In the blood smears surveyed in this study, we identified Cit-H3 in 11 patients (11/49, 22.4%). Blue, 4',6-diamidino-2-phenylindole (DAPI); red, histone H3; green, citrullinated histone H3 (Magnification ×400). Scale bar; 50 μm.

in response to various microorganisms and pathogens [14]. McDonald et al reported that NETs ensnare circulating bacteria and provide intravascular immunity that protects against bacterial dissemination during septic infection [29]. In this context, the presence of NETs and/or Cit-H3 in infected patients is to be expected. By contrast, trauma or heart disease patients were

Table 3. Comparison between patients positive and negative for neutrophil extracellular traps and/or citrullinated histone H3.

	NET and/or citrullinated histone H3		
	Positive	Negative	*p*
Number	15	34	
Age (years)	67.0 (49.0–78.0)	65.5 (56.8–75.3)	.8197
APACHE II score	20.0 (16.0–23.0)	17.5 (11.8–21.3)	.3171
SOFA score	6.0 (5.0–10.0)	5.0 (4.0–8.0)	.4062
Survivors (n)	10 (66.7%)	26 (76.5%)	.4737
SIRS patients (n)	14 (93.3%)	24 (70.6%)	.0786
The presence of bacteria in tracheal aspirate (n)	11 (73.3%)	11 (32.3%)	.0079
WBC count (/μl)	12,430 (8310.0–16510.0)	10,835 (8032.5–14307.5)	.5654
IL-8 (pg/mL)	57.6 (19.9–143.0)	65.3 (23.3–229.5)	.9136
TNF-α (pg/mL)	8.2 (6.2–21.6)	9.0 (4.8–16.3)	.9740
cf-DNA (ng/mL)	1038.3 (744.9–1329.7)	1072.7 (828.6–1770.7)	.6025
Lactate (mg/mL)	39 (11.0–71.0)	17.5 (12.0–56.3)	.5010
HMGB1 (ng/mL)	11.0 (6.8–21.5)	9.7 (5.9–16.3)	.5151

Among the factors evaluated to highlight the relation to the presence of NETs or Cit-H3 in the bloodstream, only "the presence of bacteria in tracheal aspirate" differed significantly between the NET- and/or Cit-H3-positive and -negative groups ($p<.01$). The other factors were not significantly related to the presence of NETs and/or Cit-H3. Continuous variables are presented as the median and IQR unless otherwise noted. The Wilcoxon rank-sum test and Pearson's chi-square test were used to compare two patient groups. NETs: neutrophil extracellular traps, Cit-H3: citrullinated histone H3, IQR: interquartile range, APACHE: Acute Physiological And Chronic Health Evaluation, SOFA: Sequential Organ Failure Assessment, SIRS: systemic inflammatory response syndrome, WBC: white blood cell, IL: interleukin, TNF: tumor necrosis factor, cf-DNA: circulating free DNA, HMGB1: high mobility group box-1.

Table 4. Results of single logistic regression analysis.

Variable	p
The presence of bacteria in tracheal aspirate	.0112
SIRS	.1093
cf-DNA	.3003
Lactate	.5476
WBC count	.7862
IL-8	.7875
TNF-α	.8321
HMGB1	.9439

Logistic regression analysis was performed to identify the factors related to the presence of NET and Cit-H3 in the bloodstream. Only "the presence of bacteria in tracheal aspirate" (+) at the time of intubation was a significant factor associated with the presence of NET and Cit-H3 ($p = .0112$). NETs: neutrophil extracellular traps, Cit-H3: citrullinated histone H3, SIRS: systemic inflammatory response syndrome, cf-DNA: circulating free DNA, WBC: white blood cell, IL: interleukin, TNF: tumor necrosis factor, HMGB1: high mobility group box-1.

transported to the hospital immediately after the onset of the condition, and there was no potential risk of infection on admission; this may explain why NETs and Cit-H3 were not detected in these patients.

Intriguingly, a high percentage (62.5%) of patients with CPA exhibited circulating NETs and/or Cit-H3. Acute poisoning, brain stroke, and heat stroke are clinical conditions that can cause disturbance of consciousness, which may induce aspiration. Adnet and Baud demonstrated that the risk of aspiration increases with the degree of unconsciousness (as measured by the Glasgow Coma Scale [GCS]) [32]. In the present study population, the GCS score on admission was significantly lower in the BTA (+) group than in the BTA (−) group (4 [IQR, 3–10.75] vs 13 [IQR, 7–14]; $p < .01$). Except for the infected patient group, the patients who exhibited NETs and/or Cit-H3 in their blood had a significantly lower GCS score on admission ($p = .0418$). We therefore investigated whether "the presence of bacteria in tracheal aspirate", which was represented as part of aspiration and as the presumable preclinical stage of manifested infection, was associated with the presence of NETs and/or Cit-H3, and found a significant association (odds ratio for aspiration, 5.750) (Tables 3–5). Bacteria drawn into the respiratory tract can induce epithelial injury, which provides an opportunity for bacterial translocation as well as leukocyte transmigration until completion of epithelial repair [33,34]. Concomitance of acid aspiration under impaired consciousness additionally enhances bacterial adherence to the epithelium [35]. Injured airway epithelium produces cytokines including IL-8 and alarmins such as HMGB1, both of which are representative inducers for NETs [36–39]. Next, bacteria and inflammatory

mediators infiltrating into the interstitial space secondary to epithelial injury will affect the endothelial integrity [40]. The presence of NETs in sputum following aspiration, a phenomenon that we reported previously [24], suggests breakdown of the epithelial barrier that is induced by local inflammation through direct contact between aspirated bacteria and epithelium or through activation of resident immune cells such as macrophages in the respiratory tract [41]. Such epithelial breakdown would allow influx of pathogens, pathogen-associated molecular patterns, cytokines, chemokines, and alarmins from the lumen of the respiratory tract into the circulation. These materials might stimulate the production of NETs intravenously to inhibit systemic invasion of bacteria. We assumed that NETs are induced in the respiratory tract to suppress bacterial dissemination leading to pneumonia and in the vessels to inhibit bacteremia against the invasion of bacteria into the blood and that even such colonization of bacteria in the respiratory tract could trigger citrullination of histone H3 to produce NETs in blood. Single logistic regression analyses of whether infection and/or BTA (+) were associated with the presence of NETs and/or Cit-H3 produced an odds ratio of 7.312 (Table S3). These results suggest that induction of NETs systemically through the citrullination of histone H3 in blood maybe an initial response for protection against bacterial dissemination from latent respiratory infection.

Some researchers consider cf-DNA to be equivalent to NETs in the blood [15,16]. However, our results showed that the occurrence rate of NETs and/or Cit-H3 was not significantly associated with cf-DNA concentration ($p = .6025$) (Table 3). Although the number of patients was different due to sample limitations, additional analysis by MPO-DNA ELISA (Data S1) was also performed. As a result, there was no difference in the values between the group positive for (0.076 [IQR, 0.067–0.100]; $n = 8$) and the group negative for NET and/or citrullinated histone H3 (0.078 [IQR, 0.070–0.111]; $n = 26$). We reported recently that in patients with an acute respiratory infection, NETs became fragmented during recovery from infection [24], suggesting that NETs should also be digested in the blood with time. Our method using blood smear samples cannot detect NETs that harbor inside vessels or that are already degraded. The method based on MPO-DNA ELISA might also measure neutrophil DNA fragments derived from necrosis or apoptosis and cannot detect NETs that are not truncated from the cell body. We consider that at the early phase of critical illness, i.e., when the production of NETs is just starting, the morphological approach has an advantage in being able to detect NETs that are still anchored to the cell body, in conjunction with the merit that identification of citrullination of histone H3 is possible at a stage prior to the release of NETs.

HMGB1 is a nuclear protein present in the nucleus of all nucleated cells. HMGB1 binds to DNA and acts as an inflammatory mediator once it is released extracellularly [42,43]. In this study, HMGB1 was significantly higher in SIRS patients

Table 5. Results of multiple logistic regression analysis of factors associated with the presence of neutrophil extracellular traps and/or citrullinated histone H3.

	Coeff (β)	p	OR	Lower	Upper
"the presence of bacteria in tracheal aspirate"	0.875	0.011	5.750	1.583	24.755

Two methods of multiple regression analysis, backward and forward regression, yielded similar models. "The presence of bacteria in tracheal aspirate" was the only factor that was significantly related to the presence of neutrophil extracellular traps and/or citrullinated histone H3 in the bloodstream. The odds ratio for aspiration was 5.750. Coeff (β): coefficient; OR: odds ratio, Lower: lower level of 95% confidence interval, Upper: upper level of 95% confidence interval.

than in non-SIRS patients (Table S2). Unexpectedly, however, HMGB1 was not a significant factor associated with the presence of NETs and/or Cit-H3 (Tables 3–5). NETs contain HMGB1 [44], and one possibility is that HMGB1 binding to NETs is not reflected in the amount of circulating HMGB1 measured by ELISA.

Although IL-8 and TNF-α are considered stimulatory factors that induce NET formation [14,39,45], they were not associated with the presence of NETs and/or Cit-H3 in this study (Tables 3–5). This negative result suggest the presence of an unknown complex regulatory mechanism for the production of NETs in vivo.

As limitations of this study, first, the sample size was small, and the patients were very heterogeneous. Second, we evaluated the presence of NETs and Cit-H3 and the associated factors in the bloodstream of critically ill patients only at admission. It should be investigated in the future how NETs are processed after the induction of NETosis in the circulation. It is presumable that NETs could be degraded by DNase, and the fragments would contribute partially to the formation of cf-DNA. Third, we did not rigorously quantify the amount of NETs and Cit-H3. The possibility of the degradation of NETs and the difficulty in detecting NETs, which are anchored in the vessels, might lead to underestimation of the presence of NETs in our method using blood smear samples. Further study is required to establish finer methods of quantification. We hope that future elucidation of the biological significance of NETs will lead to new strategies to treat critical illness by monitoring NET formation in blood.

Conclusions

The presence of NETs and Cit-H3 were identified immunocytochemically in the bloodstream of a subset of critically ill patients. "The presence of bacteria in tracheal aspirate" may be one important factor related to the presence of circulating NETs. NETs may play a pivotal role in biological defense in the bloodstream of infected and potentially infected patients.

Supporting Information

Figure S1   Representative images of immunostaining of isolated neutrophils that underwent drying and freezing steps before fixation. We tried to evaluate the influence of drying and freezing steps preceding paraformaldehyde fixation on the induction of NETs or citrullination of histone H3 in smear samples. For this, neutrophils separated by density gradient centrifugation from whole blood of a healthy donor were smeared on glass slides, dried, and frozen before fixation. At least through this method, the presence of NETs or citrullinated histone H3 was not identified in immunostaining. Blue, Hoechst 33342; Red, histone H3; Green, citrullinated histone H3 (left panels) or neutrophil elastase (right panels) (Magnification ×400). Scale bar; 50 μm.

Figure S2   Representative images of immunostaining for the negative control study using isotype control antibodies. To ensure accuracy for the immunoreactivity of primary antibodies against blood smear samples, whole mouse and rabbit IgG were used instead of primary antibodies in the immunostaining procedure. This control study resulted in negative signals for histone H3 and citrullinated histone H3. Blue, 4′,6-

diamidino-2-phenylindole (DAPI); Red, histone H3; Green, citrullinated histone H3. (Magnification ×200). Scale bar; 50 μm.

Figure S3   Representative images of immunostaining to detect citrullinated histone H3 (left panels) and neutrophil extracellular traps (NETs) (right panels) in the neutrophils from a healthy donor stimulated by phorbol myristate acetate. Neutrophils were isolated by density gradient centrifugation from the whole blood of a healthy donor and stimulated by phorbol myristate acetate. Citrullinated histone H3 and NETs were detected by immunohistochemistry using the same antibodies that were used against the smear samples collected from the critically ill patients. Blue, Hoechst 33342; Red, histone H3; Green, citrullinated histone H3 (left panels) or neutrophil elastase (right panels). (Magnification ×400). Scale bar; 50 μm.

Figure S4   Representative images of immunostaining to detect neutrophil extracellular traps (NETs) in the blood smear from a critically ill patient. The presence of circulating NETs was confirmed by immunohistochemistry using anti-neutrophil elastase antibody. String-like structures extending from the cell body (arrowheads) were composed of DNA and histone, and they contained neutrophil elastase. Blue, 4′,6-diamidino-2-phenylindole (DAPI); Red, histone H1; Green, Neutrophil elastase. (Magnification ×400). Scale bar; 50 μm.

Figure S5   Diff-Quik staining of a blood smear sample from the critically ill patient. Diff-Quik staining confirmed a subpopulation of cells other than neutrophils. (Magnification ×400). Scale bar; 50 μm.

Table S1   Comparison between patients presenting with and without "the presence of bacteria in tracheal aspirate". In patients classified into two groups based on the presence or absence of bacteria in tracheal aspirate, the rate of occurrence of NETs and/or Cit-H3 was significantly higher in "the presence of bacteria in tracheal aspirate" group (11/22, 50.0%) than in "the absence of bacteria in tracheal aspirate" group (4/27, 14.8%) ($p<.01$). Continuous variables are presented as the median and IQR unless otherwise noted. The Wilcoxon rank-sum test and Pearson's chi-square test were used to compare the two patient groups. NETs: neutrophil extracellular traps, Cit-H3: citrullinated histone H3, IQR: interquartile range, APACHE: Acute Physiological And Chronic Health Evaluation, SOFA: Sequential Organ Failure Assessment, SIRS: systemic inflammatory response syndrome, WBC: white blood cell, IL: interleukin, TNF: tumor necrosis factor, cf-DNA: circulating free DNA, HMGB1: high mobility group box-1.

Table S2   Comparison between patients with and without systemic inflammatory response syndrome. In patients with SIRS on admission, there was a trend toward greater expression of NETs and/or Cit-H3 ($p = .079$). Continuous variables are presented as the median and IQR unless otherwise noted. The Wilcoxon rank-sum test and Pearson's chi-square test were used to compare the two patient groups. NETs: neutrophil extracellular traps, Cit-H3: citrullinated histone H3, IQR: interquartile range, APACHE: Acute Physiological And Chronic Health Evaluation, SOFA: Sequential Organ Failure Assessment, SIRS: systemic inflammatory response syndrome,

WBC: white blood cell, IL: interleukin, TNF: tumor necrosis factor, cf-DNA: circulating free DNA, HMGB1: high mobility group box-1.

Table S3 Results of single logistic regression analysis of factors associated with the presence of neutrophil extracellular traps and/or citrullinated histone H3 according to the presence of infection and/or "the presence of bacteria in tracheal aspirate".

Single logistic regression analyses of whether infection and/or "the presence of bacteria in tracheal aspirate" were associated with the presence of NETs and/or Cit-H3 produced an odds ratio of 7.312. Coeff (β):

coefficient, OR: odds ratio, Lower: lower level of 95% confidence interval, Upper: upper level of 95% confidence interval.

Data S1 MPO-DNA ELISA.

Author Contributions

Conceived and designed the experiments: TH SH NM TI. Performed the experiments: TH SH NM TI HH NY. Analyzed the data: TH SH NM TI MS OT NY KY YA KO TS KT. Contributed reagents/materials/analysis tools: TH SH HH NY. Wrote the paper: TH SH NM.

References

1. Lekstrom-Himes JA, Gallin JI (2000) Immunodeficiency diseases caused by defects in phagocytes. New Engl J Med 343: 1703–1714.
2. Savchenko AS, Inoue A, Ohashi R, Jiang S, Hasegawa G, et al. (2011) Long pentraxin 3 (PTX3) expression and release by neutrophils in vitro and in ulcerative colitis. Pathol Int 61: 290–297.
3. Vitkov L, Klappacher M, Hannig M, Krautgartner WD (2009) Extracellular neutrophil traps in periodontitis. J Periodontal Res 44: 664–672.
4. Garcia-Romo GS, Caielli S, Vega B, Connolly J, Allantaz F, et al. (2011) Netting neutrophils are major inducers of type I IFN production in pediatric systemic lupus erythematosus. Sci Transl Med 3: 73ra20.
5. Kessenbrock K, Krumbholz M, Schonermarck U, Back W, Gross WL, et al. (2009) Netting neutrophils in autoimmune small-vessel vasculitis. Nat Med 15: 623–625.
6. Brinkmann V, Reichard U, Goosmann C, Fauler B, Uhlemann Y, et al. (2004) Neutrophil extracellular traps kill bacteria. Science 303: 1532–1535.
7. Jaillon S, Peri G, Delneste Y, Fremaux I, Doni A, et al. (2007) The humoral pattern recognition receptor PTX3 is stored in neutrophil granules and localizes in extracellular traps. J Exp Med 204: 793–804.
8. Curran CS, Demick KP, Mansfield JM (2006) Lactoferrin activates macrophages via TLR4-dependent and -independent signaling pathways. Cell Immunol 242: 23–30.
9. Zhang LT, Yao YM, Lu JQ, Yan XJ, Yu Y, et al. (2008) Recombinant bactericidal/permeability-increasing protein inhibits endotoxin-induced high-mobility group box 1 protein gene expression in sepsis. Shock 29: 278–284.
10. Urban CF, Ermert D, Schmid M, Abu-Abed U, Goosmann C, et al. (2009) Neutrophil extracellular traps contain calprotectin, a cytosolic protein complex involved in host defense against Candida albicans. PLoS Pathog 5: e1000639.
11. Cho JH, Fraser IP, Fukase K, Kusumoto S, Fujimoto Y, et al. (2005) Human peptidoglycan recognition protein S is an effector of neutrophil-mediated innate immunity. Blood 106: 2551–2558.
12. Fuchs TA, Abed U, Goosmann C, Hurwitz R, Schulze I, et al. (2007) Novel cell death program leads to neutrophil extracellular traps. J Cell Biol 176: 231–241.
13. Logters T, Margraf S, Altrichter J, Cinatl J, Mitzner S, et al. (2009) The clinical value of neutrophil extracellular traps. Med Microbiol Immunol 198: 211–219.
14. Remijsen Q, Kuijpers TW, Wirawan E, Lippens S, Vandenabeele P, et al. (2011) Dying for a cause: NETosis, mechanisms behind an antimicrobial cell death modality. Cell Death Differ 18: 581–588.
15. Margraf S, Logters T, Reipen J, Altrichter J, Scholz M, et al. (2008) Neutrophil-derived circulating free DNA (cf-DNA/NETs): A potential prognostic marker for posttraumatic development of inflammatory second hit and sepsis. Shock 30: 352–358.
16. Logters T, Paunel-Gorgulu A, Zilkens C, Altrichter J, Scholz M, et al. (2009) Diagnostic accuracy of neutrophil-derived circulating free DNA (cf-DNA/NETs) for septic arthritis. J Orthop Res 27: 1401–1407.
17. Thijssen MA, Swinkels DW, Ruers TJ, de Kok JB (2002) Difference between free circulating plasma and serum DNA in patients with colorectal liver metastases. Anticancer Res 22: 421–425.
18. Sozzi G, Conte D, Leon M, Ciricione R, Roz L, Ratcliffe C, et al. (2003) Quantification of free circulating DNA as a diagnostic marker in lung cancer. J Clin Oncol 21: 3902–3908.
19. Kamat AA, Bischoff FZ, Dang D, Baldwin MF, Han LY, et al. (2006) Circulating cell-free DNA: A novel biomarker for response to therapy in ovarian carcinoma. Cancer Biol Ther 5: 1369–1374.
20. Swarup V, Rajeswari MR (2007) Circulating (cell-free) nucleic acids—a promising, non-invasive tool for early detection of several human diseases. FEBS Lett 581: 795–799.
21. van der Vaart M, Pretorius PJ (2007) The origin of circulating free DNA. Clin Chem 53: 2215.
22. Neeli I, Khan SN, Radic M (2008) Histone deimination as a response to inflammatory stimuli in neutrophils. J Immunol 180: 1895–1902.
23. Wang Y, Li M, Stadler S, Correll S, Li P, et al. (2009) Histone hypercitrullination mediates chromatin decondensation and neutrophil extracellular trap formation. J Cell Biol 184: 205–213.
24. Hirose T, Hamaguchi S, Matsumoto N, Irisawa T, Seki M, et al. (2012) Dynamic changes in the expression of neutrophil extracellular traps in acute respiratory infections. Am J Respir Crit Care Med 185: 1130–1131.
25. Hamaguchi S, Hirose T, Akeda Y, Matsumoto N, Irisawa T, et al. (2013) Identification of neutrophil extracellular traps in blood of patients with systemic inflammatory response syndrome. J Int Med Res 41: 162–168.
26. Bone RC, Balk RA, Cerra FB, Dellinger RP, Fein AM, et al. (1992) Definitions for sepsis and organ failure and guidelines for the use of innovative therapies in sepsis. The ACCP/SCCM Consensus Conference Committee. American College of Chest Physicians/Society of Critical Care Medicine. Chest 101: 1644–1655.
27. Marik PE (2001) Aspiration pneumonitis and aspiration pneumonia. N Engl J Med 344: 665–671.
28. Massberg S, Grahl L, von Bruehl ML, Manukyan D, Pfeiler S, et al. (2010) Reciprocal coupling of coagulation and innate immunity via neutrophil serine proteases. Nat Med 16: 887–896.
29. McDonald B, Urrutia R, Yipp BG, Jenne CN, Kubes P (2012) Intravascular neutrophil extracellular traps capture bacteria from the bloodstream during sepsis. Cell Host Microbe 12: 324–333.
30. Yipp BG, Petri B, Salina D, Jenne CN, Scott BN, et al. (2012) Infection-induced NETosis is a dynamic process involving neutrophil multitasking in vivo. Nat Med 18: 1386–1393.
31. Brinkmann V, Zychlinsky A (2007) Beneficial suicide: Why neutrophils die to make NETs. Nat Rev Microbiol 5: 577–582.
32. Adnet F, Baud F (1996) Relation between Glasgow Coma Scale and aspiration pneumonia. Lancet 348: 123–124.
33. Evans SE, Xu Y, Tuvim MJ, Dickey BF (2010) Inducible innate resistance of lung epithelium to infection. Annu Rev Physiol 72: 413–435.
34. Sousa S, Lecuit M, Cossart P (2005) Microbial strategies to target, cross or disrupt epithelia. Curr Opin Cell Biol 17: 489–498.
35. Mitsushima H, Oishi K, Nagao T, Ichinose A, Senba M, et al. (2002) Acid aspiration induces bacterial pneumonia by enhanced bacterial adherence in mice. Microb Pathog 33: 203–210.
36. Hippenstiel S, Opitz B, Schmeck B, Suttorp N (2006) Lung epithelium as a sentinel and effector system in pneumonia—molecular mechanisms of pathogen recognition and signal transduction. Respir Res 7: 97.
37. Pittet JF, Koh H, Fang X, Iles K, Christiaans S, et al. (2013) HMGB1 accelerates alveolar epithelial repair via an IL-1beta- and alphavbeta6 integrin-dependent activation of TGF-beta1. PLoS One 8: e63907.
38. Tadie JM, Bae HB, Jiang S, Park DW, Bell CP, et al. (2013) HMGB1 promotes neutrophil extracellular trap formation through interactions with Toll-like receptor 4. Am J Physiol Lung Cell Mol Physiol 304: L342–L349.
39. Gupta AK, Hasler P, Holzgreve W, Gebhardt S, Hahn S (2005) Induction of neutrophil extracellular DNA lattices by placental microparticles and IL-8 and their presence in preeclampsia. Hum Immunol 66: 1146–1154.
40. Hiraiwa K, Van Eeden SF (2014) Nature and consequences of the systemic inflammatory response induced by lung inflammation. Lung Inflammation. Available: http://www.intechopen.com/books/lung-inflammation/nature-and-consequences-of-the-systemic-inflammatory-response-induced-by-lung-inflammation. Accessed 2014 Jul 4.
41. Hussell T, Bell TJ (2014) Alveolar macrophages: plasticity in a tissue-specific context. Nat Rev Immunol 14: 81–93.
42. Wang H, Bloom O, Zhang M, Vishnubhakat JM, Ombrellino M, et al. (1999) HMG-1 as a late mediator of endotoxin lethality in mice. Science 285: 248–251.
43. Wang H, Yang H, Tracey KJ (2004) Extracellular role of HMGB1 in inflammation and sepsis. J Intern Med 255: 320–331.
44. Mitroulis I, Kambas K, Chrysanthopoulou A, Skendros P, Apostolidou E, et al. (2011) Neutrophil extracellular trap formation is associated with IL-1beta and autophagy-related signaling in gout. PLoS One 6: e29318.
45. Gupta AK, Joshi MB, Philippova M, Erne P, Hasler P, et al. (2010) Activated endothelial cells induce neutrophil extracellular traps and are susceptible to NETosis-mediated cell death. FEBS Lett 584: 3193–3197.

23

The Glasgow Prognostic Score Predicts Poor Survival in Cisplatin-Based Treated Patients with Metastatic Nasopharyngeal Carcinoma

Cui Chen[1,9], **Peng Sun**[2,3,9], **Qiang-sheng Dai**[1,9], **Hui-wen Weng**[1], **He-ping Li**[1], **Sheng Ye**[1]*

1 Department of Oncology, The First Affiliated Hospital, Sun Yat-Sen University, Guangzhou, China, **2** Department of Medical Oncology, Sun Yat-sen University Cancer Center, Guangzhou, China, **3** Collaborative Innovation Center for Cancer Medicine, State Key Laboratory of Oncology in South China, Guangzhou, China

Abstract

Background: Several inflammation-based prognostic scoring systems, including Glasgow Prognostic Score (GPS), neutrophil to lymphocyte ratio (NLR) and platelet to lymphocyte ratio (PLR) have been reported to predict survival in many malignancies, whereas their role in metastatic nasopharyngeal carcinoma (NPC) remains unclear. The aim of this study is to evaluate the clinical value of these prognostic scoring systems in a cohort of cisplatin-based treated patients with metastatic NPC.

Methods: Two hundred and eleven patients with histologically proven metastatic NPC treated with first-line cisplatin-based chemotherapy were retrospectively evaluated. Demographics, disease-related characteristics and relevant laboratory data before treatment were recorded. GPS, NLR and PLR were calculated as described previously. Response to first-line therapy and survival data were also collected. Survival was analyzed in Cox regressions and stability of the models was examined by bootstrap resampling. The area under the receiver operating characteristics curve (AUC) was calculated to compare the discriminatory ability of each scoring system.

Results: Among the above three inflammation-based prognostic scoring systems, GPS ($P<0.001$) and NLR ($P=0.019$) were independently associated with overall survival, which showed to be stable in a bootstrap resampling study. The GPS consistently showed a higher AUC value at 6-month (0.805), 12-month (0.705), and 24-month (0.705) in comparison with NLR and PLR. Further analysis of the association of GPS with progression-free survival showed GPS was also associated independently with progression-free survival ($P<0.001$).

Conclusions: Our study demonstrated that the GPS may be of prognostic value in metastatic NPC patients treated with cisplatin-based palliative chemotherapy and facilitate individualized treatment. However a prospective study to validate this prognostic model is still needed.

Editor: Konradin Metze, University of Campinas, Brazil

Funding: The authors received no specific funding for this work.

Competing Interests: The authors have declared that no competing interests exist.

* Email: yes20111212@163.com

9 These authors contributed equally to this work.

Introduction

Nasopharyngeal carcinoma (NPC) is a distinct disease with unique ethnic and geographic characteristics, whose incidence varies from 0.5–3/100 000/year in North Africa to 20–30 in some areas of southern China. [1,2] Although the cure rate has been significantly improved owing to advances in diagnostic imaging, radiotherapeutic techniques and chemotherapy regimens recently, distant metastases remain the main reason for failure of treatment. [3] In these cases, palliative systemic therapy remains the primary therapeutic option and cisplatin-based combination chemotherapy is considered the standard front-line regimen for decades, offering response rates in the range of 50–80% and a significant prolongation of overall survival (OS). [4] However, there are still

wide individual differences in clinical response and outcomes. Some reports indicate that overall survival may exceed ten years for specific subgroups of patients. It is therefore of paramount interest to find an easily available model to help evaluate individual prognosis which will greatly improve the ability of clinical decision-making.

Currently, clinical characteristics are dominating indexes for judging prognosis of metastatic NPC patients, such as performance status and disease-free interval. [5] The prognostic value of circulating Epstein–Barr virus (EBV) DNA load has also been well established in various reports. [6,7] Besides aforementioned prognostic factors representing tumor status and clinical characteristics, it is now recognized that the host inflammatory response, in particular the systemic inflammatory response, plays an important role in disease development and progression by inhibition of apoptosis, promotion of angiogenesis, and damage of DNA. [8,9,10] Several inflammation-based prognostic scoring systems have been devised and found to be strongly correlated with prognosis in patients with a variety of neoplasms. These include a combination of neutrophil and lymphocyte counts as the neutrophil to lymphocyte ratio (NLR) and a combination of platelet and lymphocyte counts as the platelet to lymphocyte ratio (PLR), both of which reflect full blood count derangements induced by the acute phase reaction, while the Glasgow Prognostic Score (GPS) incorporates raised circulating C-reactive protein (CRP) and hypoalbuminemia. [11,12,13,14,15] Recently some researches have also shown that markers of systemic inflammatory response represent reliable prognostic factors in patients with early nasopharyngeal carcinoma. [16] However, to the best of our knowledge, there is no data regarding the prognostic impact of systemic inflammation-based scoring systems in metastatic NPC. In the present study, we therefore evaluated the clinical value of several inflammation-based prognostic scoring systems including GPS, NLR and PLR in a cohort of cisplatin-based treated patients with metastatic NPC.

Patients and Methods

Patient selection

From October 2005 to October 2011, 211 patients with histologically proven metastatic NPC treated with first-line cisplatin-based chemotherapy were included in the study at Sun Yat-Sen University Cancer Center. Entry criteria consisted of: (1) radiologically measurable disease; (2) treated with at least two cycles of first-line cisplatin-based palliative chemotherapy; (3) Karnofsky Performance Scores (KPS) $\geq$60; (4) normal hepatic and renal function. Exclusion criteria included: (1) patients with other types of malignancy; (2) patients with brain metastases; (3) patients with clinical evidence of infection or other inflammatory conditions. This study was approved by the institutional review board and ethics committee of Sun Yat-Sen University Cancer Center. All patients provided written informed consent to participate in this study. Parental written consent was obtained for minors in current study.

Treatment

All eligible patients received 1 of the following cisplatin-based chemotherapy regimens as the first-line treatment: (1) cisplatin (25 mg/m^2 intravenously [IV] on Days 1–3 of a 21-day cycle) plus 5-fluorouracil (500 mg/m^2 IV on Days 1–5 of a 21-day cycle), (2) paclitaxel (175 mg/m^2 IV over 3 hours with standard premedication on Day 1 of a 21-day cycle) plus cisplatin (25 mg/m^2 IV on Days 1–3 of a 21-day cycle), (3) paclitaxel (135 mg/m^2 IV over 3 hours with standard premedication on Day 1 of a 21-day cycle) plus cisplatin (25 mg/m^2 IV on Days 1–3 of a 21-day cycle) plus 5-fluorouracil (800 mg/m^2, continuous IV infusion for 24 hours, on Days 1–5 of a 21-day cycle). Of the 211 eligible patients, 78 (37.0%) patients were given the PF regimen, 24 (11.4%) patients were given the TP regimen, and 109 (51.6%) patients received the TPF regimen.

Relevant Evaluation

Basic demographics, baseline characteristics, detailed medical history as well as relevant laboratory data before treatment (C-reactive protein (CRP), Serum lactate dehydrogenase (LDH), albumin, neutrophil, lymphocyte, platelet (Plt) count and plasma EBV DNA level) were recorded. The GPS, NLR and PLR were constructed as described previously. In GPS, patients with both an elevated CRP level (>1.0 mg/dl) and hypoalbuminemia (<3.5 g/dl) were allocated a score of 2, patients with only one of these biochemical abnormalities were allocated a score of 1, and patients with neither of these abnormalities were allocated a score of 0. NLR was divided into two groups (<5 and $\geq$5) while PLR was categorized into three groups (<150, 150–300 and >300).

Progression-free survival (PFS) and overall survival (OS) were defined as the time from the first diagnosis of metastasis to the date of documented progression and to the date of death, respectively. Tumor response was evaluated according to the Response Evaluation Criteria in Solid Tumors (RECISTs) 1.0.

Table 1. Demographic and Baseline Characteristics of Patients.

Patient characteristics	Number (%)
Total evaluated	211 (100)
Age, years (median/range)	46/14–72
Gender (male/female)	181/30 (85.8/14.2)
KPS (median/range)	90/60–100
Number of involved sites (median/range)	2/1–6
Synchronous metastasis (yes/no)	53/158 (25.1/74.9)
Liver metastasis (yes/no)	73/138 (34.6/65.4)
Lung metastasis (yes/no)	97/114 (45.9/54.1)
Bone metastasis (yes/no)	88/123 (41.7/58.3)
Disease-free interval, months (median/range)	6/0–65
Chemotherapy regimen (PF/TP/TPF)	78/24/109 (37.0/11.4/51.6)
Serum LDH, U/L (median/range)	247/81–632
Pre-treatment EBV DNA, copies/mL (median/range)	$4.93 \times 10^4/0-9.73 \times 10^7$
GPS (0/1/2)	125/66/20 (59.2/31.3/9.5)
NLR (median/range)	3.12/0.81–11.03
PLR (median/range)	71.2/31.3–422.5

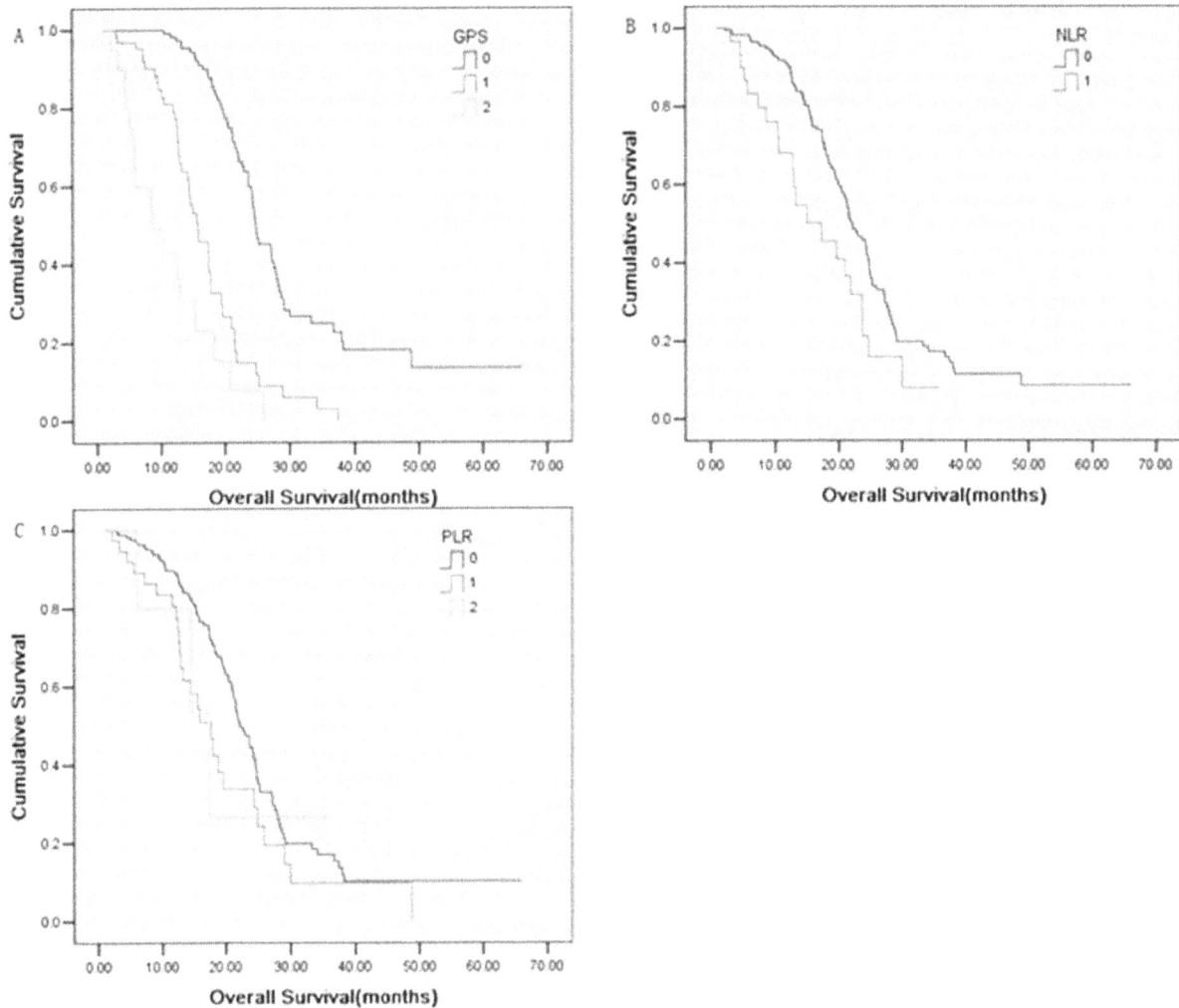

Figure 1. Comparison of overall survival according to scoring systems, GPS (A), NLR (B) and PLR (C).

Follow up

Patients were regularly followed up after chemotherapy until death or their last follow-up appointment. Physical examination and imaging studies of the relevant region(s) were performed every 3 months after the completion of the chemotherapy or when clinical indications dictated for follow-up. The start date of follow-up period was the date of initial metastatic NPC diagnosis. The time of last follow-up was 31st December 2013 or death.

Statistical analysis

All statistical analysis was performed using SPSS version 13.0 software or WinStat software. PFS and OS were obtained by using the Kaplan–Meier method and differences between the groups were compared by the log-rank test. A univariate analysis was performed for the potential prognostic factors. Age, karnofsky performance score before treatment, number of involved sites, disease-free interval, serum LDH, pre-treatment EBV DNA entered the calculations in a continuous way. NLR and PLR were also tested at first as continuous variables in order to avoid the bias induced by binarization of continuous data. And we tested the GPS and the other variables entering the analysis as categorical variables. Multivariable analysis including variables that proved to be significant in the univariate analysis was

performed subsequently using the Cox model to analyse factors related to prognosis (P<0.05 was used as the cut-off value of statistical significance). The stability of the COX model was tested by bootstrap resampling. New data sets of equal size were created by random sampling of the original data with replacement. In each new bootstrap data set, a patient may be represented once, multiple times or not at all. Cox regressions with the same conditions as in the original data set were then calculated for the new data sets in order to obtain the bootstrap parameter estimates. Descriptive statistics for the patient groups are reported as mean, median, and range. Categorical variables were presented numbers and percentages. Non-parametric test was applied for comparison of data among groups. A receiver operating characteristics (ROC) curve was also generated and the area under the curve (AUC) was calculated to evaluate the discriminatory ability of each scoring systems. A two-tailed P value less than 0.05 was considered to be statistically significant.

Results

Patient characteristics and Outcomes

A total of 211 patients with metastatic NPC were included in the present study. All of the patients were from epidemic areas in

Table 2. Univariate and Multivariate Analysis of Prognostic Factors of Overall Survival.

Variable	Univariate analysis		Multivariate analysis	
	P	HR (95% CI)	P	HR (95% CI)
Age	0.444	1.006 (0.990–1.023)		
Gender (male/female)	0.631	1.147 (0.655–2.008)		
KPS	0.934	1.020 (0.637–1.633)		
Liver metastasis (yes/no)	0.989	1.003 (0.694–1.449)		
Lung metastasis (yes/no)	0.848	1.035 (0.726–1.476)		
Number of involved sites	0.020	1.282 (1.040–1.580)	0.560	1.064 (0.864–1.310)
Synchronous metastasis (yes/no)	0.696	0.920 (0.604–1.400)		
Disease-free interval	0.278	1.218 (0.853–1.739)		
Chemotherapy regimen (PF/TP/TPF)	0.358	0.767 (0.435–1.351)		
Serum LDH	0.014	1.210 (1.040–1.409)	0.911	1.011 (0.835–1.225)
Pre-treatment EBVDNA	0.024	1.234 (1.028–1.481)	0.037	1.239 (1.013–1.515)
GPS (0/1/2)	<0.001	3.078 (2.393–3.959)	<0.001	2.520 (1.977–3.212)
NLR	0.025	1.732 (1.071–2.800)	0.019	1.800 (1.103–2.940)
PLR	0.125	1.311 (0.928–1.853)		

China, with a male predominance (85.8%). The mean age of diagnosis of metastatic NPC was 46 (range 14–72) years. About half of the patients had more than one metastatic site with lung being the most common site (45.9%). The pretreatment plasma EBV DNA ranged from 0 to 9.73×10^7 copies/mL, with a median of 4.93×10^4 copies/mL. One hundred and fifty (71.1%) patients showed an elevated pretreatment EBV DNA level ($>1 \times 10^3$ copies/mL). One hundred and twenty-five (59.2%) patients were allocated to GPS 0, 66 (31.3%) patients were allocated to GPS 1, and 20 (9.5%) patients were allocated to GPS 2, respectively. The median NLR level was 3.12 (range 0.81~11.03). Thirty patients (14.2%) had an NLR≥5 and the rest had an NLR<5. The PLR ranged from 31.3 to 422.5, with a median of 71.2. A PLR greater than 300 was seen in 5 patients (2.4%), 168 patients (79.6%) had PLR<150, and the rest had a PLR in between. Other patient characteristics are summarized in Table 1.

At the time of analysis, 124 (58.8%) patients had died, and the median PFS and OS were 7.9 and 21.6 months, respectively. The overall clinical response rate was 70.1% for all 211 patients.

Prognostic factor analysis for overall survival

Various potential prognostic factors including age, gender, karnofsky performance score before treatment, metastasis sites (liver and lung), number of involved sites, synchronous metastasis, disease-free interval, chemotherapy regimen, serum LDH, pre-treatment EBV DNA, GPS status, NLR and PLR were analyzed. Univariate analysis revealed that a larger number of involved sites ($P = 0.020$), higher baseline serum LDH level ($P = 0.014$), higher pretreatment EBV DNA level ($P = 0.024$), higher score of GPS ($P<0.001$) and higher value of NLR ($P = 0.025$) were considered adverse factors for overall survival (Table 2, Fig. 1). Age, gender, PLR and the other variables in the analysis had no prognostic relevance. In multivariate analysis, pre-treatment EBV DNA ($P = 0.037$), GPS ($P<0.001$) and NLR ($P = 0.019$) were independent prognostic factors (Table 2). The stability of this model was confirmed in a bootstrap resampling procedure. Among 1000 new

models, pre-treatment EBV DNA was present in 69%, GPS appeared in 89% and NLR in 71%.

Moreover, the two inflammation-based prognostic scoring systems constructed by categorizing the continuous variables of NLR and PLR as described before were compared with the GPS. Receiver operating characteristic curves were constructed for survival status at 6-month, 12-month, and 24-month of follow-up, and the area under the ROC curve (AUC) was compared (Fig. 2) to assess the discrimination ability of each scoring system. The GPS consistently show a higher AUC value at 6-month (0.805), 12-month (0.705), and 24-month (0.705) in comparison with other inflammation-based prognostic scores.

Association of GPS with clinicopathologic characteristics

Baseline patient and disease-related characteristics for each GPS group and comparisons between groups are depicted in Table 3. Although the difference was not statistically significant, a trend towards an association of GPS with BMI was observed. Of note, an elevated GPS was significantly associated with higher serum LDH and higher pretreatment EBV DNA.

Association of GPS with progression-free survival

GPS was further associated with PFS. Kaplan–Meier curves for PFS for the total cohort according to GPS was shown in Fig. 3. Median PFS (95% CI) was 8.73 (7.64–9.82), 5.27 (4.51–6.02) and 3.40 (1.21–5.59) months for patients with GPS 0, 1 and 2, respectively. As shown in Table 4, multivariate analysis including the aforementioned parameters and GPS revealed that GPS was also the independent predictor for PFS ($P<0.001$). The stability of this model was also confirmed in a bootstrap resampling procedure. In the bootstrap resampling, GPS entered in 100% and pre-treatment EBV DNA appeared in 25%.

Discussion

Markers of systemic inflammatory response represent reliable prognostic factors in patients with advanced cancer.

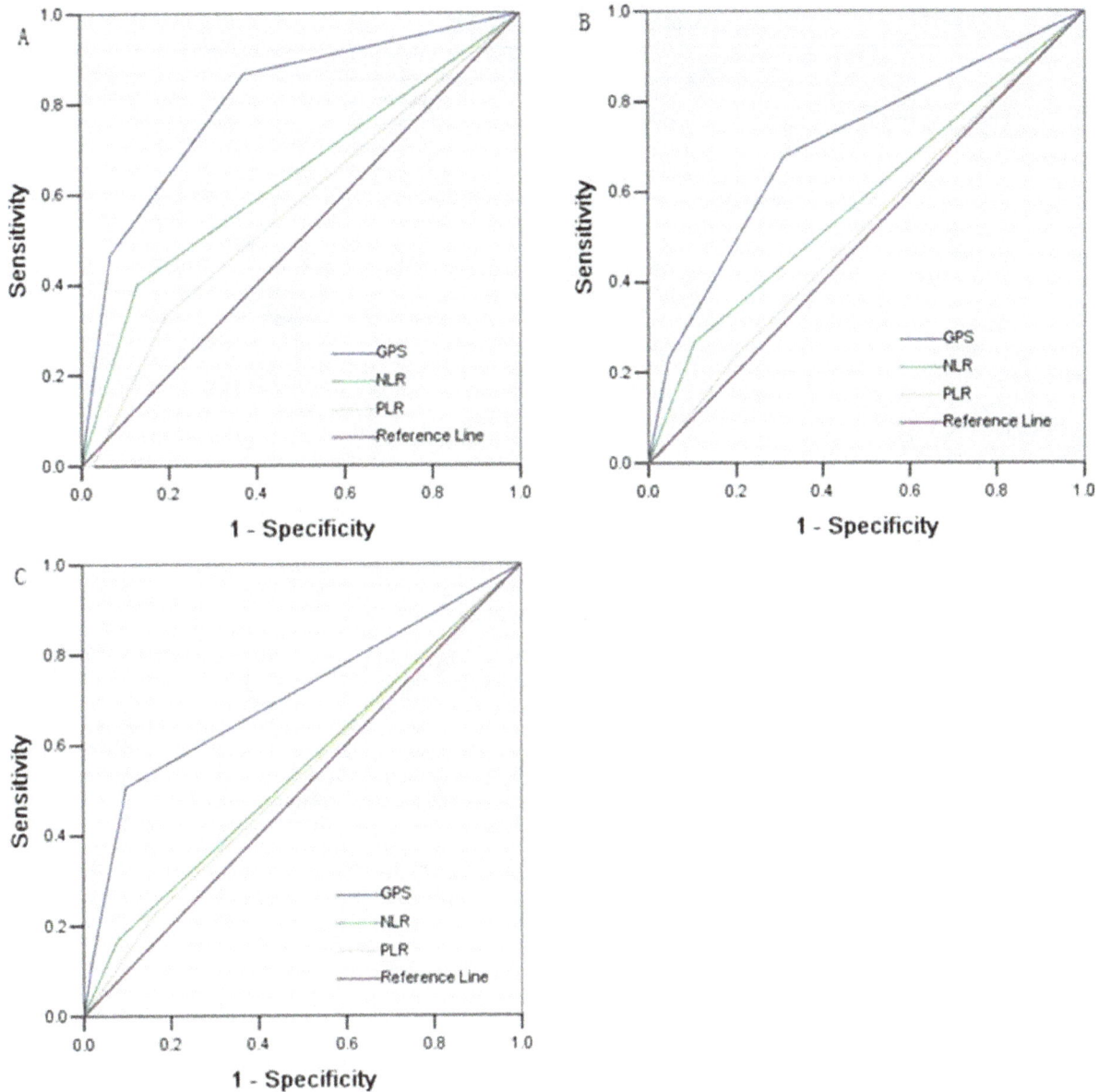

Figure 2. Comparisons of the area under the receiver operating curve for survival status between scoring systems at 6 month (A), 12 month (B) and 24 month (C).

[8,11,12,13,14,16] To the best of our knowledge, this study has firstly demonstrated that the GPS, an inflammation-based prognostic score, is an independent marker of poor prognosis in patients with metastatic NPC and is superior to the NLR in terms of prognostic ability. Furthermore, our data demonstrated a significant, independent association between GPS and PFS.

Accumulating evidence indicates the prognostic importance of GPS in various solid cancers, such as colorectal cancer, [17,18] esophageal cancer, [19] lung cancer, [13] pancreatic cancer, [12] and gastric cancer. [14] A similar result was achieved in our study. The biological basis for the correlation between the GPS and survival are not completely understood. Below are some supposed mechanisms. First, cachexia, which often manifests as nutritional depletion (weight loss, elevated resting energy expenditure and loss of lean tissue) and functional decline, is common in patients with advanced cancer and has been recognized to be associated with

poorer outcome. [20,21,22] CRP has been reported to be associated with the nutrition status and development of cachexia while albumin represents a negative acute phase protein and also represents a marker of nutritional status. [8] As we know, lower serum albumin correlates to nutritional depletion closely. Our study also shows a trend towards an association of GPS with BMI. Based on these reports, GPS, incorporating CRP and serum albumin levels, may reflect both presence of the nutritional depletion and functional decline, resulting in poor survival outcome. Second, a strong association was found between EBV infection and NPC in previous studies. [23] Plasma EBV DNA has been identified to be prognostic in metastatic NPC patients. [6,7] EBV infection stimulated the release of pro-inflammatory cytokine including IL-1, IL-6, and TNF-α from the tumor microenviron-ment, which results in the induction of CRP synthesis from the liver and the reduction of albumin by hepatocytes. [24,25] In

Table 3. Association of GPS with characteristics of patients.

characteristics	GPS = 0	GPS = 1	GPS = 2	P
Age (≤45/>45)	65/60	30/36	12/8	0.472
Gender (male/female)	103/22	60/6	18/2	0.236
KPS (≤80/>80)	24/101	12/54	4/16	0.978
BMI (≤18.5/>18.5)	21/104	20/46	6/14	0.070
Number of involved sites (1/≥2)	61/64	36/30	8/12	0.493
Synchronous metastasis (yes/no)	26/99	22/44	5/15	0.165
Liver metastasis (yes/no)	43/82	21/45	9/11	0.553
Lung metastasis (yes/no)	53/72	35/31	9/11	0.373
Bone metastasis (yes/no)	50/75	28/38	10/10	0.694
Serum LDH, U/L (<245/≥245)	83/42	27/39	8/12	0.001
Pre-treatment EBV DNA, copies/mL (<median/≥median)	99/26	5/61	2/18	0.0001

other words, GPS level may be a marker of inflammation from EBV infection and may indicate the magnitude of inflammation and the prognosis of patients as EBV DNA load. Previous studies have also indicated that inflammation in the tumor microenvironment play an important role in promoting tumor growth, invasion, and metastasis. [9,10] Our data shows that an elevated GPS is significantly associated with higher EBV-DNA level, which will, to certain extent, add further support to the proposal. In addition to these explanations, because our data find an elevated GPS is also significantly associated with elevated LDH, which has been reported to be an indicator of high tumor burden, an

elevated GPS score may indirectly reflect a high tumor burden. [26] In general, these explanations suggest that it is reasonable that GPS is a significant and independent predictor of survival outcome.

Recently a study by Wei-xiong Xia et al also showed that elevated CRP and CRP kinetics correlated with poor prognosis in patients with metastatic NPC. This study had similar aims and results compared with our study. However there are still some differences between the two studies. Firstly, the GPS incorporates CRP and hypoalbuminemia and may be more suitable to reflect systemic inflammatory response than CRP alone. Secondly, the

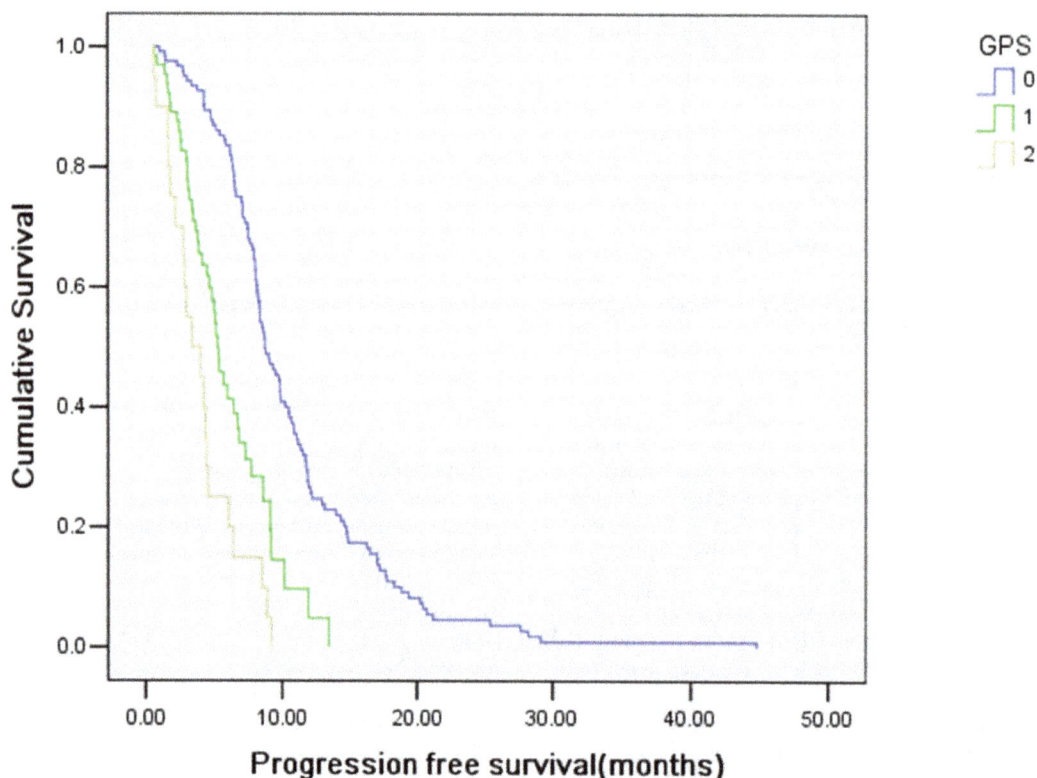

Figure 3. Kaplan–Meier estimates for progression-free survival according to GPS.

Table 4. Univariate and Multivariate Analysis of Prognostic Factors of Progression-free Survival.

Variable	Univariate analysis		Multivariate analysis	
	P	HR (95% CI)	P	HR (95% CI)
Age	0.613	0.996 (0.981–1.011)		
Gender (male/female)	0.489	1.162 (0.760–1.776)		
KPS	0.372	0.998 (0.994–1.002)		
Liver metastasis (yes/no)	0.477	0.893 (0.655–1.219)		
Lung metastasis (yes/no)	0.127	1.261 (0.936–1.698)		
Number of involved sites	0.043	1.201 (1.0066–1.435)	0.493	1.063 (0.893–1.266)
Synchronous metastasis (yes/no)	0.933	1.015 (0.719–1.434)		
Disease-free interval	0.238	1.198 (0.887–1.617)		
Chemotherapy regimen (PF/TP/TPF)	0.609	0.884 (0.552–1.417)		
Serum LDH	0.340	1.072 (0.93–1.235)		
Pre-treatment EBVDNA	<0.001	1.426 (1.170–1.739)	0.133	1.206 (0.945–1.539)
GPS (0/1/2)	<0.001	2.417 (1.916–3.050)	<0.001	2.248 (1.753–2.833)
NLR	0.054	1.400 (0.995–1.971)		
PLR	0.611	1.061 (0.844–1.334)		

eligibility criteria are different. All patients enrolled in current study received first-line cisplatin-based regimens. Thus, it is helpful to exclude the potential confounding effect of different regimens.

The GPS test is simple and based on standardized, wildly available protein assays. Therefore assessment of the GPS can be routinely in most clinical centers. Based on the present results, the significant value of GPS test is that it can identify patients at high risk of disease progression and death as a clinically convenient and useful biomarker. Thus it not only provides guidance of follow-up care at clinic but also has the potential to be a stratification factor or a selection criterion in randomized clinical trials for metastatic NPC. Moreover, in our study, most of the patients evaluated as disease progression at the end of second cycle of chemotherapy were allocated a score of 2. Patients in the good GPS group (GPS 0) had a more prolonged progression-free survival. As a consequence we believe that the presence of a systemic inflammatory response should be evaluated in the pretreatment period and might become the promising new targets of anti-tumor therapy. Nowadays there was an amount of ongoing research into the effect of non-steroidal anti-inflammatory drugs on anti-tumor treatment, including colon cancer, [27] lung cancer, [28] esophagus cancer [29] and so on. Accordingly, it is also interesting and significant to study the modification of the systemic inflammatory response in patients with metastatic nasopharyngeal carcinoma. And the GPS which is inexpensive, reliable, and widely available may have a certain guiding significance for selecting patients who might be candidates for modulation of systemic inflammatory response and provide a well defined therapeutic target for future clinical trials. Further evaluation is required to confirm this hypothesis.

In addition, the NLR and PLR have been reported to be important prognostic models in patients with a variety of solid cancers, such as colorectal cancer, esophageal cancer, gastric cancer, pancreatic cancer, and lung cancer. Several studies have also shown that an elevated NLR is associated with poor prognosis in patients with NPC. [12,14,30,31] In accord with the study of Jian-rong He et al. who tested the prognostic value of NLR in 1410 patients with various stages of NPC [32] and the study of Xin An et al. who tested the prognostic value of NLR in 363 patients with non-disseminated NPC, [16] we also found a significant association between NLR and OS. However, the COX model and the AUC analysis have shown that the GPS was superior to NLR in terms of discriminating ability and prognostic accuracy. For PLR, it was not independently associated with overall survival. In general, this study is the first to show the superior prognostic ability of the GPS over the NLR and PLR in patients with metastatic NPC.

In conclusion, our study demonstrated that the GPS may be useful to predict the prognosis of metastatic NPC patients treated with cisplatin-based palliative chemotherapy and facilitate individualized treatment. A prospective study to validate this prognostic model is needed. The mechanisms underlying the relationship between high GPS and poor prognosis in NPC still need further study.

Author Contributions

Conceived and designed the experiments: SY. Performed the experiments: CC PS HPL. Analyzed the data: CC PS QSD. Contributed reagents/materials/analysis tools: PS SY HWW. Contributed to the writing of the manuscript: CC PS.

References

1. Yu MC, Yuan JM (2002) Epidemiology of nasopharyngeal carcinoma. Semin Cancer Biol 12: 421–429.
2. Chang ET, Adami HO (2006) The enigmatic epidemiology of nasopharyngeal carcinoma. Cancer Epidemiol Biomarkers Prev 15: 1765–1777.
3. Chiesa F, De Paoli F (2001) Distant metastases from nasopharyngeal cancer. ORL J Otorhinolaryngol Relat Spec 63: 214–216.
4. Bensouda Y, Kaikani W, Ahbeddou N, Rahhali R, Jabri M, et al. (2011) Treatment for metastatic nasopharyngeal carcinoma. Eur Ann Otorhinolaryngol Head Neck Dis 128: 79–85.
5. Liu MT, Hsieh CY, Chang TH, Lin JP, Huang CC, et al. (2003) Prognostic factors affecting the outcome of nasopharyngeal carcinoma. Jpn J Clin Oncol 33: 501–508.

6. Twu CW, Wang WY, Liang WM, Jan JS, Jiang RS, et al. (2007) Comparison of the prognostic impact of serum anti-EBV antibody and plasma EBV DNA assays in nasopharyngeal carcinoma. Int J Radiat Oncol Biol Phys 67: 130–137.
7. An X, Wang FH, Ding PR, Deng L, Jiang WQ, et al. (2011) Plasma Epstein-Barr virus DNA level strongly predicts survival in metastatic/recurrent nasopharyngeal carcinoma treated with palliative chemotherapy. Cancer 117: 3750–3757.
8. McMillan DC (2009) Systemic inflammation, nutritional status and survival in patients with cancer. Curr Opin Clin Nutr Metab Care 12: 223–226.
9. Grivennikov SI, Greten FR, Karin M (2010) Immunity, inflammation, and cancer. Cell 140: 883–899.
10. Chiang AC, Massague J (2008) Molecular basis of metastasis. N Engl J Med 359: 2814–2823.
11. Kinoshita A, Onoda H, Imai N, Iwaku A, Oishi M, et al. (2013) The Glasgow Prognostic Score, an inflammation based prognostic score, predicts survival in patients with hepatocellular carcinoma. BMC Cancer 13: 52.
12. Wang DS, Luo HY, Qiu MZ, Wang ZQ, Zhang DS, et al. (2012) Comparison of the prognostic values of various inflammation based factors in patients with pancreatic cancer. Med Oncol 29: 3092–3100.
13. Gioulbasanis I, Pallis A, Vlachostergios PJ, Xyrafas A, Giannousi Z, et al. (2012) The Glasgow Prognostic Score (GPS) predicts toxicity and efficacy in platinum-based treated patients with metastatic lung cancer. Lung Cancer 77: 383–388.
14. Wang DS, Ren C, Qiu MZ, Luo HY, Wang ZQ, et al. (2012) Comparison of the prognostic value of various preoperative inflammation-based factors in patients with stage III gastric cancer. Tumour Biol 33: 749–756.
15. McMillan DC (2013) The systemic inflammation-based Glasgow Prognostic Score: a decade of experience in patients with cancer. Cancer Treat Rev 39: 534–540.
16. An X, Ding PR, Wang FH, Jiang WQ, Li YH (2011) Elevated neutrophil to lymphocyte ratio predicts poor prognosis in nasopharyngeal carcinoma. Tumour Biol 32: 317–324.
17. Maeda K, Shibutani M, Otani H, Nagahara H, Sugano K, et al. (2013) Prognostic value of preoperative inflammation-based prognostic scores in patients with stage IV colorectal cancer who undergo palliative resection of asymptomatic primary tumors. Anticancer Res 33: 5567–5573.
18. Ishizuka M, Nagata H, Takagi K, Iwasaki Y, Kubota K (2013) Inflammation-based prognostic system predicts survival after surgery for stage IV colorectal cancer. Am J Surg 205: 22–28.
19. Vashist YK, Loos J, Dedow J, Tachezy M, Uzunoglu G, et al. (2011) Glasgow Prognostic Score is a predictor of perioperative and long-term outcome in patients with only surgically treated esophageal cancer. Ann Surg Oncol 18: 1130–1138.
20. Laviano A, Meguid MM, Inui A, Muscaritoli M, Rossi-Fanelli F (2005) Therapy insight: Cancer anorexia-cachexia syndrome–when all you can eat is yourself. Nat Clin Pract Oncol 2: 158–165.
21. Donohoe CL, Ryan AM, Reynolds JV (2011) Cancer cachexia: mechanisms and clinical implications. Gastroenterol Res Pract 2011: 601434.
22. Fearon KC, Voss AC, Hustead DS (2006) Definition of cancer cachexia: effect of weight loss, reduced food intake, and systemic inflammation on functional status and prognosis. Am J Clin Nutr 83: 1345–1350.
23. Senba M, Zhong XY, Senba MI, Itakura H (1994) EBV and nasopharyngeal carcinoma. Lancet 343: 1104.
24. Eliopoulos AG, Stack M, Dawson CW, Kaye KM, Hodgkin L, et al. (1997) Epstein-Barr virus-encoded LMP1 and CD40 mediate IL-6 production in epithelial cells via an NF-kappaB pathway involving TNF receptor-associated factors. Oncogene 14: 2899–2916.
25. Pepys MB, Hirschfield GM (2003) C-reactive protein: a critical update. J Clin Invest 111: 1805–1812.
26. Liaw CC, Wang CH, Huang JS, Kiu MC, Chen JS, et al. (1997) Serum lactate dehydrogenase level in patients with nasopharyngeal carcinoma. Acta Oncol 36: 159–164.
27. Fuchs CS, Ogino S (2013) Aspirin therapy for colorectal cancer with PIK3CA mutation: simply complex!. J Clin Oncol 31: 4358–4361.
28. Gridelli C, Gallo C, Ceribelli A, Gebbia V, Gamucci T, et al. (2007) Factorial phase III randomised trial of rofecoxib and prolonged constant infusion of gemcitabine in advanced non-small-cell lung cancer: the GEmcitabine-COxib in NSCLC (GECO) study. Lancet Oncol 8: 500–512.
29. Szumilo J, Burdan F, Szumilo M, Lewkowicz D, Kedzierawska-Kurylcio A (2009) Cyclooxygenase inhibitors in chemoprevention and treatment of esophageal squamous cell carcinoma. Pol Merkur Lekarski 27: 408–412.
30. Kwon HC, Kim SH, Oh SY, Lee S, Lee JH, et al. (2012) Clinical significance of preoperative neutrophil-lymphocyte versus platelet-lymphocyte ratio in patients with operable colorectal cancer. Biomarkers 17: 216–222.
31. Feng JF, Huang Y, Chen QX (2014) Preoperative platelet lymphocyte ratio (PLR) is superior to neutrophil lymphocyte ratio (NLR) as a predictive factor in patients with esophageal squamous cell carcinoma. World J Surg Oncol 12: 58.
32. He JR, Shen GP, Ren ZF, Qin H, Cui C, et al. (2012) Pretreatment levels of peripheral neutrophils and lymphocytes as independent prognostic factors in patients with nasopharyngeal carcinoma. Head Neck 34: 1769–1776.

Permissions

All chapters in this book were first published in PLOS ONE, by The Public Library of Science; hereby published with permission under the Creative Commons Attribution License or equivalent. Every chapter published in this book has been scrutinized by our experts. Their significance has been extensively debated. The topics covered herein carry significant findings which will fuel the growth of the discipline. They may even be implemented as practical applications or may be referred to as a beginning point for another development.

The contributors of this book come from diverse backgrounds, making this book a truly international effort. This book will bring forth new frontiers with its revolutionizing research information and detailed analysis of the nascent developments around the world.

We would like to thank all the contributing authors for lending their expertise to make the book truly unique. They have played a crucial role in the development of this book. Without their invaluable contributions this book wouldn't have been possible. They have made vital efforts to compile up to date information on the varied aspects of this subject to make this book a valuable addition to the collection of many professionals and students.

This book was conceptualized with the vision of imparting up-to-date information and advanced data in this field. To ensure the same, a matchless editorial board was set up. Every individual on the board went through rigorous rounds of assessment to prove their worth. After which they invested a large part of their time researching and compiling the most relevant data for our readers.

The editorial board has been involved in producing this book since its inception. They have spent rigorous hours researching and exploring the diverse topics which have resulted in the successful publishing of this book. They have passed on their knowledge of decades through this book. To expedite this challenging task, the publisher supported the team at every step. A small team of assistant editors was also appointed to further simplify the editing procedure and attain best results for the readers.

Apart from the editorial board, the designing team has also invested a significant amount of their time in understanding the subject and creating the most relevant covers. They scrutinized every image to scout for the most suitable representation of the subject and create an appropriate cover for the book.

The publishing team has been an ardent support to the editorial, designing and production team. Their endless efforts to recruit the best for this project, has resulted in the accomplishment of this book. They are a veteran in the field of academics and their pool of knowledge is as vast as their experience in printing. Their expertise and guidance has proved useful at every step. Their uncompromising quality standards have made this book an exceptional effort. Their encouragement from time to time has been an inspiration for everyone.

The publisher and the editorial board hope that this book will prove to be a valuable piece of knowledge for researchers, students, practitioners and scholars across the globe.

List of Contributors

Shih-Ming Chu, Jen-Fu Hsu, Reyin Lien, Hsuan-Rong Huang, Ming-Chou Chiang and Ren-Huei Fu
Division of Pediatric Neonatology, Department of Pediatrics, Chang Gung Memorial Hospital, Taoyuan, Taiwan
College of Medicine, Chang Gung University, Taoyuan, Taiwan

Chiang-Wen Lee
Department of Nursing, Division of Basic Medical Sciences, and Chronic Diseases and Health Promotion Research Center, Chang Gung University of Science and Technology, Chia-Yi, Taiwan
Research Center for Industry of Human Ecology, Chang Gung University of Science and Technology, Taoyuan, Taiwan

Ming-Horng Tsai
Division of Neonatology and Pediatric Hematology/Oncology, Department of Pediatrics, Chang Gung Memorial Hospital, Yunlin, Taiwan
College of Medicine, Chang Gung University, Taoyuan, Taiwan
Department of Nursing, Division of Basic Medical Sciences, and Chronic Diseases and Health Promotion Research Center, Chang Gung University of Science and Technology, Chia-Yi, Taiwan

Stephen P. J. Macdonald
Centre for Clinical Research in Emergency Medicine, Harry Perkins Institute of Medical Research, Perth, Australia
Discipline of Emergency Medicine, School of Primary, Aboriginal and Rural Health Care, University of Western Australia, Perth, Australia
Emergency Department, Armadale Health Service, Perth, Australia

Shelley F. Stone, Claire L. Neil and Pauline E. van Eeden
Centre for Clinical Research in Emergency Medicine, Harry Perkins Institute of Medical Research, Perth, Australia
Discipline of Emergency Medicine, School of Primary, Aboriginal and Rural Health Care, University of Western Australia, Perth, Australia

Daniel M. Fatovich, Glenn Arendts and Simon G. A. Brown
Centre for Clinical Research in Emergency Medicine, Harry Perkins Institute of Medical Research, Perth, Australia, 2 Discipline of Emergency Medicine, School of Primary
Aboriginal and Rural Health Care, University of Western Australia, Perth, Australia
Emergency Department, Royal Perth Hospital, Perth, Australia

Rehan Zafar Paracha, Amjad Ali and Babar Aslam
Atta-Ur-Rahman School of Applied Biosciences (ASAB), National University of Sciences and Technology (NUST), Islamabad, Pakistan

Riaz Hussain
Shifa College of Pharmaceutical Sciences, Shifa Tameer-e-Millat University, Islamabad, Pakistan

Umar Niazi
IBERS, Aberystwyth University, Edward Llwyd Building, Penglais Campus, Aberystwyth, Ceredigion, Wales, United Kingdom

Jamil Ahmad and Samar Hayat Khan Tareen
Research Center for Modeling and Simulation (RCMS), National University of Sciences and Technology (NUST), Islamabad, Pakistan

Leonardo Lorente
Intensive Care Unit, Hospital Universitario de Canarias, La Laguna, Tenerife, Spain

María M. Martín
Intensive Care Unit, Hospital Universitario Nuestra Señora Candelaria, Santa Cruz Tenerife, Spain

Agustín F. Gonzá lez-Rivero and Juan M. Borreguero-León
Laboratory Department, Hospital Universitario de Canarias, La Laguna, Tenerife, Spain

José Ferreres
Intensive Care Unit, Hospital Clínico Universitario de Valencia, Valencia, Spain

Jordi Solé-Violán
Intensive Care Unit, Hospital Universitario Dr. Negrín, Las Palmas de Gran Canaria, Spain

Lorenzo Labarta
Intensive Care Unit, Hospital San Jorge, Huesca, Spain

César Díaz
Intensive Care Unit, Hospital Insular, Las Palmas de Gran Canaria, Spain

Alejandro Jiménez
Research Unit, Hospital Universitario de Canarias, La Laguna, Tenerife, Spain

Yu-Hua Chao
Institute of Medicine, Chung Shan Medical University, Taichung, Taiwan
Department of Pediatrics, Chung Shan Medical University Hospital, Taichung, Taiwan
School of Medicine, Chung Shan Medical University, Taichung, Taiwan

Han-Ping Wu
Department of Pediatrics, Taichung Tzuchi Hospital, the Buddhist Medical Foundation, Taichung, Taiwan
Department of Medicine, Tzu Chi University, Hualien, Taiwan

Kang-Hsi Wu
School of Chinese Medicine, China Medical University, Taichung, Taiwan
Department of Hematooncology, Children's Hospital, China Medical University Hospital, China Medical University, Taichung, Taiwan

Yi-Giien Tsai
School of Medicine, Chung Shan Medical University, Taichung, Taiwan
Departments of Pediatrics, Changhua Christian Hospital, Changhua, Taiwan
School of Medicine, Kaohsiung Medical University, Kaohsiung, Taiwan

Ching-Tien Peng
School of Chinese Medicine, China Medical University, Taichung, Taiwan
Department of Hematooncology, Children's Hospital, China Medical University Hospital, China Medical University, Taichung, Taiwan
Department of Biotechnology and Bioinformatics, Asia University, Taichung, Taiwan

Kuan-Chia Lin
School of Nursing, National Taipei University of Nursing and Health Sciences, Taipei, Taiwan
Life-Course Epidemiology and Human Development Research Group, National Taipei University of Nursing and Health Sciences, Taipei, Taiwan

Wan-Ru Chao
Institute of Medicine, Chung Shan Medical University, Taichung, Taiwan
School of Medicine, Chung Shan Medical University, Taichung, Taiwan
Department of Pathology, Chung Shan Medical University Hospital, Taichung, Taiwan

Maw-Sheng Lee
Institute of Medicine, Chung Shan Medical University, Taichung, Taiwan
Department of Obstetrics and Gynecology, Chung Shan Medical University Hospital, Taichung, Taiwan

Yun-Ching Fu
Institute of Clinical Medicine, National Yang-Ming University, Taipei, Taiwan
Department of Pediatrics, Taichung Veterans General Hospital, Taichung, Taiwan

Julie E. Goodwin, Yan Feng and Han Zhou
Department of Pediatrics, Yale University School of Medicine, New Haven, Connecticut, United States of America

Heino Velazquez
Department of Internal Medicine, Veterans Affairs Hospital, West Haven, Connecticut, United States of America

William C. Sessa
Vascular Biology and Therapeutics Program, Yale University School of Medicine, New Haven, Connecticut United States of America
Department of Pharmacology, Yale University School of Medicine, New Haven, Connecticut, United States of America

Hong Gil Jeon, Hyeong Uk Ju and Jae-Bum Jun
Department of Internal Medicine, Ulsan University Hospital, University of Ulsan College of Medicine, Ulsan, Republic of Korea

Gyu Yeol Kim
Department of Surgery, Ulsan University Hospital, University of Ulsan College of Medicine, Ulsan, Republic of Korea

Joseph Jeong
Department of Laboratory Medicine, Ulsan University Hospital, University of Ulsan College of Medicine, Ulsan, Republic of Korea

Min-Ho Kim
Biomedical Research Center, Ulsan University Hospital, University of Ulsan College of Medicine, Ulsan, Republic of Korea

Vimal Grover
Magill Department of Anaesthesia, Critical Care and Pain, Chelsea and Westminster Hospital National Health Service Foundation Trust, London, United Kingdom
Immunology Section, Department of Medicine, Imperial College, London, United Kingdom
Department of Surgery and Cancer, Imperial College, London, United Kingdom

Panagiotis Pantelidis, Don C. Henderson and Peter Kelleher
Immunology Section, Department of Medicine, Imperial College, London, United Kingdom
Department of Immunology, Imperial College Healthcare National Health Service Trust, London, United Kingdom

Neil Soni
Magill Department of Anaesthesia, Critical Care and Pain, Chelsea and Westminster Hospital National Health Service Foundation Trust, London, United Kingdom
Department of Surgery and Cancer, Imperial College, London, United Kingdom

Masao Takata
Department of Surgery and Cancer, Imperial College, London, United Kingdom

Pallav L. Shah
Department of Respiratory Medicine, Chelsea and Westminster Hospital National Health Service Foundation Trust, London, United Kingdom
Department of Respiratory Medicine, Royal Brompton & Harefield Hospitals National Health Service Foundation Trust, London, United Kingdom

Athol U. Wells
Department of Respiratory Medicine, Royal Brompton & Harefield Hospitals National Health Service Foundation Trust, London, United Kingdom

Suveer Singh
Magill Department of Anaesthesia, Critical Care and Pain, Chelsea and Westminster Hospital National Health Service Foundation Trust, London, United Kingdom
Department of Surgery and Cancer, Imperial College, London, United Kingdom
Department of Respiratory Medicine, Chelsea and Westminster Hospital National Health Service Foundatio n Trust, London, United Kingdom

Luuk Wieske
Department of Intensive Care Medicine, Academic Medical Center, Amsterdam, the Netherlands
Department of Neurology, Academic Medical Center, Amsterdam, the Netherlands
Laboratory of Experimental Anesthesiology and Intensive Care (LNENINCNA), Academic Medical Center, Amsterdam, the Netherlands

Esther Witteveen and Marcus J. Schultz
Department of Intensive Care Medicine, Academic Medical Center, Amsterdam, the Netherlands
Laboratory of Experimental Anesthesiology and Intensive Care (LNENINCNA), Academic Medical Center, Amsterdam, the Netherlands

Camiel Verhamme and Ivo N. van Schaik
Department of Neurology, Academic Medical Center, Amsterdam, the Netherlands

Daniela S. Dettling-Ihnenfeldt and Marike van der Schaaf
Department of Rehabilitation, Academic Medical Center, Amsterdam, the Netherlands

Janneke Horn
Department of Intensive Care Medicine, Academic Medical Center, Amsterdam, the Netherlands

Gareth R. Davies
Institute of Life Science, College of Medicine, Swansea University, Singleton Park, Swansea, Wales, United Kingdom

Gavin M. Mills
NISCHR Haemostasis Biomedical Research Unit (HBRU), Morriston Hospital, Swansea, Wales, United Kingdom

Matthew Lawrence, Karl Hawkins and Phillip Adrian Evans
NISCHR Haemostasis Biomedical Research Unit (HBRU), Morriston Hospital, Swansea, Wales, United Kingdom
Institute of Life Science, College of Medicine, Swansea University, Singleton Park, Swansea, Wales, United Kingdom

Ceri Battle
NISCHR Haemostasis Biomedical Research Unit (HBRU), Morriston Hospital, Swansea, Wales, United Kingdom
Intensive Therapy Unit, Abertawe Bro Morgannwg University Health Board, Swansea, Wales, United Kingdom

Keith Morris
NISCHR Haemostasis Biomedical Research Unit (HBRU), Morriston Hospital, Swansea, Wales, United Kingdom
School of Applied Science, University of Wales Institute Cardiff, Cardiff, Wales, United Kingdom

Phylip Rhodri Williams
College of Engineering, Swansea University, Singleton Park, Swansea, Wales, United Kingdom

Simon Davidson
Department of Haematology, Royal Brompton and Harefield NHS Foundation Trust, London, United Kingdom

Dafydd Thomas
NISCHR Haemostasis Biomedical Research Unit (HBRU), Morriston Hospital, Swansea, Wales, United Kingdom
Cardiac Intensive Care Unit, Abertawe Bro Morgannwg University Health Board, Swansea, Wales, United Kingdom

Elise Launa
CHU Nantes, Hôpital de la Mère et de l'Enfant, Clinique médicale pédiatrique, Facultéde médecine de Nantes, Nantes, France
Inserm U1153, Obstetrical, Perinatal and Pediatric Epidemiology Research Team, Research Center for Epidemiology and Biostatistics Sorbonne Paris Cité (CRESS), Paris Descartes University, Paris, France

Christèle Gras-Le Guen
CHU Nantes, Hôpital de la Mère et de l9Enfant, Clinique médicale pédiatrique, Facultéde médecine de Nantes, Nantes, France
CHU Nantes, Hôpital de la Mère et de l9Enfant, Urgences pédiatriques, Faculté de médecine de Nantes, Nantes, France

Alain Martinot
CHU de Lille, Hôpital R. Salengro, Unité d'urgences pédiatriques et de maladies infectieuses, Université de Lille-Nord de France, Lille, France

Rémy Assathiany
Association pour le Recherche et l'Enseignement en Pédiatrie Générale
(AREPEGE); Association Franc̦aise de Pédiatrie Ambulatoire (AFPA), Cabinet de Pédiatrie, Issy-les-Moulineaux, France

Elise Martin and Thomas Blanchais
CHU Nantes, Hôpital de la Mère et de l9Enfant, Clinique médicale pédiatrique, Facultéde médecine de Nantes, Nantes, France

Catherine Deneux-Tharaux
Inserm U1153, Obstetrical, Perinatal and Pediatric Epidemiology Research Team, Research Center for Epidemiology and Biostatistics Sorbonne Paris Cité (CRESS), Paris Descartes University, Paris, France

Jean-Christophe Rozé
CHU Nantes, Hôpital de la Mère et de l'Enfant, Réanimation pédiatrique et néonatale, Facultéde médecine de Nantes, Nantes, France

Martin Chalumeau
Inserm U1153, Obstetrical, Perinatal and Pediatric Epidemiology Research Team, Research Center for Epidemiology and Biostatistics Sorbonne Paris Cité (CRESS), Paris Descartes University, Paris, France
Hôpital Necker Enfants Malades, AP-HP, Service de pédiatrie générale, Paris Descartes University, Paris, France

Luke T. Lavallée and Rodney H. Breau
Division of Urology, Department of Surgery, The Ottawa Hospital, University of Ottawa, Ottawa, Ontario, Canada
Clinical Epidemiology Program, Ottawa Hospital Research Institute, Ottawa, Ontario, Canada

David Schramm
Clinical Epidemiology Program, Ottawa Hospital Research Institute, Ottawa, Ontario, Canada
Department of Otolaryngology, The Ottawa Hospital, University of Ottawa, Ottawa, Ontario, Canada

Kelsey Witiuk, Ranjeeta Mallick and Dean Fergusson
Clinical Epidemiology Program, Ottawa Hospital Research Institute, Ottawa, Ontario, Canada

Christopher Morash and Ilias Cagiannos
Division of Urology, Department of Surgery, The Ottawa Hospital, University of Ottawa, Ottawa, Ontario, Canada

Aleksander Krag
Department of Gastroenterology, Odense University Hospital, Odense, Denmark
Gastro Unit, Medical Division, Hvidovre Hospital, University of Copenhagen, Copenhagen, Denmark

Flemming Bendtsen
Gastro Unit, Medical Division, Hvidovre Hospital, University of Copenhagen, Copenhagen, Denmark

Emilie Kristine Dahl
Department of Gastroenterology, Odense University Hospital, Odense, Denmark

Andreas Kjær
Hvidovre Hospital, Department of Clinical Physiology Nuclear Medicine & PET, Rigshospitalet, Hvidovre Hospital, University of Copenhagen, Copenhagen, Denmark

Claus Leth Petersen and Søren Møller
Centre of Functional Imaging and Research, Department of Clinical Physiology and Nuclear Medicine, Hvidovre Hospital, University of Copenhagen, Copenhagen, Denmark

Cheng-Ming Tsao
Department of Anesthesiology, Taipei Veterans General Hospital, and National Yang-Ming University, Taipei, Taiwan, R.O.C.
Department of Anesthesiology, Tri-Service General Hospital, National Defense Medical Center, Taipei, Taiwan, R.O.C.

Jhih-Gang Jhang
Department of Pharmacology, National Defense Medical Center, Taipei, Taiwan, R.O.C.

Shiu-Jen Chen
Department of Nursing, Kang-Ning Junior College of Medical Care and Management, Taipei, Taiwan, R.O.C.
Department of Physiology, National Defense Medical Center, Taipei, Taiwan, R.O.C.

Shuk-Man Ka
Graduate Institute of Aerospace and Undersea Medicine, National Defense Medical Center, Taipei, Taiwan, R.O.C.

Tao-Cheng Wu
Division of Cardiology, Department of Medicine, Taipei Veterans General Hospital, Taipei, Taiwan, R.O.C., 8 Cardiovascular Research Center, National Yang-Ming University, Taipei, Taiwan, R.O.C.

Wen-Jinn Liaw
Department of Anesthesiology, Tri-Service General Hospital, National Defense Medical Center, Taipei, Taiwan, R.O.C.

Hsieh-Chou Huang
Department of Anesthesiology, Cheng-Hsin General Hospital, Taipei, Taiwan, R.O.C.

Chin-Chen Wu
Department of Pharmacology, National Defense Medical Center, Taipei, Taiwan, R.O.C.
Department of Pharmacology, Taipei Medical University, Taipei, Taiwan, R.O.C.

Hongyan Hou, Weiyong Liu, Shiji Wu, Yanjun Lu, Jing Peng, Yaowu Zhu, Yanfang Lu, Feng Wang and Ziyong Sun
Department of Clinical Laboratory, Tongji Hospital, Tongji Medical College, Huazhong University of Science and Technology, Wuhan, China

Kun Wang
Department of Mathematics, Colorado State University, Fort Collins, Colorado, United States of America
Department of Mechanical Engineering & Materials Science, Yale University, New Haven, Connecticut, United States of America

Vineet Bhandari and John S. Giuliano Jr
Department of Pediatrics, Yale University School of Medicine, New Haven, Connecticut, United States of America

Corey S. ÓHern
Department of Mechanical Engineering & Materials Science, Yale University, New Haven, Connecticut, United States of America
Department of Applied Physics, Department of Physics, and Graduate Program in Computational Biology & Bioinformatics, Yale University, New Haven, Connecticut, United States of America

Mark D. Shattuck
Benjamin Levich Institute and Physics Department, The City College of New York, New York, New York, United States of America

Michael Kirby
Department of Mathematics, Colorado State University, Fort Collins, Colorado, United States of America

Mônica Andrade de Carvalho, Hélio Tedesco Silva Junior and José Osmar Medina Pestana
Unidade de Transplante, Disciplina de Nefrologia, Universidade Federal de São Paulo, São Paulo, SP, Brazil

Flávio Geraldo Rezende Freitas and Antônio Toneti Bafi
Unidade de Transplante, Disciplina de Nefrologia, Universidade Federal de São Paulo, São Paulo, SP, Brazil
Disciplina de Anestesiologia, Dor e Terapia Intensiva. Universidade Federal de São Paulo, São Paulo, SP, Brazil

Flávia Ribeiro Machado
Disciplina de Anestesiologia, Dor e Terapia Intensiva. Universidade Federal de São Paulo, São Paulo, SP, Brazil

Matthias Kott, Gunnar Elke, Dirk Schädler, Günther Zick, Inéz Frerichs and Norbert Weiler
Department of Anesthesiology and Intensive Care Medicine, University Medical Center Schleswig-Holstein, Campus Kiel, Kiel, Germany

Maike Reinicke
Department of Anesthesiology and Intensive Care Medicine, University Medical Center Schleswig-Holstein, Campus Kiel, Kiel, Germany

Institute of Immunology, University Medical Center Schleswig-Holstein, Campus Kiel, Kiel, Germany

Supandi Winoto-Morbach and Stefan Schütze
Institute of Immunology, University Medical Center Schleswig-Holstein, Campus Kiel, Kiel, Germany

Katherine Shortt, Dmitry Grigoryev and Shui Q. Ye
Department of Pediatrics, Division of Experimental and Translational Genetics, Children's Mercy Hospital, University of Missouri - Kansas City School of Medicine, Kansas City, Missouri, United States of America
Department of Biomedical and Health Informatics, University of Missouri - Kansas City School of Medicine, Kansas City, Missouri, United States of America

Daniel P. Heruth, Suman Chaudhary and Li Q. Zhang
Department of Pediatrics, Division of Experimental and Translational Genetics, Children's Mercy Hospital, University of Missouri - Kansas City School of Medicine, Kansas City, Missouri, United States of America

Lakshmi Venkitachalam
Department of Biomedical and Health Informatics, University of Missouri - Kansas City School of Medicine, Kansas City, Missouri, United States of America

Michiel B. Haeseker and Cathrien A. Bruggeman
Department of Medical Microbiology, Maastricht University Medical Center, Maastricht, the Netherlands
Care and Public Health Research Institute (CAPHRI), Maastricht, the Netherlands,

Sander Croes, Cees Neef and Leo M. L. Stolk
Department of Clinical Pharmacy and Toxicology, Maastricht University Medical Center, Maastricht, the Netherlands

Annelies Verbon
Department of Medical Microbiology, Maastricht University Medical Center, Maastricht, the Netherlands
Department of Internal Medicine, Erasmus Medical Center, Rotterdam, the Netherlands

Saswati Datta, Subhasree Roy, Somdatta Chatterjee and Sulagna Basu
Division of Bacteriology, National Institute of Cholera and Enteric Diseases, Kolkata, West Bengal, India

Anindya Saha, Barsha Sen and Tapas Som
Department of Neonatology, Institute of Postgraduate Medical Education & Research, SSKM Hospital, Kolkata, West Bengal, India

Titir Pal
AbsolutData Research and Analytics, Gurgaon, Haryana, India

Tomoya Hirose, Naoya Matsumoto, Taro Irisawa, Hideo Hosotsubo and Takeshi Shimazu
Department of Traumatology and Acute Critical Medicine, Osaka University Graduate School of Medicine, Osaka, Japan

Masafumi Seki, Shigeto Hamaguchi, Norihisa Yamamoto and Kazunori Tomono
Division of Infection Control and Prevention, Osaka University Graduate School of Medicine, Osaka, Japan

Osamu Tasaki
Department of Emergency Medicine, Unit of Clinical Medicine, Nagasaki University Graduate School of Biomedical Sciences, Nagasaki, Japan

Kouji Yamamoto
Department of Medical Innovation, Osaka University Hospital, Osaka, Japan

Yukihiro Akeda and Kazunori Oishi
International Research Center for Infectious Diseases, Research Institute for Microbial Diseases, Osaka University, Osaka, Japan

Cui Chen, Qiang-sheng Dai, Hui-wen Weng, He-ping Li and Sheng Ye
Department of Oncology, The First Affiliated Hospital, Sun Yat-Sen University, Guangzhou, China

Peng Sun
Department of Medical Oncology, Sun Yat-sen University Cancer Center, Guangzhou, China
Collaborative Innovation Center for Cancer Medicine, State Key Laboratory of Oncology in South China, Guangzhou, China

Index